ANNALS OF
THE NEW YORK ACADEMY
OF SCIENCES

Volume 922

EDITORIAL STAFF

Executive Editor
BARBARA M. GOLDMAN

Managing Editor
JUSTINE CULLINAN

Associate Editor
ANGELA FINK
LINDA HOTCHKISS MEHTA

The New York Academy of Sciences
2 East 63rd Street
New York, New York 10021

THE NEW YORK ACADEMY OF SCIENCES
(Founded in 1817)

BOARD OF GOVERNORS, September 2000 – September 2001

BILL GREEN, *Chairman of the Board*
TORSTEN WIESEL, *Vice Chairman of the Board*
RODNEY W. NICHOLS, *President and CEO* [ex officio]

Honorary Life Governors
WILLIAM T. GOLDEN   JOSHUA LEDERBERG

JOHN T. MORGAN, *Treasurer*

Governors

ELEANOR BAUM	D. ALLAN BROMLEY	KAREN BURKE
LAWRENCE B. BUTTENWIESER	PRAVEEN CHAUDHARI	
MICHAEL GOLDEN	JOHN H. GIBBONS	RONALD L. GRAHAM
ROBERT G. LAHITA	JACQUELINE LEO	WILLIAM J. McDONOUGH
JOHN F. NIBLACK	SANDRA PANEM	RICHARD RAVITCH
RICHARD A. RIFKIND	SARA LEE SCHUPF	JAMES H. SIMONS

HELENE L. KAPLAN, *Counsel* [ex officio]   PETER H. KOHN, *V.P. & Secretary* [ex officio]

THE CAMPTOTHECINS
UNFOLDING THEIR ANTICANCER POTENTIAL

ANNALS OF THE NEW YORK ACADEMY OF SCIENCES
Volume 922

THE CAMPTOTHECINS
UNFOLDING THEIR ANTICANCER POTENTIAL

*Edited by Joachim G. Liehr, Beppino C. Giovanella,
and Claire F. Verschraegen*

The New York Academy of Sciences
New York, New York
2000

Copyright © 2000 by the New York Academy of Sciences. All rights reserved. Under the provisions of the United States Copyright Act of 1976, individual readers of the Annals are permitted to make fair use of the material in them for teaching or research. Permission is granted to quote from the Annals provided that the customary acknowledgment is made of the source. Material in the Annals may be republished only by permission of the Academy. Address inquiries to the Permissions Department (editorial@nyas.org) at the New York Academy of Sciences.

Copying fees: For each copy of an article made beyond the free copying permitted under Section 107 or 108 of the 1976 Copyright Act, a fee should be paid through the Copyright Clearance Center, Inc., 222 Rosewood Drive, Danvers, MA 01923 (www.copyright.com).

♾ The paper used in this publication meets the minimum requirements of the American National Standard for Information Sciences—Permanence of Paper for Printed Library Materials, ANSI Z39.48-1984.

Library of Congress Cataloging-in-Publication Data

The camptothecins : unfolding their anticancer potential / editors, Joachim G. Liehr, Beppino C. Giovanella, Claire F. Verschraegen.
    p. cm. — (Annals of the New York Academy of Sciences ; v. 922)
    Includes bibliographical references and indexes.
    ISBN 1-57331-291-6 (cloth : alk. paper) — ISBN 1-57331-292-4 (pbk. : alk. paper)
    1. Camptothecin—Congresses. 2. Camptothecin—Derivatives—Congresses. 3. Cancer—Chemotherapy—Congresses. I. Liehr, Joachim G. II. Giovanella, Beppino C. III. Verschraegen, Claire F. IV. Series

Q11.N5 vol. 922
[RC271.C35]
500 s—dc21
[616.99'4061]   00-051567

GYAT / PCP
Printed in the United States of America
ISBN 1-57331-291-6 (cloth)
ISBN 1-57331-292-4 (paper)
ISSN 0077-8923

ANNALS OF THE NEW YORK ACADEMY OF SCIENCES

Volume 922
December 2000

THE CAMPTOTHECINS
UNFOLDING THEIR ANTICANCER POTENTIAL

Editors and Conference Organizers
JOACHIM G. LIEHR, BEPPINO C. GIOVANELLA, AND
CLAIRE F. VERSCHRAEGEN

[This volume is the result of a conference entitled **The Camptothecins: Unfolding Their Anticancer Potential** held by the New York Academy of Sciences and Pharmacia & Upjohn on March 17–20, 2000 in Arlington, Virginia.]

CONTENTS

Introduction. *By* JOACHIM G. LIEHR AND BEPPINO GIOVANELLA xi

Keynote Lecture

Mechanism of Action of Camptothecin. *By* LEROY F. LIU, SHYAMAL D.
 DESAI, TSAI-KUN LI, YONG MAO, MEI SUN, AND SAI-PENG SIM 1

Part I. Mechanism of Action of Camptothecins

Molecular and Biological Determinants of the Cytotoxic Actions of Camptothecins. Perspective for the Development of New Topoisomerase I
 Inhibitors. *By* KURT W. KOHN AND YVES POMMIER 11

Dependence of Anticancer Activity of Camptothecins on Maintaining Their
 Lactone Function. *By* B.C. GIOVANELLA, N. HARRIS, J. MENDOZA,
 Z. CAO, J. LIEHR, AND J.S. STEHLIN 27

Camptothecin Design and Delivery Approaches for Elevating Anti-
 Topoisomerase I Activities *in Vivo*. *By* THOMAS G. BURKE AND
 DAVID BOM 36

Mechanisms of Resistance to Camptothecins. *By* AHAMED SALEEM, TROY K.
 EDWARDS, ZESHAAN RASHEED, AND ERIC H. RUBIN 46

Part II. Mechanism-Based Design and Synthesis of Novel Camptothecins

Structure-Based Analysis of the Effects of Camptothecin on the Activities of
 Human Topoisomerase I. *By* JAMES J. CHAMPOUX 56

Mechanisms of DNA Topoisomerase I-Induced Cell Killing in the Yeast *Saccharomyces cerevisiae*. By PAOLA FIORANI AND MARY-ANN BJORNSTI 65

Camptothecins as Probes of the Microenvironments of Topoisomerase I – DNA Complexes. By SIDNEY M. HECHT 76

Part III. Novel Topoisomerase I Inhibitors

Preclinical and Clinical Trials of Topoisomerase Inhibitors. By NAGAHIRO SAIJO 92

Homocamptothecins: E-Ring Modified CPT Analogues. By OLIVIER LAVERGNE, DANIELE DEMARQUAY, PHILIP G. KASPRZYK, AND DENNIS C.H. BIGG 100

The Cascade Radical Annulation Approach to New Analogues of Camptothecins. Combinatorial Synthesis of Silatecans and Homosilatecans. By DENNIS P. CURRAN, HUBERT JOSIEN, DAVID BOM, ANA E. GABARDA, AND WU DU 112

Part IV. New Camptothecin Derivatives and Formulations

Structure–Activity Relationship of Alkyl Camptothecin Esters. By ZHISONG CAO, PANAYOTIS PANTAZIS, JOHN MENDOZA, JANET EARLY, ANTHONY KOZIELSKI, NICK HARRIS, DANA VARDEMAN, JOACHIM LIEHR, JOHN S. STEHLIN, AND BEPPINO GIOVANELLA 122

Conjugation of Camptothecins to Poly-(L-Glutamic Acid). By JACK W. SINGER, PETER DE VRIES, RAMA BHATT, JOHN TULINSKY, PETER KLEIN, CHUN LI, LUKA MILAS, ROBERT A. LEWIS, AND SIDNEY WALLACE ... 136

9-Nitrocamptothecin Liposome Aerosol Treatment of Human Cancer Subcutaneous Xenografts and Pulmonary Cancer Metastases in Mice. By VERNON KNIGHT, EUGENIE S. KLEINERMAN, J. CLIFFORD WALDREP, BEPPINO C. GIOVANELLA, BRIAN E. GILBERT, AND NADEZHDA V. KOSHKINA 151

Modified Lactone/Carboxylate Salt Equilibria *in Vivo* by Liposomal Delivery of 9-Nitro-Camptothecin. By DIANA S-L. CHOW, LING GONG, MICHAEL D. WOLFE, AND BEPPINO C. GIOVANELLA 164

New Analogues of Camptothecins. Activity and Resistance. By EPIE BOVEN, ANNEMARIE H. VAN HATTUM, ILSE HOOGSTEEN, HENNIE M.M. SCHLÜPER, AND H.M. PINEDO 175

Intraperitoneal Topoisomerase-I Inhibitors. Preliminary Findings with 9-Aminocamptothecin. By FRANCO MUGGIA, LEONARD LIEBES, MILAN POTMESIL, ANNE HAMILTON, HOWARD HOCHSTER, GILA HORNREICH, JOAN SORICH, ANDREA DOWNEY, AND HEATHER WASSERSTROM 178

Part V. Pharmacology

Transport of Topoisomerase I Inhibitors by the Breast Cancer Resistance Protein. Potential Clinical Implications. By JAN H.M. SCHELLENS, MARC MALIEPAARD, RIK J. SCHEPER, GEORGE L. SCHEFFER, JOHAN W. JONKER, JOHAN W. SMIT, JOS H. BEIJNEN, AND ALFRED H. SCHINKEL 188

Pharmacokinetics of Orally Administered Camptothecins. *By* ELORA GUPTA, VIRAL VYAS, FARHEENA AHMED, PATRICK SINKO, THOMAS COOK, AND ERIC RUBIN 195

Metabolism of CPT-11. Impact on Activity. *By* LAURENT P. RIVORY 205

Pharmacology of Camptothecin Esters. *By* JOACHIM G. LIEHR, NICK J. HARRIS, JOHN MENDOZA, AHMED E. AHMED, AND BEPPINO C. GIOVANELLA 216

Part VI. Clinical Trials I, Newer Analogues

The Clinical Development of 9-Aminocamptothecin. *By* CHRIS H. TAKIMOTO AND REBECCA THOMAS 224

Alternative Administration of Camptothecin Analogues. *By* C.F. VERSCHRAEGEN, K. JAECKLE, B. GIOVANELLA, V. KNIGHT, AND B.E. GILBERT 237

Topotecan (Hycamptin) and Topotecan-Containing Regimens in the Treatment of Hematologic Malignancies. *By* MILOSLAV BERAN AND HAGOP M. KANTARJIAN 247

DX-8951f: Summary of Phase I Clinical Trials. *By* R. DE JAGER, P. CHEVERTON, K. TAMANOI, J. COYLE, M. DUCHARME, N. SAKAMOTO, M. SATOMI, M. SUZUKI, AND THE DX-8951f INVESTIGATORS 260

Part VII. Clinical Trials II, Combination Therapy

Cellular and Molecular Responses to Topoisomerase I Poisons. Exploiting Synergy for Improved Radiotherapy. *By* SHIGEKI MIYAMOTO, TONY T. HUANG, SHELLY WUERZBERGER-DAVIS, WILLIAM G. BORNMANN, JOHN J. PINK, COLLEEN TAGLIARINO, TIMOTHY J. KINSELLA, AND DAVID A. BOOTHMAN 274

In Vitro Antitumor Activity of 9-Nitro-Camptothecin as a Single Agent and in Combination with other Antitumor Drugs. *By* RALPH J. BERNACKI, PAULA PERA, PETER GAMBACORTA, YSEULT BRUN, AND WILLIAM R. GRECO 293

p53 and p21 Are Major Cellular Determinants for DNA Topoisomerase I-Mediated Radiation Sensitization in Mammalian Cells. *By* ALLAN Y. CHEN, PAUL B. SCRUGGS, LING GENG, MACE L. ROTHENBERG, AND DENNIS E. HALLAHAN 298

Part VIII. Poster Papers

The Homocamptothecin, BN 80927, Is a Potent Topoisomerase I Poison and Topoisomerase II Catalytic Inhibitor 1. *By* DANIÈLE DEMARQUAY, HÉLÈNE COULOMB, MARION HUCHET, LAURENCE LESUEUR-GINOT, JOSÉ CAMARA, OLIVIER LAVERGNE, AND DENNIS BIGG 301

The Dual Topoisomerase Inhibitor, BN 80927, Is Highly Potent against Cell Proliferation and Tumor Growth. *By* MARION HUCHET, DANIÈLE DEMARQUAY, HÉLÈNE COULOMB, PHILIP KASPRZYK, MARK CARLSON, JEFFREY LAUER, OLIVIER LAVERGNE, AND DENNIS BIGG .. 303

Ubiquitin, SUMO-1, and UCRP in Camptothecin Sensitivity and Resistance. *By* SHYAMAL D. DESAI, YONG MAO, MEI SUN, TSAI-KUN LI, JIAXI WU, AND LEROY F. LIU 306

A Spectrophotometric Study of the pH-Dependent and DNA Binding
Properties of Topotecan. *By* STEVEN E. MILLER AND DANIEL S. PILCH . 309

Kinetics of *in Vitro* Hydrolysis of Homocamptothecins As Measured by
Fluorescence. *By* D. CHAUVIER, I. CHOURPA, D.C.H. BIGG, AND
M. MANFAIT 314

The Combinatorial Synthesis of Racemic Homosilatecan Libraries via a
Cascade Radical Annulation. *By* WU DU, ANA E. GABARDA, DAVID
BOM, AND DENNIS P. CURRAN 317

Combined Radiation and 9-Nitrocamptothecin (Rubitecan) in the Treatment
of Locally Advanced Pancreatic Cancer. *By* K.R. KEMP, J.G. LIEHR,
AND B. GIOVANELLA 320

Preclinical and Phase I Clinical Studies with Ckd-602, a Novel Camptothecin
Derivative. *By* J.H. LEE, J.M. LEE, K.H. LIM, J.K. KIM, S.K. AHN, Y.J.
BANG, AND C.I. HONG 324

Action of Topoisomerase Targeting Drugs on Non-Hodgkin's Lymphoma and
Leukemia. Correlation of Clinical and Cell Culture Studies. *By*
J.S. NAIR, R. KANCHERLA, K. SEITER, F. TRAGANOS, AND
Y.-C. TSE-DINH 326

Improvement of Therapeutic Index of Low-Dose Topotecan Delivered per os.
By GRAZIELLA PRATESI, MICHELANDREA DE CESARE, AND
FRANCO ZUNINO 330

Camptothecin Dose, Schedule, and Timing of Administration for Clinical
Radiation Sensitization. *By* TYVIN A. RICH AND ALEXANDER V.
KIRICHENKO 334

Rapid Chromatin Reorganization Induced by Topoisomerase I-Mediated
DNA Damage. *By* MEI SUN, PU DUANN, CHIN-TAI LIN, HUI ZHANG,
AND LEROY F. LIU 340

NF-κB Activation in Topoisomerase I Inhibitor-Induced Apoptotic Cell Death
in Human Non-Small Cell Lung Cancer. *By* MASAHIRO TABATA AND
RAM GANAPATHI 343

Phase I Study of 9-Nitro-20(S)-Camptothecin in Combination with Cisplatin
for Patients with Advanced Malignancies. *By* C.F. VERSCHRAEGEN,
M. VINCENT, J.L. ABBRUZZESE, D. SIEGLER, J.J. KAVANAGH,
E. LOYER, A.P. KUDELKA, AND E. RUBIN 345

Phase II Study of Intravenous DX-8951f in Patients with Advanced Ovarian,
Tubal, or Peritoneal Cancer Refractory to Platinum, Taxane, and
Topotecan. *By* C.F. VERSCHRAEGEN, C. LEVENBACK, M. VINCENT, J.
WOLF, M. BEVERS, E. LOYER, A.P. KUDELKA, AND J.J. KAVANAGH . . 349

Feasibility, Phase I, and Pharmacological Study of Aerosolized Liposomal 9-
Nitro-20(S)-Camptothecin in Patients with Advanced Malignancies in
the Lungs. *By* C.F. VERSCHRAEGEN, B.E. GILBERT, A.J. HUARINGA,
R. NEWMAN, N. HARRIS, F.J. LEYVA, L. KEUS, K. CAMPBELL,
T. NELSON-TAYLOR, AND V. KNIGHT 352

Inhibition of DNA Replication in Camptothecin-Treated Cells Is Regulated by
Protein Kinases. *By* XIANG-YANG ZHOU AND YA WANG 355

Part IX. Concluding Remarks

Concluding Remarks. *By* CLAIRE VERSCHRAEGEN 360

Index of Contributors 361

Financial assistance was received from:

Co-sponsor
- PHARMACIA & UPJOHN

Supporters
- AVENTIS PHARMAS SA
- BIONUMERIK PHARMACEUTICALS, INC.
- DAIICHI PHARMACEUTICAL CORPORATION
- SMITHKLINE BEECHAM PHARMACEUTICALS
- SUPERGEN

Contributors
- BAYER CORPORATION
- BRISTOL-MYERS SQUIBB COMPANY
- CELL THERAPEUTICS, INC.
- INSTITUT HENRI BEAUFOUR
- ORTHO BIOTECH
- XECHEM, INC.
- YAKULT HONSHA CO., LTD

The New York Academy of Sciences believes it has a responsibility to provide an open forum for discussion of scientific questions. The positions taken by the participants in the reported conferences are their own and not necessarily those of the Academy. The Academy has no intent to influence legislation by providing such forums.

Introduction

JOACHIM G. LIEHR AND BEPPINO GIOVANELLA
The Stehlin Foundation for Cancer Research at Christus St. Joseph Hospital, 1918 Chenevert, Houston, Texas 77003, USA

Camptothecin derivatives are among the most promising anticancer drugs in development today. Two derivatives, CPT-11 and topotecan, are already available for cancer treatment. Several other derivatives are at various stages of clinical development and are expected to come to market within the next 2–4 years. Mechanistic aspects of the action of these topoisomerase I inhibitors are also becoming clearer. In an effort to focus attention on the preclinical and clinical development of effective cancer chemotherapeutic drugs based on camptothecin, this volume is presented as a summary of the state of the art in this field of research. The chapters in this volume are based on presentations at a conference entitled "The Camptothecins: Unfolding Their Anticancer Potential" (March 2000, Arlington, Virginia). The text summarizes the progress in this area of drug development with a focus on advances made since the last conference on this topic entitled "The Camptothecins: From Discovery to the Patient" (Annals of the New York Academy of Sciences, volume 803).

Despite the potential of camptothecins in cancer treatment, research in this area has not increased steadily, but has proceeded in several stages. Initially, extracts with antitumor activity were isolated from the leaves of *Camptotheca acuminata* in the 1950s by Monroe E. Wall and Mansukh C. Wani. These scientists subsequently isolated the pharmacologically active substance, camptothecin, from such extracts and determined the structure of this compound. They developed several promising camptothecin derivatives as drug candidates in the subsequent years. Dr. Wall and Dr. Wani received the General Motors Cancer Research Charles F. Kettering Prize for their efforts in this and other areas of cancer chemotherapy research.

Camptothecin was rapidly entered into a clinical trial in the late 1960s soon after its discovery and it also failed rapidly. The reason for this failure was the utilization in this trial not of the water-insoluble camptothecin, but of the hydrophilic carboxylate salt form of camptothecin. Unfortunately, this carboxylate salt form of camptothecin barely has 10% of the anticancer activity of camptothecin. Interest in this class of chemotherapeutic agents was revived in the mid-1980s, when the potent activity of camptothecin as a topoisomerase I inhibitor was detected. This discovery led to rapid advances in camptothecin research in the late 1980s and early 1990s. Camptothecin and many of its analogues are potent antitumor agents against human tumor xenografts in nude mice. Drs. Beppino Giovanella and John Stehlin of the Stehlin Foundation for Cancer Research in Houston, Texas, demonstrated the complete eradication of human tumors in nude mice by camptothecin, 9-aminocamptothecin, 9-nitrocamptothecin, and other derivatives. Dr. Stehlin also entered camptothecin and 9-nitrocamptothecin into clinical trials. As a result of this work, 9-nitrocamptothecin is being developed as chemotherapy for pancreatic cancer.

Many newer derivatives of camptothecin are undergoing preclinical evaluations at this time. Several of these compounds have entered clinical trials. Other promising avenues include combination therapy of a camptothecin-based drug with radiation or another chemotherapeutic agent. Novel forms of administration of the drug are also being explored. The chapters in this volume are designed to give the reader an overview of the status of the preclinical and clinical development of camptothecin-based anticancer therapy. The texts represent the frontier in this area of cancer research.

Mechanism of Action of Camptothecin

LEROY F. LIU,[a] SHYAMAL D. DESAI, TSAI-KUN LI, YONG MAO, MEI SUN, AND SAI-PENG SIM

Department of Pharmacology, UMDNJ-Robert Wood Johnson Medical School, Piscataway, New Jersey 08854, USA

ABSTRACT: Camptothecin (CPT) class of compounds has been demonstrated to be effective against a broad spectrum of tumors. Their molecular target has been firmly established to be human DNA topoisomerase I (topo I). CPT inhibits topo I by blocking the rejoining step of the cleavage/religation reaction of topo-I, resulting in accumulation of a covalent reaction intermediate, the cleavable complex. The primary mechanism of cell killing by CPT is S-phase–specific killing through potentially lethal collisions between advancing replication forks and topo-I cleavable complexes. Collisions with the transcription machinery have also been shown to trigger the formation of long-lived covalent topo-I DNA complexes, which contribute to CPT cytotoxicity. Two novel repair responses to topo-I-mediated DNA damage involving covalent modifications of topo-I have been discovered. The first involves activation of the ubiquitin/26S proteasome pathway, leading to degradation of topo-I (CPT-induced topo-I downregulation). The second involves SUMO conjugation to topo-I. The potential roles of these new mechanisms for repair of topo-I-mediated DNA damage in determining CPT sensitivity/resistance in tumor cells are discussed.

FORMATION OF THE COVALENT TOPO-I–CPT–DNA TERNARY COMPLEX: THE CLEAVABLE COMPLEX

The primary cellular DNA lesion induced by camptothecin (CPT) has been established to be the reversible human DNA topoisomerase (topo)-I–CPT–DNA covalent complexes, the cleavable complexes.[1-4] The properties of these complexes have been studied extensively *in vitro*. Biochemical studies have suggested that CPT binds at the interface between topo I and DNA and inhibits specifically the religation step in the cleavage/religation reaction.[3,5] The molecular mechanism of inhibition appears to be of the uncompetitive type, because CPT binds neither the enzyme nor the DNA substrate, but interacts with the enzyme-DNA complex to form a reversible nonproductive complex.[3,6] X-ray crystallographic studies of topo I and topo I–DNA complexes have revealed multiple interactions between the DNA substrate and topo I in both the cleavable and the noncleavable complex forms.[7,8] A drug intercalation model has been suggested in which CPT interacts with the DNA by intercalation at

---

[a]Address for correspondence: Dr. Leroy F. Liu, Department of Pharmacology, UMDNJ-Robert Wood Johnson Medical School, 675 Hoes Lane, Piscataway, NJ 08854. Voice: 732-235-4592; fax: 732-235-4073.
  lliu@umdnj.edu

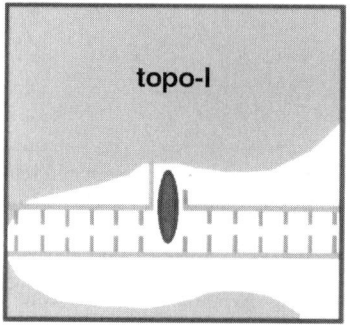
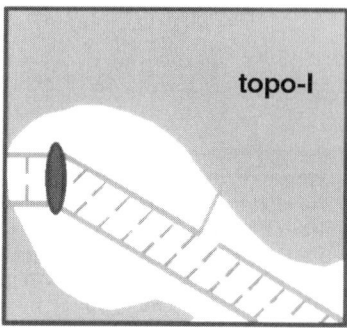

FIGURE 1. Two proposed models for ligand-induced trapping of topo-I cleavable complexes. (**A**) A drug intercalation model for CPT. In this model, CPT is presumed to bind at the interface between topo-I and DNA. CPT interacts with both DNA and topo-I. CPT presumably intercalates between the bases of DNA at the site of cleavage. The +1 base has been suggested to flip out of the helical stack to accommodate CPT intercalation.[7] (**B**) A DNA bending model for nogalamycin. Nogalamycin binds DNA with a footprint of 3–6 bases upstream of the site of cleavage. Nogalamycin binding induces local DNA bending which favors topo-I binding/cleavage.

the site of cleavage (FIG. 1A). Additional interactions between CPT and topo-I, and CPT and a flipped base at the +1 position have also been suggested.[7] However, in the absence of the co-crystal structure of the ternary topo I-CPT-DNA complex, the molecular details of the interactions remain uncertain.

In addition to CPTs, an increasing list of agents has been shown to trap covalent topo-I–DNA complexes (reviewed in ref. 1). Many of these agents are DNA binders, suggesting that ligand-DNA interaction may be a key component in the formation of the ternary cleavable complex.[9–15] For examples, studies with DNA minor groove binding bi- and ter-benzimidazoles as well as protoberberines have strongly suggested that DNA binding is tightly linked to trapping of topo-I cleavable complexes.[11–13,16] More recent studies with nogalamycin have demonstrated that ligand binding 3–6 bases upstream of the site of DNA cleavage is responsible for trapping topo-I cleavable complexes (ref. 17; S.P. Sim and L.F. Liu, unpublished results). In this case, ligand-induced DNA bending at a distal site has been suggested to be the mechanism for trapping topo-I cleavable complexes. Consistent with the notion that DNA structural changes induced by ligand binding can trap topo-I cleavable complexes, certain DNA structural perturbations due to covalent modifications of DNA or DNA structural changes (e.g., benz[a]pyrene adducts, base mismatches, 8-oxoguanine, and UV dimers) have also been shown to trap covalent topo-I cleavable complexes.[18–21] These studies highlight the importance of altered DNA structures and the possibility of multiple mechanisms for trapping topo-I cleavable complexes.

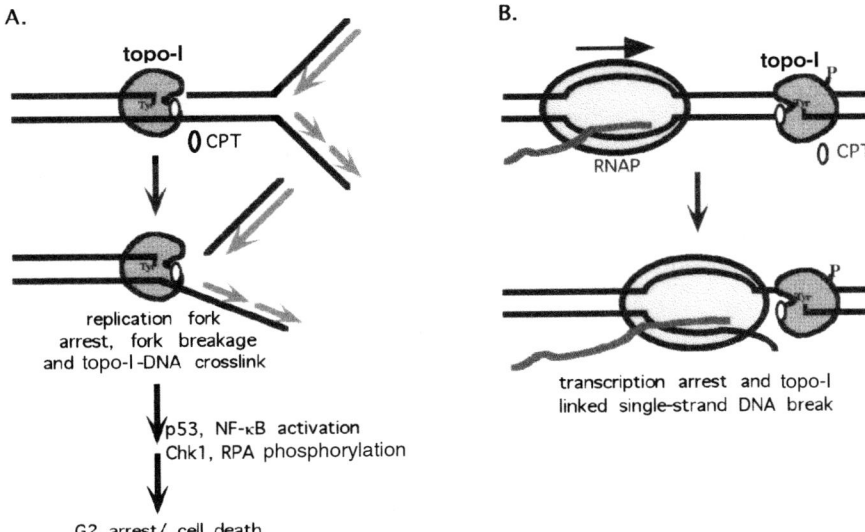

FIGURE 2. Cellular processing of topo-I cleavable complexes. The collision models. (**A**) A replication fork collision model. This orientation-specific collision between the replication fork and the topo-I cleavable complex results in irreversible arrest of the replication fork, formation of a double-strand break and the conversion of the reversible cleavable complex into a topo-I-linked DNA break. (**B**) An RNA polymerase collision model. The collision between the elongating RNA polymerase complex and the topo-I cleavable complex results in transcription arrest and the formation of topo-I-linked single-strand break. A small fraction of topo-I-linked double-strand breaks could occur.

COLLISION BETWEEN THE TOPO-I–CPT–DNA CLEAVABLE COMPLEX AND THE REPLICATION FORK

The primary mechanism by which CPT kills cells is through S-phase–specific cytotoxicity. The mechanism of S-phase–specific cytotoxicity has been studied extensively,[22–25] and a replication fork collision model has been established, which is shown in FIGURE 2A.[26] The reversible topo I–CPT–DNA cleavable complexes are nonlethal by themselves. However, upon their collisions with the advancing replication forks, cell death ensues. Three biochemical events have been identified *in vitro* following collision: the formation of a double-strand break, irreversible arrest of the replication fork, and the formation of topo-I-linked DNA break at the site of collision.[23–25] The relative contribution of each of these three events in cell death is not known. However, studies in yeast have suggested the importance of the double-strand break in CPT cytotoxicity.[27] This potentially lethal collision has been shown to be dependent on the orientation of the cleavable complex relative to the replication fork.[25] The collision is potentially lethal only if the cleavable complex is formed on the strand complementary to the leading strand of DNA synthesis.[25] In addition to cell death, this potentially lethal collision is also responsible for G2 arrest/delay, stabilization of p53, activation of NF-κB, activation/phosphorylation of Chk1, and phosphorylation of RPA.[28–30]

At higher concentrations of CPT, non–S-phase cells can also be killed by CPT. Unlike S-phase–specific cytotoxicity, S-phase–independent cytotoxicity of CPT is unaffected by inhibitors of DNA replication.[31,32] S-phase–independent cytotoxicity of CPT appears to be apoptotic.[33] Involvement of transcription has been suggested.[33]

COLLISION BETWEEN THE TOPO-I–CPT–DNA CLEAVABLE COMPLEX AND THE TRANSCRIPTION MACHINERY

One of the prominent cellular effects of CPT is arrest of RNA synthesis.[34–37] Arrest of RNA synthesis occurs at the level of transcription elongation, leading to the accumulation of RNA polymerase elongation complexes at the 5′ ends of the transcribed genes.[36,37] The inhibitory effect of topo-I-CPT-DNA cleavable complexes on transcription elongation has been studied *in vitro*.[38] Using T7 RNA polymerase, topo-I cleavable complexes were shown to arrest transcription causing premature termination. Surprisingly, as in the case of replication fork collision, arrest of transcription depends on the orientation of the cleavable complex relative to the transcribing RNA polymerase. Arrest of transcription occurs only if the topo-I cleavable complex is formed on the template strand of transcription. In addition to arrest of RNA transcription, topo-I cleavable complexes can also produce irreversible topo-I-linked single-strand breaks on the template but not the nontemplate strand.[38] A small fraction of irreversible double-strand breaks have also been demonstrated to occur near the promoter region.[38] Based on these results, an RNA polymerase collision model was proposed in which the collisions between the RNA polymerase complex and the topo-I cleavable complexes on the template strand of transcription arrest the RNA transcription and concomitantly convert the reversible topo-I cleavable complexes into irreversible topo-I-linked single-strand breaks[38] (FIG. 1B).

CPT INDUCES TOPO-I DOWNREGULATION VIA A UBIQUITIN/26S PROTEASOME PATHWAY

The involvement of transcription-coupled repair (TCR) in the repair of topo-I-mediated DNA damage has been suggested from studies of Cockayne syndrome (CS) cells.[39] However, removal of such a bulky protein adduct from DNA is conceptually challenging. Recent studies have suggested that repair of topo-I-mediated DNA damage may involve topo-I degradation.[40,41] CPT-induced topo-I degradation was shown to depend on E1 and 26S proteasome, suggesting involvement of the ubiquitin/26S proteasome pathway.[41] The involvement of RNA transcription in topo-I downregulation has also been suggested from studies with DRB and α-amanitin (S.D. Desai and L.F. Liu, unpublished results). A model for transcription-dependent topo-I downregulation is shown in FIGURE 3. In this model, the collision between the elongating RNA polymerase complex and the topo-I cleavable complex (on the template strand) results in transcription arrest and the formation of a topo-I-linked single-strand break (a long-lived topo-I-DNA covalent complex). This colli-

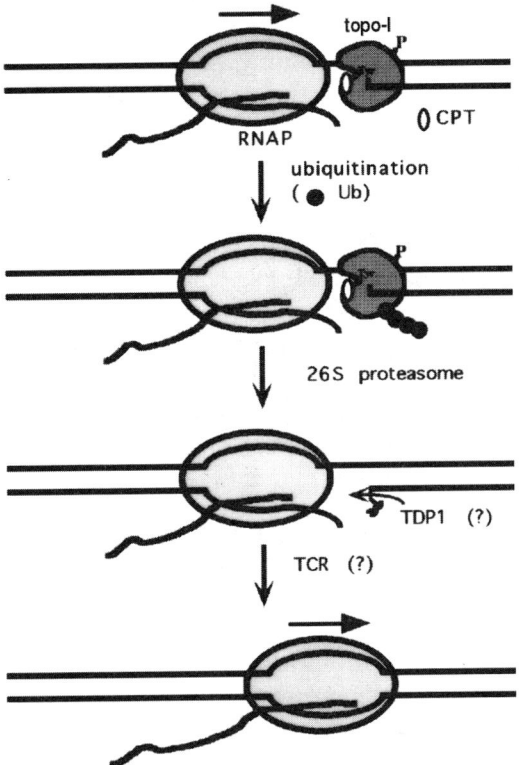

FIGURE 3. CPT-induced topo-Itopo-I downregulation. Roles of RNA transcription and ubiquitin/26S proteasome. The major mechanism for topo-I downregulation is collisions between the RNA polymerase complexes and topo-I cleavable complexes. Such collisions trigger multi-ubiquitination of topo-I and subsequent 26S proteasome-dependent degradation of topo-I. Downregulation of topo-I could precede repair of topo-I-mediated DNA damage by TCR or other repair machineries. A potential role for tyrosyl-DNA phosphodiesterase (TDP1) could be the removal of the residual peptide.

sion triggers ubiquitin/26S proteasome-dependent degradation of topo-I. Subsequent to topo-I destruction, repair of the single-strand break can presumably occur. It could be speculated that prior to TCR, the enzyme, tyrosyl-DNA phosphodiesterase (TDP1),[42] may be involved in the removal of the residual peptide which is still covalently linked to DNA following 26S proteasome-mediated degradation of topo-I. Alternatively, TCR and other repair processes may be able to repair the damage independent of TDP1.

SUMO/UBC9-DEPENDENT MODIFICATION OF TOPO-I

CPT has also been shown to induce rapid conjugation of SUMO-1 (also SUMO-2/3) to topo I.[43] Human SUMO-1 (Small Ubiquitin-like MOdifier) (also named UBL1,[44] PIC1,[45] GMP1,[46] SMT3C,[47] and sentrin[48] in the literature) is a ubiquitin-

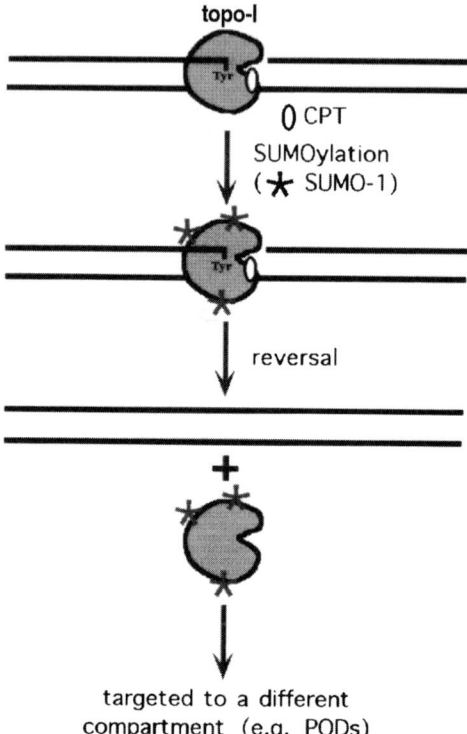

FIGURE 4. Speculation on the possible role(s) of CPT-induced SUMO conjugation of topo-I. The formation of topo-I cleavable complexes triggers SUMO (SUMO-1 and SUMO-2/3) conjugations to topo-I by UBC9. The formation of SUMO-topo-I conjugates is independent of transcription and is specific for dephosphorylated topo-I. SUMO-topo-I conjugates can dissociate from DNA (e.g., due to the reversibility of the conjugates) and be targeted to a different cellular compartment (e.g., PODs). Removal of topo-I from DNA by SUMOylation can effectively reduce the amount of topo-I cleavable complexes.

like protein that shares about 18% identity to ubiquitin.[49] They share a similar activation and conjugation pathway with ubiquitin, but employ distinct sets of E1 and E2 enzymes.[50] UBC9 is the only E2 identified for SUMO-1, whereas a dozen E2 enzymes have been identified for ubiquitin in yeast.[51,52] While the primary role of ubiquitin-protein conjugation is to facilitate protein degradation by 26S proteasome,[53] the role of SUMO-1–protein conjugation is not clear. SUMOylation has been suggested to be involved in diverse biological functions such as regulation of ubiquitin conjugation in the case of IκBα,[54] regulation of protein transport in the case of RanGAP1,[55–57] the formation of PODs (nuclear bodies) in the case of PML,[58,59] regulation of transcriptional activation in the case of p53,[60,61] and regulation of apoptosis in the case of the FAS ligand.[48]

Ubiquitination and SUMOylation of topo I share some reaction characteristics. For example, both reactions are dependent on the formation of topo-I cleavable complexes, and both are unaffected by treatment with the replication inhibitor aphidicolin or the poly (ADP-ribose) polymerase inhibitor, 3-amino-benzamide (3AB).[41,43] However, the two reactions differ in the following ways: (1) Ubiquitination/proteolysis but not SUMOylation of topo I is transcription dependent. (2) Ubiquitination/proteolysis appears to be specific for the phosphorylated topo-I population, whereas SUMOylation appears to be specific for the dephosphorylated topo-I. Phosphorylated topo-I has been shown to be associated with transcription.[62] (3) Ubiquitination/proteolysis of topo I appears to be defective in most human tumor cells, while SUMOylation of topo-I appears to be normal in both tumor and normal cells. Currently, the function of SUMOylation of topo I in response to CPT is still unclear. It is possible that SUMOylation of topo I represents a distinct cellular response to CPT from ubiquitination. Ubiquitination of phosphorylated topo-I may occur within the transcribed regions, while SUMOylation of topo-I may occur outside of the transcribed regions. The speculation is that SUMOylation of topo I may target topo I to a different cellular compartment (e.g., PODs), so that relocated topo I cannot participate in the formation of topo-I cleavable complexes (FIG. 4). In this view, both downregulation and relocation of topo I can be effective ways to deal with topo-I-mediated DNA damage.

DEFECT OF CPT-INDUCED TOPO-I DOWNREGULATION IN TUMOR CELLS: IMPLICATION IN TREATMENT

Studies of a panel of breast, colon, and leukemia cell lines have demonstrated that CPT-induced topo-I downregulation is defective in most tumor cell lines (ref. 63; S.D. Desai and L.F. Liu, unpublished results). The defect in topo-I downregulation in tumor cells has also been correlated with CPT hypersensitivity (S.D. Desai and L.F. Liu, unpublished results). The molecular mechanism for altered regulation of topo-I downregulation in many tumor cells is still unclear. However, the 26S proteasome pathway appears normal, since ubiquitin/26S proteasome-dependent degradation of topo IIβ occurs efficiently in tumor cells defective in CPT-induced topo I downregulation (Y. Mao and L.F. Liu, unpublished results). It seems possible that a specific E2 or E3 enzyme, which is responsible for conjugating ubiquitin to topo I, is defective in these tumor cells. The suggestion that E2 or E3 is altered during tumorigenesis is consistent with the results that 26S-proteasome–dependent protein degradation can be either up- or downregulated in tumor cells depending on the protein target.[64]

Topo-I downregulation in peripheral blood mononuclear cells has been observed in patients treated with CPT.[65,66] It remains to be established whether patients undergoing CPT treatment can downregulate topo I in all cells in their bodies except tumor cells. If this is the case, CPT-induced downregulation of topo-I could result in protection of normal cells from CPT toxicity, while tumor cells remain sensitive to CPT during prolonged exposure to CPT. Studies *in vitro* have demonstrated that topo-I downregulation depends on the continued presence of CPT. Complete repopulation of topo I occurs within 24 hours of CPT removal (S.D. Desai and L.F. Liu, unpublished results). Consequently, intermittent CPT treatment in patients could result in rapid rebound of topo I in normal cells, and concomitant sensitization of normal cells to the toxic side effects of CPT. On the other hand, treatment protocols that can maintain sufficient CPT levels may benefit from lower toxic side effects and hence an improved therapeutic index. The defect of topo-I downregulation in many tumor cells suggests that the antitumor activity of CPT is at least in part determined by the tumorigenesis process itself.

ACKNOWLEDGMENT

This work was supported by National Institutes of Health grants CA 39662 and CA77433.

REFERENCES

1. GATTO, B. & L.F. LIU. 1998. Topoisomerase I-targeting drugs: new developments in cancer pharmacology. *In* Advances in DNA Sequence-Specific Agents. M. Palumbo *et al.*, Eds. **8**: 39–66. CRC Press, Inc. Boca Raton, FL.
2. CHEN, A.Y. & L.F. LIU. 1994. DNA topoisomerases: essential enzymes and lethal targets. Annu. Rev. Pharmacol. Toxicol. **34**: 191–218.
3. HSIANG, Y.H. *et al.* 1985. Camptothecin induces protein-linked DNA breaks via mammalian DNA topoisomerase I. J Biol. Chem. **260**: 14873–14878.
4. HSIANG, Y.H. & L.F. LIU. 1988. Identification of mammalian DNA topoisomerase I as an intracellular target of the anticancer drug camptothecin. Cancer Res. **48**: 1722–1726.
5. SVEJSTRUP, J.Q. *et al.* 1991. New technique for uncoupling the cleavage and religation reactions of eukaryotic topoisomerase I. The mode of action of camptothecin at a specific recognition site. J Mol. Biol. **222**: 669–678.
6. HERTZBERG, R.P. *et al.* 1989. On the mechanism of topoisomerase I inhibition by camptothecin: evidence for binding to an enzyme-DNA complex. Biochemistry **28**: 4629–4638.
7. REDINBO, M.R. *et al.* 1998. Crystal structures of human topoisomerase I in covalent and noncovalent complexes with DNA [see comments]. Science **279**: 1504–1513.
8. STEWART, L. *et al.* 1998. A model for the mechanism of human topoisomerase I. Science **279**: 1534–1541.
9. CHEN, A.Y. *et al.* 1993. DNA minor groove-binding ligands: a different class of mammalian DNA topoisomerase I inhibitors. Proc. Natl. Acad. Sci. USA **90**: 8131–8135.
10. LETEURTRE, F. *et al.*1994. Saintopin, a dual inhibitor of DNA topoisomerases I and II, as a probe for drug-enzyme interactions. J Biol. Chem. **269**: 28702–28707.
11. PILCH, D.S *et al.* 1996. Characterizing the DNA binding modes of a topoisomerase I-poisoning terbenzimidazole: evidence for both intercalative and minor groove binding properties. Drug Des. Discov. **13**: 115–133.
12. PILCH, D.S *et al.* 1997. A terbenzimidazole that preferentially binds and conformationally alters structurally distinct DNA duplex domains: a potential mechanism for topoisomerase I poisoning. Proc. Natl. Acad. Sci. USA **94**:13565–13570.
13. PILCH, D.S *et al.* 1997. Minor groove-directed and intercalative ligand-DNA interactions in the poisoning of human DNA topoisomerase I by protoberberine analogs. Biochemistry **36**: 12542–12553.
14. PODDEVIN, B. *et al.* 1993. Dual topoisomerase I and II inhibition by intoplicine (RP-60475), a new antitumor agent in early clinical trials. Mol. Pharmacol. **44**: 767–774.
15. YOSHINARI, T. *et al.* 1993. Induction of topoisomerase I-mediated DNA cleavage by a new indolocarbazole, ED-110. Cancer Res. **53**: 490–494.
16. XU, Z. *et al.* 1998. DNA minor groove binding-directed poisoning of human DNA topoisomerase I by terbenzimidazoles. Biochemistry **37**: 3558–3566.
17. SIM, S.P. *et al.* 1997. Differential poisoning of topoisomerases by menogaril and nogalamycin dictated by the minor groove-binding nogalose sugar. Biochemistry **36**: 13285–13291.

18. POMMIER, Y.G. et al. 2000. Benzo[a]pyrene diol epoxide adducts in DNA are potent suppressors of a normal topoisomerase I cleavage site and powerful inducers of other topoisomerase I cleavages. Proc. Nat. Acad. Sci. USA **97**: 2040–2045.
19. POURQUIER, P. et al. 1997. Effects of uracil incorporation, DNA mismatches, and abasic sites on cleavage and religation activities of mammalian topoisomerase I. J Biol. Chem. **272**: 7792–7796.
20. POURQUIER, P. et al. 1997. Trapping of mammalian topoisomerase I and recombinations induced by damaged DNA containing nicks or gaps. Importance of DNA end phosphorylation and camptothecin effects. J Biol. Chem. **272**: 26441–26447.
21. POURQUIER, P. et al. 1999. Induction of reversible complexes between eukaryotic DNA topoisomerase I and DNA-containing oxidative base damages. 7, 8-dihydro-8-oxoguanine and 5-hydroxycytosine. J Biol. Chem. **274**: 8516–8523.
22. D'ARPA, P. et al. 1990. Involvement of nucleic acid synthesis in cell killing mechanisms of topoisomerase poisons. Cancer Res. **50**: 6919–6924.
23. HSIANG, Y.H. et al. 1989. Arrest of replication forks by drug-stabilized topoisomerase I-DNA cleavable complexes as a mechanism of cell killing by camptothecin. Cancer Res. **49**: 5077–5082.
24. TSAO, Y.P. et al. 1992. The involvement of active DNA synthesis in camptothecin-induced G2 arrest: altered regulation of p34cdc2/cyclin B. Cancer Res. **52**: 1823–1829.
25. TSAO, Y.P. et al. 1993. Interaction between replication forks and topoisomerase I-DNA cleavable complexes: studies in a cell-free SV40 DNA replication system. Cancer Res. **53**: 5908–5914.
26. ZHANG, H. et al. 1990. A model for tumor cell killing by topoisomerase poisons. Cancer Cells **2**: 23–27.
27. NITISS, J. & J.C. WANG. 1988. DNA topoisomerase-targeting antitumor drugs can be studied in yeast. Proc. Natl. Acad. Sci. USA **85**: 7501–7505.
28. HUANG, T.T. et al. 2000. NF-kappaB activation by camptothecin. A linkage between nuclear DNA damage and cytoplasmic signaling events. J. Biol. Chem. **275**: 9501–9509.
29. PIRET, B. & J. PIETTE. 1996. Topoisomerase poisons activate the transcription factor NF-kappaB in ACH-2 and CEM cells. Nucleic Acids Res. **24**: 4242–4248.
30. SHAO, R.G. et al. 1999. Replication-mediated DNA damage by camptothecin induces phosphorylation of RPA by DNA-dependent protein kinase and dissociates RPA:DNA-PK complexes. EMBO J. **18**: 1397–1406.
31. GOLDWASSER, F. et al. 1995. Topoisomerase I-related parameters and camptothecin activity in the colon carcinoma cell lines from the National Cancer Institute anticancer screen. Cancer Res. **55**: 2116–2121.
32. LIU, L.F. et al. 1996. Mechanism of action of camptothecin. Ann. N.Y. Acad. Sci. **803**: 44–49.
33. MORRIS, E.J. & H..M. GELLER. 1996. Induction of neuronal apoptosis by camptothecin, an inhibitor of DNA topoisomerase-I: evidence for cell cycle-independent toxicity. J. Cell Biol. **134**: 757–770.
34. HORTWIZ, S.B. et al. 1972. Studies on camptothecin I: effect on nucleic acid and protein synthesis. Mol. Pharmacol. **7**: 632–644.
35. KANN, H.E. & K.W. KURT. 1972. Effect of DNA-reactive drugs on RNA synthesis patterns in L1210 cells. Mol. Pharmacol. **8**: 551–560.
36. LJUNGMAN, M. & P.C. HANAWALT. 1996. The anti-cancer drug camptothecin inhibits elongation but stimulates initiation of RNA polymerase II transcription. Carcinogenesis **17**: 31–35.
37. ZHANG, H. et al. 1988. Involvement of DNA topoisomerase I in transcription of human ribosomal RNA genes. Proc. Natl. Acad. Sci. USA **85**: 1060–1064.
38. WU, J. & L.F. LIU. 1997. Processing of topoisomerase I cleavable complexes into DNA damage by transcription. Nucleic Acids Res. **25**: 4181–4186.
39. SQUIRES, S. et al. 1993. Hypersensitivity of Cockayne's syndrome cells to camptothecin is associated with the generation of abnormally high levels of double strand breaks in nascent DNA. Cancer Res. **53**: 2012–2019.
40. BEIDLER, D.R. & Y.C. CHENG. 1995. Camptothecin induction of a time- and concentration-dependent decrease of topoisomerase I and its implication in camptothecin activity. Mol. Pharmacol. **47**: 907–914.

41. DESAI, S.D. et al. 1997. Ubiquitin-dependent destruction of topoisomerase I is stimulated by the antitumor drug camptothecin. J. Biol. Chem. **272:** 24159–24164.
42. POULIOT, J.J. et al. 1999. Yeast gene for a Tyr-DNA phosphodiesterase that repairs topoisomerase I complexes. Science **286:** 552–555.
43. MAO, Y. et al. 2000. SUMO-1 conjugation to topoisomerase I: a possible repair response to topoisomerase-mediated DNA damage. Proc. Natl. Acad. Sci. USA **97:** 4046–4051.
44. SHEN, Z. et al. 1996. UBL1, a human ubiquitin-like protein associating with human RAD51/RAD52 proteins. Genomics **36:** 271–279.
45. BODDY, M.N. et al. 1996. PIC 1, a novel ubiquitin-like protein which interacts with the PML component of a multiprotein complex that is disrupted in acute promyelocytic leukaemia. Oncogene **13:** 971–982.
46. MATUNIS, M.J. et al. 1996. A novel ubiquitin-like modification modulates the partitioning of the Ran-GTPase-activating protein RanGAP1 between the cytosol and the nuclear pore complex. J. Cell Biol. **135:** 1457–1470.
47. LAPENTA, V. et al. 1997. SMT3A, a human homologue of the S. cerevisiae SMT3 gene, maps to chromosome 21qter and defines a novel gene family. Genomics **40:** 362–366.
48. OKURA, T. et al. 1996. Protection against Fas/APO-1 and tumor necrosis factor-mediated cell death by a novel protein, sentrin. J. Immunol. **157:** 4277–4281.
49. MAHAJAN, R. et al. 1997. A small ubiquitin-related polypeptide involved in targeting RanGAP1 to nuclear pore complex protein RanBP2. Cell **88:** 97–107.
50. DESTERRO, J.M. 1999. Identification of the enzyme required for activation of the small ubiquitin-like protein SUMO-1. J. Biol. Chem. **274:** 10618–10624.
51. CHEN, P. et al. 1993. Multiple ubiquitin-conjugating enzymes participate in the *in vivo* degradation of the yeast MAT alpha repressor. Cell **74:** 357–369.
52. GILON, T. et al. 1998. Degradation signals for ubiquitin system proteolysis in *Saccharomyces cerevisiae*. EMBO J. **17:** 2759–2766.
53. HOCHSTRASSER, J. 1996. Ubiquitin-dependent protein degradation. Annu. Rev. Genet. **30:** 405–439.
54. DESTERRO, J.M. et al. 1998. SUMO-1 modification of IkappaB-alpha inhibits NF-kappaB activation. Mol. Cell. **2:** 233–239.
55. MAHAJAN, R. et al. 1998. Molecular characterization of the SUMO-1 modification of RanGAP1 and its role in nuclear envelope association. J. Cell. Biol. **140:** 259–270.
56. MATUNIS, M.J. et al. 1998. SUMO-1 modification and its role in targeting the Ran GTPase-activating protein, RanGAP1, to the nuclear pore complex. J. Cell. Biol. **140:** 499–509.
57. SAITOH, H. et al. 1998. Ubc9p and the conjugation of SUMO-1 to RanGAP1 and RanBP2. Curr. Biol. **8:** 121–124.
58. KAMITANI, T. et al. 1998. Identification of three major sentrinization sites in PML. J. Biol. Chem. **273:** 26675–26682.
59. MULLER, S. & A. DEJEAN. 1999. Viral immediate-early proteins abrogate the modification by SUMO-1 of PML and Sp100 proteins, correlating with nuclear body disruption. J. Virol. **73:** 5137–5143.
60. GOSTISSA, M. et al. 1999. Activation of p53 by conjugation to the ubiquitin-like protein SUMO-1. EMBO J. **18:** 6462–6471.
61. RODRIGUEZ, M.S et al. 1999. SUMO-1 modification activates the transcriptional response of p53. EMBO J. **18:** 6455–6461.
62. D'ARPA, P. & L.F. LIU. 1995. Cell cycle-specific and transcription-related phosphorylation of mammalian topoisomerase I. Exp. Cell Res. **217:** 125–131.
63. LEROY, L.F. et al. 1999. The roles of ubiquitin-dependent proteolysis in determining the sensitivity/resistance of tumor cells to topoisomerase inhibitors. Proc. Am. Assoc. Cancer Res **40:** 775.
64. SPATARO, V. et al. 1998. The ubiquitin-proteasome pathway in cancer. Br. J. Cancer **77:** 448–455.
65. GUPTA, E. et al. 1998. Clinical evaluation of sequential topoisomerase targeting in the treatment of advance maligancy. Cancer Ther. **1:** 292–302.
66. MURREN, J.R. et al. 1996. Camptothecin resistance related to drug-induced down-regulation of topoisomerase I and to steps occurring after the formation of protein- linked DNA breaks. Ann. N.Y. Acad. Sci. **803:** 74–92.

Molecular and Biological Determinants of the Cytotoxic Actions of Camptothecins

Perspective for the Development of New Topoisomerase I Inhibitors

KURT W. KOHN[a] AND YVES POMMIER

Laboratory of Molecular Pharmacology, Division of Basic Sciences, National Cancer Institute, National Institutes of Health, Bethesda, Maryland 20892, USA

ABSTRACT: Camptothecin, originally discovered in 1957 as an antitumor activity in plant extracts, has recently become one of the most promising leads to new anticancer drugs. After lingering for many years, interest in camptothecin was revitalized in 1985 upon discovery of its specific action on topoisomerase I. Detailed elucidation of action mechanisms at the molecular, cellular, and pharmacologic levels has made camptothecin and its congeners perhaps the best understood among clinical anticancer drugs. Promising chemical variants of camptothecin, and recently other chemical categories of topoisomerase I-targeted drugs, provide unusually rich opportunities for rational drug selection and design. This is made possible by current concepts based, for the most part, on a sound experimental foundation, which points the way towards optimally effective therapy.

HISTORICAL INTRODUCTION

Camptothecin illustrates some of the opportunities and difficulties experienced in the development of clinically useful antitumor drugs from plant materials. Although it was discovered and chemically characterized in the 1960s, two decades elapsed before its clinical potential was realized. Camptothecin was the active component in an alcoholic extract of leaves from the Chinese tree *Camptotheca accuminata*, which gave one of the first strongly positive results in an antitumor screen of natural products from plants, initiated by the Cancer Chemotherapy National Service Center (CCNSC) under the direction of Jonathan Hartwell in the early 1950s. This extract stood out among many plant extracts submitted in 1957 by Monroe E. Wall. The details of the discovery and isolation of camptothecin were recounted by Wall and Wani in these *Annals*,[1] as well as elsewhere.[2,3] In 1963, a sufficient sample of the wood and bark of the tree became available for fractionation, which was conducted by Wall and his associate, Mansukh C. Wani, in collaboration with the CCNSC using the murine leukemia L1210 tumor as bioassay. Despite the long time delay of this assay, pure compound was soon obtained. The activity of an extract against the L1210 tumor was highly unusual. Isolation was aided by the very low solubility of camptothecin in most solvents, which caused the compound to crystallize out at an

---

[a]Voice: 301-496-2769; fax: 301-402-0752.
kohnk@dc37a.nci.nih.gov

TABLE 1. CPT action mechanism (current picture)

- Topo I-blocking activity is necessary (but not sufficient) for antitumor activity.
- Activity resides in the lactone form of the drug, which undergoes a slow pH-dependent interconversion with the inactive salt form of the drug.
- Active camptothecin derivatives with modified properties and solubilities can be designed based on structure-activity data.
- Camptothecins stabilize topo I-DNA cleavage complexes, which are spontaneously reversible and not in themselves cytotoxic.
- A CPT-stabilized DNA cleavage complex can become fixed and potentially cytotoxic when encountered by a progressing DNA replication fork or transcription complex.
- Processing of such fixed DNA lesions may lead to successful or unsuccessful repair.
- Cell survival depends also on controls of cell cycle and apoptosis.

early stage of fractionation. By 1966, the chemical structure of camptothecin was solved with the aid of X-ray crystallography.[4]

Early development of the drug, however, was hampered by the insolubility of the compound and by the difficulty of obtaining large amounts of plant material. Moreover, early clinical trials (reported in 1972) had disappointing results, because they used the soluble sodium salt of camptothecin, which later turned out to be an inactive form of the drug (refs. 2 and 3 and references cited therein).

Interest in camptothecin then lingered until dramatically revived by the discovery in 1985 of its specific action on topoisomerase I (topo I).[5] The subsequent flurry of chemical and biological investigations stimulated by this seminal finding soon uncovered the key facts needed for successful clinical application of this new class of drugs. The key findings, which constitute the current picture of the camptothecin action mechanism, are summarized in TABLE 1.

PERSPECTIVE ON THE DEVELOPMENT OF NOVEL TOPO I INHIBITORS

Structure-activity studies in biochemical systems with purified topo I and with blood components, as well as in tissue culture and in animal studies are being used to improve the activity of camptothecins and to discover novel topo I inhibitors.

Structure-Activity Relationships

Many CPT derivatives, prepared by Wall and Wani, led to a coherent structure-activity picture, which was derived first on the basis of murine antitumor data and later by assays of the effects on topo I. The biochemical and antitumor data were in excellent agreement with each other and provided the first strong indication that topo I is the antitumor target of these drugs.

It was of particular importance to determine where substituents could be added on the CPT structure without diminution of activity ("bulk tolerance"). Bulk tolerance was found at positions 7, 9, 10, and, to some degree, position 11 (FIG. 1). Many active derivatives were obtained substituted at these positions. Position 12, on the

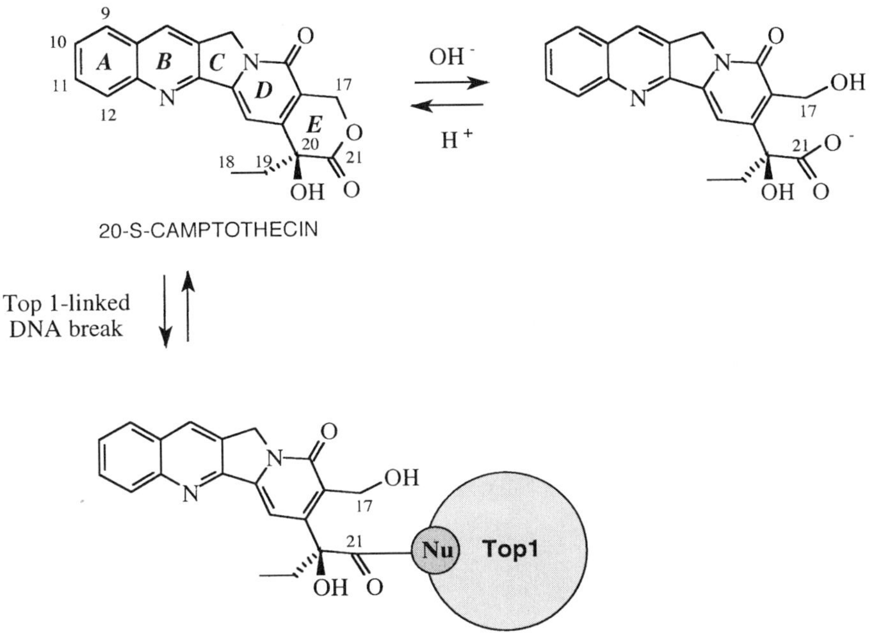

FIGURE 1. Camptothecin structure, activity, and reactivity. Bulk tolerance for topo I inhibition and cytotoxicity exists at the 7, 9, 10, and, to some extent, the 11-position, but not at the 12-position. The stereoconfiguration of the 20-hydroxyl must be *S* for activity. The lactone in the E-ring undergoes a pH-dependent interconversion to the inactive carboxylate (*right*). A nucleophilic site on topo I may react with the lactone to form a covalent bond, which could be spontaneously reversible (*below*).

other hand, did not tolerate the addition of any substituents. A notable early observation concerned positions 10 and 11.[6] The addition of methylenedioxy to form a 5-membered ring joined to these positions yielded a compound of increased potency in both antitumor and topo I assays. However, the addition of methoxy groups simultaneously to both positions abolished activity, whereas the addition of a methoxy group to either one or the other position did not. The inactivity of the dimethoxy derivative was attributed to steric encroachment into the neighborhood of the 12 position. It was surmised that extension on the A-ring could increase activity, provided that it did not encroach upon the region of the 12 position.[6]

The E-ring was thought to be sacrosanct. Any alteration, such as replacement of the lactone by an amide group, reduction of the lactone, removal of the carbonyl oxygen, or removal of the 20-hydroxyl, inactivated the molecule[7]. Moreover, the stereochemistry of the 20-position was critical: the 20(S) hydroxy compound was active whereas the 20(R) was inactive. It was assumed that activation of the lactone by the α-hydroxy configuration was required. One of the themes of this Conference was homocamptothecin (hCPT) and its derivatives, which violate this E-ring paradigm. Next, we present a current view of the role of the E-ring.

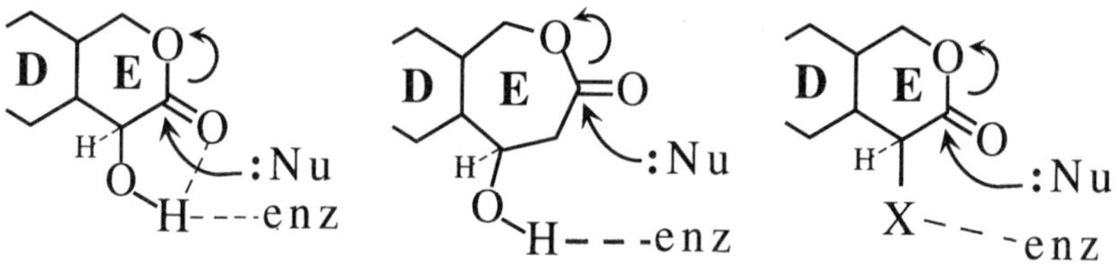

Effect on Top1 binding

	CPT	hCPT	\multicolumn{3}{c}{Substituent on CPT 20-position}
			Cl	Br	H
H-bond to enzyme	+	++	...	...	...
Intramolecular H-bond	−	...	...	...	...
Electron withdrawal	++	...	+	±	...
Polarizability bond	...	...	+	++	...
Net Top1 binding	++	++	+	+	...

FIGURE 2. The activity of E-ring congeners affecting the 20-hydroxyl is not inconsistent with covalent lactone-enzyme reaction (see text).

Hypothesis of Covalent Interaction between the E-ring Lactone and the topo I-DNA Complex

The reactivity of the E-ring lactone with nucleophiles was noted early by Wall and Wani, who suggested that the compound could function as an alkylating agent.[8] This gave rise to the hypothesis of labile covalent bond formation between the camptothecin lactone and the enzyme. The alpha-hydroxy configuration was presumed necessary to enhance the reactivity of the lactone. Recently, however, the covalency model was challenged by the unexpectedly potent activity of hCPT.[9,10] In this molecule, a methylene group is inserted between the lactone and the 20-hydroxyl in CPT (FIG. 2), as a result of which the reactivity of the lactone is diminished (although not abolished).

The activity of hCPT, however, can be rationalized in a manner that preserves the covalency hypothesis. First, the stereospecificity of the CPT 20-hydroxyl suggests that the hydroxy group interacts with the topo I protein. Intramolecular H-bonding between the hydroxyl and the lactone then would not only activate the lactone but also diminish the interaction with the enzyme. In hCPT, the lactone has relatively low reactivity, but the hydroxyl is free to interact optimally with topo I (FIG. 2). Second, the reactivity of the lactone in hCPT could be facilitated in the topo I complex. Third, low reactivity would retard both the formation and the reversal of the covalent bond between drug and enzyme. The net effect could be to maintain, or even increase, the steady-state level of topo I-DNA cleavage complexes. Moreover, longer persistence of cleavage complexes could increase their cytotoxic potential.

It is notable that hCPT exhibits a pattern of topo I-DNA cleavage sites distinct from that of other camptothecins.[11]

TABLE 2. Why develop new topo I inhibitors?

- Within each class of anticancer drugs, different drugs have different activity spectra (example: top2 inhibitors).
- Limitations of camptothecins:

    General limitations:

        Rapid reversibility of the topo I-DNA cleavage complexes

        E-ring opening ($\rightarrow$ inactive carboxylate)

        Poor solubility

        High binding to human serum albumin

    Drug-specific limitations:

      CPT-11

        Prodrug that needs activation by esterase(s)

        Cholinesterase inhibition

      10-hydroxy-derivatives

        Glucuronidation

        MXR (BCRP)-mediated efflux

Another recent surprise regarding the E-ring was the activity (albeit reduced potency) of CPT derivatives in which the 20-hydroxyl was replaced by Cl or Br.[12] The presumed essentiality of the 20-hydroxyl, which had been based in part on the inactivity of deoxy derivative, was thus contradicted. The polarizability of the halogen may allow an interaction sufficient to stabilize the complex with the enzyme. A framework to account for the E-ring structure-activity dependence is suggested in FIGURE 2.

Rationale for Developing Novel topo I Inhibitors (TABLE 2)

The activity of camptothecin derivatives validates topo I as an anticancer target. Two camptothecins were recently approved by the Food and Drug Administration (FDA) for clinical use in the United States. Topotecan (Hycamtin^R, SmithKline Beecham) is used for the treatment of cisplatin-refractory ovarian carcinoma and for second-line therapy in small-cell lung cancer (SCLC). Irinotecan (CPT-11, Camptosar^R, Pharmacia Upjohn) has been approved for treatment of colorectal cancer. (See FIGURE 3 for structures.) Ongoing clinical trials indicate that camptothecin derivatives will be useful in a variety of other human malignancies.

New topo I inhibitors with different activity profiles probably can be developed, as has been the case for other cancer chemotherapy targets. In the case of topoisomerase II inhibitors, for example, amsacrine and etoposide (VP16) both are potent inhibitors of the enzyme, whereas the latter has much broader antitumor activity.[13] Hence, having one class of active topo I inhibitors should not preclude but rather foster the search for other inhibitors.

Although camptothecins are very potent and selective topo I inhibitors, they suffer from limitations (TABLE 2). Complexes of camptothecin and topo I-DNA, possibly through labile covalent linkage to the camptothecin E-ring (see preceding text and FIGURE 1), reverse within minutes after camptothecin removal.[14,15] For this reason, clinical protocols use prolonged drug infusions.

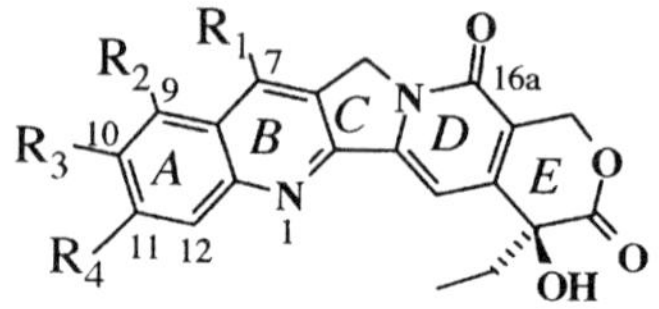

Camptothecin Derivative	R_1	R_2	R_3	R_4
Camptothecin	H	H	H	H
Topotecan	H	$-CH_2-N(CH_3)_2$	-OH	H
Irinotecan (CPT-11)	$-CH_2-CH_3$	H	A	H
SN-38	$-CH_2-CH_3$	H	-OH	H
Exatecan (DX-8951f)	—— B ——		$-CH_3$	-F
Rubitecan (9-nitroCPT)	H	$-NO_2$	H	H
9-aminoCPT	H	$-NH_2$	H	H
Lurtotecan (GI-147211)	C	H	—— D ——	

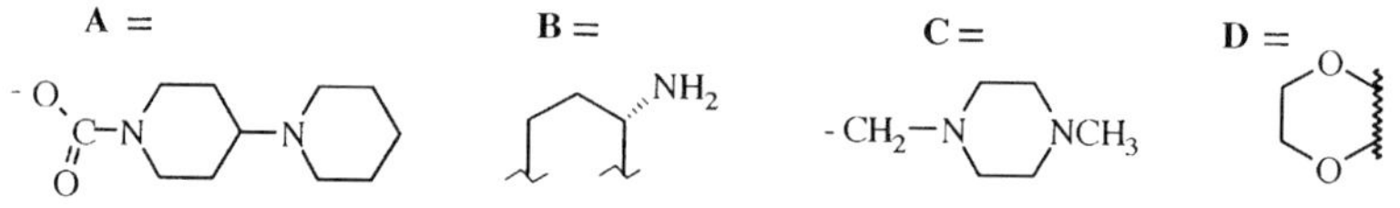

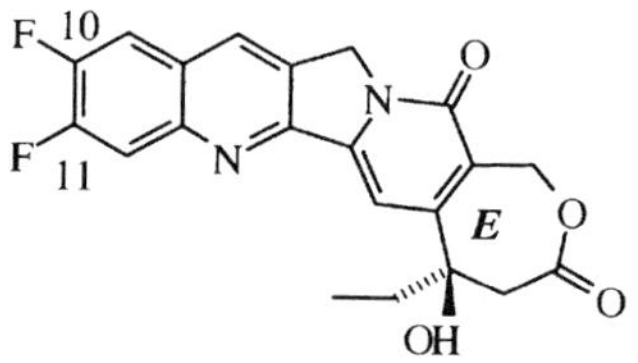

FIGURE 3. Structures of camptothecins in clinical use.

E-ring opening leads to the watersoluble carboxylate forms of camptothecins, which are inactive against topo I[6] and bind with high affinity to human serum albumin.[16] This E-ring opening occurs readily at physiological pH and can be reversed at acidic pH (FIG. 1).

Some limitations of camptothecins are drug-specific (TABLE 2). Irinotecan is a prodrug that needs to be activated to SN-38 by carboxylesterases.[17] Irinotecan also binds and inhibits cholinesterase, which may account for the cholinergic diarrhea often associated with this drug.[18]

Camptothecin derivatives are substrates for the newly described transporter BCRP/MXR/ABCP.[19–21] This ATP cassette transporter confers resistance to topote-

TABLE 3. Development of novel camptothecins

- Knowledge of the limitations of camptothecins (see TABLE 2).
- Detailed structure-activity data with respect to topo I and pharmacokinetics.[22]
- Relatively facile synthesis of derivatives.
- Biochemical assays to quantitate topo I inhibition.
- Availability of camptothecin-resistant and/or topo I-deficient cells to test cellular pharmacology.

can, mitoxantrone, and doxorubicin. Cells overexpressing the MXR protein appear most resistant to the 10-hydroxy–substituted camptothecin derivatives possibly after drug glucuronidation,[21] and some cell lines made resistant to topotecan were reported to overexpress the BCRP/MXR/ABCP membrane transporter.[20]

Novel Camptothecins

The rational development of camptothecins is facilitated by detailed (albeit incomplete) knowledge of the structure and function of its specific pharmacologic target, the biological consequences of this interaction, and the coordinated efforts of biochemists, cell biologists, medicinal chemists, pharmacologists, and clinicians, combining capabilities from academia, government, and industry. TABLE 3 summarizes factors that contribute to the successful development of novel camptothecins.

The following novel derivatives are under development:

(1) Homocamptothecins, in which the E-ring is 7-membered due to the insertion of a methylene group between the hydroxyl and lactone moieties of camptothecin (FIG. 2). As just discussed, this E-ring modification provides a less reactive lactone with enhanced stability and decreased protein binding in human plasma.[10] Homocamptothecin is more potent than camptothecin in biochemical assays with purified topo I and is also more active against preclinical tumors.[10] The topo I-DNA cleavage complexes trapped by homocamptothecin are less reversible than those induced by camptothecin.[11] The 10,11-difluoro derivative (BN-80915) is in clinical development.

(2) 7-Substituted 10,11-methylenedioxy and 10,11-ethylenedioxy-camptothecins (Exatecan and Lurtotecan; see FIG. 3). Both the 7-substitution and the 10,11-methylenedioxy or ethylenedioxy substitutions increase the potency of the drugs against topo I.[14,15,23,24] They also confer enhanced stabilization of the topo I-DNA cleavage complexes, which become less reversible. The 7-substitutions can be used to increase solubility.

(3) 7-Silyl-camptothecins (DB67, kareniticins), which have less reversible topo I-DNA cleavage complexes (Pommier, Curran, & Burke, unpublished results). Their E-ring is more stable than that in camptothecin (although less than for homocamptothecins). They bind less to human serum albumin and are liposoluble, a property that is useful for formulation but can also influence organ distribution.[25]

Non-Camptothecin topo I Inhibitors

Because of the limitations of the known camptothecins, other chemical classes of topo I poisons have been sought and recently discovered. The assays used to discover

FIGURE 4. Structures of indolocarbazoles.

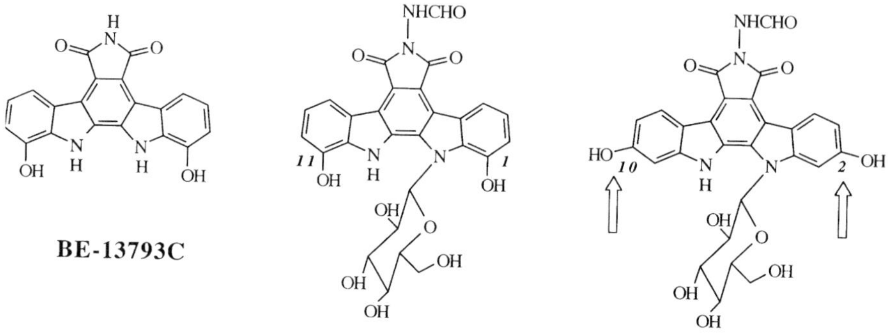

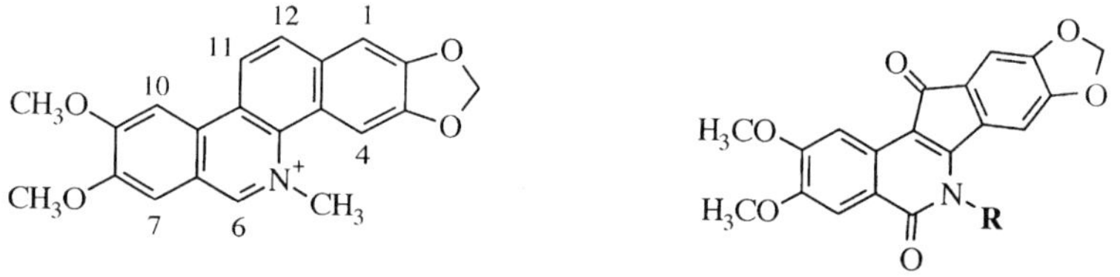

FIGURE 5. Structures of non-camptothecin topo I poisons.

these compounds include biochemical assays with eukaryotic topo I,[26] yeast screening with strains that overexpress or are defective in topo I,[27] and statistical analysis of drug databases (NCI Compare[R]).[28]

Indolocarbazoles were initially discovered in actinomycete extracts.[26] To increase the watersolubility of these compounds (BE-13793C; FIG. 4), sugar derivatives were obtained, leading to NB-506,[29] which until recently was in clinical trial. These indolocarbazoles are also DNA intercalators and probably target other DNA metabolizing and binding proteins. Recently, moving the hydroxyls from the 1 and 11 positions to the 2 and 10 positions led to weaker DNA intercalators with high topo I inhibitory activity (see ED-571 in FIG. 8).[30] Such derivatives are presently being developed for clinical trials (see chapter by Saijo, this volume).

A number of other non-camptothecin topo I inhibitors were recently identified (for review see ref. 31). FIGURE 5 shows examples of two classes of inhibitors, the benzophenanthridine, nitidine,[32,33] and the indenoisoquinolines (NSC314622 and MJ-III-65). The indenoisoquinolines were discovered by searching the NCI database

TABLE 4. Possible modes of processing or repair of DNA replication- or transcription-encounter lesions

- Enzymatic cleavage of the phosphotyrosyl ester between topo I and DNA.[35]
- Ubiquitination[36] or SUMO-lation,[37] followed by degradation or repair of the DNA-linked topo I complex.
- Nucleotide excision repair.
- Recombination.
- Removal of the newly replicated DNA segment by means of helicase and exonuclease action.

of approximately 40,000 compounds with cytotoxicity profiles similar to those of other known topo I inhibitors (NCI compare analysis[34]). The first compound identified was NSC 314622. More potent inhibitors have now been synthesized, including MJ-III-65 (FIG. 5).

CELLULAR RESPONSES DOWNSTREAM FROM TOPO I-DNA CLEAVAGE COMPLEXES

Replication-Encounter and Transcription-Encounter Lesions

CPT-stabilized DNA cleavage complexes reverse spontaneously within minutes both *in vivo* and *in vitro* and are not in themselves cytotoxic. When encountered by a replication fork or a transcription process, however, a less easily reversible lesion is thought to result, characterized by a terminated DNA double-strand or DNA-RNA hybrid (FIG. 6). The manner in which these potentially cytotoxic lesions may be processed or repaired was discussed during the conference and is summarized in TABLE 4.

The importance of replication-encounter lesions was shown by the ability of DNA synthesis inhibitors, such as aphidicolin or hydroxyurea, to prevent the cytotoxicity of CPT when DNA synthesis inhibitor and CPT were administered concurrently.[38–41] This protection was complete in some lines, but only partial in others. Cell lines that were only partially protected could be more fully protected by additionally inhibiting RNA synthesis, thus suggesting that encounters with transcription complexes also could have cytotoxic consequences. The cytotoxicity of CPT to non-replicating cells was clearly demonstrated in differentiated neuronal cells, which could be protected by RNA synthesis inhibitors, but not by DNA synthesis inhibitors.[42] It is not clear why some cell lines can be fully protected by DNA synthesis inhibitors, whereas others exhibit only partial protection.

The production and/or repair of replication-encounter or transcription-encounter lesions may depend on the persistence time (e.g., stability) of the topo I-DNA cleavage complexes.[15] It may be that transcription-encounter lesions require longer persistence or greater stability of topo I-DNA cleavage complexes than do replication-encounter lesions. Because most clinical tumors have a very low fraction of replicating cells, the ability to kill cells by means of a transcription encounter mechanism may be important. Therefore, the stability of topo Itopo I-DNA cleavage complexes formed by different CPT derivatives may critically affect their therapeutic potential.

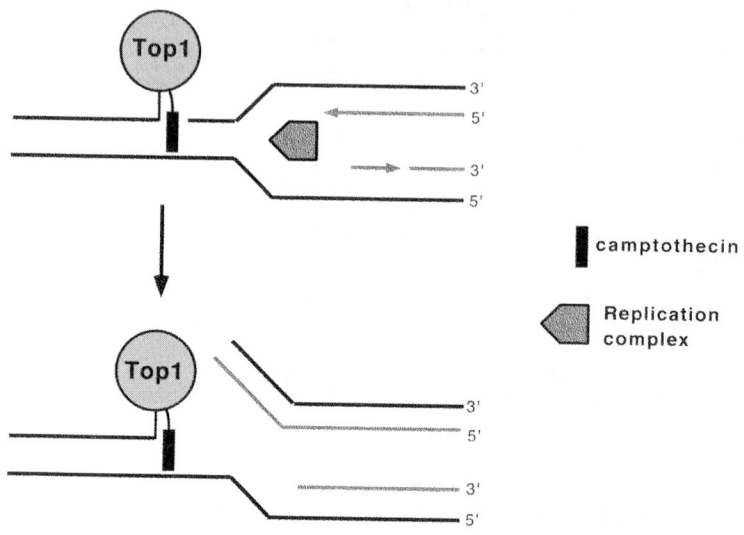

FIGURE 6. Model of how a potentially lethal DNA lesion may result from encounter of a DNA replication fork or transcription process with a CPT-stabilized topo I-DNA cleavage complex. The potentially lethal lesion includes a double-strand terminus, produced by the forward replicating or transcribing strand, and a DNA single-stranded region in the complementary DNA strand.

Signaling of DNA Lesions to the Cell Cycle and Apoptosis Control Systems

Cell cycle arrest and apoptosis are common responses to a variety of DNA damaging agents, including CPT. The manner in which the presence of DNA damage is signaled to the relevant control systems, however, remains unknown.

We recently reported the phosphorylation of RPA in CPT-treated cells, probably due to the action of DNA-PK, which we believe to be a possible component of this signaling process.[43] RPA binds to DNA single-stranded regions and would be expected to bind to such regions associated with replication-encounter lesions. As expected, DNA-PK in association with Ku was found to associate with and be activated by DNA double-strand ends,[44] which may form at replication-encounter lesions. In this way, DNA-PK may become juxtaposed to RPA and facilitate its phosphorylation. This model is diagrammed in FIGURE 7. A DNA damage signal might be generated and amplified if phosphorylated RPA dissociates from the lesions. Several RPA molecules might associate, become phosphorylated, and dissociate sequentially. The signal possibly could go by way of p53, which can bind RPA.[45] This binding may be disrupted when RPA becomes hyperphosphorylated in response to DNA damage[46] and thus could facilitate or further amplify signaling via p53.

A commonly observed response to CPT, as well as other DNA damaging agents, is cell cycle arrest in G2. Recent evidence has begun to show how this cell cycle checkpoint operates. The published evidence so far concerns mainly DNA damage produced by ionizing radiation and UV, which produce different types of DNA damage. Nevertheless, aside from the initiating steps, ionizing radiation and UV utilize

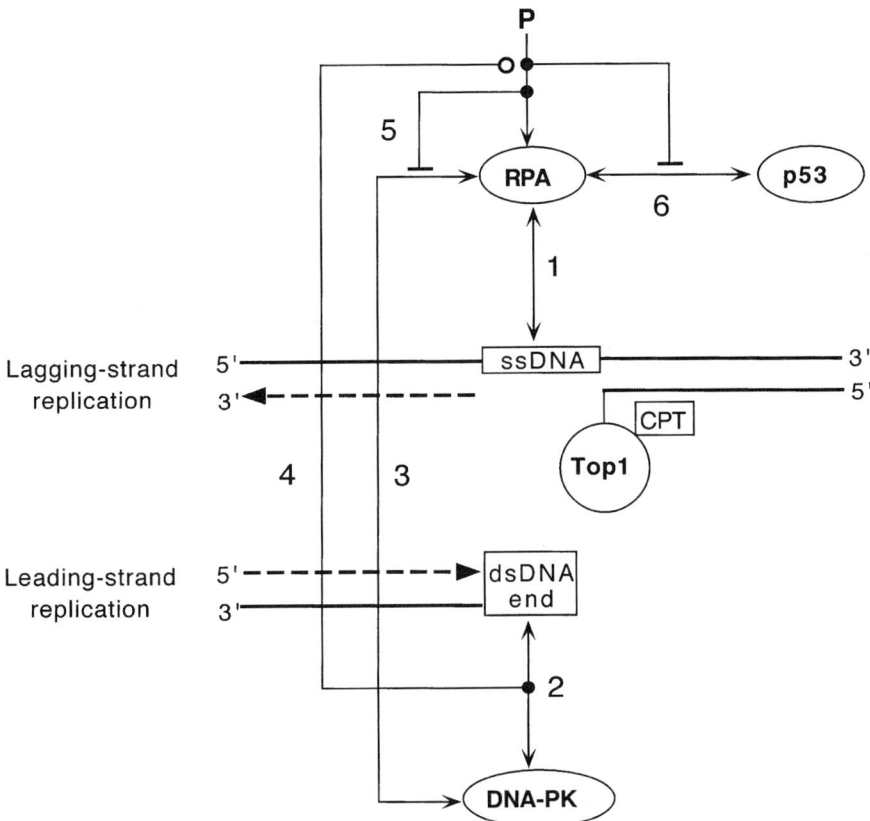

FIGURE 7. Proposed model of RPA and DNA-PK interactions at a replication-encounter lesion.[43] Diagram symbols utilize the conventions described[50] (see website http://discover.nci.nih.gov). RPA can bind to a DNA single-stranded segment (*1*), and DNA-PK can bind to a DNA double-strand end (*2*). (Non-covalent binding is represented by a line having *barbed arrowheads* at both ends.) RPA and DNA-PK thus may colocalize at or near the lesions, thereby facilitating their interaction (*3*) and the phosphorylation of RPA by DNA-PK (*4*). (Protein modification, for example by phosphorylation, is represented by a line having a *barbed arrowhead* at one end.) Phosphorylated RPA may dissociate from the complex (*5*). RPA binding to p53 (*6*) also may play a role in the signaling.

the same pathways to signal G2 arrest. This is probably true also for their stimulation of apoptosis. We anticipate that the response to CPT will also go by the same pathways, although the initiating steps may differ. A diagram summarizing the current picture of these signaling pathways is presented in FIGURE 8. Because of the rapid accumulation of new evidence, this picture is likely to be out of date by the time this article is published. An updated version of the diagram will be available at http://discover.nci.nih.gov.

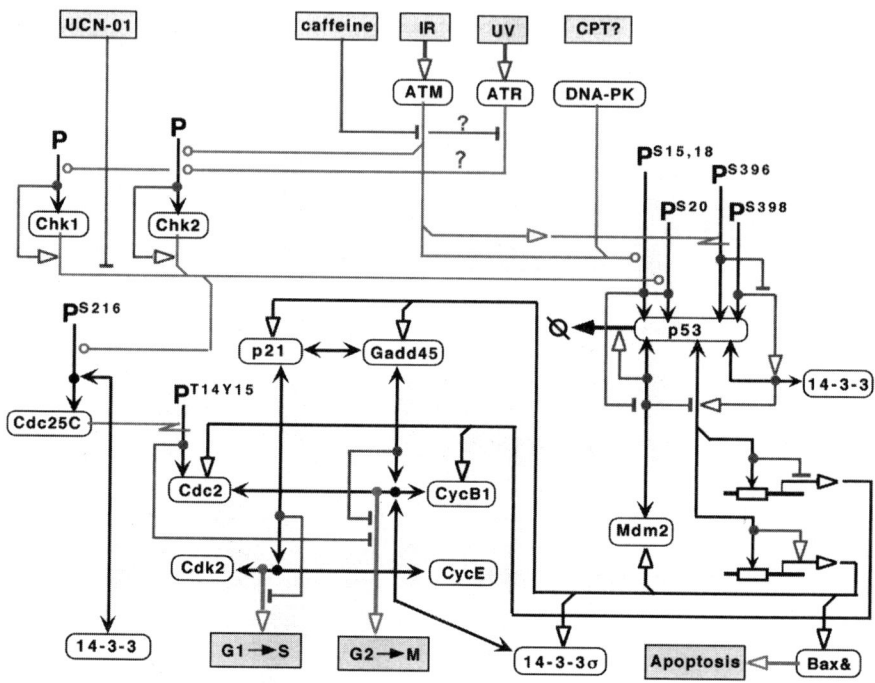

FIGURE 8. Current picture of signaling pathways from DNA damage to G2 arrest. (Paths to G1 arrest and apoptosis are indicated in abbreviated form.) The diagram utilizes the conventions previously described[50] (see website http://discover.nci.nih.gov). Signals from ionizing radiation (IR) go by way of ATM, whereas signals from UV-induced DNA lesions may go largely by way of ATR (references cited in 51 and 52). The path from CPT is not yet clear, although our preliminary findings suggest that DNA-PK may be involved. From ATM/ATR, the signals branch into two paths. One leads to phosphorylation of p53 at Ser15, permitting phosphorylation of Ser18 by casein kinase I (or a related kinase), which inhibits Mdm2-induced p53 degradation.[53] The second branch proceeds to Chk1 and/or Chk2, from which it again branches. One branch (from Chk2) leads to p53 phosphorylation at Ser20,[52] which is also reported to inhibit Mdm2–induced p53 degradation.[54] The other branch from Chk2 leads to phosphorylation of Cdc25C which then binds to and is sequestered by 14-3-3. All of these paths then come together in inhibiting Cdc2-Cyclin B (refs. 55 and 56 and references cited therein). The accumulation of p53 transcriptionally activates 14-3-3σ and Gadd45, both of which inhibit Cdc2-Cyclin B1, and transcriptionally inhibit the production of Cdc2 and Cyclin B1.[57] This network exemplifies a pattern of coherent actions, leading by several paths to a similar outcome.

Effects of p53 on the Survival of CPT-Treated Cells

Studies of the effects of normal p53 function on the sensitivity of cells to various DNA-targeted drugs have yielded conflicting results. This may be due to the multiple actions of p53, which include both protective and proapoptotic effects. The protective effects include activation of cell cycle checkpoints at G1/S and G2/M as well as stimulation of DNA repair. In many cell types, and depending on the circumstances of the study system, however, these potentially protective actions appear to be

TABLE 5. Determinants of camptothecin cytotoxicity

Topoisomerase I
- Topo I protein expression
- Topo I mutation

Drug-Topo I-DNA interactions
- Thermodynamic and kinetic parameters of complex formation and dissociation
- Preferred interaction sites depending on DNA sequence and chromatin structure

DNA lesion fixation
- DNA replication fork encounters
- Transcription process encounters

DNA lesion processing
- See TABLE 4.

Cell cycle checkpoint and apoptosis controls
- DNA-PK and RPA; possible signal to p53
- Determinants of apoptosis

Pharmacologic factors
- Structure-activity relationships
- Distribution in tissues and cells
- Metabolic conversion (e.g. of pro-drugs)
- Solubility and formulation

---

overridden by the p53-dependent sensitization to apoptosis.[47] In some systems, however, a protective effect of p53 on CPT-treated cells can be demonstrated.[48]

Determinants of CPT Cytotoxicity

Although topo I may be the primary or even sole biological target of action of camptothecins and may be an important cytotoxicity determinant, the cytotoxic actions of the drugs depend also on biochemical and metabolic factors. For example, a recent structure-activity study of a series of terbenzimidazole-type of topo I blockers bearing substituents of various lipophilicity at a given position revealed a correlation with cytotoxic activity, but not with topo I blocking activity.[49] This example illustrates one way in which clues might be obtained to chemical factors that play a role in topo I blocking activity, as opposed to other cytotoxicity determinants.

The various factors that come into play to determine the sensitivity of particular cell types to camptothecins are outlined in TABLE 5. In some cells, sensitivity is directly related to the expression of topo I protein. Several topo I point mutations have been observed to convey specific resistance to these drugs. The stability and persistence time of the complex may be important factors, as already discussed, influencing the formation and potential recovery of potentially lethal lesions generated by encounters with the replication or transcription machinery. The genomic sites of lesion formation, depending on local DNA sequence and chromatin structure, could have diverse cytotoxic potential. The ability of cells to process or repair the potentially lethal lesions is of obvious importance. The final life-or-death consequence to a cell then depends on the complex functions of the cell cycle and apoptosis control systems; the final outcome may be stochastic, that is, unpredictable in detail for any given cell, meaning that responses can fundamentally only be evaluated statistically. A thorough understanding of these factors, as well as pharmacological and molecular structural principles, will be essential for the optimal clinical application of topo I-targeted drugs.

REFERENCES

1. WALL, M.E. & M.C. WANI. 1996. Camptothecin. Ann. N.Y. Acad. Sci. **803:** 1–12.
2. WALL, M.E. & M.C. WANI. 1995. Camptothecin and taxol: discovery to clinic. Thirteenth Bruce F. Cain Memorial Award Lecture. Cancer Res. **55:** 753–760.
3. WALL, M.E. 1998. Camptothecin and taxol: discovery to clinic. Medicinal Res. Rev. **18:** 299–314.
4. WALL, W.E., M.C. WANI, C.C.E., K.H. PALMER, et al. 1966. Plant antitumor agents. I. The isolation and structure of camptothecin, a novel alkaloidal leukemia and tumor inhibitor from *Camptotheca accuminata*. J. Am. Chem Soc. **88:** 3888–3890.
5. HSIANG, Y. H., R. HERTZBERG, S. HECHT & L.F. LIU. 1985. Camptothecin induces protein-linked DNA breaks via mammalian DNA topoisomerase I. J. Biol. Chem. **260:** 14873–14878.
6. JAXEL, C., K.W. KOHN, M.C. WANI, et al. 1989. Structure-activity study of the actions of camptothecin derivatives on mammalian topoisomerase I: evidence for a specific receptor site and a relation to antitumor activity. Cancer Res. **49:** 1465–1469.
7. HERTZBERG, R.P., M.F. CARANFA, K.G. HOLDEN, et al. 1989. Modification of the hydroxy lactone ring of camptothecin: inhibition of mammalian topoisomerase I and biological activity. J. Med. Chem. **32:** 715–720.
8. WALL, M.E. & M.C. WANI. 1977. Antineoplastic agents from plants. Ann. Rev. Pharmacol. Toxicol. **17:** 117–132.
9. LAVERGNE, O., L. LESUEUR-GINOT, F.P. RODAS, et al. 1998. Homocamptothecins: synthesis and antitumor activity of novel E-ring-modified camptothecin analogues. J. Med. Chem. **41:** 5410–5419.
10. LESUEUR-GINOT, L., D. DEMARQUAY, R. KISS, et al. 1999. Homocamptothecin, an E-ring modified camptothecin with enhanced lactone stability, retains topoisomerase I-targeted activity and antitumor properties. Cancer Res. **59:** 2939–2943.
11. BAILLY, C., A. LANSIAUX, L. DASSONNEVILLE, et al. 1999. Homocamptothecin, an E-ring-modified camptothecin analogue, generates new topoisomerase I-mediated DNA breaks. Biochemistry **38:** 15556–15563.
12. WANG, X., X. ZHOU & S.M. HECHT. 1999. Role of the 20-hydroxyl group in camptothecin binding by the topoisomerase I-DNA binary complex. Biochemistry **38:** 4374–4381.
13. POMMIER, Y., M.R. FESEN & F. GOLDWASSER. 1996. Topoisomerase II inhibitors: the epipodophyllotoxins, *m*-AMSA, and the ellipticine derivatives. *In* Cancer Chemotherapy and Biotherapy: Principles and Practice. B.A. Chabner & D.L. Longo, Eds. :435–461. Lippincott – Raven. Philadelphia.
14. TANIZAWA, A., A. FUJIMORI, Y. FUJIMORI & Y. POMMIER. 1994. Comparison of topoisomerase I inhibition, DNA damage, and cytotoxicity of camptothecin derivatives presently in clinical trials. J. Natl. Cancer Inst. **86:** 836–842.
15. TANIZAWA, A., K.W. KOHN, G. KOHLHAGEN, et al. 1995. Differential stabilization of eukaryotic DNA topoisomerase I cleavable complexes by camptothecin derivatives. Biochemistry **34:** 7200–7206.
16. MI, Z. & T.G. BURKE. 1994. Differential interactions of camptothecin lactone and carboxylate forms with human blood components. Biochemistry **33:** 10325–10336.
17. HUMERICKHOUSE, R., K. LOHRBACH, L. LI, et al. 2000. Characterization of CPT-11 hydrolysis by human liver carboxylesterase isoforms hCE-1 and hCE-2. Cancer Res. **60:** 1189–1192.

18. DODDS, H.M. & L.P. RIVORY. 1999. The mechanim for the inhibition of acetylcholinesterases by irinotecan (CPT-11). Mol. Pharmacol. **56:** 1346–1353.
19. MALIEPAARD, M., M.A. VAN GASTELEN, L.A. DE JONG, et al. 1999. Overexpression of the BCRP/MXR/ABCP gene in a topotecan-selected ovarian tumor cell line. Cancer Res. **59:** 4559–4563.
20. ALLEN, J.D., R.F. BRINKHUIS, J. WIJNHOLDS & A.H. SCHINKEL. 1999. The mouse Bcrp1/Mxr/Abcp gene: amplification and overexpression in cell lines selected for resistance to topotecan, mitoxantrone, or doxorubicin. Cancer Res. **59:** 4237–4241.
21. BRANGI, M., T. LITMAN, M. CIOTTI, et al. 1999. Camptothecin resistance: role of the ATP binding cassette (ABC) half-transporter, mitoxantrone-resistance (MXR), and potential for glucuronidation in MXR-expressing cells. Cancer Res. **59:** 5938–5946.
22. POMMIER, Y. & A. TANIZAWA. 1994. Camptothecins: mechanism of action and resistance. Cancer Invest. **11:** 3–6.
23. O'CONNOR, P.M., D. KERRIGAN, R. BERTRAND, et al. 1990. 10,11-Methylenedioxycamptothecin, a topoisomerase I inhibitor of increased potency: DNA damage and correlation to cytotoxicity in human colon carcinoma (HT-29) cells. Cancer Commun. **2:** 395–400.
24. VALENTI, M., W. NIEVES-NEIRA, G. KOHLHAGEN, et al. 1997. Novel 7-alkyl methylenedioxycamptothecin derivatives exhibit increased cytotoxicity and induce persistent cleavable complexes both with purified mammalian topoisomerase I and in human colon carcinoma SW620 cells. Mol. Pharmacol. **52:** 82–87.
25. BOM, D., D.P. CURRAN, A.J. CHAVAN, et al. 1999. Novel A,B,E-ring-modified camptothecins displaying high lipophilicity and markedly improved human blood stabilities. J. Med. Chem. **42:** 3018–3022.
26. YOSHINARI, T., A. YAMADA, D. UEMURA, et al. 1993. Induction of topoisomerase I-mediated DNA cleavage by a new indolocarbazole, ED-110. Cancer Res. **53:** 490–494.
27. NITISS, J.L., A. ROSE, K.C. SYKES, et al. 1996. Using yeast to understand drugs that target topoisomerases. Ann. N.Y. Acad. Sci. **803:** 32–43.
28. KOHLHAGEN, G., K. PAULL, M. CUSHMAN, et al. 1998. Protein-linked DNA strand breaks induced by NSC 314622, a non-camptothecin topoisomerase I poison. Mol. Pharmacol. **54:** 50–58.
29. YOSHINARI, T., M. MATSUMOTO, H. ARAKAWA, et al. 1995. Novel antitumor indolocarbazole compound 6-N-formylamino-12, 13-dihydro-1, 11-dihydroxy-13-(ß-D-glucopyranosyl)-5H-indolo[2, 3-a] pyrrolo[3,4-c] carbazole-5,7(6H)-dione (NB-506): induction of Topoisomerase I-mediated DNA cleavage and mechanisms of cell line-selective cytotoxicity. Cancer Res. **55:** 1310–1315.
30. BAILLY, C., L. DASSONNEVILLE, P. COLSON, et al. 1999. Intercalation into DNA is not required for inhibition of topoisomerase I by indolocarbazole antitumor agents. Cancer Res. **59:** 2853–2860.
31. POMMIER, Y., P. POURQUIER, Y. URASAKI, et al. 1999. Topoisomerase I inhibitors: selectivity and cellular resistance. Drug Resistance Update **2:** 307–318.
32. WANG, L.-K., R.K. JOHNSON & S.M. HECHT. 1993. Inhibition of topoisomerase I function by nitidine and fagaronine. Chem. Res. Toxicol. **6:** 813–818.
33. HOLDEN, J.A., M.E. WALL, M.C. WANI & G. MANIKUMAR. 1999. Human DNA topoisomerase I: quantitative analysis of the effects of camptothecin analogs and the benzophenanthridine alkaloids nitidine and 6-ethoxydihydronitidine on DNA topoisomerase I-induced DNA strand breakage [In Process Citation]. Arch. Biochem. Biophys. **370:** 66–76.
34. PAULL, K.D., E. HAMEL & L. MALPEIS. 1995. Prediction of biochemical mechanism of action from the in vitro antitumor screen of the National Cancer Institute. In Cancer Chemotherapeutic Agents. W.O. Foye, Ed. : 8–45. ACS. Washington, DC.
35. POULIOT, J.J., K.C. YAO, C.A. ROBERTSON & H.A. NASH. 1999. Yeast gene for a Tyr-DNA phosphodiesterase that repairs topoisomerase I complexes. Science **286:** 552–555.
36. DESAI, S.D., L.F. LIU, D. VAZQUEZ-ABAD & P. D'ARPA. 1997. Ubiquitin-dependent destruction of topoisomerase I is stimulated by the antitumor drug camptothecin. J. Biol. Chem. **272:** 24159–24164.

37. MAO, Y., M. SUN, S.D. DESAI & L.F. LIU. 2000. SUMO-1 conjugation to topoisomerase 1: A possible repair response to topoisomerase-mediated DNA damage. Proc. Natl. Acad. Sci. USA **97**: 4046–4051.
38. HOLM, C., J.M. COVEY, D. KERRIGAN & Y. POMMIER. 1989. Differential requirement of DNA replication for the cytotoxicity of DNA topoisomerase I and II inhibitors in Chinese hamster DC3F cells. Cancer Res. **49**: 6365–6368.
39. HSIANG, Y., M.G. LIHOU & L.F. LIU. 1989. Arrest of replication forks by drug-stabilized topoisomerase I-DNA cleavable complexes as a mechanism of cell killing by camptothecin. Cancer Res. **49**: 5077–5082.
40. GOLDWASSER, F., T. SHIMIZU, J. JACKMAN, et al. 1996. Correlations between S and G2 arrest and the cytotoxicity of camptothecin in human colon carcinoma cells. Cancer Res. **56**: 4430–4437.
41. BOROVITSKAYA, A.E. & P. D'ARPA. 1998. Replication-dependent and -independent camptothecin cytotoxicity of seven human colon tumor cell lines. Oncol. Res. **10**: 271–276.
42. MORRIS, E.J. & H.M. GELLER. 1996. Induction of neuronal apoptosis by camptothecin, an inhibitor of DNA topoisomerase-I: evidence for cell cycle-independent toxicity. J. Cell. Biol. **134**: 757–770.
43. SHAO, R.-G., C.-X. CAO, H. ZHANG, et al. 1999. Replication-mediated DNA damage by camptothecin induces phosphorylation of RPA by DNA-dependent protein kinase and dissociates DNA-PK/RPA complexes. EMBO J. **18**: 1397–1406.
44. YANEVA, M., R. KOWALEWSKI & M.R. LIEBER. 1997. Interaction of DNA-dependent protein kinase with DNA and with Ku: biochemical and atomic-force microscopy studies. EMBO J. **16**: 5098–5112.
45. WOLD, M.S. 1997. Replication protein A: A heterotrimeric, single-stranded DNA-binding protein required for eukaryotic DNA metabolism. Annu. Rev. Biochem. **66**: 61–92.
46. ABRAMOVA, N.A., J. RUSSELL, M. BOTCHAN & R. LI. 1997. Interaction between replication protein A and p53 is disrupted after UV damage in a DNA repair-dependent manner. Proc. Natl. Acad. Sci. USA **94**: 7186–7191.
47. O'CONNOR, P.M., J. JACKMAN, I. BAE, et al. 1996. Characterization of the p53 tumor suppressor pathway in cell lines of the NCI anticancer drug screen and relationships with chemosensitivity. Cancer Res. **57**: 4285–4300.
48. GUPTA, M., S. FAN, Q. ZHAN, et al. 1997. Inactivation of p53 increases the cytotoxicity of camptothecin in human colon HCT116 and breast MCF-7 cancer cells. Clin. Cancer Res. **3**: 1653–1660.
49. KIM, J.S., Q. SUN, C. YU, et al. 1998. Quantitative structure activity relationships on 5-substituted terbenzimidazoles as topoisomerase I poisons and antitumor agents. Bioorg. Med. Chem. **6**: 163–172.
50. KOHN, K.W. 1999. Molecular interaction map of the mammalian cell cycle control and DNA repair systems. *Mol. Biol. Cell* **10**: 2703–2734.
51. CHEHAB, N.H., A. MALIKZAY, M. APPEL & T.D. HALAZONETIS. 2000. Chk2/hCds1 functions as a DNA damage checkpoint in G1 by stabilizing p53. Genes Dev. **14**: 278–288.
52. HIRAO, A., Y.-Y. KONG, S. MATSUOKA, et al. 2000. DNA damage-induced activation of p53 by the checkpoint kinase Chk2. Science **287**: 1824–1827.
53. SAKAGUCHI, K., S. SAITO, Y. HIGASHIMOTO, et al 2000. Damage-mediated phosphorylation of human p53 threonine 18 through a cascade mediated by a casein 1-like kinase. J. Biol. Chem. **275**: 9278–9283.
54. CHEHAB, N.H., A. MALIKZAY, E.S. STAVRIDI & T.D. HALAZONETIS. 1999. Phosphorylation of Ser-20 mediates stabilization of human p53 in response to DNA damage. Proc. Natl. Acad. Sci. USA **96**: 13777–13782.
55. PIWNICA-WORMS, H. 1999. Fools rush in (News and Views). Nature **401**: 535–537.
56. CHAN, T.A., H. HERMEKING, C. LENGAUER, et al. 1999. 14-3-3σ is required to prevent mitotic catastrophe after DNA damage. Nature **401**: 616–620.
57. INNOCENTE, S.A., J.L.A. ABRAHAMSON, J.P. COGSWELL & J.M. LEE. 1999. p53 regulates a G2 checkpoint through cyclin B1. Proc. Natl. Acad. Sci. USA **96**: 2147–2152.

Dependence of Anticancer Activity of Camptothecins on Maintaining Their Lactone Function

B.C. GIOVANELLA, N. HARRIS, J. MENDOZA, Z. CAO, J. LIEHR, AND J.S. STEHLIN

The Stehlin Foundation for Cancer Research, 1918 Chenevert, Houston, Texas 77003, USA

ABSTRACT: Camptothecins contain a lactone ring that exists in the closed form below ph 7. Above 7, the open (CPT$^+$) and the closed (CPT) form coexist in a 50-50 ratio in mouse plasma and in a 90-10 ratio in human plasma due to the high affinity of human serum albumin (HSA) for CPT$^+$. CPT$^+$ is much less toxic than CPT and it is excreted much faster. In complete RPMI 1640 culture medium, the equilibrium CPT$^+$-CPT is 50-50. If 4% HSA is added, it moves to 90-10 modeling for the human physiological situation.

INTRODUCTION

Camptothecin (CPT), a naturally occurring alkaloid of plant origin (*Camptotheca acuminata*), was found in the 1960s to have very high anticancer activity.[1–3] Shortly afterwards, it was introduced into clinical trial. However, the results were very disappointing,[4–6] and the trials were therefore discontinued. The reason for the discrepancy between experimental and clinical results was that in order to use the i.v. route in human patients, CPT, which is water-insoluble, was converted to its sodium salt, which is very soluble, but it unfortunately has very little anticancer activity.[7,8] Camptothecin and its derivatives were eventually rediscovered as inhibitors of topoisomerase I[9–14] and as potent anticancer agents against human tumor xenografts in nude mice.[7,15] Clinical trials again indicated that CPT exhibited strong anticancer activity; however, the results obtained were always inferior to those obtained with the same camptothecin or derivative administered to nude mice carrying human cancer xenografts.[15,16]

It was soon realized that the reason for such discrepancy was the opening of the lactone ring of CPT (present also in all of its derivatives[15]). The anticancer activity of CPT is mediated through "inhibition" of topoisomerase I, an enzyme that relieves supercoiling of DNA necessary for cell division and other physiological activities.[10–14] In the open lactone form, CPT causes only 10% of the inhibition produced by the corresponding closed ring CPT.

The lactone ring exists in the closed form at or below pH 7.[8,15] Above it, it opens and the two forms at physiological pH 7.4 coexist in a 50–50% equilibrium[15] in the plasma of mice.

Human serum albumin, however, has a strong affinity for the open form and binds to it avidly, moving the equilibrium between the two forms from 50–50 to 90–10, in favor of the open lactone form.[17,18] Hence, there is a large difference in results between the sensitivity to CPT of human tumors when treated in nude mice (where 50% of the drug is in the closed lactone form, ie, the active form) and the results obtained in clinical trials in humans (where only 10% or less is in the active form).

These facts are well known by now, but what is still lacking is a systematic comparison between the biological activities of the two forms to assess their respective contribution to toxicity and their conversion kinetics according to routes of administration and excretion.

MATERIALS AND METHODS

Camptothecin lactone was obtained from several commercial sources and purified to 98% standards in our laboratory. Camptothecin sodium salt was prepared from CPT in our laboratory, as were 9 nitrocamptothecin (9NC; Rubitecan), 9NC potassium salt, and the propionate ester of CPT (CZ48).

The animals used were Swiss nude NIH high fertility strain mice aged approximately 3 months. Human tumors serially transplanted subcutaneously in our laboratory were used throughout. Tissue cultured cells of human cancers growing in RPMI plus 10% fetal calf serum (FCS) and other additives as noted were also used throughout. Camptothecin, 9NC, and their salts (CPT^+ and $9NC^+$) were suspended in cottonseed oil and injected into the thigh muscles or directly into the stomach of mice. The same substances were dissolved in ethanol and added to the tissue culture medium for treatment of cultured cells.

RESULTS

First, we investigated the toxicity of CPT^+ compared to that of CPT in nude mice. Remember that when CPT or 9NC is administered orally or intramuscularly to a mouse, the serum contains the two forms roughly in a 1:1 proportion.[15] It is also important to keep in mind that both forms are always present and the equilibrium between the two can easily be changed by pH changes in the medium and other factors. In man, the $9NC-9NC^+$ ratio in the serum is approximately 1:9, but when the drug reaches the urine (pH <7), this ratio becomes 2:3 and sometimes even 2:1.

FIGURES 1 and 2 show the concentration of CPT and CPT^+ in function of time after i.m. injection of CPT and CPT^+, respectively, in a mouse. Comparing these two graphs, it is evident that with injection of CPT, the closed lactone form and the open one are in equilibrium at approximately a 1:1 ratio. Instead, when CPT^+ is administered i.m., most of the drug is present in the serum as open lactone form. It is interesting that if CPT^+ is administered in the stomach instead of intramuscularly, the percentage of the closed (FIG. 3) lactone form in the serum is increased considerably from 11% to 24%. Thus, to compare the toxicity and the antitumor effect of the two forms, we used the intramuscular route that offered the largest quantitative differences between CPT and CPT^+. FIGURE 4 shows an experiment in which the toxicity of increasing amounts of CPT^+ (8 to 15 mg/kg) is expressed as body weight loss and animal survival, compared to a fixed dose of CPT–8 mg/kg both administered i.m. twice a week. It is immediately evident that CPT–8 mg/kg is very toxic, but no tox-

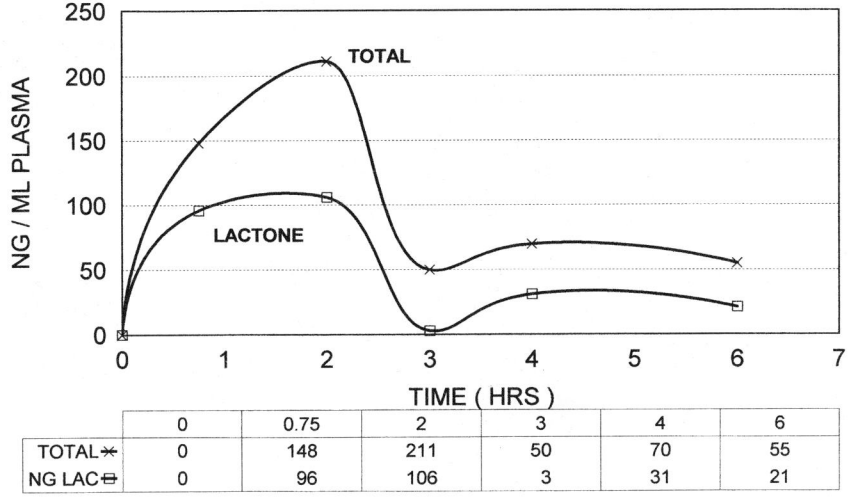

FIGURE 1. Intramuscular administration of CPT in nude mice.

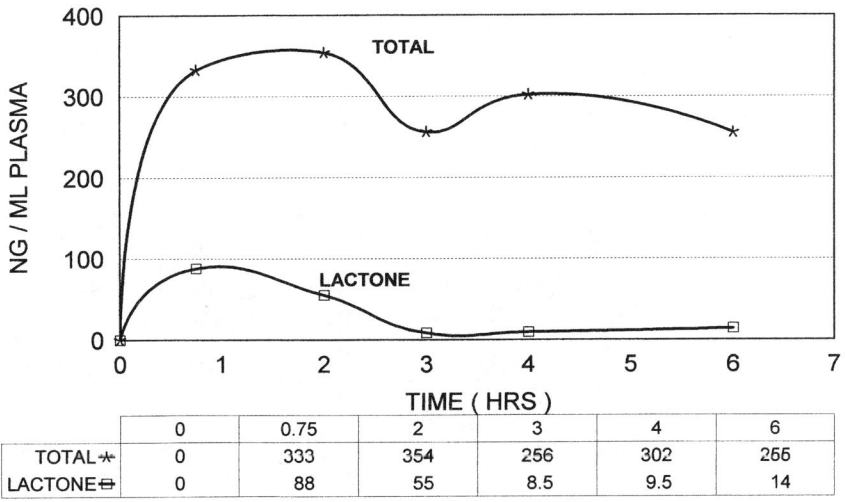

FIGURE 2. Intramuscular administration of Na-CPT in nude mice.

icity is observed even with 15 mg/kg of CPT$^+$. Only when the dose was above 40 mg/kg did toxicity appear. From our observations, the toxicity of CPT injected i.m. is 5- to 10-fold higher than that of CPT$^+$. Similar results were observed with 9NC (Rubitecan) and 9NC$^+$. The anticancer activity of the two forms was compared using the same experimental setup. FIGURE 5 shows clearly that 9NC$^+$ has no effect on a tumor that is totally inhibited by 9NC at the same dose. If, however, 9NC$^+$ is admin-

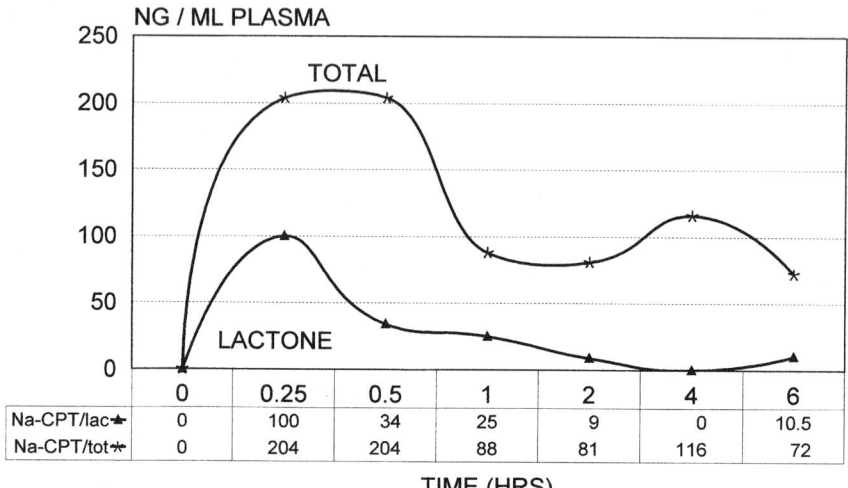

FIGURE 3. Administration of H^3-Na CPT in the stomach of mice.

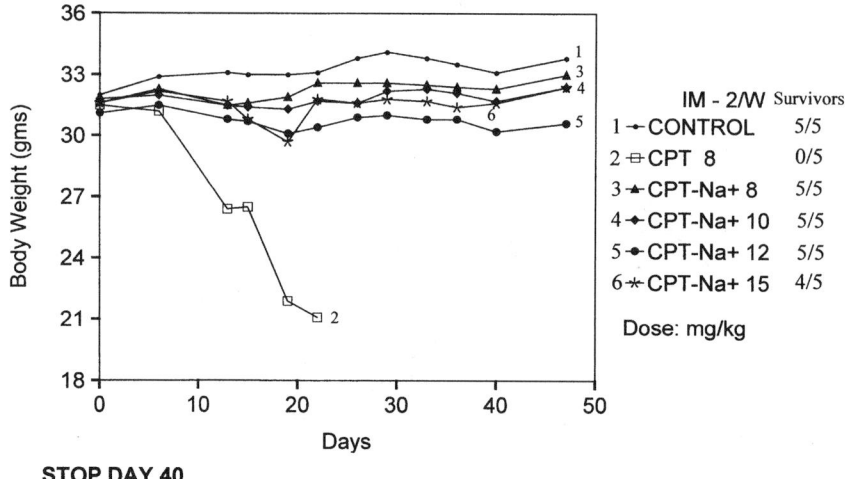

FIGURE 4. TX 1296–body weight CPT vs CPT–Na⁺–toxicity.

istered in the stomach, which, as we have already seen, increases the percentage of the active closed ring form in the serum, a very modest anticancer effect is obtained (FIG. 6). Having determined these parameters *in vivo*, we proceeded to study them in tissue culture.

FIGURE 7 shows the stability of CPT in RPMI 1640 medium supplemented with 10% FCS. The 50% lactone is reached about 32 hours after the drug has been added.

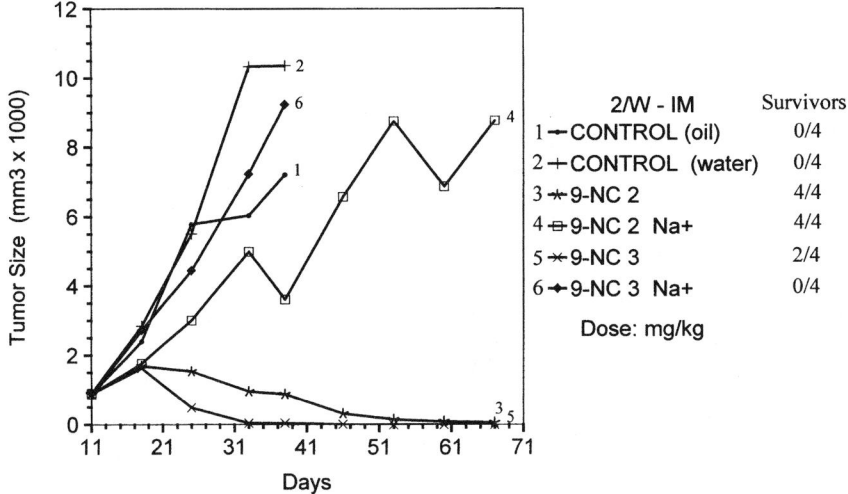

FIGURE 5. Tumor size. DOY-Lung Ca.

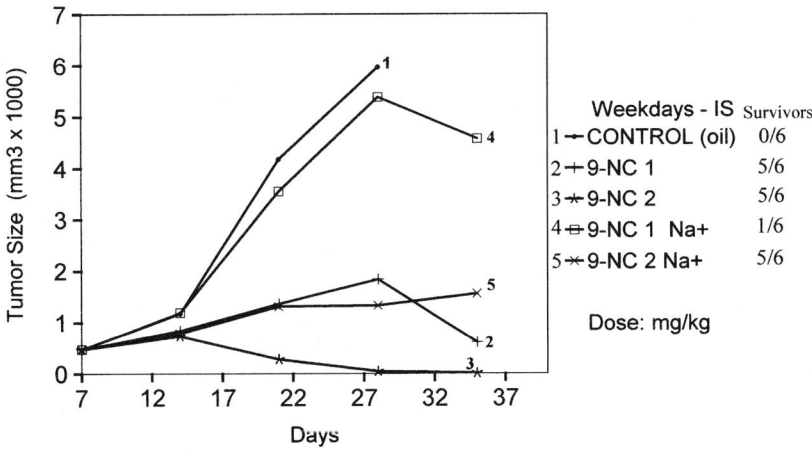

STOP. SAC Day 38

FIGURE 6. Tumor size. DOY-Lung Ca.

If, however, 4% human albumin is added to the culture medium, the concentration of CPT after the addition drops precipitously to 50% within an hour and a half versus 32 hours in the medium alone (FIG. 8).

The lactone versus the open form of CPT is at roughly the same level of equilibrium in complete tissue culture medium and in the cells growing in it.

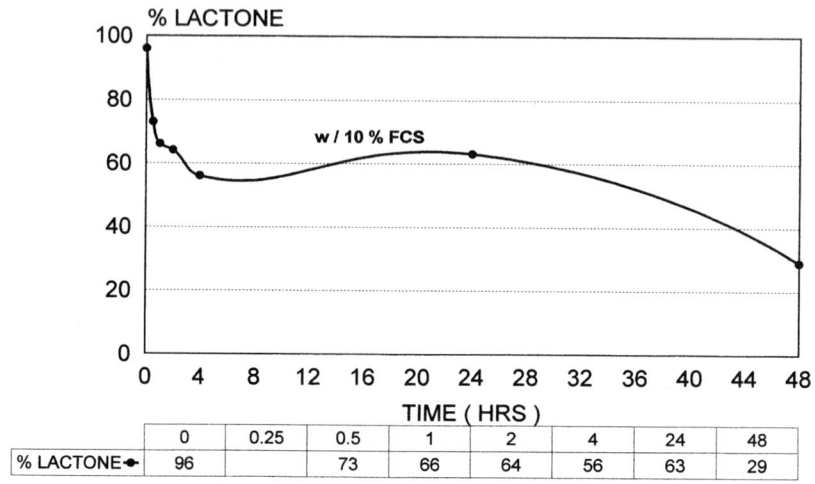

FIGURE 7. Stability of CPT in RPMI 1640.

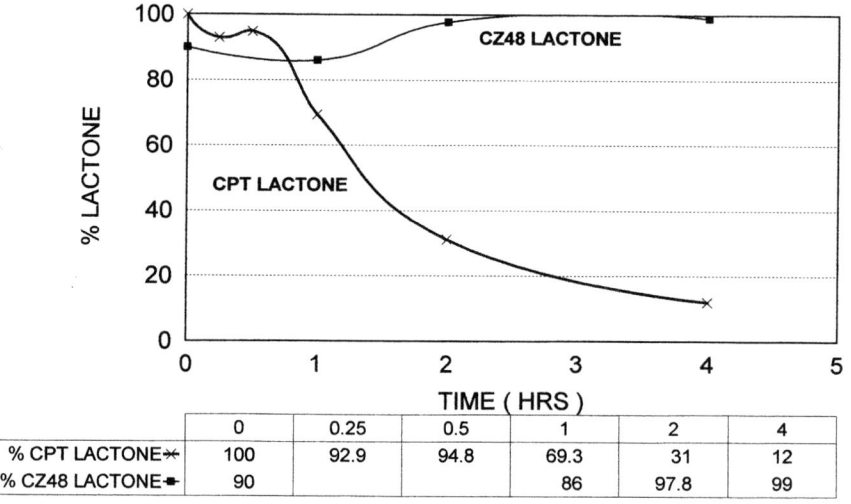

FIGURE 8. Stability in PBS w/4% human serum albumin: 1 µg/ml.

We are now investigating the possible explanation for the different biological behavior of CPT versus CPT$^+$. The first question is, Is there a difference in cell permeability between CPT and CPT$^+$? It is too soon to reach any conclusions, but the initial results show that the two forms are taken up by tumor cells about equally at very low levels (FIG. 9).

	30' CPT	24 hrs.	30' CPT$^+$	24 hrs.
HT29	127	231	73	227
BRO	112	94	122	180
CLO	71	52	48	117

DPM/cell

FIGURE 9. Uptake of tritiated CPT and CPT$^+$ in three human tumors.

DISCUSSION

From our findings, it is clear that the salts of CPT and its derivatives have much less biological activity than do their closed lactone ring counterparts. Specifically, CPT$^+$ is about 10-fold less toxic in mice than is CPT. CPT$^+$ also has much less anticancer activity, but it is difficult to establish exactly how much less. In mouse plasma, the CPT ⇆ CPT$^+$ is at equilibrium at 50:50, which means that there will always be a certain concentration of CPT in the blood even administering CPT$^+$. Also, to complicate things further, CPT$^+$ is excreted much more rapidly than is CPT.

When CPT is administered *in vitro* to cells in tissue culture, the equilibrium is again at around 50%, making the *in vitro* system very similar to the mouse system. Not surprisingly, the results obtained with these two systems are generally in good agreement with each other.

To render the *in vitro* system capable of modeling the human situation, it has been found that adding 4% human serum albumin (HSA) to complete RPMI 1640 plus 10% FCS produces a curve of CPT–CPT$^+$ very similar to the one obtained in human serum. We are now planning to repeat our *in vitro* anticancer activity experiment using medium plus HSA in order to have a better model for the human situation.

In vivo attempts will be made to utilize the nude rat xenografted with human tumors as a temporary model for the human condition. Rat albumin is about midway between mouse serum albumin (MSA) and HSA in the ability to accelerate the opening of the ring of CPT. Our final goal, for a really functional model of the human situation, is a nude animal having human liver parenchyma secreting HSA. We are working at it from multiple approaches.

Finally, FIGURE 10 summarizes what we currently know about the transit of CPT through the human body. From this it is evident that only small amounts of CPT reach tissues and target tumors. Direct measurements, rendered possible by the availability of stably tritium-labeled CPT, confirm that the rates of uptake of radioactive CPT by various tumors are very low. However, even these low uptakes are effective; at the doses administered, total kill of neoplastic cells was achieved.

Further studies are in progress to determine the minimum amount of CPT necessary to totally inhibit growth of most human tumors and the best way for it to reach the tumor target in the active form.

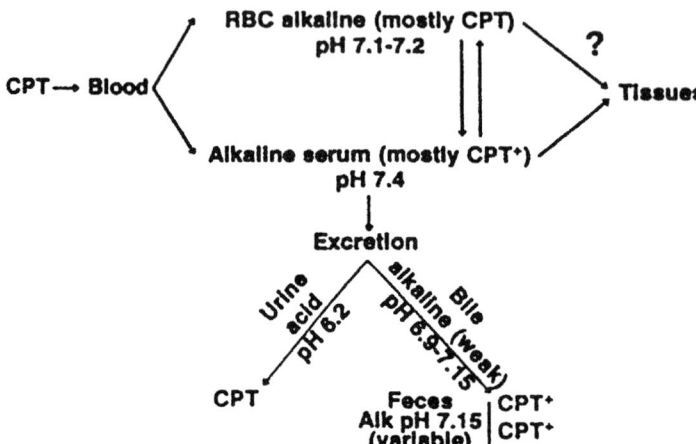

FIGURE 10. CPT and CPT⁺ in the blood circulation and excretion of humans receiving oral CPT.

ACKNOWLEDGMENTS

The authors wish to thank Betty Harris for preparation of the manuscript and Dr. Z. Cao for assistance with FIGURE 1. Funding by The Stehlin Foundation and by SuperGen, Inc. is gratefully acknowledged.

REFERENCES

1. WALL, M.E., M.C. WANI, C.E. COOK, et al. 1966. Plant antitumor agents. I. The isolation and structure of camptothecin, a novel alkaloidal leukemia and tumor inhibitor from *Camptotheca acuminata*. J. Am. Chem. Soc. **88**: 3888–3890.
2. WALL, M.E. 1969. Alkaloids with antitumor activity. *In* International Symposium on Biochemistry and Physiology of the Alkaloids. K. Mothes, K. Schreiber, & H.R. Schutte, Eds. : 77-87. Academie-Verlag. Berlin.
3. DEWYS, W.D., S.R. HUMPHREYS & A. GOLDIN. 1968. Studies on the therapeutic effectiveness of drugs with tumor weight and survival time indices of Walker 256 carcinosarcoma. Cancer Chemother. Rep. **52**: 229–242.
4. GOTTLIEB, J.A. & J.K. LUCE. 1972. Treatment of malignant melanoma with camptothecin (NSC-100880). Cancer Chemother. Rep. Part I **56**: 515–521.
5. MUGGIA, F.M., P.J. CREAVEN, H.H. HANSON, et al. 1972. Phase I clinical trial of weekly and daily treatment with camptothecin (NSC-100880); correlation with preclinical studies. Cancer Chemother. Rep. **56**: 515–521.
6. MOERTEL, C.G., A.J. SCHUTT, R.C. REITEMERER, & R.G. HAHN. 1972. Phase II study of camptothecin (NSC-100880) in the treatment of advanced gastrointestinal cancer. Cancer Chemother. Rep. Part I **56**: 95.
7. GIOVANELLA, B.C., H.R. HINZ, A.J. KOZIELSKI, et al. 1991. Complete growth inhibition of human cancer xenografts in nude mice by treatment with 20-(S)-camptothecin. Cancer Res. **51**: 3052–3055.
8. KINGSBURY, W.C., J. BOEHM, D.R. JAKAS, et al. 1991. Synthesis of water-soluble (aminoalkyl) camptothecin analogues: inhibition of Topoisomerase I and antitumor activity. J. Med. Chem. **35**: 98–107.

9. LI, L., H.T.J. FRASER & B.K. OLIN BHUYAN. 1972. Action of camptothecin on mammalian cells in culture. Cancer Res. **32:** 2643–2650.
10. HOLM, C., J.M. COVEY, D. KERRIGAN & Y. POMMIER. 1989. Differential requirement of DNA replication for the cytotoxicity of DNA Topoisomerase I and to II inhibitors in Chinese hamster DC3F cells. Cancer Res. **49:** 6365–6368.
11. D'ARPA, P., C. BEARDMORE & L.F. LIU. 1990. Involvement of nucleic acid synthesis in cell killing mechanisms of Topoisomerase poisons. Cancer Res. **50:** 6919–6924.
12. ZHANG, H., P. D'ARPA & L.F. LIU. 1990. A model for tumor cell killing by Topoisomerase poisons. Cancer Cells **2:** 23–27.
13. TSAO, Y.-P., A. RUSSO, G. NYAMUSWA, et al.. 1993. Interaction between replication forks and Topoisomerase I-DNA cleavable complexes: studies in a cell-free SV40 DNA replication system. Cancer Res. **53:** 1–8.
14. HSIANG, Y.H., M.G. LIHOU & L.F. LIU. 1989. Arrest of replication forks by drug-stabilized topoisomerase I-DNA cleavable complexes as a mechanism of cell killing by camptothecin. Cancer Res. **49:** 5077–5082.
15. GIOVANELLA, B.C., J.S. STEHLIN, M.E. WALL, et al. 1989. DNA Topoisomerase I-targeted chemotherapy of human colon cancer in xenografts. Science **246:** 1046–1048.
16. STEHLIN, J.S., B.C. GIOVANELLA, E.A. NATELSON, et al. 1999. A study of 9-nitrocamptothecin (RFS-2000) in patients with advanced pancreatic cancer. Int. J. Oncol. **14:** 821–832.
17. MI, Z. & T.G. BURKE. 1994. Differential interactions of camptothecin lactone and carboxylate forms with human blood components. Biochemistry **33:** 10325–10336.
18. MI, Z. & T.G. BURKE. 1994. Marked interspecies variations concerning interactions of camptothecin with serum albumin. Biochemistry **33:** 12540–12545.

Camptothecin Design and Delivery Approaches for Elevating Anti-Topoisomerase I Activities *in Vivo*

THOMAS G. BURKE[a] AND DAVID BOM

Department of Pharmaceutical Sciences, College of Pharmacy, and The Experimental Therapeutics Program, Lucille P. Markey Cancer Center, University of Kentucky Medical Center, Lexington, Kentucky 40506, USA

ABSTRACT: The camptothecins as a class have exhibited unique dynamics and reactivity *in vivo*, with respect to both drug hydrolysis and blood protein interactions. These factors have confounded their pharmaceutical development and clinical implementation. Recent bench and clinical research alike indicates that the combination of medicinal chemical and drug delivery approaches has been and will continue to be highly valuable in improving the overall therapeutic indices of camptothecin-based anti-topoisomerase I therapies. In the future the development of camptothecin analogues that exhibit highly specific human albumin interactions will likely be avoided, and agents such as the highly lipophilic DB-67 analogue with improved tissue stability will be evaluated. Drug delivery scientists will also devise better ways of targeting camptothecin therapies to solid tumors by using carriers such as tumor-targeted long-circulating liposomes.

INTRODUCTION

Anti-Topoisomerase I Activity Lost Through Lactone Ring Hydrolysis

Camptothecin (CPT, FIG. 1) and related analogues represent an important class of agents useful in the treatment of cancer.[1-11] Widespread clinical interest in the camptothecins stems from their unique mechanism of action: they stabilize the covalent binding of the enzyme topoisomerase I (topo I), an intranuclear enzyme that is overexpressed in a variety of tumor lines, to DNA.[5,12] This drug/enzyme/DNA complex leads to reversible, single-strand nicks that, according to the fork collision model, are converted to irreversible and lethal double-strand DNA breaks during replication. Therefore, due to the mechanism of its cytotoxicity, CPT is S-phase specific, indicating that it is only toxic to cells that are undergoing DNA synthesis.[13,14] Rapidly replicating cells, such as cancerous cells, spend more time in the S-phase relative to most healthy tissues. Thus, overexpression of topo I, combined with the faster rate of cell replication, provides a limited basis for selectivity via which camptothecins can effect cytotoxicity on cancerous cells rather than on healthy host tissues.

As a class, the camptothecins have exhibited unique dynamics and reactivity *in vivo* with respect to both drug hydrolysis and blood protein interactions. These fac-

---

[a]The University of Kentucky, ASTeCC Building, Lexington, KY 40506. Voice: 859-257-2300, ext. 255; fax: 859-257-2489.
tgburke@pop.uky.edu

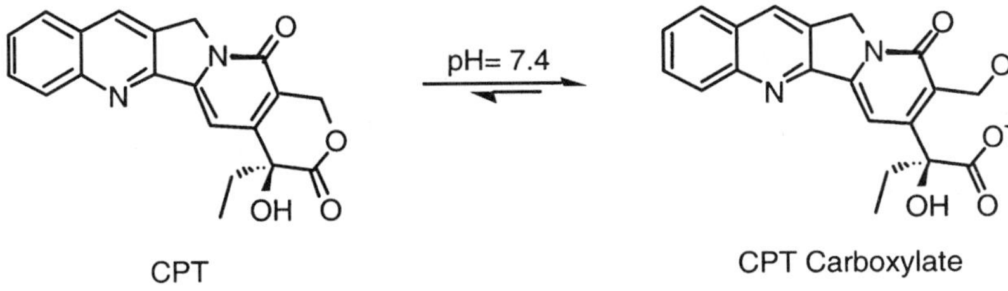

FIGURE 1. CPT hydrolysis at physiological pH.

tors have confounded their pharmaceutical development and clinical implementation. In terms of hydrolysis, each of the clinically relevant camptothecins shown in FIGURE 2 contains an α-hydroxy-δ-lactone pharmacophore; at pH 7 and above, this functionality is highly reactive and readily converts to the "ring opened" carboxylate form. Unfortunately, the carboxylate form of the camptothecin agent is inactive.[15–17] Thus, as a result of the labile α-hydroxy-δ-lactone pharmacophore, camptothecins exist in an equilibrium consisting of two distinct drug species: (1) the biologically active lactone form in which the lactone ring is closed; and (2) a biologically inactive carboxylate form generated upon the hydrolysis of the lactone ring of the parent drug.[11,15]

Unfortunately, the hydrolysis problem with CPT and many analogues (e.g., 9-aminocamptothecin, 9-nitrocamptothecin) is exacerbated in human blood. In human blood and tissues, the CPT equilibrium of active lactone form versus inactive carboxylate form can be greatly affected by the presence of human serum albumin (HSA). Time-resolved fluorescence spectroscopic measurements taken on the intensely fluorescent CPT lactone and CPT carboxylate species have yielded direct information on the differential nature of these interactions with HSA.[18] The lactone form of CPT binds to HSA with moderate affinity, yet the carboxylate form of CPT binds tightly to HSA, displaying a 150-fold enhancement in its affinity for this highly abundant serum protein. Thus, when the lactone form of CPT is added to a solution containing HSA, the preferential binding of the carboxylate form to HSA drives the chemical equilibrium to the right, resulting in the lactone ring hydrolyzing more rapidly and completely than when CPT is in an aqueous solution without HSA. These dynamic processes present a major hurdle to achieving successful chemotherapy of a cancerous disease state.

For example, the carboxylate forms of CPT, 9-aminocamptothecin and 9-nitrocamptothecin, exhibit a very high and species-specific affinity for human serum albumin. Perhaps as a result of these species-specific interactions, the clinical translation of the impressive biological activities observed in murine models has been very difficult to achieve. The interspecies variations in albumin binding noted for these camptothecins may in part explain why 9-aminocamptothecin (9-AC) was highly effective against human cancer in xenograft models[5] but has performed poorly in humans trials.[19,20] In addition to modulating human blood stability, the presence of physiologically relevant concentrations of HSA can greatly attenuate (by orders of magnitudes) the anticancer activities (IC_{50} values) of these agents.[21,22] In

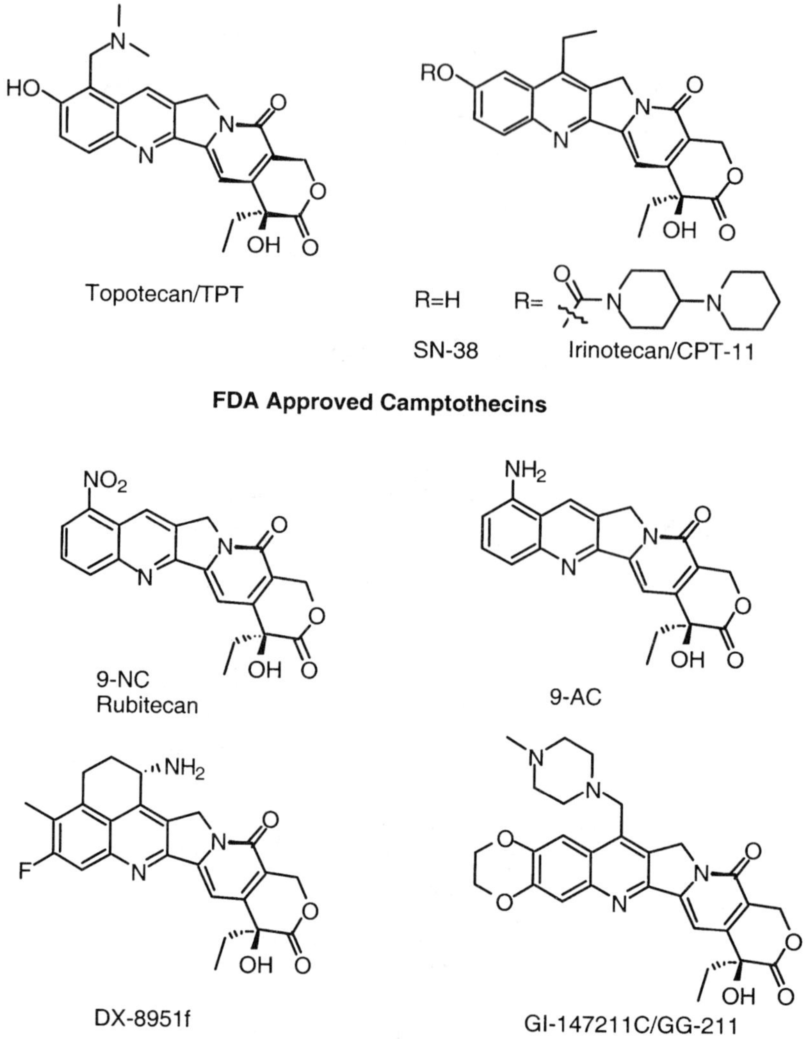

FIGURE 2. Clinical candidates and FDA-approved analogues in the camptothecin family of antitumor agents.

humans it appears that protein binding interactions make it difficult to achieve therapeutically effective unbound lactone levels of these agents, particularly when we consider that *continuous* exposures (for tumors cells to cycle through S-phase) of the active lactone form are requisite for efficacy purposes.

STRUCTURE–STABILITY–ACTIVITY RELATIONSHIPS AND THE RATIONAL DESIGN OF POTENT CAMPTOTHECINS DISPLAYING MARKEDLY IMPROVED HUMAN BLOOD STABILITIES

Camptothecin was first administered to patients in its initial clinical debut in 1972 as the "ring-opened" carboxylate (sodium salt form). This trial was initiated without the knowledge of the ultimate biological target (topo I) of CPT and without the awareness that an intact lactone functionality was required for anti-topoisomerase I activity.[2,3,15] Since the discovery that the "closed-ring" lactone form of CPT is responsible for its anti-topoisomerase I activity, drug development efforts in the CPT field have focused on water-soluble "closed-ring" congeners. These agents, typically developed for administration by intravenous bolus injection, were substituted in the A and B rings (at the opposite end of the molecule and away from the lactone moiety) with water-solubilizing groups. With the expanded synthetic efforts in the 1980s, it became apparent that the A and B rings of CPT are tolerant of modification, with a variety of substitutions allowing the anti-topoisomerase I activity to be conserved. In marked contrast to the ease by which A,B-ring modification results in conservation of activity, changes in the C-, D-, and E-rings typically resulted in reduced anti-topoisomerase I and anticancer activity.

Although the anti-topoisomerase I activities of camptothecins are frequently retained with A,B-ring modification, human plasma and blood stabilities can be strongly modulated through A,B-ring substitution. For example, >99.5% of CPT and 9-AC convert to carboxylate in human plasma, whereas the plasma stabilities of topotecan, CPT-11, and SN-38 are vastly improved (with lactone levels enhanced 10-fold or more).[21,23] In a similar fashion, <0.5% and 1% are the fractions of 9-AC and CPT, respectively, that remain in the lactone form at equilibrium in whole human blood.[24] Topotecan (12%), CPT-11 (21%), and SN-38 (20%) all display markedly improved human blood stabilities relative to CPT. The significant gains in the relative stabilities of topotecan, CPT-11, and SN-38 relative to CPT and 9-AC can be correlated to their favorable interactions with HSA. Topotecan, SN-38, and CPT-11 contain structural changes in the A,B-rings that effectively hinder and prevent high affinity binding of the carboxylate drug forms by HSA. Clearly, HSA plays an important role in determining the relative human blood stabilities of the camptothecins. In the cases of CPT and 9-AC, high affinity binding of the carboxylate species shifts the lactone-carboxylate equilibria in favor of the carboxylate. For topotecan, CPT-11, and SN-38, no such preferential binding of the carboxylate drug form by HSA is observed because of key structural changes in the A,B-rings.

The complications of markedly reduced blood lactone levels, together with loss of anticancer activities, indicate that agents with improved activities could be attained through reduction of the high affinity drug–HSA interactions. Recent rational design efforts have resulted in the identification of A,B-ring modified camptothecins displaying improved human blood stabilities combined with potent anti-topoisomerase I activities. Bioanalytical measurements have shown that dual 7,10-substitution (where the 10-substituent is a hydroxy group) result in camptothecins displaying vastly improved human blood stabilities.[25] SN-38 contains this dual 7-alkyl-10-hydroxy substitution pattern, and in 1994 these changes were shown to block SN-38 from associating with the high affinity CPT carboxylate binding pocket on HSA.[23]

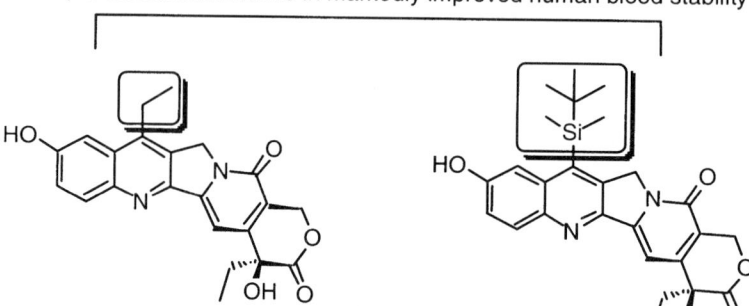

FIGURE 3. Structural comparison of SN-38 and DB-67.

More recently, the design of another dual 7,10-modified CPT was described; this agent displays markedly improved human blood stability and potent antitopoisomerase I anticancer activity.[26] The new agent, shown in FIGURE 3, is 7-*t*-butyldimethylsilyl-10-hydroxycamptothecin (DB-67). DB-67 was prepared using the radical cascade approach developed by Curran and colleagues at the University of Pittsburgh,[27,28] and its design was based on the following two considerations: (1) dual 7,10-substitution patterns eliminate the highly specific binding of the carboxylate form over the lactone form by HSA[18,23,24,29,30]; and (2) lactone stabilization is further promoted by enhanced lipophilicity or lipid bilayer partitioning.[18,31,32] We showed previously that lipophilicity promotes CPT drug stability by favoring lactone partitioning into blood cells, thereby protecting the active lactone forms from hydrolysis. The key α-hydroxy-δ-lactone pharmacophore in DB-67 displays superior stability in human blood when compared with FDA-approved topotecan, CPT-11, and several other clinically relevant CPT analogues.[26] DB-67 displayed a $t_{1/2}$ of 130 minutes and a % lactone at equilibrium value of 30 in human blood; the *t*-butyldimethylsilyl group enhances lipophilicity and thereby promotes drug associations with blood cells. DB-67 is 25 times more lipophilic than CPT and readily incorporates as its active lactone form into cellular and liposomal bilayers. Equally important, the dual 7-alkylsilyl and 10-hydroxy substitution in DB-67 blocks the associations of the carboxylate form of DB-67 with the high affinity carboxylate binding pocket on HSA. Together, the enhanced lipophilicity and altered HSA interactions combine to provide DB-67 with the highest human blood stability when compared with clinically relevant camptothecins containing the conventional α–hydroxy-δ-lactone pharmacophore.

In vitro cytotoxicity assays have shown that DB-67 is of comparable potency relative to CPT and 10-hydroxycamptothecin as well as to the FDA-approved CPT analogues topotecan and CPT-11. Cell-free cleavage assays reveal that DB-67 forms more stable topo I cleavage complexes than does CPT or SN-38. DB-67 was recently shown to display activity against human glioma in a murine model. Overall, the fa-

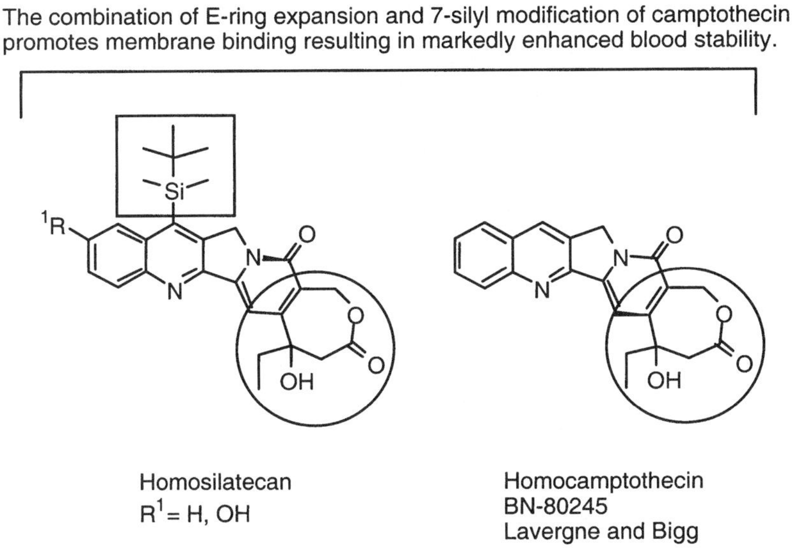

The combination of E-ring expansion and 7-silyl modification of camptothecin promotes membrane binding resulting in markedly enhanced blood stability.

Homosilatecan
R^1 = H, OH

Homocamptothecin
BN-80245
Lavergne and Bigg

FIGURE 4. Structural comparison of the homosilatecans and homocamptothecin.

vorable stability and activity profiles of DB-67 indicate how rational drug design can result in new agents displaying improved pharmacological properties.

A second medicinal chemical approach to enhancing lactone ring stability was developed in 1997 by Lavergne, Bigg, and collaborators.[33] They reported that an E-ring expanded analogue of CPT (or hCPT), prepared by homologation of the α-hydroxy lactone to a β-hydroxy lactone, exhibited enhanced human plasma stability and high anti-topoisomerase I activity.[33,34] Whereas the α-hydroxy lactone of CPT activates the pharmacophore for opening by nucleophilic attack, the β-hydroxy lactone does not exhibit this type of activation. As a result, the β-hydroxy lactone is dramatically more stable over a period of several hours. The finding that activity can be conserved through E-ring modification came as a significant surprise in light of the years of work suggesting that any change to this part of the molecule would result in loss of activity.[11,15,16,35]

Following the publication of the provocative data concerning the favorable biological characteristics of hCPT, the rational design and total synthesis of A,B,E-ring modified camptothecins displaying significantly higher lipophilicity than CPT or hCPT (FIG. 4) were described. The new agents, which combine E-ring expansion (or homologation of the α-hydroxy lactone to a β-hydroxy lactone as described by Lavergne, Bigg, and co-workers) with A,B-ring modifications, are the most blood-stable camptothecins (over several hour time periods) yet to be identified.[36] Our new homosilatecan compounds contain a silyl group at position 7 and, in some cases, modifications at the 10-position. The agents were prepared by total synthesis using the cascade radical annulation approach.[27] The resulting homosilatecans displayed markedly enhanced human blood stabilities relative to clinically relevant camptothecins; the greater than 80% lactone levels following 3 hours of incubation for the homosilatecans in human blood are many-fold in excess of the corresponding lactone levels in human blood observed for clinically relevant camptothecins. In addition, the new homosilatecans do not display the marked interspecies variations in blood stabilities previously noted for agents such as CPT and 9-AC. Thus, it seems likely that successful treatment strategies achieved in animal models with homosilatecans may be more readily translated to a clinical setting. The IC_{50} cytotoxicity values of the homosilatecans against MDA-MB-435 tumorigenic metastatic human breast cancer cells, following 72-hour exposure times, were in the 20- to 100-nM range. Thus, our results clearly indicate that rational design efforts can lead to the development of new analogues with markedly improved blood stabilities and high intrinsic potencies.

LACTONE STABILIZATION ACHIEVED THROUGH LIPOSOMAL FORMULATION

Liposomes contain both aqueous and lipid bilayer compartments, and in 1992 it was demonstrated that both of these compartments could be utilized for stabilizing the lactone form of camptothecins.[31,32,37,38] Each camptothecin is capable of associating with membranes,[31,32,37] and some fraction of a liposomally formulated drug will locate within the lipid bilayer (high fraction for lipophilic drugs such as DB-67; lower fraction for water-soluble agents such as topotecan). Bilayer-localized camptothecins preferentially partition as the active lactone form; in this manner, bilayer associations can promote and stabilize the active lactone forms of camptothecins. For the agents displaying reduced lipophilicity, drug stabilization can also be achieved by reducing the pH of the internal aqueous core.[37] By reducing the pH of the internal core, drugs localizing in the internal aqueous compartments and not within the bilayer compartment can be stabilized.[37]

The dynamic nature of camptothecins under physiological conditions exemplifies how liposomal delivery systems can be utilized both to control drug reactivity and to improve therapeutic efficacy. Drug-laden liposomal particles can be administered to patients, and prolonged plasma exposure can be achieved.[39] Liposomal particles can be passively or actively targeted to tumor and, as a consequence, elevated active lactone levels of the drug can be attained at tumor sites. Liposomes that target tumors and slowly release drug (so that tumor cells are continuously exposed to drug) appear to be attractive drug delivery systems to pursue due to the S-phase specificity of camptothecins. Overall, interest in using liposomes to stabilize camptothecins and target their delivery to specific tissues has grown, and many preclinical and clinical investigations of liposomal CPT products are ongoing.

Interest in liposomal camptothecins has also promoted a demand for tailoring camptothecins for liposomal delivery systems. For long-circulating liposomal CPT products it is important to have agents that predominantly localize in the core of the particle. This core localization allows the bilayer membrane to act as a barrier and to provide a means of promoting drug retention within the particle. An area of current interest in the liposomal CPT field is the control or minimization of drug leakage from the particle while in circulation. Intrinsically potent camptothecins displaying improved retention properties within the core of liposomal particles are now being sought.

In summary, recent bench and clinical research alike indicates that the combination of medicinal chemical and drug delivery approaches has been and will continue to be highly valuable in improving the overall therapeutic index of CPT therapy. In the future the development of CPT analogues that exhibit highly specific human albumin interactions will likely be avoided, and a greater number of lactone-stable agents will likely emerge. Targeted and long-circulating liposomal drug products are on the rise, and it is likely that camptothecins displaying improved retention and release characteristics in these carrier systems will be developed. Medicinal chemical and drug delivery systems have contributed and will continue to contribute to the advancement of oral CPT therapy, an important route of delivery gaining in acceptance because it offers a convenient means of achieving protracted dosing. Finally, in the coming years, medicinal chemical and drug delivery scientists will likely devise better ways of targeting CPT therapy to tumor sites while engineering in drug features that minimize the toxicological potential of the agents.

REFERENCES

1. WALL, M.E., M.C. WANI, C.E. COOK & K.H. PALMER. 1966. Plant antitumor agents. I. The isolation and structure of camptothecin, a novel alkaloidal leukemia and tumor inhibitor from *Camptotheca acuminata*. J. Am. Chem. Soc. **88:** 3888–3889.
2. WANI, M.C., A.W. NICHOLAS, G. MANIKUMAR & M.E. WALL. 1987. Plant antitumor agents. 25. Total synthesis and antileukemic activity of ring A substituted camptothecin analogues. Structure-activity correlations. J. Med. Chem. **30:** 1774–1779.
3. WANI, M.C., A.W. NICHOLAS & M.E. WALL. 1987. Plant antitumor agents. 28. Resolution of a key tricyclic synthon, 5′(RS)-1,5-dioxo-5′-ethyl-5′-hydroxy-2′H,5′H,6′H-6′-oxopyrano[3′,4′- f]delta 6,8-tetrahydro-indolizine: total synthesis and antitumor activity of 20(S)- and 20(R)-camptothecin. J. Med. Chem. **30:** 2317–2319.
4. KANEDA, N., H. NAGATA, T. FURUTA & T. YOKOKURA. 1990. Metabolism and pharmacokinetics of the camptothecin analogue CPT-11 in the mouse. Cancer Res. **50:** 1715-1720.
5. GIOVANELLA, B.C., J.S. STEHLIN, M.E. WALL, *et al.* 1989. DNA topoisomerase I--targeted chemotherapy of human colon cancer in xenografts. Science **246:** 1046-1048.
6. KINGSBURY, W.D., J.C. BOEHM, D.R. JAKAS, *et al.* 1991. Synthesis of water-soluble (aminoalkyl)camptothecin analogues: inhibition of topoisomerase I and antitumor activity. J. Med. Chem. **34:** 98-107.
7. ROWINSKY, E.K., L.B. GROCHOW, C.B. HENDRICKS, *et al.* 1992. Phase I and pharmacologic study of topotecan: a novel topoisomerase I inhibitor. J. Clin. Oncol. **10:** 647-656.
8. HOUGHTON, P.J., P.J. CHESHIRE, L. MYERS, *et al.* 1992. Evaluation of 9-dimethylaminomethyl-10-hydroxycamptothecin against xenografts derived from adult and childhood solid tumors. Cancer Chemother. Pharmacol. **31:** 229-239.
9. BLANEY, S.M., F.M. BALIS, D.E. COLE, *et al.* 1993. Pediatric phase I trial and pharmacokinetic study of topotecan administered as a 24-hour continuous infusion. Cancer Res. **53:** 1032-1036.
10. SLICHENMYER, W.J., W.G. NELSON, R.J. SLEBOS & M.B. KASTAN. 1993. Loss of a p53-associated G1 checkpoint does not decrease cell survival following DNA damage. Cancer Res. **53:** 4164-4168.
11. HSIANG, Y.H., R. HERTZBERG, S. HECHT & L.F. LIU. 1985. Camptothecin induces protein-linked DNA breaks via mammalian DNA topoisomerase I. J. Biol. Chem. **260:** 14873-14878.

12. POTMESIL, M., Y.H. HSIANG, L.F. LIU, et al. 1988. Resistance of human leukemic and normal lymphocytes to drug-induced DNA cleavage and low levels of DNA topoisomerase II. Cancer Res. **48:** 3537-3543.
13. KESSEL, D., H.B. BOSMANN & K. LOHR. 1972. Camptothecin effects on DNA synthesis in murine leukemia cells. Biochim. Biophys. Acta **269:** 210-216.
14. LI, L.H., T.J. FRASER, E.J. OLIN & B.K. BHUYAN. 1972. Action of camptothecin on mammalian cells in culture. Cancer Res. **32:** 2643-2650.
15. JAXEL, C., K.W. KOHN, M.C. WANI, et al. 1989. Structure-activity study of the actions of camptothecin derivatives on mammalian topoisomerase I: evidence for a specific receptor site and a relation to antitumor activity. Cancer Res. **49:** 1465-1469.
16. HERTZBERG, R.P., M.J. CARANFA, K.G. HOLDEN, et al. 1989. Modification of the hydroxy lactone ring of camptothecin: inhibition of mammalian topoisomerase I and biological activity. J. Med. Chem. **32:** 715-720.
17. HSIANG, Y.H. & L.F. LIU. 1988. Identification of mammalian DNA topoisomerase I as an intracellular target of the anticancer drug camptothecin. Cancer Res. **48:** 1722-1726.
18. MI, Z. & T.G. BURKE. 1994. Differential interactions of camptothecin lactone and carboxylate forms with human blood components. Biochemistry **33:** 10325-10336.
19. HOCHBERG, F., S.A. GROSSMAN, T. MIKKELSON, et al. 1998. For the NABTT CNS Consortium, Baltimore, MD. Efficacy of 9-aminocamptothecin (9-AC) in adults with newly diagnosed glioblastoma multiforme (GBM) and recurrent high grade astrocytomas (HGA). Proc. Am. Soc. Clin. Oncol. **17:** 388.
20. TAKIMOTO, C.H., W. DAHUT, N. HAROLD, et al. 1996. Clinical pharmacology of 9-aminocamptothecin. Ann. N.Y. Acad. Sci. **803:** 324-329.
21. MI, Z., H. MALAK & T.G. BURKE. 1995. Reduced albumin binding promotes the stability and activity of topotecan in human blood. Biochemistry **34:** 13722-13728.
22. ZIMMER, S.G. & T.G. BURKE. 2000. Human serum albumin markedly diminishes the blood stabilities and anticancer activities of several clinically relevant camptothecins. Proc. Am. Soc. Clin. Oncol. **19:** 200A.
23. BURKE, T.G. Z. MI. 1994. The structural basis of camptothecin interactions with human serum albumin: impact on drug stability. J. Med. Chem. **37:** 40-46.
24. BURKE, T.G. & Z. MI. 1993. Preferential binding of the carboxylate form of camptothecin by human serum albumin. Anal. Biochem. **212:** 285-287.
25. BURKE, T.G. & Z. MI. 1993. Ethyl substitution at the 7 position extends the half-life of 10-hydroxycamptothecin in the presence of human serum albumin. J. Med. Chem. **36:** 2580-2582.
26. BOM, D., D.P. CURRAN, S. KRUSZEWSKI, et al. 2000. The novel silatecan 7-*tert*-butyldimethylsilyl-10-hydroxycamptothecin displays high lipophilicity, improved human blood stability, and potent anticancer activity. J. Med. Chem. **43:** 3970–3980.
27. JOSIEN, H., S.-B. KO, D. BOM & D.P. CURRAN. 1998. A general synthetic approach to the (20s)-camptothecin family of antitumor agents by a regiocontrolled cascade radical cyclization of aryl isonitriles. Chem. Eur. J. **4:** 67-83.
28. JOSIEN, H., D. BOM, D.P. CURRAN, et al. 1997. 7-Silylcamptothecins (silatecans): a new family of camptothecin antitumor agents. Bioorg. Med. Chem. Lett. **7:** 3189-3194.
29. BURKE, T.G., C.B. MUNSHI, Z. MI & Y. JIANG. 1995. The important role of albumin in determining the relative human blood stabilities of the camptothecin anticancer drugs [letter] [published erratum appears in J. Pharm. Sci. 1995. **84:** 1492]. J. Pharm. Sci. **84:** 518-519.
30. MI, Z. & T.G. BURKE. 1994. Marked interspecies variations concerning the interactions of camptothecin with serum albumins: a frequency-domain fluorescence spectroscopic study. Biochemistry **33:** 12540-12545.
31. BURKE, T.G., A.E. STAUBUS & A.K. MISHRA. 1992. Liposomal stabilization of camptothecin's lactone ring. J. Am. Chem. Soc. **114:** 8318-8319.
32. BURKE, T.G., A.K. MISHRA, M.C. WANI & M.E. WALL. 1993. Lipid bilayer partitioning and stability of camptothecin drugs. Biochemistry **32:** 5352-5364.
33. LAVERGNE, O., L. LESUEUR-GINOT, F. PLA RODAS & D.C.H. BIGG. 1997. BN80245: an e-ring modified camptothecin with potent antiproliferative and topoisomerase I inhibitory activities. Bioorg. Med. Chem. Lett. **7:** 2235-2238.

34. LAVERGNE, O., L. LESUEUR-GINOT, F. PLA RODAS, et al. 1998. Homocamptothecins: synthesis and antitumor activity of novel E-ring-modified camptothecin analogues. J. Med. Chem. **41:** 5410-5419.
35. HSIANG, Y.H., L.F. LIU, M.E. WALL, et al. 1989. DNA topoisomerase I-mediated DNA cleavage and cytotoxicity of camptothecin analogues [published erratum appears in Cancer Res. 1989. **49:** 6868]. Cancer Res. **49:** 4385-4389.
36. BOM, D., D.P. CURRAN, A.J. CHAVAN, et al. 1999. Novel A,B,E-ring-modified camptothecins displaying high lipophilicity and markedly improved human blood stabilities. J. Med. Chem. **42:** 3018-3022.
37. BURKE, T.G. 1996. Liposomal and micellar stabilization of camptothecin drugs. U.S. Patent 5,552,156.
38. BURKE, T.G. & X. GAO. 1994. Stabilization of topotecan in low pH liposomes composed of distearoylphosphatidylcholine. J. Pharm. Sci. **83:** 967-969.
39. COLBERN, G.T., D.J. DYKES, C. ENGBERS, et al. 1998. Encapsulation of the topoisomerase I inhibitor GL147211C in pegylated (STEALTH) liposomes: pharmacokinetics and antitumor activity in HT29 colon tumor xenografts. Clin. Cancer Res. **4:** 3077-3082.

Mechanisms of Resistance to Camptothecins

AHAMED SALEEM, TROY K. EDWARDS, ZESHAAN RASHEED, AND ERIC H. RUBIN[a]

Departments of Medicine and Pharmacology, The Cancer Institute of New Jersey, RWJMS-UMDNJ, New Brunswick, New Jersey 08901, USA

ABSTRACT: Camptothecins are broad-spectrum anticancer drugs that specifically target DNA topoisomerase I. Although the availability of camptothecins has had a significant impact on cancer therapeutics, de novo or acquired clinical resistance to camptothecins is common. Studies of camptothecin resistance using yeast and mammalian cell culture models suggest three general mechanisms of resistance: (1) reduced cellular accumulation of camptothecins, (2) alteration in the structure or location of topoisomerase I, and (3) alterations in the cellular response to camptothecin-DNA-ternary complex formation. The relevance of these mechanisms to clinical drug resistance is not yet known, but evaluation of these models in clinical specimens should enhance the use of camptothecins both as single agents and in combination with other anticancer drugs.

CLINICAL RESISTANCE TO CAMPTOTHECINS

Camptothecin is a naturally occurring alkaloid that was identified in the 1960s by Wani and Wall in a screen of plant extracts for antineoplastic drugs.[1] Currently, two camptothecin analogues, topotecan and irinotecan, are approved for the treatment of cancer in the United States. Topotecan contains a 10-hydroxyl modification of the parent compound that enhances water solubility (FIG. 1). Irinotecan is essentially a prodrug that is converted to the active compound SN-38 by plasma and cellular carboxylesterases (FIG. 1). For topotecan, the initial U.S. (FDA) approvals were based on antitumor responses obtained in patients with previously treated ovarian cancer who were treated with daily infusions of 1.5 mg/m^2 drug for 5 days every 3 weeks.[2] Similarly, irinotecan was approved as a result of response data in patients with previously treated colon cancer who received an infusion of 125 mg/m^2 of drug each week for 4 weeks, followed by a 2-week rest period.[3] However, using these schedules of administration, for both drugs the response rates in these diseases are below 50%, which is somewhat disappointing relative to the curative potential of camptothecin analogues observed in xenograft models.[4] The mechanisms underlying this apparent de novo clinical resistance to camptothecins (and the disparity between the xenograft and clinical studies) are not known, but cell culture and yeast models continue to provide information that can be evaluated clinically. As with other drugs, resistance to camptothecins potentially may involve alterations in cellular drug accumulation, alterations in the drug target, or alterations in the response to the drug-target interaction.

[a]Voice: 732-235-7955; fax: 732-235-7493.
ehrubin@umdnj.edu

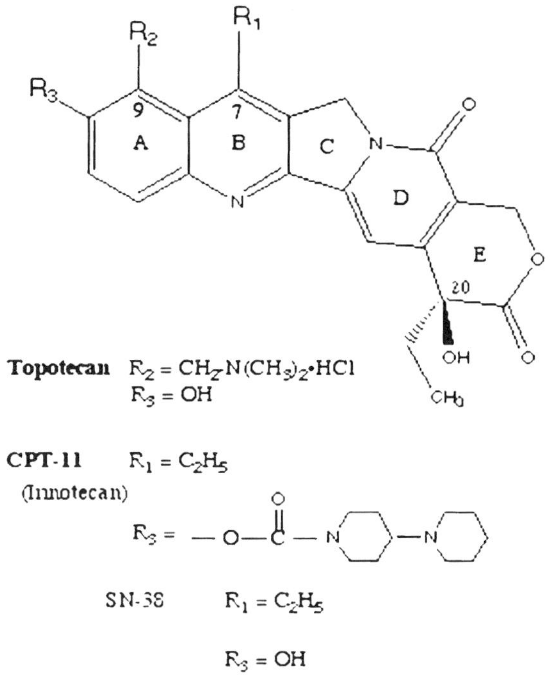

FIGURE 1. Structures of the FDA-approved camptothecins, topotecan and irinotecan. The structure of the active irinotecan metabolite, SN-38, is also shown.

CELLULAR ACCUMULATION OF CAMPTOTHECINS

Cell culture data indicate that brief exposures to submicromolar concentrations of camptothecin (in the range of 1 h) are sufficient to destroy proliferating neoplastic cells.[5] Thus, relatively low sustained cellular concentrations of camptothecin should be sufficient for antineoplastic activity. As with other drugs, cellular accumulation of camptothecin is dependent upon uptake, metabolism, and efflux. Little is known regarding cellular metabolism of camptothecins, although differences in cellular carboxylesterase activity may confer differential sensitivity to irinotecan.[6] In addition, recent data suggest that glucuronidation of certain camptothecin derivatives may occur intracellularly and may affect cellular sensitivity to these compounds.[7]

With regard to cellular uptake, although passive diffusion may play a role, recent studies suggest that energy-requiring transport processes are involved in the cellular uptake of camptothecin.[8,9] In addition, data from both yeast and mammalian cells indicate that several ATP-binding cassette (ABC) proteins can efflux camptothecins. Overexpression of the ABC protein Mdr1 (P-glycoprotein), which has been implicated in resistance to many natural product antineoplastic drugs,[10] can confer resistance to camptothecins, although to a lesser degree than that observed for topoisomerase II–targeting drugs such as doxorubicin or etoposide.[11] A screen for mutations that suppress the cytotoxic effects of camptothecin in yeast cells implicated two ABC proteins, Snq2 and Pdr5, in resistance to camptothecin.[12] Similarly, overexpression of the recently identified Bcrp/Mxr protein is associated with resistance to topotecan, 9-aminocamptothecin, and SN-38, suggesting that this ABC protein can also bind and efflux camptothecins.[7,13,14] In addition, since antisense oligonucleotides directed against the *MRP2* gene increase cellular sensitivity to irinotecan and SN-38, the Mrp2 protein, which is an ABC protein known to transport organic anions, may also efflux camptothecin.[15]

ALTERATIONS IN TOPOISOMERASE I, THE CELLULAR TARGET OF CAMPTOTHECINS

As with many antineoplastic drugs, camptothecins were used clinically before their mechanism was understood. Early mechanistic studies indicated that cells treated with camptothecin accumulated DNA strand breaks,[16] with subsequent work indicating that camptothecin damages DNA by stabilizing a normally transient covalent complex between topo I and DNA.[17] Genetic studies in yeast indicate that topoisomerase I is a unique cellular target for camptothecins.[18–20] Therefore, it is not surprising that several studies of camptothecin-resistant mammalian or yeast cells identified point mutations in the topoisomerase I gene, most of which have been shown *in vitro* to confer enzymatic drug resistance.[21] The recent availability of crystals of topoisomerase I-DNA covalent complexes allowed structural mapping of these mutations (FIG. 2).[22] Not surprisingly, many of the mutations are found near tyrosine 723, the residue involved in the covalent linkage of the enzyme to DNA that occurs transiently during the topoisomerase I catalytic cycle. Particularly helpful from the structural analysis was the finding that mutations involving amino acids 361–364 and 533 localize to two "lip" domains that bind DNA and are likely to undergo conformational changes during enzyme catalysis.[23,24] Additional work is required to clarify the function of these "lip" regions in topoisomerase I catalysis. Nevertheless, a model of the putative camptothecin–topo I–ternary complex proposes specific interactions between amino acids in these two regions and the drug molecule, providing an explanation for the resistance conferred by mutations involving these residues.[22] A additional structural perturbation of topo I was identified recently in a murine cell line resistant to the indolocarbazole NB-506.[25] This cell line expresses a mutant topo I that contains an internal duplication of residues 20–609. Analyses of a recombinant form of the mutant protein indicate that this alteration is sufficient to confer enzymatic resistance, although the mechanism is not yet clear.[25]

Recent studies indicate that interactions between topo I and other proteins may affect cellular sensitivity to camptothecins. For example, the topo I-binding protein nucleolin may recruit topo I to the nucleolus as a result of the high rate of transcription in this region.[26] Nucleolin binds the N-terminus of topo I and is known to shuttle between the nucleus and cytoplasm.[27] Studies of a yeast nucleolin orthologue, Nsr1p, indicate that in the absence of this protein, topo I relocalizes from a predominantly nucleolar localization to a diffuse nuclear localization (FIG. 3).[28] Further-

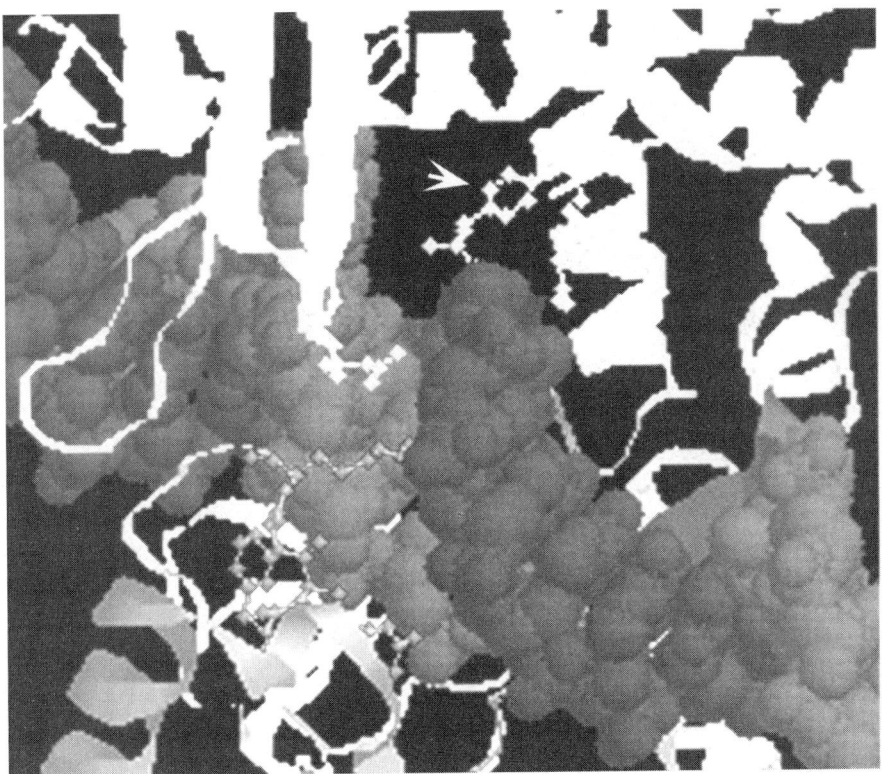

FIGURE 2. Location of amino acids involved in camptothecin resistance in a topoisomerase I-DNA covalent complex. The figure was produced using RasMac software and coordinates obtained from the Protein Data Bank (http://www.rcsb.org/pdb/). DNA is shown in the center of the image. Tyrosine-723, involved in the phosphodiester bond with DNA, is indicated by the *white arrow*. Nearby residues implicated in resistance to camptothecin are also shown as white ball-and-stick images. Aspartate-533, part of one "lip" region, is shown in a white ball-and-stick configuration near the center of the image. Residues 361-364, part of the other "lip" region, are shown as gray ball-and-stick representations.

more, loss of Nsr1p results in resistance to camptothecin.[28] Although altered localization of topo I in resistant mammalian cells has not been reported, topo I is known to move rapidly from the nucleolus to the nucleus or even cytoplasm after cellular exposure to camptothecin.[29,30] This relocalization may decrease topo I-DNA interactions and thus minimize topo I-mediated DNA damage induced by camptothecin. Notably, altered localization of Top2α (as a result of loss of nuclear localization sequences) was identified in mammalian cell lines resistant to the Top2-targeting drugs etoposide and mitoxantrone.[31–33] In these cases, the mutant Top2α localizes to the cytoplasm, which presumably results in resistance to Top2-targeting drugs by decreasing interactions between the enzyme and DNA.

NSR1⁺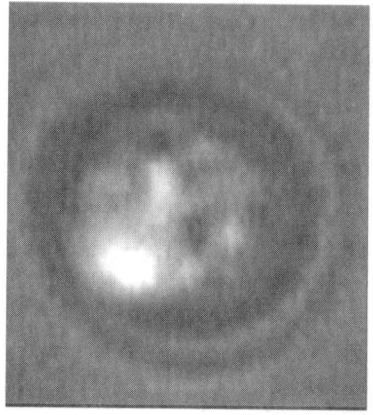

△*nsr1*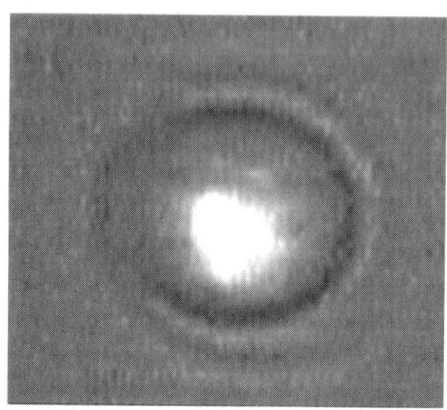

FIGURE 3. Relocalization of yeast topoisomerase I in a strain lacking the nucleolin orthologue *NSR1*. The pictures represent merged phase contrast and fluorescent images of representative cells from *Saccharomyces cerevisiae* strains that are genetically identical with the exception of the *NSR1* gene. Both cells express a green fluorescent protein-topoisomerase I fusion protein, allowing visualization of the localization of topoisomerase I. In these images, the green fluorescence exhibited by the fusion protein appears white.

TABLE 1. Cellular processes implicated in the response to ternary complex formation

Process	Mutated gene[a]	Reference
Checkpoint	ATM, MEC1, MEC2	43, 44
	CHK1	37
	RAD9, RAD17	44, 45
DNA repair	CSA, CSB	36
	RAD6	44
	TDP	38
	TRF4[b]	46
DNA replication	CDC45, DPB11	39
	WRN	47
Unknown	UBP11	40

[a]With the exception of *UBP11*, this refers to loss-of-function mutants that have been shown to confer hypersensitivity to camptothecin.

[b]TRF4 has been shown to function in chromatin condensation and is speculated to function in repair of DNA damage.

ALTERATIONS IN THE CELLULAR RESPONSE TO TERNARY CAMPTOTHECIN– TOPO I–DNA COMPLEX FORMATION

Relatively little is known about events occurring after formation of camptothecin– topo I–DNA complexes. Liu and colleagues demonstrated that collision of replication forks with ternary complexes results in destruction of these forks and DNA double-strand breaks.[34] Moreover, camptothecins selectively target S-phase cells, and the DNA polymerase inhibitor aphidicolin can ameliorate camptothecin cytotoxicity,[35] suggesting that replication fork collisions may be important in the cytotoxic effects of camptothecin.

Genetic studies implicate several DNA damage checkpoint and repair proteins in the cellular response to ternary complex formation (TABLE 1). Cells deficient in double-strand break repair or transcription-coupled repair are known to be hypersensitive to camptothecin.[20,36] In fission yeast, loss of the G2 checkpoint protein Chk1 also results in hypersensitivity to camptothecin.[37] In addition, Nash and colleagues recently identified a phosphodiesterase that can specifically repair topo I-DNA covalent complexes.[38] However, despite the importance of these DNA repair and checkpoint proteins in cellular camptothecin sensitivity, alteration of these proteins in camptothecin-resistant cells has not been reported.

Yeast genetic models have been very useful in identifying cellular processes that are involved in the response to ternary complex formation. A search for yeast mutants with enhanced sensitivity to topo I-mediated DNA damage yielded two genes, *CDC45* and *DPB11*, that are involved in processive DNA replication.[39] Based on these data, a role for properly ligated Okazaki fragments in the repair of topo I-mediated DNA damage has been proposed.[39] Another yeast genetic screen, involving suppressors of topo I-mediated DNA damage, indicated that overexpression of Ubp11, a ubiquitin-specific protease, can confer resistance to topo I-mediated DNA damage.[40] Additional data that support an important role for ubiquitination in the cellular response to camptothecin include the following: (1) mammalian topo I is ubiquitinated and degraded after camptothecin exposure,[41] (2) topo I binds Topors, a RING domain protein that is homologous to proteins known to function in ubiquitin conjugation,[42] and (3) studies of mammalian cell lines suggest that the camptothecin-induced degradation of topo I correlates with cellular resistance to camptothecin (S.D. Desai and L.F. Liu, personal communication). Elucidation of the machinery by which topo I is ubiquitinated and degraded after drug exposure may identify other cellular proteins involved in the response to ternary complex formation.

BIOCHEMICAL STUDIES OF CLINICAL SPECIMENS OBTAINED BEFORE OR DURING THERAPY WITH CAMPTOTHECINS

Studies of clinical specimens before and after camptothecin therapy are required to determine whether resistance mechanisms identified in yeast and cell culture models are clinically relevant. Currently, only a few studies have reported these kinds of data. Although not thoroughly investigated, topo I mutations have not been reported in clinical specimens. A resistance-conferring mutation in Top2α was reported in 1 of 13 small-cell lung cancer biopsy specimens, most obtained after treatment of patients with a Top2-targeting drug.[48] The frequency of resistance-conferring Top2 mutations in clinical specimens is unknown. Notably, yeast genetic studies indicate that resistance-conferring topo I alterations can produce genetic instability,[49] a phenotype that is selected for early in carcinogenesis. Thus, it is possible that resistance-conferring topoisomerase mutations are present prior to drug exposure and may contribute to de novo clinical resistance to camptothecins. This conjecture is supported by the recent finding that topo I is involved in a t(11;20) translocation implicated in the pathogenesis of therapy-induced myelodysplasia.[50]

With regard to topo I downregulation, comparative studies of nonmalignant and malignant tissues, albeit in separate groups of patients, support a role for topo I degradation in drug resistance. Analysis of nonmalignant peripheral blood cells in patients treated with a 72-hour infusion of 9-aminocamptothecin identified decreases in topo I protein at 48 or 72 hours in two of three patients.[51] This decrease in topo I was accompanied by reciprocal increases in Top2α. Further analyses in another clinical study indicated that these topo I decreases are not due to cleavable complex formation, suggesting that topo I is degraded after drug exposure in nonmalignant peripheral blood cells.[52] By contrast, in malignant blast cells obtained from patients with leukemia who received the same schedule of 9-AC administration, topo I protein levels did not change, and in two of four patients studied, decreases in Top2α were identified (FIG. 4). While the mechanisms underlying these different effects of 9-aminocamptothecin on topoisomerase protein levels in leukemic versus normal blood cells are not known, it is tempting to speculate that ubiquitin/proteasome pathways are involved. This hypothesis is supported by recent data indicating that malignant and nonmalignant cells differ in their capacity to ubiquitinate and degrade topo I (S.D. Desai and L.F. Liu, personal communication).

Mechanisms of resistance to camptothecin identified more recently in yeast and cell culture systems have not been evaluated clinically. In particular, the role of topo I localization and specific repair processes (such as removal of topo I-DNA adducts by a specific phosphodiesterase) need to be investigated as potential mechanisms of

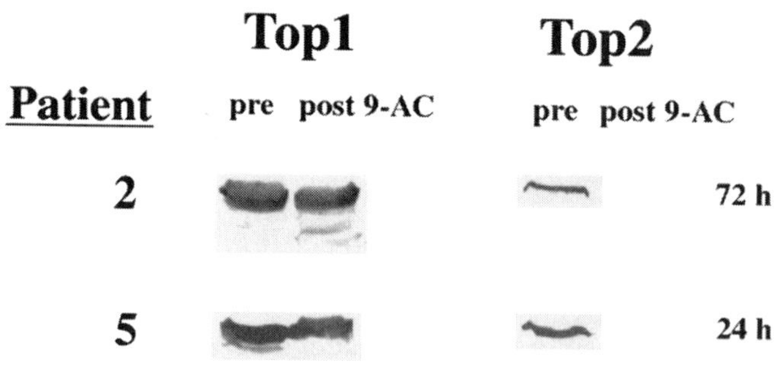

FIGURE 4. Analysis of topo I and Top2α proteins in leukemic blasts obtained from two patients before and after initiation of a 72-hour 9-AC infusion. Cell lysates were prepared from circulating leukemic cells obtained before and at the indicated time after initiation of a 72-hour 9-aminocamptothecin infusion. Equal amounts of protein were subjected to sequential immunoblotting using antibodies recognizing topo I and Top2α.

clinical drug resistance. With this knowledge, attempts to improve the clinical utility of camptothecins can be approached mechanistically.

ACKNOWLEDGMENTS

This work was supported by Public Health Service Grants CA70981 and GM59170.

REFERENCES

1. WALL, M.E. & M.C. WANI. 1995. Camptothecin and taxol: discovery to clinic. Thirteenth Bruce F. Cain Memorial Award lecture. Cancer Res. **55:** 753–760.
2. TEN BOKKEL HUININK, W., M. GORE, J. CARMICHAEL, et al. 1997. Topotecan versus paclitaxel for the treatment of recurrent epithelial ovarian cancer [see comments]. J. Clin. Oncol. **15:** 2183–2193.
3. ROTHENBERG, M.L., J.R. ECKARDT, J.G. KUHN, et al. 1996. Phase II trial of irinotecan in patients with progressive or rapidly recurrent colorectal cancer. J. Clin. Oncol. **14:** 1128–1135.
4. GIOVANELLA, B.P., J.S. STEHLIN, M.E. WALL, et al. 1989. DNA topoisomerase I-targeted chemotherapy of human colon cancer in xenografts. Science **246:** 1046–1048.
5. GOLDWASSER, F., I. BAE, M. VALENTI, et al. 1995. Topoisomerase I-related parameters and camptothecin activity in the colon carcinoma cell lines from the National Cancer Institute Anticancer Screen. Cancer Res. **55:** 2116–2121.
6. DANKS, M.K., C.L. MORTON, C.A. PAWLIK, et al. 1998. Overexpression of a rabbit liver carboxylesterase sensitizes human tumor cells to CPT-11. Cancer Res. **58:** 20–22.
7. BRANGI, M., T. LITMAN, M. CIOTTI, et al. 1999. Camptothecin resistance: role of the ATP-binding cassette (ABC), mitoxantrone-resistance half-transporter (MXR), and potential for glucuronidation in MXR-expressing cells. Cancer Res. **59:** 5938–5946.
8. MA, J., M. MALIEPAARD, K. NOOTER, et al. 1998. Reduced cellular accumulation of topotecan: a novel mechanism of resistance in a human ovarian cancer cell line. Br. J. Cancer **77:** 1645–1652.
9. GUPTA, E., F. LUO, A. LALLO, et al. 2000. The intestinal transport of campothecin, a higly lipophilic drug, across Caco-2 cells is mediated by active transporters. Anticancer Res. **20.** In press.
10. FORD, J.M., J.M. YANG, & W.N. HAIT. 1996. P-glycoprotein-mediated multidrug resistance: experimental and clinical strategies for its reversal. Cancer Treat. Res. **87:** 3–38.
11. CHEN, A.Y., C. YU, M. POTMESIL, et al. 1991. Camptothecin overcomes MDR1-mediated resistance in human KB carcinoma cells. Cancer Res. **51:** 6039–6044.
12. REID, R.J.D., E.A. KAUH, & M.-A. BJORNSTI. 1997. Camptothecin sensitivity is mediated by the pleiotropic drug resistance network in yeast. J. Biol. Chem. **272:** 12091–12099.
13. ALLEN, J.D., R.F. BRINKHUIS, J. WIJNHOLDS, et al. 1999. The mouse Bcrp1/Mxr/Abcp gene: amplification and overexpression in cell lines selected for resistance to topotecan, mitoxantrone, or doxorubicin. Cancer Res. **59:** 4237–4241.
14. MALIEPAARD, M., M.A. VAN GASTELEN, L.A. DE JONG, et al. 1999. Overexpression of the BCRP/MXR/ABCP gene in a topotecan-selected ovarian tumor cell line. Cancer Res. **59:** 4559–4563.
15. KOIKE, K., T. KAWABE, T. TANAKA, et al. 1997. A canalicular multispecific organic anion transporter (cMOAT) antisense cDNA enhances drug sensitivity in human hepatic cancer cells. Cancer Res. **57:** 5475–5479.
16. HORWITZ, S.B. & M.S. HORWITZ. 1973. Effects of camptothecin the breakage and repair of DNA during the cell cycle. Cancer Res. **33:** 2834–2836.
17. HSIANG, Y., R. HERTZBERG, S. HECHT, et al. 1985. Camptothecin induces protein-linked DNA breaks via mammalian DNA topoisomerase I. J. Biol. Chem. **260:** 14873–14878.

18. BJORNSTI, M., P. BENEDETTI, G. VIGILANTI, et al. 1989. Expression of human DNA topoisomerase I in yeast cells lacking yeast DNA topoisomerase I: restoration of sensitivity of the cells to the antitumor drug camptothecin. Cancer Res. **49:** 6318–6323.
19. ENG, W.K., L. FAUCETTE, R.K. JOHNSON, et al. 1988. Evidence that DNA topoisomerase I is necessary for the cytotoxic effects of camptothecin. Mol. Pharmacol. **34:** 755–760.
20. NITISS, J. & J.C. WANG. 1988. DNA topoisomerase-targeting antitumor drugs can be studied in yeast. Proc. Natl. Acad. Sci. USA **85:** 7501–7505.
21. RUBIN, E.H., T. LI, P. DUAN, et al. 1996. Cellular resistance to topoisomerase poisons, *In* Drug Resistance. W.N. Hait, Ed. :243–260. Kluwer Academic Publishers. Norwell, MA.
22. REDINBO, M.R., L. STEWART, P. KUHN, et al. 1998. Crystal structure of human topoisomerase I in covalent and noncovalent complexes with DNA. Science **279:** 1504–1513.
23. STEWART, L., M.R. REDINBO, X. QIU, et al. 1998. A model for the mechanism of human topoisomerase I. Science **279:** 1534–1541.
24. POND, C.D., X.G. LI, E.H. RUBIN, et al. 1999. Effects of mutations in the F361 to R364 region of topoisomerase I (Topo I), in the presence and absence of 9-aminocamptothecin, on the Topo I-DNA interaction. Anticancer Drugs **10:** 647–653.
25. KOMATANI, H., M. MORITA, N. SAKAIZUMI, et al. 1999. A new mechanism of acquisition of drug resistance by partial duplication of topoisomerase I. Cancer Res. **59:** 2701–2708.
26. BHARTI, A.K., M.O.J. OLSON, D.W. KUFE, et al. 1996. Identification of a nucleolin binding site in human topoisomerase I. J. Biol. Chem. **271:** 1993–1997.
27. BORER, R.A., C.F. LEHNER, H.M. EPPENBERGER, et al. 1989. Major nulceolar proteins shuttle between nucleus and cytoplasm. Cell **56:** 379–390.
28. EDWARDS, T.K., A. SALEEM, J.A. SHAMAN, et al. 1999. Role for nucleolin/Nsr1 in the cellular localization of topoisomerase I. Submitted.
29. BUCKWALTER, C.A., A.H. LIN, A. TANIZAWA, et al. 1996. RNA synthesis inhibitors alter the subnuclear distribution of DNA topoisomerase I. Cancer Res. **56:** 1674–1681.
30. DANKS, M.K., K.E. GARRETT, R.C. MARION, et al. 1996. Subcellular redistribution of DNA topoisomerase I in anaplastic astrocytoma cells treated with topotecan. Cancer Res. **56:** 1664–1673.
31. MIRSKI, S.E.L. & S.P.C. COLE. 1995. Cytoplasmic localization of a mutant M_r 160,000 topoisomerase IIa is associated with the loss of putative bipartite nuclear localization signals in a drug-resistant human lung cancer cell line. Cancer Res. **55:** 2129–2134.
32. HARKER, W.G., D.L. SLADE, R.L. PARR, et al. 1995. Alterations in the topoisomerase IIα gene, messenger RNA, and subcellular protein distribution as well as reduced expression of the DNA topoisomerase IIβ enzyme in a mitoxantrone-resistant HL-60 human leukemia cell line. Cancer Res. **55:** 1707–1716.
33. WESSEL, I., P.B. JENSEN, J. FALCK, et al. 1997. Loss of amino acids 1490Lys-Ser-Lys1492 in the COOH-terminal region of topoisomerase IIalpha in human small cell lung cancer cells selected for resistance to etoposide results in an extranuclear enzyme localization. Cancer Res. **57:** 4451–4454.
34. HSIANG, Y., M. LIHOU, & L. LIU. 1989. Arrest of replication forks by drug-stabilized topoisomerase I-DNA cleavable complexes as a mechanism of cell killing by camptothecin. Cancer Res. **49:** 5077–5082.
35. D'ARPA, P., C. BEARDMORE, & L.F. LIU. 1990. Involvement of nucleic acid synthesis in cell killing mechanisms of topoisomerase poisons. Cancer Res. **50:** 6919–6924.
36. SQUIRES, S., A.J. RYAN, H.L. STRUTT, et al. 1993. Hypersensitivity of Cockayne's syndrome cells to camptothecin is associated with the generation of abnormally high levels of double strand breaks in nascent DNA. Cancer Res. **53:** 2012–2019.
37. WAN, S., H. CAPASSO & N.C. WALWORTH. 1999. The topoisomerase I poison camptothecin generates a Chk1-dependent DNA damage checkpoint signal in fission yeast. Yeast **15:** 821–828.
38. POULIOT, J.J., K.C. YAO, C.A. ROBERTSON, et al. 1999. Yeast gene for a tyr-DNA phosphodiesterase that repairs topoisomerase I complexes [In Process Citation]. Science **286:** 552–555.

39. REID, R.J., P. FIORANI, M. SUGAWARA, et al. 1999. CDC45 and DPB11 are required for processive DNA replication and resistance to DNA topoisomerase I-mediated DNA damage. Proc. Natl. Acad. Sci. USA **96:** 11440–11445.
40. REID, R.J.D., H. ASKARI, P. FIORANI, et al. 1998. Novel genes affecting DNA topoisomerase I poison sensitivity. Proc. Am. Assoc. Cancer Res. **39:** a546.
41. DESAI, S.D., L.F. LIU, D. VAZQUEZ-ABAD, et al. 1997. Ubiquitin-dependent destruction of topoisomerase I is stimulated by the antitumor drug camptothecin. J. Biol. Chem. **272:** 24159–24164.
42. HALUSKA, P.H., A. SALEEM, Z. RASHEED, et al. 1999. Interaction between human topoisomerase I and a novel RING finger/arginine-serine protein. Nucleic Acids Res. **27:** 2538–2544.
43. SMITH, P.J., T.A. MAKINSON, & J.V. WATSON. 1989. Enhanced sensitivity to camptothecin in ataxia-telangiectasia cells and its relationship with the expression of DNA topoisomerase I. Int. J. Radiat. Biol. **55:** 217–231.
44. SIMON, J.A., P. SZANKASI, D.K. NGUYEN, et al. 2000. Differential toxicities of anticancer agents among DNA repair and checkpoint mutants of *Saccharomyces cerevisiae*. Cancer Res. **60:** 328–333.
45. MEGONIGAL, M.D., J. FERTALA, & M.-A. BJORNSTI. 1997. Alterations in the catalytic activity of yeast DNA topoisomerase I result in cell cycle arrest and cell death. J. Biol. Chem. **272:** 12801–12808.
46. WALOWSKY, C., D.J. FITZHUGH, I.B. CASTANO, et al. 1999. The topoisomerase-related function gene TRF4 affects cellular sensitivity to the antitumor agent camptothecin. J. Biol. Chem. **274:** 7302–7308.
47. LEBEL, M. & P. LEDER. 1998. A deletion within the murine Werner syndrome helicase induces sensitivity to inhibitors of topoisomerase and loss of cellular proliferative capacity. Proc. Natl. Acad.Sci. USA **95:** 13097–13102.
48. KUBO, A., A. YOSHIKAWA, T. HIRASHIMA, et al. 1996. Point mutations of the topoisomerase IIa gene in patients with small cell lung cancer treated with etoposide. Cancer Res. **56:** 1232–1236.
49. LEVIN, N.A., M.-A. BJORNSTI, & G.R. FINK. 1993. A novel mutation in DNA topoisomerase I of yeast causes DNA damage and RAD9-dependent cell cycle arrest. Genetics **133:** 799–814.
50. AHUJA, H.G., C.A. FELIX, & P.D. APLAN. 1999. The t(11;20)(p15;q11) chromosomal translocation associated with therapy-related myelodysplastic syndrome results in an NUP98-TOP1 fusion [In Process Citation]. Blood **94:** 3258–3261.
51. RUBIN, E., V. WOOD, A. BHARTI, et al. 1995. A phase I and pharmacokinetic study of a new camptothecin derivative, 9-aminocamptothecin. Clin. Cancer Res. **1:** 269–276.
52. GUPTA, E., D. TOPPMEYER, R. ZAMEK, et al. 1998. Clinical evaluation of sequential topoisomerase targeting in the treatment of advanced malignancy. Cancer Therapeutics **1:** 292–301.

Structure-Based Analysis of the Effects of Camptothecin on the Activities of Human Topoisomerase I

JAMES J. CHAMPOUX[a]

Department of Microbiology, Box 357242, University of Washington, Seattle, Washington 98195-7242, USA

ABSTRACT: The sole target for the anticancer drug camptothecin (CPT) is the type I topoisomerase. The drug poisons the topoisomerase by slowing the religation step of the reaction, thereby trapping the enzyme in a covalent complex on the DNA. In addition, CPT has been shown to inhibit plasmid DNA relaxation *in vitro*. The structural bases for these two activities of CPT are explored in relation to the recently published crystal structure of the enzyme with bound DNA.

INTRODUCTION

Human topoisomerase I relieves torsional tension in duplex DNA by introducing a temporary, enzyme-bound, single-strand break in the DNA (FIG. 1). Cleavage involves nucleophilic attack by the O4-oxygen of the active site tyrosine on a phosphodiester bond in the DNA that results in the covalent attachment of the protein to the 3′ phosphate at the site of the break.[1,2] The resulting nick permits rotation of the downstream helix about one or more bonds in the intact strand that is driven by the free energy associated with DNA supercoiling. Restoration of the DNA backbone and release of the enzyme are accomplished by nucleophilic attack by the 5′ hydroxyl of the broken strand on the phosphodiester bond between the enzyme tyrosine and the DNA. The amount of covalent intermediate in a topoisomerase I-catalyzed reaction can be estimated by trapping the complexes using a protein denaturant such as SDS (FIG. 1). Based on assays of enzyme activity *in vitro*, the enzyme is processive under physiological conditions and completely relaxes a plasmid DNA through multiple cycles of cleavage and religation before dissociating from the DNA.[3,4] Although detailed kinetic analyses have not been carried out for the human enzyme under processive conditions, the rate of religation for the structurally related vaccinia topoisomerase[5] is approximately 10-fold faster than the rate of cleavage,[6] and thus the equilibrium level of nicked intermediate is expected to be low.

A combination of biochemical analyses and structural studies has identified four distinct domains within the topoisomerase I protein.[2,4,7–9] The relatively disordered, protease-sensitive and poorly conserved NH$_2$-terminal domain ends at approximately residue 214 and is dispensable for enzyme activity *in vitro*. The highly conserved

---

[a]Voice: 206-543-8574; fax: 206-543-8297.
champoux@u.washington.edu

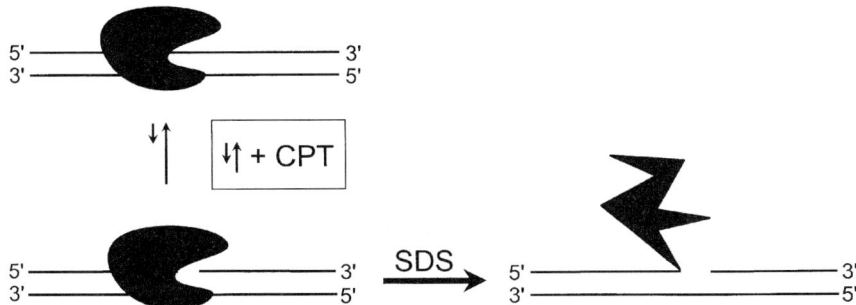

FIGURE 1. Topoisomerase I reaction and detergent-trapping of the covalent complex. A schematic shows topoisomerase I catalyzing the cleavage and religation of duplex DNA. The enzyme becomes covalently attached to the 3' end of the cleaved strand in the cleavage reaction. Religation restores continuity to the DNA strand and releases the enzyme. Addition of a detergent such as SDS denatures the enzyme and irreversibly traps the covalent complex.

core domain (residues 215-635) contains most of the amino acid residues responsible for binding DNA and catalysis. A second unconserved and protease-sensitive domain, termed the linker, extends from residues 636 to 712 and connects the core domain to the COOH-terminal domain (residues 713-765) (FIG. 2). The linker domain comprises two antiparallel α helices (α18 and α19) and, like the NH_2-terminal domain, is dispensable for enzyme activity *in vitro*.[10–13] Although the function of the linker domain is unknown, the presence of numerous basic amino acid side chains on the DNA-proximal face of the coiled-coil structure (FIG. 2) and the protection from proteolysis by bound DNA suggest that the linker interacts with DNA. The active site tyrosine residue that becomes covalently attached to the 3' end of the broken strand is located at position 723 within the COOH-terminal domain (FIG. 2).

EFFECTS OF CAMPTOTHECIN ON HUMAN TOPOISOMERASE I

The sole intracellular target of the anticancer drug camptothecin is topoisomerase I.[14–19] Camptothecin has been shown to have two biochemical effects on reactions catalyzed by human topoisomerase I. First, camptothecin binds to the enzyme DNA covalent complex, and by reducing the rate of religation,[20–25] it prolongs the lifetime of the nicked intermediate (FIG. 1). This activity of the drug results in enhancement of cleavage *in vitro* when topoisomerase I reactions are terminated with a detergent such as SDS.[20,21,26] It is generally believed that the major cytotoxic effects of the drug are mediated through stabilization of topoisomerase-DNA covalent complexes that produce potentially lethal double-strand breaks when encountered by the DNA replication machinery.[27–32]

Based on the crystal structure of the covalent topoisomerase I-DNA complex, a hypothetical model for the binding of CPT has been proposed.[7] The model attempts to take into account (1) the essential nature of the 20(S)-hydroxyl, pyridone and the lactone moieties of the drug, (2) the tolerance of additions to positions 7, 9, 10, and

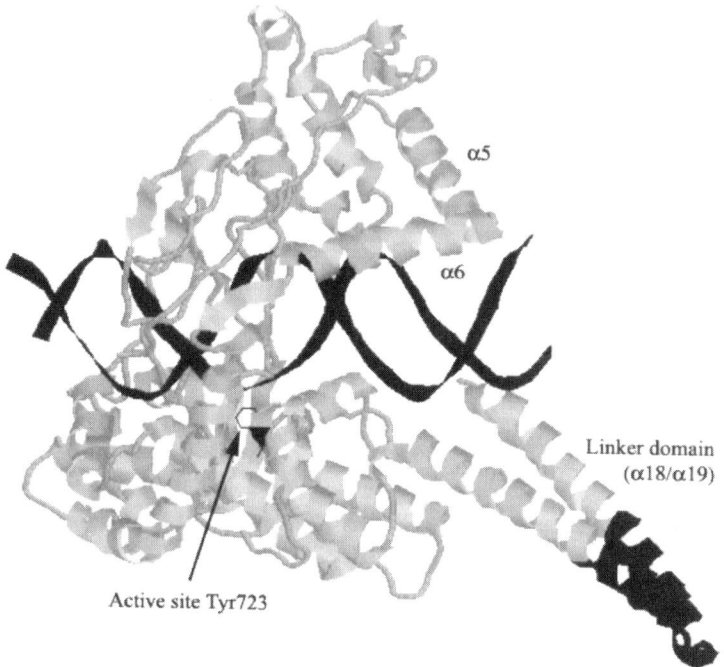

FIGURE 2. Crystal structure of human topoisomerase I with bound DNA. The polypeptide chain is rendered as a grey ribbon except for the distal 29 amino acids of the linker region (residues 660-688 of α helices 18 and 19 missing in topo70ΔL) which are shown in *black*. The two α helices that form the V-shaped structure to one side of the DNA (α5 and α6) are labeled. The amino acids that connect α18 of the linker region to the core domain (residues 634 to 640) are disordered in the crystal and therefore not included in the diagram. The location of the active site tyrosine (residue 723) is indicated by an *arrow*.

11 of the A and B rings, (3) the reactivity of substituents at the 7 position with the +1 guanine base in the DNA,[33] and (4) the locations of amino acids that, when mutated, confer resistance to CPT. The model proposes that CPT partially inserts into the DNA helix and displaces the +1 guanine base away from its normal base-paired position with the opposing cytosine. This configuration stacks the guanine base on top of CPT and places the C-7 position of the drug in close proximity to the guanine N-3 nitrogen. The model also proposes a series of interactions with the amino acid side chains of Arg364, Asp533, and Asn722 that are required for CPT sensitivity. The proposed hydrogen bonding between the 20(S)-hydroxyl and Asp 533 requires revision in light of the recent finding that the hydroxyl can be replaced by either chlorine or bromine without loss of the binding activity of the drug.[34] Importantly, this model proposes that bound CPT moves the free 5′ hydroxyl end of the DNA 4.5 Å away from the scissile phosphate and thereby provides a structural basis for the inhibition of religation. An alternative computational model for the binding of CPT has been suggested that involves intercalation of the drug into the DNA in the opposite orientation and proposes that hydrogen-bonding interactions occur between the drug and both the side

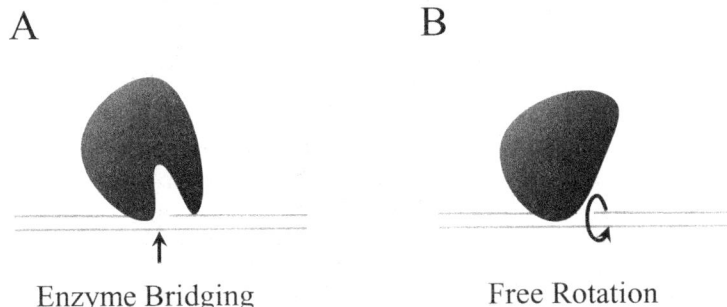

FIGURE 3. Alternative mechanisms of DNA relaxation. (**A**) In the enzyme-bridging model for DNA relaxation, the enzyme is both covalently attached to the 3′ end at the site of the nick and noncovalently attached to the 5′ end of the broken strand. Relaxation is accomplished by passage of the intact strand through the enzyme-bridged gate in the broken strand. (**B**) In the free rotation model for DNA relaxation, the DNA helix downstream of the enzyme is free to rotate during the lifetime of the enzyme-catalyzed break.

chain of Asn722 and the 5′ hydroxyl on the end of the broken strand.[35] A crystal structure with bound drug will be invaluable in distinguishing between these and possibly other models for the binding of CPT to the enzyme-DNA complex.

A second and less-well characterized activity of CPT is the inhibition of plasmid DNA relaxation by topoisomerase I.[20,23,25,36,37] An explanation for this activity of the drug requires knowledge about the mechanism of relaxation by the enzyme. For the linking number of a closed circle to be changed by topoisomerase I, the winding of the DNA helix must be changed during the lifetime of the enzyme-induced single-strand break. Topologically, such changes are equivalent to the passage of one strand of the DNA through the nick in the other strand one or more times. Two alternative mechanisms have been proposed for the change in the helical properties of the DNA that leads to the relaxation of DNA supercoils (FIG. 3).[1] The enzyme-bridging mechanism hypothesizes that the topoisomerase not only attaches covalently to the 3′ end of the broken strand, but also binds tightly noncovalently to the DNA downstream to form a bridge (FIG. 3A). Relaxation is accomplished by the passage of the intact strand through the enzyme-bridged gate in the broken strand. By this mechanism, only one supercoil can be relaxed per cleavage event because once the intact strand has passed through the gate, the enzyme must religate the DNA before carrying out another cycle of nicking and closing. Were this to be the mechanism of plasmid DNA relaxation, it is relatively straightforward to account for the inhibition of relaxation by CPT, because a reduction in the rate of religation mediated by the drug would prolong each cleavage-religation cycle and thus slow the overall rate of DNA relaxation.

The co-crystal structure of human topoisomerase I containing bound DNA[2,7] appears to be incompatible with the enzyme-bridging model for DNA relaxation. Although the enzyme wraps completely around the DNA and makes over 35 close contacts to the DNA backbone, there is a paucity of enzyme-DNA contacts downstream of the cleavage site that could serve to anchor the enzyme and form a stable bridge once cleavage has occurred (FIG. 2). Furthermore, the crystal structure of the covalent complex is virtually superimposable on the structure of the noncovalent complex,[7] indicating that no conformational changes accompany the cleavage reaction to create a tight binding interaction with the DNA downstream of the nick. Therefore, we provisionally ruled out the enzyme-bridging mechanism for DNA relaxation and therefore must seek an explanation for the inhibitory effects of CPT on relaxation in other models.

The free rotation hypothesis for DNA relaxation supposes that once the DNA is nicked, the downstream helix is free to rotate around some combination of bonds in the intact strand (FIG. 3B).[1] Using the crystal structure of the enzyme-DNA covalent complex, we previously attempted to model rotation of the DNA downstream of the cleavage site in the opening of the protein that is bounded by the V-shaped α helices (α5 and α6) on one side and the coiled-coil linker region (α18 and α19) on the other side (FIG. 2).[2] By assuming some flexibility in the DNA and tilting the DNA axis by ~10° away from the V-shaped helices, this model permitted complete rotation of the DNA without significant clash between the DNA and the protein. However, it appeared likely that the DNA backbone would be in close proximity to both the V-shaped α helices and the coiled-coil linker region during rotation. Furthermore, the fact that the DNA-proximal surfaces of both of these regions are rich in basic amino acids suggests that protein-DNA contacts may indeed accompany the rotation process. To distinguish this type of mechanism in which the rotation is hindered or guided by the protein from the aforementioned free rotation mechanism, the term "controlled rotation" was proposed.[2]

With the controlled mechanism for DNA relaxation by human topoisomerase I, it is not obvious how CPT inhibits plasmid DNA relaxation. If CPT prolongs the nicked state by slowing religation, then the number of supercoils released per nicking-closing cycle under processive reactions conditions should be increased relative to the no-drug control, and the rate of relaxation should be increased rather than decreased. Because the rate of DNA relaxation should be a function of the rate of cleavage, the finding that CPT not only slows religation, but also inhibits the cleavage reaction by topoisomerase I[38,39] could provide a solution to this dilemma. However, these studies have only reported inhibition of cleavage by CPT for oligonucleotide suicide substrates in which the DNA downstream of the cleavage site is either single-stranded or relatively unstable. When completely duplex DNA is used as a substrate, inhibition of cleavage is lost.[39] Thus, it is unlikely that an effect of CPT on cleavage is the basis for the inhibitory effects of the drug observed with the duplex substrates used routinely in plasmid DNA relaxation assays. Therefore, we have proposed that in addition to slowing religation, CPT also hinders or blocks DNA rotation.[25] If rotation is severely impeded by bound CPT such that little or no rotation occurs during some nicking-closing cycles, then the rate of DNA relaxation would be reduced. Clearly, additional experiments are necessary to validate this hypothesis.

THE LINKER AND CAMPTOTHECIN INHIBITION OF RELAXATION

The linker region in human topoisomerase I is an intriguing coiled-coil structure 77 amino acids in length that protrudes conspicuously from the body of the protein (FIG. 2). The linker region is dispensable for enzyme activity, because protein reconstituted from separately isolated core and COOH-terminal domains is enzymatically active,[4] as is a deletion of 29 amino acids from the distal part of the structure (topo70ΔL).[40] Although the linker appears to make only minimal contacts with DNA in the crystal structure,[2] several observations support a role for the linker in DNA binding. First, the reconstituted enzymes lacking a functional linker bind DNA with a 20-fold reduced affinity relative to the wild-type enzyme.[4] Second, protection of the linker from proteolysis by bound DNA[8] and the distribution of basic amino acids on the DNA proximal surface of the linker are also consistent with an interaction between the linker and the bound DNA. Finally, the source of substantial crystal-to-crystal nonisomorphism has been traced, at least in part, to an inherent flexibility of the linker region,[41] suggesting that failure of the crystal structure to reveal an intimate association between the linker and the bound DNA might be due to a crystal packing artifact.

Although the lack of a functional linker in the reconstituted enzymes and topo70ΔL does not impair their catalytic activity, these enzymes exhibit two unusual properties. First, the cleavage-religation equilibrium is shifted towards religation, reflecting an increase in the rate of religation rather than a decrease in the rate of cleavage.[4,40] The corollary to this conclusion is that one role of the linker in the wild-type enzyme is to prolong the lifetime of the nicked intermediate, perhaps through direct interaction with the cleaved DNA, as just described.

The second unusual property is that without a functional linker, the enzymes are nearly unaffected by CPT in a plasmid DNA relaxation assay.[4,40] What is the basis for this loss of sensitivity to CPT? A number of CPT-resistant mutants of eukaryotic topoisomerase I have been identified that reduce or eliminate binding of the drug to the enzyme-DNA complex.[42–47] Because CPT enhances cleavage by the mutant enzymes lacking a functional linker to approximately the same extent as for the wild-type enzyme, loss of drug binding cannot explain the lack of inhibition of DNA relaxation.[25,40] Moreover, the shift in cleavage-religation equilibrium towards religation by loss of the linker is likely to be approximately offset by the decrease in the rate of religation by the bound CPT. In support of this suggestion, we found that the amount of SDS-induced cleavage of a duplex oligonucleotide substrate was approximately the same for the mutant enzyme lacking a complete linker (topo70ΔL) in the presence of CPT as for the wild-type enzyme in the absence of the drug.[40] It was proposed above that CPT inhibits DNA relaxation, not by prolonging the lifetime of the nicked intermediate, but rather by hindering DNA rotation such that little or no rotation occurs during some cycles of cleavage and religation. If we further propose that the linker is necessary for the proposed slowing of DNA rotation, then in the absence of the linker, the amount of rotation per cleavage-religation cycle might be increased such that relaxation is nearly completed with each cleavage-religation cycle. The reduction in the DNA affinity of the enzymes lacking a functional linker[4,40] may make the enzymes less processive and also contribute to increasing the rate of relaxation under conditions of substrate excess. A combination of these two effects may be the underlying basis for the lack of inhibition of DNA relaxation by CPT when the linker is absent.

CONCLUSIONS

A hypothetical model for the binding of CPT to the topoisomerase I-DNA covalent complex can explain several observations concerning the nature of the drug-enzyme interaction and provides a plausible model for how bound drug slows the religation process. Given that DNA relaxation likely occurs by a rotational mechanism, inhibition of DNA relaxation by CPT is apparently unrelated to the effects of the drug on religation. Instead, it is proposed that the bound drug also hinders DNA rotation and that this effect requires the presence of a functional linker in the enzyme.

ACKNOWLEDGMENTS

I thank Sharon Schultz, Lance Stewart, Greg Ireton, Zheng Yang, and Heidrun Interthal for their contributions to the work discussed here. The work described here was supported by National Institutes of Health Grant GM49156.

REFERENCES

1. CHAMPOUX, J.J. 1990. Mechanistic aspects of type-i topoisomerases. *In* DNA Topology and Its Biological Effects. N.R. Cozzarelli & J.C. Wang, Eds. :217-242. Cold Spring Harbor Laboratory Press. Cold Spring Harbor, NY.
2. STEWART, L., M.R. REDINBO, X. QIU, *et al.* 1998. A model for the mechanism of human topoisomerase I. Science **279:** 1534–1541.
3. MCCONAUGHY, B.L., L.S. YOUNG & J.J. CHAMPOUX. 1981. The effect of salt on the binding of the eucaryotic DNA nicking-closing enzyme to DNA and chromatin. Biochim. Biophys. Acta **655:** 1–8.
4. STEWART, L., G.C. IRETON & J.J. CHAMPOUX. 1997. Reconstitution of human topoisomerase I by fragment complementation. J. Mol. Biol. **269:** 355–372.
5. CHENG, C., P. KUSSIE, N. PAVLETICH & S. SHUMAN. 1998. Conservation of structure and mechanism between eukaryotic topoisomerase I and site-specific recombinases. Cell **92:** 841–850.
6. STIVERS, J.T., S. SHUMAN & A.S. MILDVAN. 1994. Vaccinia DNA topoisomerase I: single-turnover and steady-state kinetic analysis of the DNA strand cleavage and ligation reactions. Biochemistry **33:** 327–339.
7. REDINBO, M.R., L. STEWART, P. KUHN, *et al.* 1998. Crystal structures of human topoisomerase I in covalent and noncovalent complexes with DNA. Science **279:** 1504–1513.
8. STEWART, L., G.C. IRETON & J.J. CHAMPOUX. 1996. The domain organization of human topoisomerase I. J. Biol. Chem. **271:** 7602–7608.
9. CHAMPOUX, J.J. 1998. Domains of human topoisomerase I and associated functions. Prog. Nucleic Acid Res. Mol. Biol. **60:** 111–132.
10. LIU, L.F. & K.G. MILLER. 1981. Eukaryotic DNA topoisomerases: two forms of type I DNA topoisomerases from HeLa cell nuclei. Proc. Natl. Acad. Sci. USA **78:** 3487–3491.
11. ALSNER, J., J.Q. SVEJSTRUP, E. KJELDSEN, *et al.* 1992. Identification of an N-terminal domain of eukaryotic DNA topoisomerase I dispensable for catalytic activity but essential for in vivo function. J. Biol. Chem. **267:** 12408–12411.
12. BJORNSTI, M.A. & J.C. WANG. 1987. Expression of yeast DNA topoisomerase I can complement a conditional- lethal DNA topoisomerase I mutation in *Escherichia coli*. Proc. Natl. Acad. Sci. USA **84:** 8971–8975.
13. STEWART, L., G.C. IRETON & J.J. CHAMPOUX. 1996. Biochemical and biophysical analyses of recombinant forms of human topoisomerase I. J. Biol. Chem. **271:** 7593–7601.
14. ANDOH, T., K. ISHII, Y. SUZUKI, *et al.* 1987. Characterization of a mammalian mutant with a camptothecin-resistant DNA topoisomerase I. Proc. Natl. Acad. Sci. USA **84:** 5565–5569.
15. HSIANG, Y.H. & L.F. LIU. 1988. Identification of mammalian DNA topoisomerase I as an intracellular target of the anticancer drug camptothecin. Cancer Res. **48:** 1722–1726.

16. NITISS, J. & J.C. WANG. 1988. DNA topoisomerase-targeting antitumor drugs can be studied in yeast. Proc. Natl. Acad. Sci. USA **85:** 7501–7505.
17. ENG, W.K., L. FAUCETTE, R.K. JOHNSON & R. STERNGLANZ. 1988. Evidence that DNA topoisomerase I is necessary for the cytotoxic effects of camptothecin. Mol. Pharmacol. **34:** 755–760.
18. MADDEN, K.R. & J.J. CHAMPOUX. 1992. Overexpression of human topoisomerase I in baby hamster kidney cells: hypersensitivity of clonal isolates to camptothecin. Cancer Res. **52:** 525–532.
19. BJORNSTI, M.A., P. BENEDETTI, G.A. VIGLIANTI & J.C. WANG. 1989. Expression of human DNA topoisomerase I in yeast cells lacking yeast DNA topoisomerase I: restoration of sensitivity of the cells to the antitumor drug camptothecin. Cancer Res. **49:** 6318–6323.
20. HSIANG, Y.H., R. HERTZBERG, S. HECHT & L.F. LIU. 1985. Camptothecin induces protein-linked DNA breaks via mammalian DNA topoisomerase I. J. Biol. Chem. **260:** 14873–14878.
21. PORTER, S.E. & J.J. CHAMPOUX. 1989. The basis for camptothecin enhancement of DNA breakage by eukaryotic topoisomerase I. Nucleic Acids Res. **17:** 8521–8532.
22. SVEJSTRUP, J.Q., K. CHRISTIANSEN, I.I. GROMOVA, et al. 1991. New technique for uncoupling the cleavage and religation reactions of eukaryotic topoisomerase I. The mode of action of camptothecin at a specific recognition site. J. Mol. Biol. **222:** 669–678.
23. HERTZBERG, R.P., M.J. CARANFA & S.M. HECHT. 1989. On the mechanism of topoisomerase I inhibition by camptothecin: evidence for binding to an enzyme-DNA complex. Biochemistry **28:** 4629–4638.
24. HERTZBERG, R.P., R.W. BUSBY, M.J. CARANFA, et al. 1990. Irreversible trapping of the DNA-topoisomerase I covalent complex. Affinity labeling of the camptothecin binding site. J. Biol. Chem. **265:** 19287–19295.
25. STEWART, L., G.C. IRETON & J.J. CHAMPOUX. 1999. A functional linker in human topoisomerase I is required for maximum sensitivity to camptothecin in a DNA relaxation assay. J. Biol. Chem. **274:** 32950–32960.
26. CHAMPOUX, J.J. & R. ARONOFF. 1989. The effects of camptothecin on the reaction and the specificity of the wheat germ type I topoisomerase. J. Biol. Chem. **264:** 1010–1015.
27. COVEY, J.M., C. JAXEL, K.W. KOHN & Y. POMMIER. 1989. Protein-linked DNA strand breaks induced in mammalian cells by camptothecin, an inhibitor of topoisomerase I. Cancer Res. **49:** 5016–5022.
28. D'ARPA, P., C. BEARDMORE & L.F. LIU. 1990. Involvement of nucleic acid synthesis in cell killing mechanisms of topoisomerase poisons. Cancer Res. **50:** 6919–6924.
29. HSIANG, Y.H., M.G. LIHOU & L.F. LIU. 1989. Arrest of replication forks by drug-stabilized topoisomerase I-DNA cleavable complexes as a mechanism of cell killing by camptothecin. Cancer Res. **49:** 5077–5082.
30. HSIANG, Y.H., L.F. LIU, M.E. WALL, et al. 1989. DNA topoisomerase I-mediated DNA cleavage and cytotoxicity of camptothecin analogues. Cancer Res. **49:** 4385–4389.
31. MATTERN, M.R., S.M. MONG, H.F. BARTUS, et al. 1987. Relationship between the intracellular effects of camptothecin and the inhibition of DNA topoisomerase I in cultured L1210 cells. Cancer Res. **47:** 1793–1798.
32. TSAO, Y.P., A. RUSSO, G. NYAMUSWA, et al. 1993. Interaction between replication forks and topoisomerase I-DNA cleavable complexes: studies in a cell-free SV40 DNA replication system. Cancer Res. **53:** 5908–5914.
33. POMMIER, Y., G. KOHLHAGEN, K.W. KOHN, et al. 1995. Interaction of an alkylating camptothecin derivative with a DNA base at topoisomerase I-DNA cleavage sites. Proc. Natl. Acad. Sci. USA **92:** 8861–8865.
34. WANG, X., X. ZHOU & S.M. HECHT. 1999. Role of the 20-hydroxyl group in camptothecin binding by the topoisomerase I-DNA binary complex. Biochemistry **38:** 4374–4381.
35. FAN, Y., J.N. WEINSTEIN, K.W. KOHN, et al. 1998. Molecular modeling studies of the DNA-topoisomerase I ternary cleavable complex with camptothecin. J. Med. Chem. **41:** 2216–2226.

36. JAXEL, C., K.W. KOHN, M.C. WANI, *et al.* 1989. Structure-activity study of the actions of camptothecin derivatives on mammalian topoisomerase I: evidence for a specific receptor site and a relation to antitumor activity. Cancer Res. **49:** 1465–1469.
37. HOLDEN, J.A., M.E. WALL, M.C. WANI & G. MANIKUMAR. 1999. Human DNA topoisomerase I: quantitative analysis of the effects of camptothecin analogs and the benzophenanthridine alkaloids nitidine and 6-ethoxydihydronitidine on DNA topoisomerase I-induced DNA strand breakage. Arch. Biochem. Biophys. **370:** 66–76.
38. POMMIER, Y., G. KOHLHAGEN, P. POURQUIER, *et al.* 2000. Benzo[a]pyrene diol epoxide adducts in DNA are potent suppressors of a normal topoisomerase I cleavage site and powerful inducers of other topoisomerase I cleavages. Proc. Natl. Acad. Sci. USA **97:** 2040–2045.
39. KJELDSEN, E., J.Q. SVEJSTRUP, I.I. GROMOVA, *et al.* 1992. Camptothecin inhibits both the cleavage and religation reactions of eukaryotic DNA topoisomerase I. J. Mol. Biol. **228:** 1025–1030.
40. IRETON, G.C., L. STEWART, L.H. PARKER & J.J. CHAMPOUX. 2000. Expression of human topoisomerase I with a partial deletion of the linker region yields monomeric and dimeric enzymes that respond differently to camptothecin. Submitted.
41. REDINBO, M.R., L. STEWART, J.J. CHAMPOUX & W.G. HOL. 1999. Structural flexibility in human topoisomerase I revealed in multiple non-isomorphous crystal structures. J. Mol. Biol. **292:** 685–696.
42. KNAB, A.M., J. FERTALA & M.A. BJORNSTI. 1993. Mechanisms of camptothecin resistance in yeast DNA topoisomerase I mutants. J. Biol. Chem. **268:** 22322–22330.
43. RUBIN, E., P. PANTAZIS, A. BHARTI, *et al.* 1994. Identification of a mutant human topoisomerase I with intact catalytic activity and resistance to 9-nitro-camptothecin. J. Biol. Chem. **269:** 2433–2439.
44. TAMURA, H., C. KOHCHI, R. YAMADA, *et al.* 1991. Molecular cloning of a cDNA of a camptothecin-resistant human DNA topoisomerase I and identification of mutation sites. Nucleic Acids Res. **19:** 69–75.
45. KUBOTA, N., F. KANZAWA, K. NISHIO, *et al.* 1992. Detection of topoisomerase I gene point mutation in CPT-11 resistant lung cancer cell line. Biochem. Biophys. Res. Comm. **188:** 571–577.
46. BENEDETTI, P., P. FIORANI, L. CAPUANI & J.C. WANG. 1993. Camptothecin resistance from a single mutation changing glycine 363 of human DNA topoisomerase I to cysteine. Cancer Res. **53:** 4343–4348.
47. LI, X.G., P. HALUSKA, JR., Y.H. HSIANG, *et al.* 1997. Involvement of amino acids 361 to 364 of human topoisomerase I in camptothecin resistance and enzyme catalysis. Biochem. Pharmacol. **53:** 1019–1027.

Mechanisms of DNA Topoisomerase I- Induced Cell Killing in the Yeast *Saccharomyces cerevisiae*

PAOLA FIORANI AND MARY-ANN BJORNSTI[a]

Department of Molecular Pharmacology, St. Jude Children's Research Hospital, Memphis, Tennessee 38103, USA

ABSTRACT: DNA topoisomerase I (Top1) catalyzes the relaxation of supercoiled DNA by a mechanism of transient DNA strand cleavage characterized by the formation of a phosphotyrosyl bond between the DNA end and active site tyrosine. Camptothecin reversibly stabilizes the covalent enzyme-DNA intermediate by inhibiting DNA religation. During S-phase, collisions with advancing replication forks convert these complexes into potentially lethal lesions. To define the DNA damage induced by alterations in Top1p catalysis and the cellular processes that mediate the repair of such lesions, the yeast *Saccharomyces cerevisiae* was used. Substitution of conserved residues N-terminal to the active site tyrosine (Tyr-727) produced alterations in the camptothecin sensitivity or catalytic cycle of DNA Top1. For example, substituting Ala for Thr-722 in Top1T722A increased the stability of the covalent enzyme DNA intermediate. As with camptothecin, Top1T722A-induced cytotoxicity was ascribed to a reduction in DNA religation. By contrast, enhanced covalent complex formation by Top1N726H resulted from a relative increase in the rate of DNA cleavage. Conditional yeast mutants were also selected that exhibit temperature-sensitive growth only in the presence of the self-poisoning Top1T722A enzyme. Subsequent analyses of these *tah* mutants identified 9 genes whose function suppresses the cytotoxic action of camptothecin and Top1T722A. These include genes encoding essential DNA replication proteins (*CDC45* and *DPB11*) and proteins involved in SUMO- or ubiquitination (*UBC9* and *DOA4*).

INTRODUCTION

Eukaryotic DNA topoisomerase I (Top1) catalyzes changes in DNA topology and plays an important role in cellular processes involving DNA, including replication, recombination, transcription, and chromosome condensation.[1–3] This monomeric enzyme is encoded by the *TOP1* gene and is highly conserved in terms of amino acid sequence, reaction mechanism, and sensitivity to anticancer agents, such as camptothecin (CPT).[1,2,4,5] Topoisomerase I binds duplex DNA and transiently cleaves a single DNA strand.[3,6,7] A phosphodiester bond in the DNA undergoes nucleophilic attack by the active tyrosine to generate a phosphotyrosyl linkage between the enzyme and the 3' phosphate of the nicked DNA. The noncovalently bound end of

---

[a]Department of Molecular Pharmacology, St. Jude Children's Research Hospital, 332 N. Lauderdale, Memphis, TN 38103. Voice: 901-495-2315; fax: 901-521-1668.
Mary-Ann.Bjornsti@stjude.org

DNA presumably rotates around the intact, nonscissile strand to affect changes in the linkage of the DNA strands. The formation of the covalent enzyme-DNA intermediate conserves the energy of the phosphodiester bond, so that religation of the nicked DNA via a second transesterification reaction does not require ATP.

Camptothecin interferes with the catalytic cycle of DNA Top1 by reversibly stabilizing the covalent enzyme-DNA intermediate.[1,4,5] However, the formation of this ternary drug–enzyme–DNA complex is insufficient to cause cell death. Rather, the collision of advancing replication forks with these drug-stabilized intermediates appears to produce the cytotoxic DNA lesions that signal cell cycle arrest and cause cell death. Such a model is further supported by numerous studies establishing the S-phase specificity of CPTs at pharmacologically relevant doses and the ability of replication inhibitors, such as aphidicolin, to suppress CPT cytotoxicity.[4,8–11]

In contrast to *Drosophila* and mouse, the *TOP1* gene in the budding yeast *Saccharomyces cerevisiae* is nonessential.[12–15] Genetic studies have established that other gene products, such as DNA topoisomerase II and Trf4p, can compensate for the loss of Top1p function. Nevertheless, DNA topoisomerase I is required for the cytotoxic action of CPT.[16–18] Yeast cells deleted for *TOP1* (*top1Δ*) are resistant to CPT, while expression of yeast or human *TOP1* sequences from plasmids is sufficient to restore drug sensitivity. These data establish DNA topoisomerase I as the cellular target of CPT and confirm that drug cytotoxicity results from the stabilization of the covalent complex, rather than the inhibition of a nonessential enzyme. Thus, camptothecins have been described as topoisomerase I poisons to contrast their action on enzyme function with drugs that inhibit catalytic activity. Although CPT inhibits the relaxation of supercoiled DNA catalyzed by human DNA topoisomerase I, the concentrations of drug needed exceeds those required to stabilize the covalent enzyme-DNA intermediate or induce cell death.[4,19] Moreover, CPT does not inhibit the catalytic activity of yeast Top1, yet expression of the yeast enzyme is sufficient to restore CPT sensitivity to *top1Δ* yeast cells and enhance CPT cytotoxicity in mammalian cells.[19, 20]

MUTATIONS IN DNA TOPOISOMERASE I

The phenotypic consequences of CPT treatment are faithfully reiterated in yeast.[1,21,22] As in mammalian cells, drug treatment induces sister chromatid exchange and cell cycle arrest in G2. The enhanced CPT sensitivity of cells defective in double-strand break repair (due to deletion of the *RAD52* gene) argues for the involvement of DNA recombination in the repair of drug-induced DNA lesions.[16,17] The cytotoxic action of the drug is also highly S-phase dependent, as the DNA replication inhibitor, aphidicolin, abrogates CPT-induced cell killing.[10] However, in terms of investigating the cytotoxic mechanism of camptothecins, the genetically tractable yeast system offers the added advantage that the *TOP1* gene is dispensable for mitotic cell growth, yet essential for drug action.[13] Thus, the regulated expression of yeast or human *TOP1* from plasmid-borne sequences in *top1Δ* strains enables direct assessment of specific amino acid substitutions on DNA topoisomerase I function and CPT sensitivity in the absence of the endogenous enzyme.[1, 21]

The structures of an N-terminal deletion of human DNA topoisomerase I, in covalent and noncovalent complexes with DNA, were recently reported.[7,23,24] As with

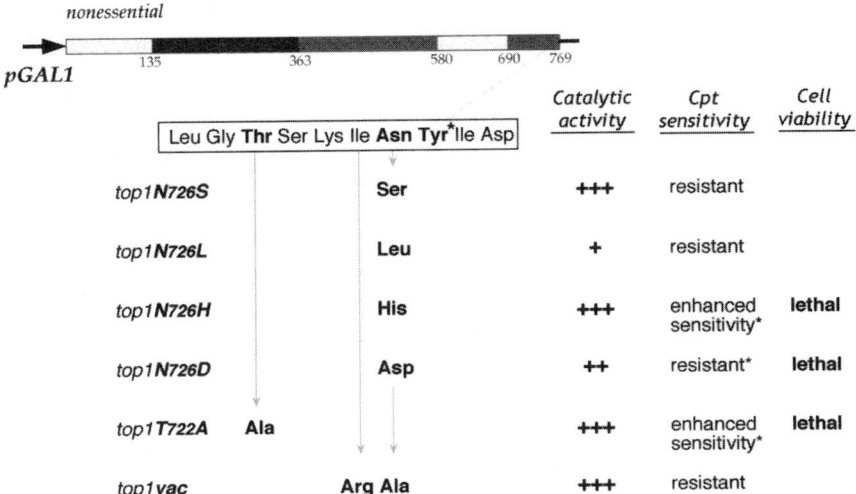

FIGURE 1. Substitutions of conserved residues around the active site tyrosine affect the catalytic activity and camptothecin sensitivity of DNA topoisomerase I. Conserved central and C-terminal domains of eukaryotic DNA topoisomerase I, essential for enzyme activity, are indicated by *gray shading*. The *boxed residues* around the active site tyrosine* (Tyr-727) in yeast Top1 are identical to those found at the corresponding position in the human enzyme, with the exception of isoleucine to leucine changes. The amino acid substitutions in each *top1* mutant are indicated with the allele designations on the left. For each *top1* mutant, any affects on cell viability or camptothecin sensitivity were assessed following galactose-induced expression of plasmid-borne sequences in *top1*Δ cells, in the presence or absence of camptothecin. Following protein purification, the specific activity of equal concentrations of the mutant enzymes was determined in plasmid DNA relaxation assays. Each + indicates a 10-fold difference in activity relative to wild-type Top1 (+++). The ability of camptothecin to stabilize the covalent enzyme-DNA complex was also determined in DNA cleavage assays. In the case of the lethal *top1* mutants, *top1N726H*, *top1N726D*, and *top1T722A*, galactose induced a greater than 3-log drop in cell viability in the absence of camptothecin. Thus, relative enzyme sensitivity to camptothecin was solely defined *in vitro*.

other DNA topoisomerases, this eukaryotic type IB enzyme forms a protein clamp that circumscribes the DNA duplex. Several amino acid substitutions have been reported to affect the CPT sensitivity of yeast or human Top1.[1,4,7,25] Although widely scattered among conserved sequences, these residues cluster near the active site of the enzyme, along one face of the DNA in the crystal structures.

The conservation in enzyme mechanism and CPT sensitivity among cellular type IB enzymes is also reflected in amino acid sequence.[1,4,26] As shown in FIGURE 1, the residues immediately N-terminal to the active site tyrosine (Tyr727 in yeast and Tyr723 in human) are mostly identical. Indeed, substitution of these residues has profound effects on the catalytic activity and CPT sensitivity of DNA topoisomerase I. For instance, substituting Arg-Ala for the two residues preceding the active site tyrosine in yeast or human Top1 rendered the mutant enzymes resistant to CPT.[19,27] In these experiments, *top1*Δ strains were transformed with a single copy yeast vector expressing the indicated *top1* allele from the galactose-inducible *GAL1* promoter.

Cells expressing wild-type *TOP1* exhibit a greater than 3-log drop in viability when plated on selective media containing galactose and CPT. In contrast, cells expressing the yeast or human *top1vac* mutant were unaffected by the drug. Comparisons of wild-type and mutant proteins purified from these cells indicated that enzyme specific activities were indistinguishable in plasmid DNA relaxation assays. However, relative to wild-type Top1, the levels of CPT-stabilized, covalent enzyme-DNA complexes were dramatically diminished in DNA cleavage assays containing the mutant enzymes. Thus, the levels of drug-stabilized enzyme-DNA complexes *in vitro* corresponded with the cytotoxic activity of CPT in cells expressing the particular *top1* mutant.

Mutation of the conserved Thr-722 to Ala in yeast *top1T722A* had the surprising effect of mimicking the action of CPT, by increasing the stability of the covalent enzyme-DNA intermediate.[28,29] *GAL1*-promoted expression of *top1T722A* induced a rapid drop in cell viability and a terminal G2-arrested phenotype in the absence of CPT. Although the mutant enzyme was catalytically active, biochemical studies indicated a defect in DNA religation, resulting in higher concentrations of the covalent intermediate. This mirrors the cytotoxic mechanism ascribed to CPT.[30] The analogous substitution in human *top1T718A* produces similar alterations in enzyme function.[31]

To further investigate the contribution of active site residues to DNA topoisomerase I catalysis and drug sensitivity, we focused on several substitutions of Asn-726. In the active site of the human enzyme, this Asn is one of a few residues to interact with phosphate groups in the scissile DNA strand. In addition to studies of the *top1vac* and *top1N726L* mutants,[19,27] substitution of this residue with Ser in the human enzyme conferred CPT resistance with little affect on enzyme activity.[32] More recently, Asn-726 was mutated to His, Ser, or Asp in yeast Top1N726H, Top1N726S, and Top1N726D, respectively.[33] As described above for the *top1vac*, *top1N726L*, and *top1T722A* mutants, the consequences of these substitutions on cell viability, drug sensitivity, and enzyme function were assayed in *top1Δ* cells and in DNA relaxation and cleavage assays *in vitro*.

As summarized in FIGURE 1, each mutations had profound effects on various aspects on DNA topoisomerase I function.[33] In terms of DNA relaxation, substitution of Asn with an aliphatic residue (Leu) or an acidic residue (Asp) produced a 20–100-fold drop in specific activity. In contrast, a hydroxyl residue (Ser) or basic residue (His) had little effect on enzyme-catalyzed relaxation of supercoiled DNA. However, the requirements for CPT sensitivity were more stringent. Only enzymes containing the basic His (Top1N726H) or polar Asn (wild-type Top1) exhibited CPT-enhanced DNA cleavage *in vitro*. The presence of an acidic residue (Asp), aliphatic (Leu) or hydroxyl (Ser) residue immediately N-terminal to the active site tyrosine (Tyr-727) abrogated the ability of CPT to stabilize the covalent enzyme-DNA intermediate *in vitro*.

In *top1Δ* cells, galactose-induced expression of the CPT resistant Ser and Leu mutants also conferred a drug-resistant phenotype.[27,33] However, despite differences in specific enzyme activity and drug sensitivity *in vitro*, *GAL1*-promoted expression of the His and Asp mutants (*top1N726H* and *top1N726D*, respectively) induced cell death in the absence of CPT. Detailed biochemical studies of enzyme-DNA complexes in DNA cleavage assays, using full-length DNA substrates, suicide DNA substrates, or nicked DNA molecules, indicated distinct mechanisms of enzyme-induced lethality. The His mutant (Top1N726H) exhibited increased covalent complex formation in the absence of CPT. However, in contrast to the decrease in DNA religation attributed to camptothecin or Top1T722A,[28,30] the His mutant exhibited increased rates of DNA scission.[33]

With Top1N726D, the presence of Asp at position 726 diminished enzyme binding of DNA.[33] Whereas this did not produce an increment in covalent complexes, the introduction of nicks in the nonscissile strand, downstream of the cleavage site, selectively destabilized the covalent enzyme-DNA intermediate. Wild-type and His mutant complexes were not affected. These data suggest that once the covalent linkage is formed between the Asp mutant enzyme and DNA, the deficit in DNA binding is localized to the noncovalently bound DNA, 3' to the cleavage site. As a consequence, protein assemblies tracking along the DNA (such as replication forks) would have a greater probability of displacing the noncovalently bound DNA end before the phosphotyrosyl linkage is resolved.

Although additional studies are necessary to test various aspects of this model, the data clearly indicate novel mechanisms of DNA topoisomerase I-induced DNA damage result from single residue changes in the active site. Related questions concerning cellular responses to these lesions have also to addressed. Nevertheless, these findings suggest an opportunity to develop novel DNA topoisomerase I poisons that interfere with aspects of the catalytic cycle, distinct from that targeted by camptothecins.

CELLULAR FACTORS THAT MODULATE CAMPTOTHECIN SENSITIVITY

Yeast has also proven a valuable model to investigate cellular processes that function in modulating cellular responses to camptothecins.[1,10,21] Genetic and biochemical studies established DNA topoisomerase I as the cellular target of these drugs. Furthermore, in isogenic cell lines or yeast strains, the relative levels of DNA topoisomerase I correlate with the cytotoxic action of CPT.[20,22,27,34] However, in genetically diverse backgrounds, such as tumor cells or yeast strains defective in various aspects of DNA repair or DNA damage checkpoints, enzyme levels are not predictive of drug sensitivity.[11,16,28,35,36] For example, yeast cells defective in double-strand break repair (rad52Δ strains) or the DNA damage checkpoint (rad9Δ strains) are hypersensitive to CPT as well as the damage induced by the top1T722A mutant.[16–18,28] Furthermore, CPT-resistant mammalian cell lines have been isolated with no apparent alteration in DNA topoisomerase I activity.[4,11] Experiments in yeast and mammalian cells implicate recombinational repair in the resolution of CPT-induced DNA lesions during S-phase. Yet, the specific drug-induced DNA lesions and the cellular processes involved in the recognition and repair of such lesions remain poorly defined. These issues are of critical importance for the effective clinical application of camptothecins and in the development of more potent DNA topoisomerase I poisons.

To define cellular factors that modulate cell sensitivity to CPT, we previously reported a yeast screen to identify mutations in genes other than *TOP1* that confer resistance to CPT.[22] In these studies, wild-type *TOP1* was expressed from the *GAL1* promoter on a single copy vector, in *top1Δ* cells. Following mutagenesis and selection of drug-resistant colonies on galactose-containing media, the mutants were cured of the original vector and transformed with a plasmid that constitutively expressed *TOP1*. A secondary screen for CPT resistance eliminated *TOP1* mutants or mutations affecting efficient expression of the *GAL1* promoter. Each mutant strain contained a dominant mutation in the *PDR1* gene, resulting in a pleiotropic drug resistant phenotype.[35] *PDR1* encodes a transcription factor that regulates the expression of a network of yeast genes encoding ATP binding cassette (ABC) transport proteins.[37] These membrane-spanning proteins form membrane channels that transport a variety of molecules. Overexpression of ABC transporters has been linked to cytotoxic drug resistance, although CPT is not an effective substrate for p-glycoprotein or MRP. Only modest effects have been seen with topotecan and SN-38[5,21]; however, anion transporters have been implicated in the renal clearance of the carboxylate form of topotecan.[38] The ~1,000-fold CPT resistance of the yeast *PDR1* mutants required a specific transporter, Snq2.[35] Although ABC transporters exhibit some substrate specificity, 50-fold overexpression of a heterologous transporter also conferred CPT resistance. This raises the intriguing possibility that other, as yet unknown, transporters will be identified that modulate tumor cell sensitivity to various CPT analogues. Indeed, overexpression of the ABC transporter BCRP in ovarian cell lines selected for resistance to topotecan or mitoxantrone was recently shown to promote efficient efflux of topotecan.[39]

Although potential mechanisms of drug uptake/efflux are important considerations, this approach failed to illuminate events that occur downstream of the covalent complex. So to avoid the complications attendant with drug transport, we initiated a genetic screen for mutations that enhance cell sensitivity to the damage induced by DNA topoisomerase I mutant (*top1T722A*) that mimics the cytotoxic action of CPT.[36] The rationale for these studies was that low, constitutive levels of *top1T722A* expression, just like sublethal doses of CPT, still induce DNA damage. This is evidenced by increased rates of DNA recombination in repair-proficient strains and the inability of repair defective strains (i.e, *rad52Δ* cells) to tolerate even low levels of Top1T722A.[28,36] Thus, we reasoned that cellular processes that normally protect cells from DNA topoisomerase-I mediated DNA damage could be identified by isolating yeast mutants that exhibit temperature-dependent sensitivity to *top1T722A* (called *tah* mutants).

As depicted in FIGURE 2, *tah* mutants tolerate *top1T722A*-induced DNA damage at the permissive temperature (26°C).[36] However, at the high temperature (35°C), *tah* gene function is lost or diminished, and the cells are unable to survive the lesions induced by the Top1T722A mutant enzyme. To ensure that the *tah* temperature-sensitive (*tah*^{ts}) phenotype was plasmid linked, the cells were cured of the original *top1T722A* vector and rescreened for viability at 35°C. Only those cells exhibiting a *tah*^{ts} phenotype, whose viability at 35°C was unaffected by the expression of wild-type *TOP1* or the absence of DNA topoisomerase I function were selected. Twelve mutants were isolated exhibiting a stable *tah*^{ts} phenotype that segregated as a single, recessive gene mutation and enhanced sensitivity to CPT. This validated the use of *top1T722A* as a drug mimetic. Moreover, the large budded terminal phenotypes observed at 35°C were indicative of S-phase-induced lesions.

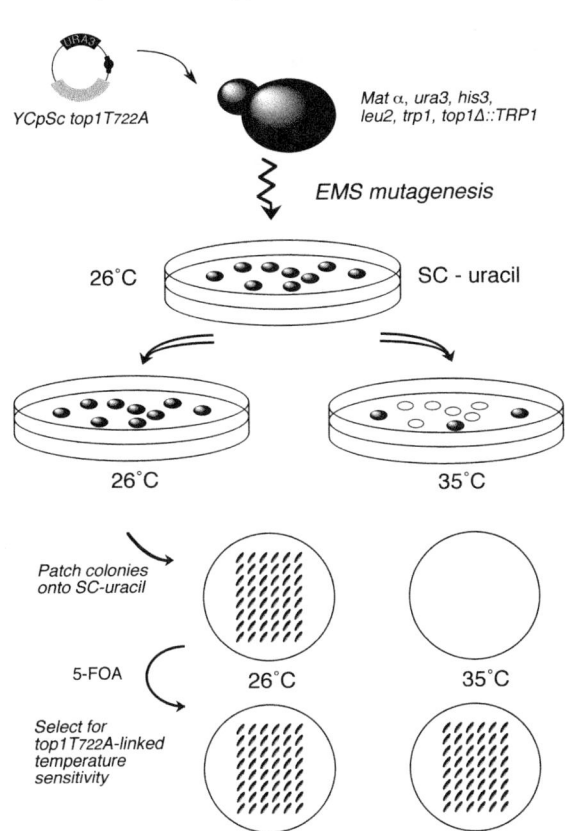

FIGURE 2. Isolation of *top1T722A* hypersensitive (*tah*) mutants.

The *tah* mutants exhibited a pleiotropic pattern of hypersensitivity to other forms of DNA damage at the nonpermissive temperature, in the absence of *top1T722A*. Most showed enhanced sensitivity to the inhibition of DNA replication induced by hydroxyurea (HU), consistent with the S-phase toxicity of CPT. Some were also hypersensitive to the alkylating agent MMS and UV irradiation. However, the spectrum of alterations in drug sensitivity was confined to DNA damaging agents. Furthermore, the temperature-sensitive phenotypes could not be attributed to alterations in DNA topoisomerase I function, as drug sensitivity was assessed in the absence of *TOP1*.

Wild-type *TAH* alleles were cloned by complementation. A yeast genomic DNA library in a single copy vector was transformed into individual mutants and plasmids capable of suppressing the *tah*[ts], or HU hypersensitive phenotypes were isolated. Subsequent subcloning identified individual *TAH* genes. These studies were facilitated by annotated databases containing the sequence of the yeast genome (*Saccha-*

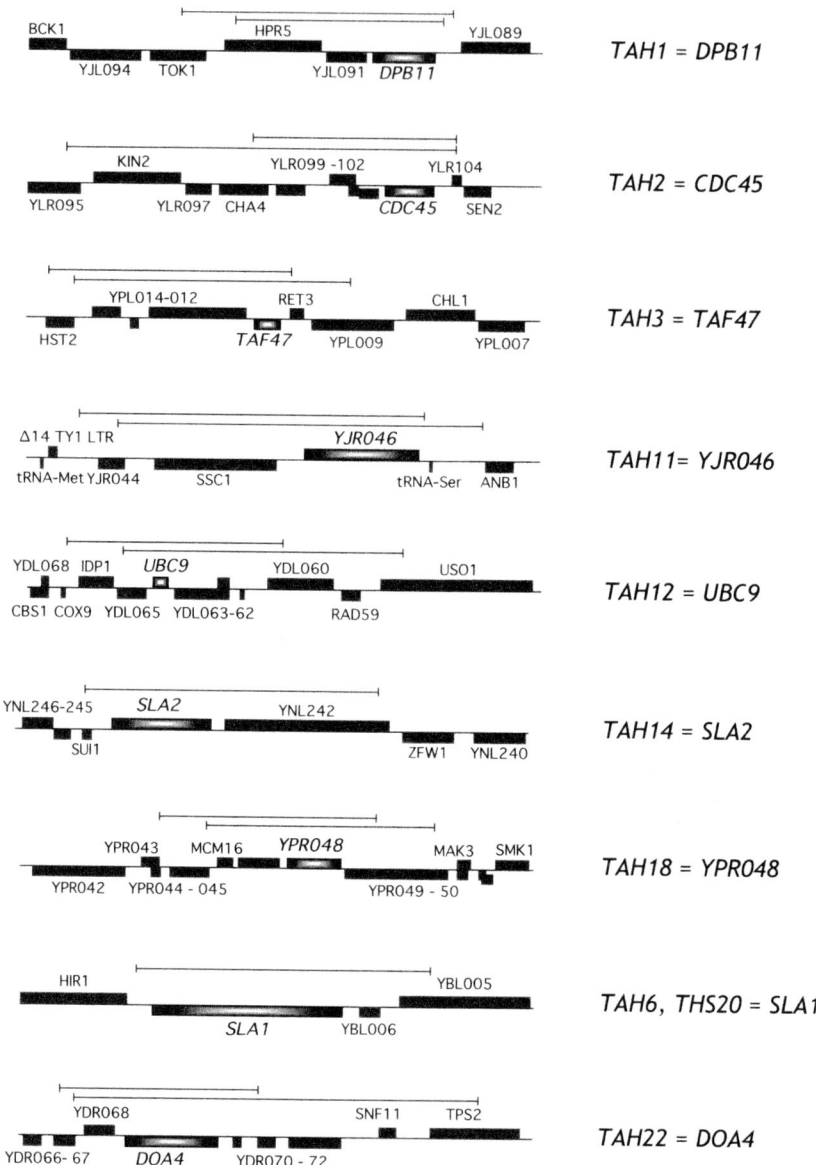

FIGURE 3. Wild-type *TAH* alleles cloned by complementation. Inserts of plasmids containing yeast genomic DNA capable of restoring tah mutant cell growth at the nonpermissive temperature in the presence of either *top1T722A* or HU are shown relative to their location on the indicated yeast chromosome. Subcloning and subsequent genetic studies confirmed the identity of the wild-type *TAH* gene within each plasmid.

romyces Genome Database [http://genome-www.stanford.edu/Saccharomyces/]. As depicted in FIGURE 3, the *TAH* genes encode proteins involved in DNA replication (*CDC45*–initiation of DNA replication,[40,41] *DPB11*–DNA replication, and the S-phase checkpoint[43]), SUMO- or ubiquitination (*UBC9*, *DOA4*) and transcription (*TAF47*), as well as cortical actin components (*SLA1*, *SLA2*) and two unknowns (*TAH11* and *TAH18*).

Experiments are currently underway to define the specific role that each gene product plays in modulating cell sensitivity to CPT. However, in the case of the *cdc45-10* and *dpb11-10* mutants, the construction of strains bearing both mutations (*cdc45-10, dpb11-10* cells) revealed a synthetic lethal interaction.[36] At 35°C, in the absence of *top1T722A* or any other DNA damaging agent, the double mutants were inviable. In synchronized cultures at the nonpermissive temperature, each of the single mutants (*cdc45-10* or *dpb11-10*) exhibited a delay in early S-phase transit. This coincided with a transient accumulation of Okazaki-sized DNA fragments in asynchronous cultures. Yet, the S-phase checkpoint was functional in each mutant. In contrast, the double *cdc45-10, dpd11-10* mutant exhibited a persistent accumulation of Okazaki-sized DNA fragments and a drop in viability as the cells transited S-phase. Taken together, these data suggest that *CDC45* and *DPB11* are required for processive DNA replication, possibly in mediating the switch from priming to processive DNA polymerases. In terms of CPT sensitivity, the accumulation of Okazaki fragments behind the advancing replication fork would preclude recombinational repair of the lesions resulting from collision of the fork with the drug-stabilized enzyme-DNA complexes.

Further genetic analyses will decipher the function of other *TAH* genes in modulating cell sensitivity to CPT-induced DNA damage. Despite the apparent complexity of gene functions uncovered in this screen, similarities in terminal phenotype suggest common action during S-phase, consistent with the cytotoxic action of CPT. However, preliminary studies also suggest that the DNA damage induced by the different self-poisoning forms of DNA topoisomerase I described above[33] may involve distinct signaling or repair processes. Thus, despite a unique cellular target (DNA topoisomerase I), various CPT analogues or structurally unrelated Top1 poisons may elicit DNA lesions with distinct cellular consequences, which may be exploited in the development of new antitumor agents.

ACKNOWLEDGMENTS

Many thanks to past and present members of the lab for their many contributions to this work and to D.J. Hall, P. Benedetti, Y. Pommier, and M. Redinbo. This work was supported in part by Fellowship 203.04.15 from the C.N.R., Italy (to P.F.), National Institutes of Health Grants CA58755 and CA70406 to (M.-A.B.), CA21675 Cancer Center Grant, and the American Lebanese Syrian Associated Charities (ALSAC).

REFERENCES

1. REID, R.J.D., P. BENEDETTI & M.A. BJORNSTI. 1998. Yeast as a model organism for studying the actions of DNA topoisomerase-targeted drugs. Biochem. Biophys. Acta **1400:** 289–300.

2. NITISS, J. 1998. Investigating the biological functions of DNA topoisomerases in eukaryotic cells. Biochem. Biophys. Acta **1400:** 63–82.
3. WANG, J.C. 1996. DNA topoisomerases. Ann. Rev. Biochem. **65:** 635–692.
4. POMMIER, Y., P. POURQUIER, Y. FAN, et al. 1998. Mechanism of action of eukaryotic DNA topoisomerase I and drugs targeted to the enzyme. Biochem. Biophys. Acta **1400:** 83–106.
5. CHEN, A. & L.F. LIU. 1994. DNA topoisomerases: essential enzymes and lethal targets. Ann. Rev. Pharmacol. Toxicol. **34:** 191–218.
6. CHAMPOUX, J. 1990. Mechanistic aspects of type-I topoisomerases. In DNA Topology and Its Biological Effects. N. Cozzarelli & J.C. Wang, Eds.: 217–242. Cold Spring Harbor Lab Press. Cold Spring Harbor, NY.
7. REDINBO, M.R., J.J. CHAMPOUX & W.G. HOL. 1999. Structural insights into the function of typeIB topoisomerases. Curr. Opin. Struct. Biol. **9:** 29–36.
8. HSIANG, Y., M.G. LIHOU & L.F LIU. 1989. Arrest of replication forks by drug-stabilized topoisomerase I-DNA cleavable complexes as a mechanism of cell killing by camptothecin. Cancer Res. **49:** 5077–5082.
9. HOLM, C., J.M. COVEY, D. KERRIGAN, et al. 1989. Differential requirement of DNA replication for the cytotoxicity of DNA topoisomerase I and II inhibitors in Chinese hamster DC3F cells. Cancer Res. **49:** 6365–6368.
10. NITISS, J.L. & J.C. WANG. 1991. Yeast as a genetic system in the dissection of the mechanism of cell killing by topoisomerase-targeting anticancer drugs. In DNA Topoisomerases in Cancer. M. Potmesil & K.W. Kohn, Eds.:77–92. Oxford University Press. Oxford, UK.
11. KAUFMANN, S.H. 1998. Cell death induced by topoisomerase-targeted drugs: more questions than answers. Biochem. Biophys. Acta **1400:** 195–212.
12. MORHAM, S.G., K.D. KLUCKMAN, N. VOULOMANOS, et al. 1996. Targeted disruption of the mouse topoisomerase I gene by camptothecin selection. Mol. Cell. Biol. **16:** 6804–6809.
13. GOTO, T. & J.C. WANG. 1985. Cloning of yeast TOP1, the gene encoding DNA topoisomerase I, and construction of mutants defective in both DNA topoisomerase I and DNA topoisomerase II. Proc. Natl. Acad. Sci. USA **82:** 7178–7182.
14. CASTANO, I.B., S. HEATHPAGLIUSO, B.U. SADOFF, et al. 1996. A novel family of Trf (DNA topoisomerase I-related function) genes required for proper nuclear segregation. Nucl. Acids Res. **24:** 2404–2410.
15. LEE, M.P., S.D. BROWN, A. CHEN, et al. 1993. DNA topoisomerase I is essential in Drosophila melanogaster. Proc. Natl. Acad. Sci. USA **90:** 6656–6660.
16. NITISS, J.L. & J.C. WANG 1988. DNA topoisomerase-targeting antitumor drugs can be studied in yeast. Proc. Natl. Acad. Sci. USA **85:** 7501–7505.
17. ENG, W.K., L. FAUCETTE, R.K. JOHNSON, et al. 1988. Evidence that DNA topoisomerase I is necessary for the cytotoxic effects of camptothecin. Mol. Pharmacol. **34:** 755–760.
18. BJORNSTI, M.A., P. BENEDETTI, G.A. VIGLIANTI, et al. 1989. Expression of human DNA topoisomerase I in yeast cells lacking yeast DNA topoisomerase I: restoration of sensitivity of the cells to the antitumor drug camptothecin. Cancer Res. **49:** 6318–6323.
19. KNAB, A.M., J. FERTALA & M.A. BJORNSTI. 1995. A camptothecin-resistant DNA topoisomerase I mutant exhibits altered sensitivities to other DNA topoisomerase poisons. J. Biol. Chem. **270:** 6141–6148.
20. HANN, C., D.L. EVANS, J. FERTALA, et al. 1998. Increased camptothecin toxicity in mammalian cells expressing Saccharomyces cerevisiae DNA topoisomerase I. J. Biol. Chem. **273:** 8425–8433.
21. BENEDETTI, P., Y. BENCHOKROUN, Y, P.J. HOUGHTON, et al. 1998. Analysis of camptothecin resistance in yeast: relevance to cancer. Drug Res. Updates **1:** 176–183.
22. KAUH, E.A. & M.-A. BJORNSTI. 1995. SCT1 mutants suppress the camptothecin sensitivity of yeast cells expressing wild-type DNA topoisomerase I. Proc. Natl. Acad. Sci. USA **92:** 6299–6303.
23. REDINBO, M.R., L. STEWART, P. KUHN, et al. 1998. Crystal structures of human topoisomerase I in covalent and noncovalent complexes with DNA. Science **279:** 1504–1513.

24. STEWART, L., M.R. REDINBO, X. QIU, et al. 1998. A model for the mechanism of human topoisomerase I. Science **279:** 1534–1541.
25. BENEDETTI, P., P. FIORANI, L. CAPUANI, et al. 1993. Camptothecin resistance from a single mutation changing glycine 363 of human DNA topoisomerase I to cysteine. Cancer Res. **53:** 4343–4348.
26. CARON, P. 1999. Compendium of DNA topoisomerase sequences. In DNA Topoisomerase Protocols: DNA Topology and Enzymes. M.A. Bjornsti & N. Osheroff, Eds.:279–316. Humana Press, Inc. Totowa, NJ.
27. KNAB, A.M., J. FERTALA & M.A. BJORNSTI. 1993. Mechanisms of camptothecin resistance in yeast DNA topoisomerase I mutants. J. Biol. Chem. **268:** 22322–22330.
28. MEGONIGAL, M.D., J. FERTALA & M.A. BJORNSTI. 1997. Cell cycle arrest and lethality produced by alterations in the catalytic activity of yeast DNA topoisomerase I mutants. J. Biol. Chem. **272:** 12801–12808.
29. HANN, C.L., A.L. CARLBERG & M.A. BJORNSTI. 1998. Intragenic suppressors of mutant DNA topoisomerase I-induced lethality diminish enzyme binding of DNA. J. Biol. Chem. **273:** 31519–31527.
30. PORTER, S.E. & J.J. CHAMPOUX. 1989. The basis for camptothecin enhancement of DNA breakage by eukaryotic topoisomerase I. Nucl. Acids Res. **17:** 8521–8532.
31. FIORANI, P., J.F. AMATRUDA, A. SILVESTRI, et al. 1999. Domain interactions affecting human DNA topoisomerase I catalysis and camptothecin sensitivity. Mol. Pharmacol. **56:** 1105–1115.
32. FUJIMORI, A., W.G. HARKER, G. KOHLHAGEN, et al. 1995. Mutation at the catalytic site of topoisomerase I in CEM/C2, a human leukemia cell line resistant to camptothecin. Cancer Res. **55:** 1339–1346.
33. FERTALA, J., J.R. VANCE, P. POURQUIER, et al. 2000. Substitutions of Asn-726 in the active site of yeast DNA topoisomerase I define novel mechanisms of stabilizing the covalent-enzyme DNA intermediate. J. Biol. Chem. In press.
34. MADDEN, K.R. & J.J. CHAMPOUX. 1992. Overexpression of human topoisomerase I in baby hamster kidney cells: hypersensitivity of clonal isolates to camptothecin. Cancer Res. **52:** 525–532.
35. REID, R.J.D., E.A. KAUH & M.A. BJORNSTI. 1997. Camptothecin sensitivity is mediated by the pleiotropic drug resistance network in yeast. J. Biol. Chem. **272:** 12091–12099.
36. REID, R.J.D., P. FIORANI, M. SUGAWARA, et al. 1999. CDC45 and DPB11 are required for processive DNA replication and resistance to DNA topoisomerase I-mediated DNA damage. Proc. Natl. Acad. Sci. USA **96:** 11440–11445.
37. BAUER, B.E., H. WOLFGER & K. KUCHLER. 1999. Inventory and function of yeast ABC proteins: about sex, stress, pleiotropic drug and heavy metal resistance. Biochem. Biophys. Acta **1461:** 217–236.
38. ZAMBONI, W.C., P.J. HOUGHTON, R.K. JOHNSON, et al. 1998. Probenecid alters topotecan systemic and renal disposition by inhibiting renal tubular secretion. J. Pharm. Exp. Ther. **284:** 89–94.
39. MALIEPAARD, M., M.A. VAN GASTELEN, L.A. DE JONG, et al. 1999. Overexpression of the BCRP/MXR/ABCP gene in a topotecan-selected ovarian tumor cell line. Cancer Res. **59:** 4559–4563.
40. ZOU, L., J. MITCHELL & B. STILLMAN. 1997. CDC45, a novel yeast gene that functions with the origin recognition complex and Mcm proteins in initiation of DNA replication. Mol. Cell. Biol. **17:** 553–563.
41. ZOU, L. & B. STILLMAN. 1998. Formation of a preinitiation complex by S-phase cyclin CDK-dependent loading of Cdc45p onto chromatin. Science **280:** 593–596.
42. ARAKI, H., S.H. LEEM, A. PHONGDARA, et al. 1995. Dpb11, which interacts with DNA polymerase II(e) in Saccharomyces cerevisiae, has a dual role in S-phase progression and at a cell cycle checkpoint. Proc. Natl. Acad. Sci. USA **92:** 11791–11795.

Camptothecins as Probes of the Microenvironments of Topoisomerase I – DNA Complexes

SIDNEY M. HECHT[a]

Departments of Chemistry and Biology, University of Virginia, Charlottesville, Virginia 22901, USA

ABSTRACT: By uncoupling the cleavage and ligation reactions of DNA oligonucleotides mediated by topoisomerase I, it has been possible to demonstrate modification of DNA oligonucleotide structure by the enzyme. These modifications indicate an unusual flexibility inherent in the behavior of topoisomerase I and may reflect some of the cellular roles played by the enzyme. The ability of individual camptothecin analogues to inhibit these modification processes differentially provides insight into the relative nature of the microenvironments present. To the extent that these enzyme-mediated structural modifications do constitute models of cellular roles for the enzyme, the observed differential inhibition also provides a potential strategy for assessing the function and importance of such modifications.

INTRODUCTION

While the function of DNA topoisomerase I in DNA relaxation has been the subject of detailed biochemical investigation and has helped to define the role of the enzyme in DNA replication and transcription, it now seems clear that the enzyme plays additional roles. These may include functions in DNA recombination,[1–14] nuclear segregation,[15] and regulation of gene expression.[16–19]

At a chemical level, the mechanism(s) by which topoisomerase I functions is less well understood, although significant progress has been made in recent years in defining both the structure and the function of the enzyme.[20–23] An important motivation for more precise definition of topoisomerase I structure and function derives from the identification of specific inhibitors of topoisomerase function,[24–35] some of which have been found to have utility as antitumor agents. Understanding the molecular mechanism(s) by which such agents exert these antitumor effects is an important goal, as it may facilitate a more detailed understanding of enzyme function and lead to anticancer agents with improved properties.

This report is concerned with the characterization of topoisomerase I behavior and function and the use of DNA topoisomerase I inhibitors as probes of enzyme function. Of particular importance is the finding that the enzyme exhibits uncommon flexibility in mediating DNA relaxation and structure modification, perhaps reflecting its several putative cellular functions.

---

[a]Voice: 804-924-3906; fax: 804-924-7856.
sidhecht@virginia.edu

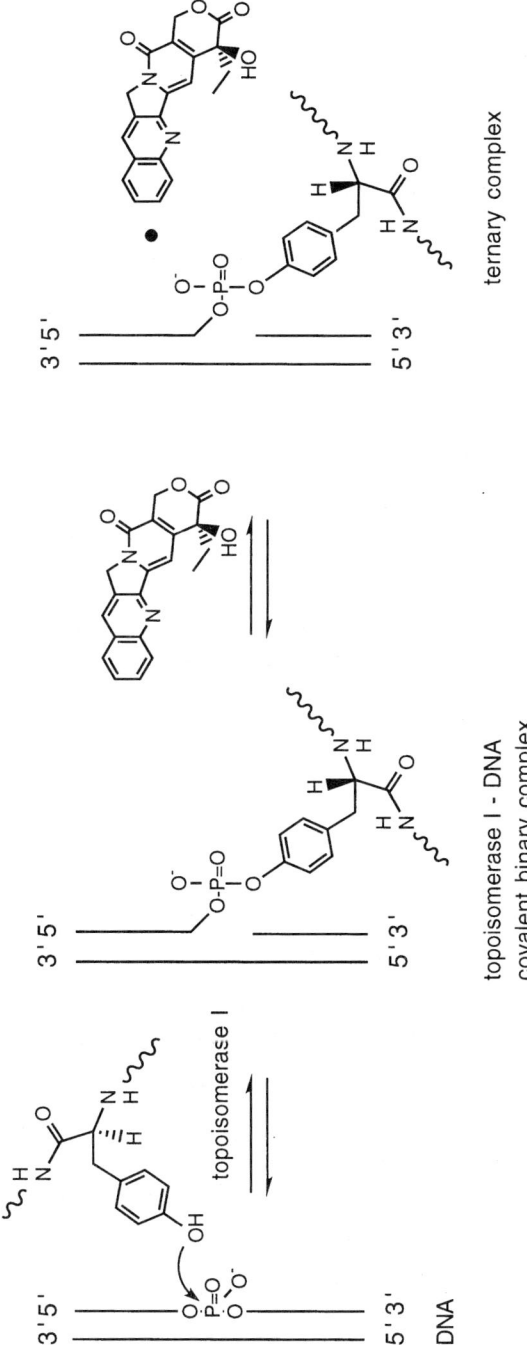

FIGURE 1. Equilibrium between free DNA and the topoisomerase I-DNA covalent binary complex (*left*) and between the covalent binary complex and a noncovalent ternary complex formed with the alkaloid camptothecin (CPT) (*right*).

DNA RELAXATION BY TOPOISOMERASE I

As shown in FIGURE 1, topoisomerase I-mediated DNA relaxation involves the nucleophilic attack of an active site tyrosine phenolic OH group on the phosphodiester backbone of one strand of DNA. This results in covalent attachment of the enzyme to its DNA substrate with concomitant breakage of the DNA backbone. The enzyme becomes attached to the DNA substrate through a 3'-phosphate ester, with concomitant release of a free DNA strand having a 5'-OH terminus.[36] Where the substrate DNA is supercoiled, relaxation can occur by passage of the free DNA strand around the unbroken one. Religation of the broken DNA strand then occurs with release of topoisomerase I by a process that can be regarded superficially as a reversal of the cleavage reaction. It may be noted, however, that at least for vaccinia topoisomerase I the rate-determining steps in the forward and reverse directions would seem to be different.[37]

DNA cleavage by topoisomerase I is facile and exhibits sequence selectivity characteristic of the specific enzyme. An important technical advance for the study of topoisomerase I was realized by Westergaard and coworkers[11,38,39] who found that the enzyme was capable of cleaving a partial DNA duplex. By utilizing a partial DNA duplex having only a few nucleotides downstream from the preferred cleavage site for the enzyme, it was possible to release a free DNA oligonucleotide whose affinity for the uncleaved strand based on H-bonding interactions was insufficient to maintain the duplex structure (FIG. 2). The enzyme–DNA covalent binary complex lacking the cleaved oligonucleotide (AGAGA in this example) retains its catalytic competence, as shown by its ability to utilize another acceptor oligonucleotide in the religation reaction (FIG. 2).

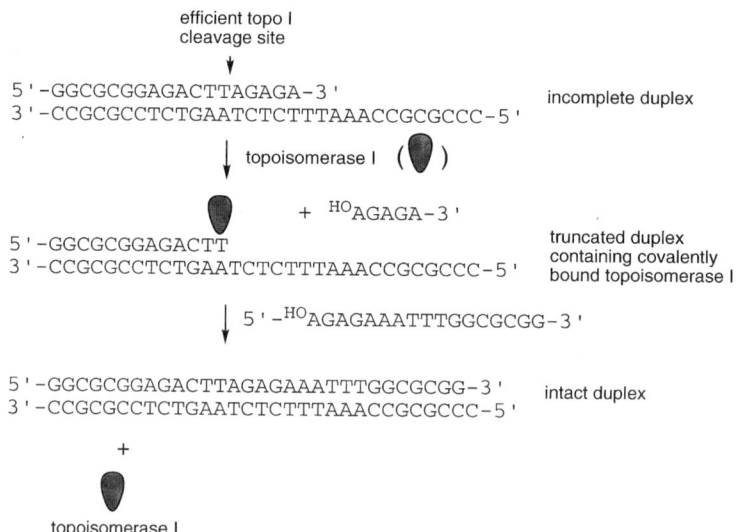

FIGURE 2. Uncoupling of the cleavage and ligation reactions mediated by topoisomerase I through the use of a partial DNA duplex substrate.

TABLE 1. Ligation yields obtained with modified acceptor oligonucleotides[a]

5'-Terminus of acceptor	pH	Ligation (%)
X = O	7.5	100
X = OCH$_2$	7.5	32.8
X = S	7.5	3.8
X = NH	7.5	2.6
	8.0	4.0
	8.5	8.4
	9.0	12.0

[a]Yields of full-length products resulting from ligation of the donor and acceptor oligonucleotides in FIGURE 3.

The uncoupling of the forward (cleavage) and reverse (religation) reactions mediated by topoisomerase I has provided some important opportunities for characterizing enzyme function. These include the actual chromatographic purification of the intermediate enzyme–DNA covalent binary complex[40]; because substrate cleavage ordinarily proceeds only in low yield, access to the purified intermediate greatly facilitated study of the religation reaction. Uncoupling of the forward and reverse reactions also permitted the use of structurally modified acceptors, which have allowed definition of the degree of flexibility exhibited by the enzyme.[12,38,41]

An interesting application is illustrated in FIGURE 3, which posits the ability of the covalent topoisomerase I-DNA binary complex to react with acceptor oligonucleotides having nucleophilic groups other than the usual OH group at their 5'-termini.[40] As shown in TABLE 1, the introduction of an additional methylene group at

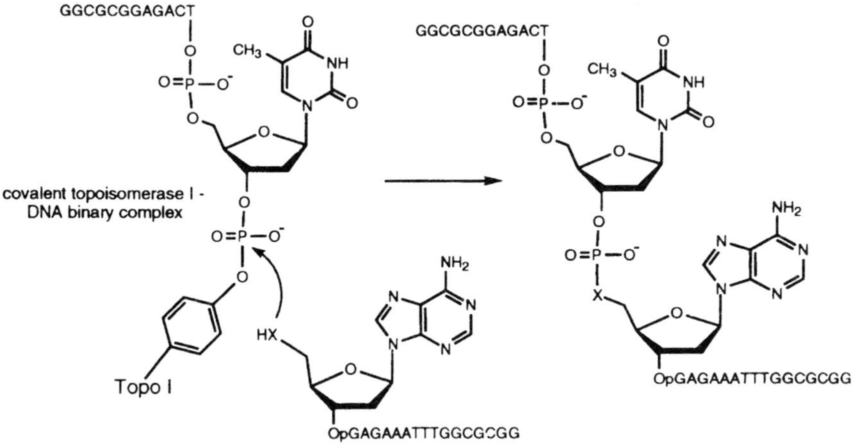

FIGURE 3. Reaction of the topoisomerase I-DNA covalent binary complex with acceptor oligonucleotides altered at their 5'-termini.

the 5′-terminus resulted in a threefold reduction in ligated product, whereas replacement of the OH group by SH or NH_2 functionalities further reduced, but did not eliminate, the ability of the enzyme to effect ligation of the donor and acceptor oligonucleotides. Interestingly, an increase in the pH of the system greatly potentiated the ability of the acceptor nucleotide having a 5′-NH_2 group to undergo ligation, presumably reflecting increased nucleophilicity at higher pH, in parallel with decreased protonation of this functional group. As anticipated, the other three acceptor oligonucleotides in the table exhibited no comparable pH dependence.

The surprising flexibility of the enzyme with regard to tolerance of alteration of substrate structure was also reflected in studies in which a 3′-deoxynucleotide was introduced at different sites in proximity to a high efficiency topoisomerase I cleavage site.[42,43]

TOPOISOMERASE I-MEDIATED REORGANIZATION OF DNA STRUCTURE

To develop a system to model the possible participation of topoisomerase I in nonhomologous or illegitimate recombination, a few modified DNA duplexes were explored as substrates for the enzyme.

As shown in FIGURE 4, cleavage of a partial DNA duplex produced two enzyme–DNA covalent binary complexes initially, one of which was at the anticipated high efficiency cleavage site and the other was two nucleotides upstream.[44] The inclusion of overlapping (branched) acceptor oligonucleotide substrates complementary to the single-stranded regions of the two enzyme–DNA binary complexes afforded the anticipated (cf FIG. 2) DNA duplex products. The 17-mer acceptor mediated religation with the complex formed at the high efficiency site, whereas the 19-mer acceptor afforded a duplex derived from the binary complex two nucleotides farther upstream. Of greater interest was the outcome of adding a complementary acceptor oligonucleotide 18 nucleotides in length. As shown in the figure, two new products were formed. DNA sequence analysis revealed that the shorter of the two products was a 1-nucleotide deletion product resulting from ligation of the 18-mer acceptor to the binary complex formed at site 2. The other was a 1-nucleotide addition product resulting from ligation at site 1. Conceptually, this finding is of great interest both because it demonstrates the ability of topoisomerase I to mediate the alteration of DNA structure and because it represents a clear example of the generation of diversity: one set of reactants afforded two products.

Shown in FIGURE 5 are two more examples of topoisomerase I-mediated rearrangement of DNA structure. In one, a nicked DNA substrate was found to undergo cleavage-ligation to afford a DNA duplex having a 3-nucleotide deletion on one strand. The other illustrates the formation of an 18-nucleotide deletion product, the formation of which seems remarkable even when one recognizes the potential for extrusion of a hairpin from the formed topoisomerase I-DNA covalent binary complex (FIG. 6). This transformation proceeded in 8% overall yield with the calf thymus enzyme,[44] but in yields up to 80% when human topoisomerase I was employed.[45]

Since the rearrangements shown in FIGURES 5 and 6 were intended to model the putative participation of DNA topoisomerase I in illegitimate recombination, a pro-

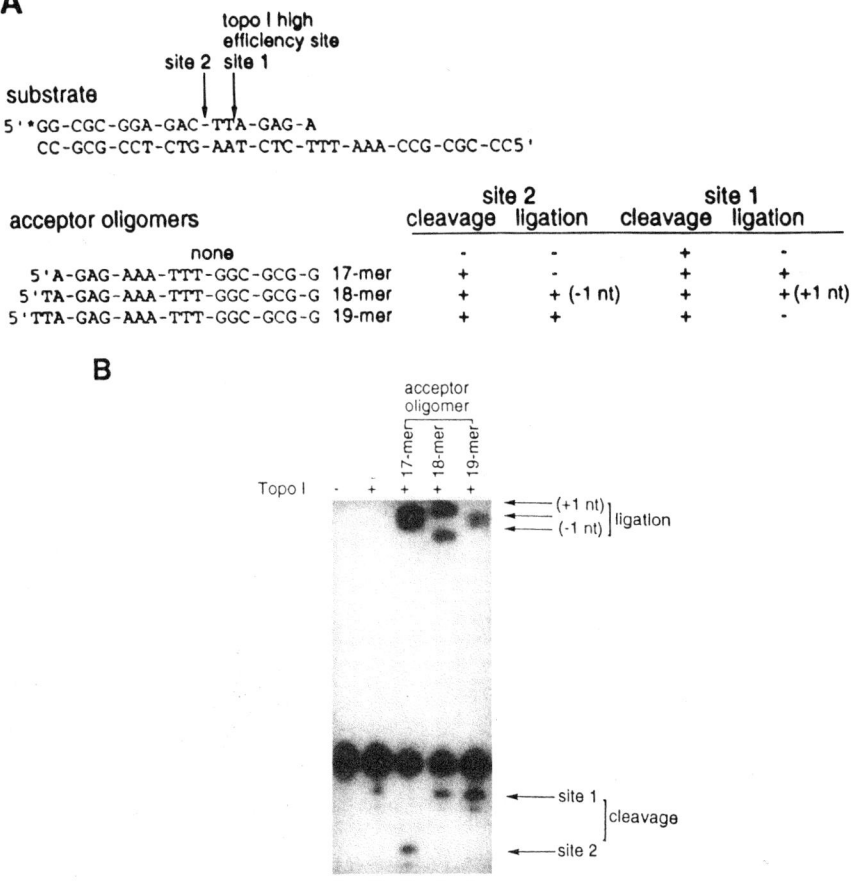

FIGURE 4. Topoisomerase I-mediated cleavage and ligation of a branched DNA substrate.

cess that has been linked to cancer and genetic diseases,[46–48] it seemed of interest to determine whether the topoisomerase I inhibitor camptothecin and its structural analogues would inhibit these rearrangements and especially whether inhibition would occur in a fashion different from that observed in the presence of normal DNA duplexes.

As shown in FIGURE 1, camptothecin (CPT) is an alkaloid that binds noncovalently to the covalent binary complex formed between topoisomerase I and DNA. While the equilibrium between free and covalently bound enzyme normally strongly favors free enzyme, in the presence of CPT or its analogues the equilibrium is rapidly shifted towards the ternary complex shown in the figure. The consequence of this shift for cells treated with CPT is eventual cell death, undoubtedly due to the

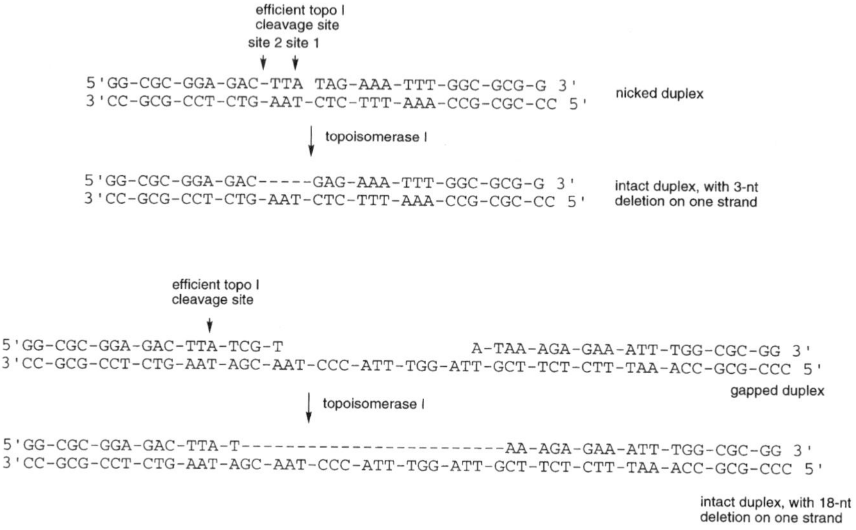

```
                    efficient topo I
                     cleavage site
                    site 2 site 1
                      ↓     ↓
       5'GG-CGC-GGA-GAC-TTA TAG-AAA-TTT-GGC-GCG-G 3'
       3'CC-GCG-CCT-CTG-AAT-CTC-TTT-AAA-CCG-CGC-CC 5'    nicked duplex

                    ↓ topoisomerase I

       5'GG-CGC-GGA-GAC-----GAG-AAA-TTT-GGC-GCG-G 3'    intact duplex, with 3-nt
       3'CC-GCG-CCT-CTG-AAT-CTC-TTT-AAA-CCG-CGC-CC 5'   deletion on one strand


              efficient topo I
               cleavage site
                    ↓
5'GG-CGC-GGA-GAC-TTA-TCG-T                   A-TAA-AGA-GAA-ATT-TGG-CGC-GG 3'
3'CC-GCG-CCT-CTG-AAT-AGC-AAT-CCC-ATT-TGG-ATT-GCT-TCT-CTT-TAA-ACC-GCG-CCC 5'
                                                                           gapped duplex
                    ↓ topoisomerase I

5'GG-CGC-GGA-GAC-TTA-T----------------------AA-AGA-GAA-ATT-TGG-CGC-GG 3'
3'CC-GCG-CCT-CTG-AAT-AGC-AAT-CCC-ATT-TGG-ATT-GCT-TCT-CTT-TAA-ACC-GCG-CCC 5'

                                                 intact duplex, with 18-nt
                                                 deletion on one strand
```

FIGURE 5. Two examples of topoisomerase I-mediated rearrangement of DNA structure.

TABLE 2. Inhibition of human topoisomerase I-mediated rearrangements of DNA substrate structures[a]

CPT analogue	Inhibition of rearrangements (%)			
	DNA duplex	Branched substrate	Nicked substrate	Gapped substrate
—	2 ± 1			
1	56 ± 2	64 ± 1	56 ± 1	7 ± 1
2	63 ± 3	76 ± 2	75 ± 1	29 ± 5
3	24 ± 5	56 ± 1	54 ± 1	2 ± 1
4	8 ± 1	42 ± 2	80 ± 1	24 ± 6
5	59 ± 5	83 ± 1	70 ± 3	25 ± 1
6	30 ± 1	42 ± 1	8 ± 1	< 1
7	60 ± 1	57 ± 2	44 ± 1	< 1
8	58 ± 7	71 ± 1	54 ± 6	6 ± 1
9	6 ± 1	31 ± 1	15 ± 2	< 1
10	56 ± 1	70 ± 2	43 ± 1	3 ± 1
11	68 ± 1	74 ± 1	62 ± 1	46 ± 3

[a]The DNA duplex had the sequence 5'-GGCGCGGAGACTTGGAGAAATTTGGCGCGG-3' on the scissile strand. The other substrates had the structures shown in FIGURES 5 and 6.

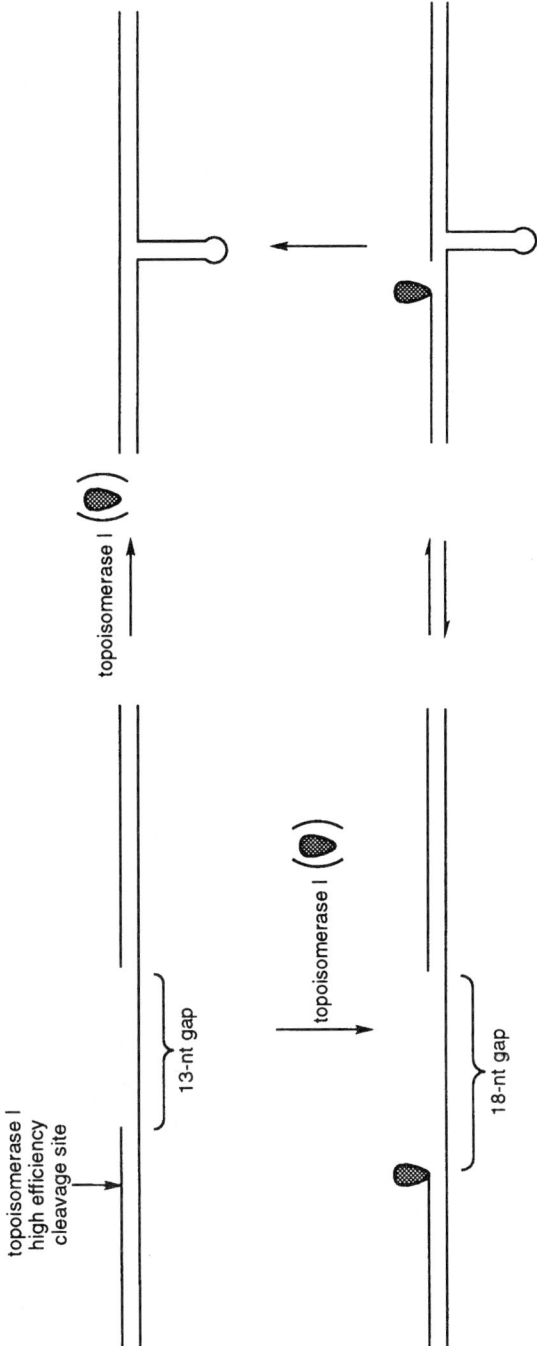

FIGURE 6. Putative mechanism of topoisomerase I-mediated ligation across a formed 18-nucleotide gap.

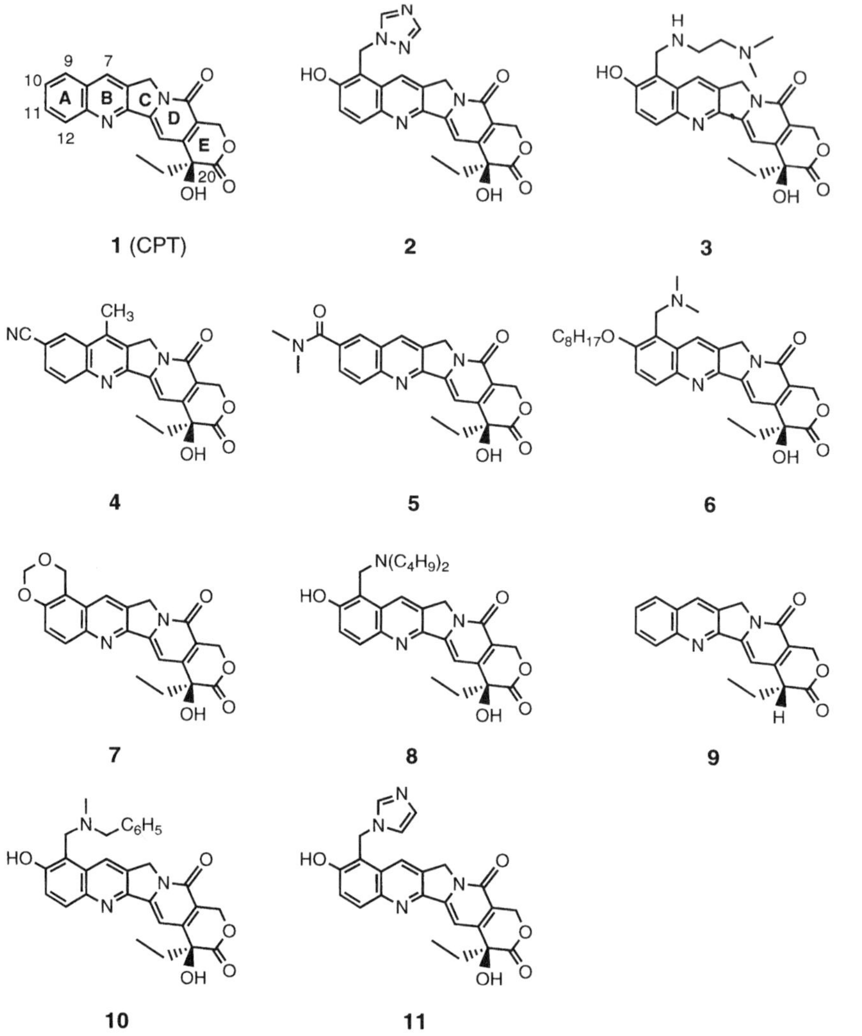

FIGURE 7. Eleven CPT congeners used to study selective inhibition of topoisomerase I-mediated DNA rearrangements.

inability of cells to deal adequately with the formed DNA lesion involving this essential enzyme.[49,50]

A set of CPT analogues (FIG. 7) was then employed to study the effect of these inhibitors on the rearrangements shown in FIGURES 5 and 6. As shown in FIGURE 8, these compounds exhibited a range of inhibitory effects when employed in the presence of the nicked DNA substrate shown in FIGURE 5. Quantification of the effects of 11 CPT analogues is shown in TABLE 2. As indicated in the table, individual CPT analogues could exhibit very different inhibitory potencies towards single topo-

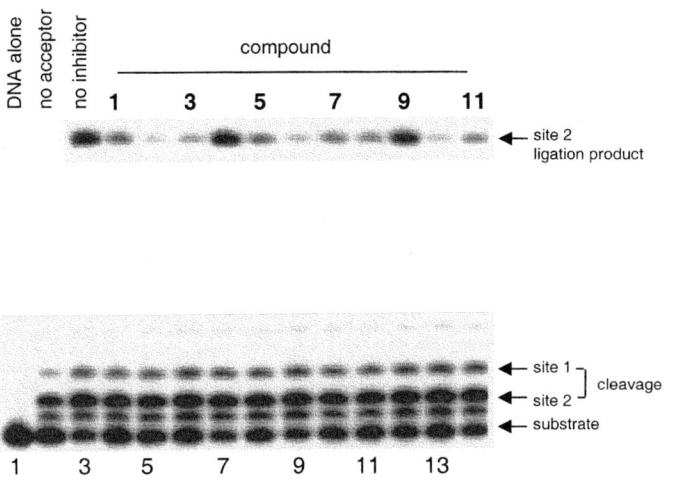

FIGURE 8. Effect of CPT analogues on the topoisomerase I-mediated ligation across a formed 3-nucleotide gap.

isomerase I-mediated rearrangements of DNA structure. A particularly interesting example was 20-deoxycamptothein (**9**) which has minimal activity as an inhibitor of enzyme function in the presence of normal DNA duplexes, but exhibited much more significant inhibition of rearrangement of the branched substrate studied.[51,52]

These findings indicate that it should be possible to identify small molecules that inhibit a given topoisomerase I-mediated transformation. Assuming that topoisomerase I actually does participate in multiple cellular process, this implies that individual functions should be amenable to selective inhibition. From the perspective of topoisomerase I function, the findings in TABLE 2 also constitute strong evidence that the microenvironments of individual types of topoisomerase I-DNA covalent binary complexes are unique and distinguishable chemically. It is interesting that differential effects for a given DNA substrate could also be demonstrated for the calf thymus versis human enzymes,[52] again implying substantial uniqueness of individual enzyme–DNA binary complex structures.

MODELS OF THE TOPOISOMERASE I-DNA COVALENT BINARY COMPLEX

Recently, two laboratories have proposed structures that describe the molecular nature of the ternary complex formed between topoisomerase I, DNA, and camptothecin. One of these, shown in part in FIGURE 9A, is based on extrapolation of X-ray crystallographic data obtained for reconstituted and truncated human topoisomerases I which were determined in covalent and noncovalent complexes with a DNA substrate.[53,54] The part of that model illustrated in FIGURE 9A emphasizes the proposed interactions of the enzyme with the E-ring of CPT. These include H-bonding

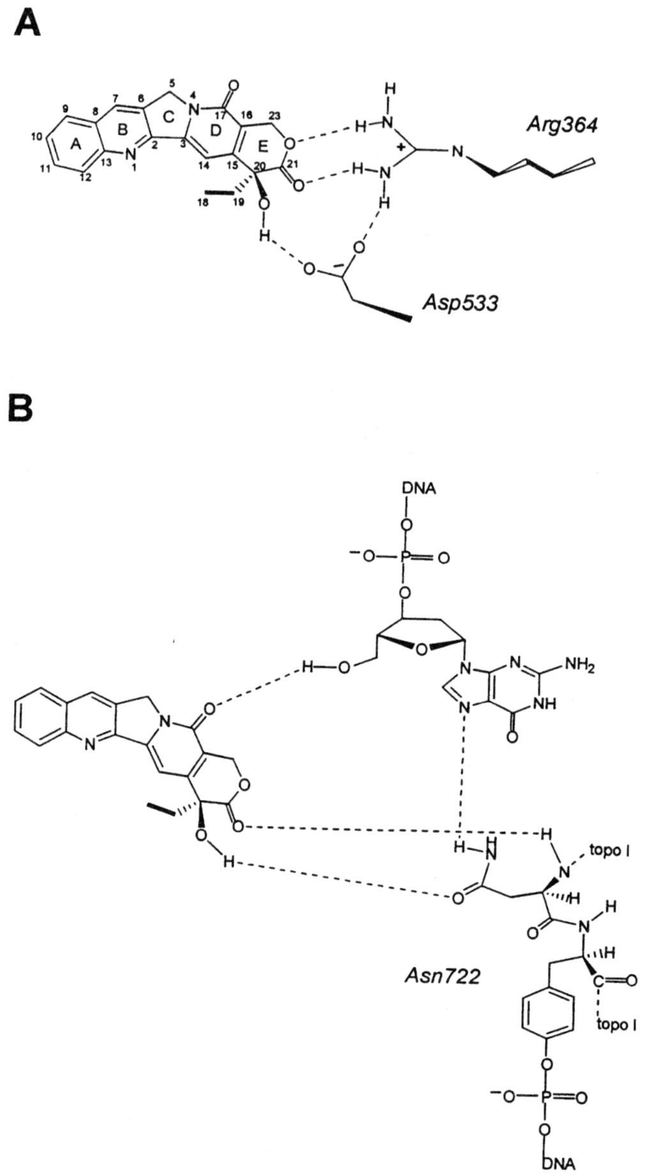

A

B

FIGURE 9. Models of CPT binding to the topoisomerase I-DNA covalent binary complex.

interactions with Arg364 and Asp533 of topoisomerase I. It may be noted that the latter of these is proposed to interact with the 20-OH group of CPT.

A second model of the topoisomerase I–DNA–CPT ternary complex has been proposed by Fan et al.[55] based on computational studies. This model involves pro-

TABLE 3. Participation of CPT analogues in topoisomerase I-DNA-CPT ternary complexes[a]

	Duplex DNA cleavage (%)		
CPT analogue	50 μM CPT	20 μM CPT	Dissociation rate constant k ($\times 10^{-3}$ s^{-1})
CPT	82	78	23.4
20-ChloroCPT	26	29	18.2
20-BromoCPT	33	24	20.0
20-AminoCPT	34	21	> 139

[a]The DNA duplex employed has the same sequence as that described in TABLE 2. Off-rate studies were carried out in the presence of 50 μM CPT analogues.

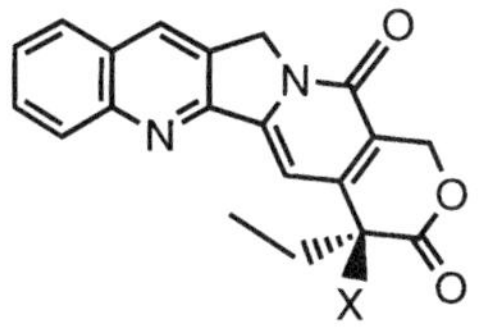

X = OH camptothecin (CPT)
X = Cl 20-chloroCPT
X = Br 20-bromoCPT
X = NH$_2$ 20-aminoCPT

FIGURE 10. CPT analogues modified at the 20-position, used to study the mechanistic role of the 20-OH group in CPT.

posed pseudointercalation of CPT at the topoisomerase I-linked DNA cleavage site and is consistent with numerous pertinent experimental observations, notably the rank order potencies of a number of CPT analogues and the fact that replacement of Asp722 in topoisomerase I with Ser afforded a mutant enzyme resistant to CPT. As shown in FIGURE 9B, Asn722 is proposed to participate as an H-bond acceptor from the 20-OH group of CPT.

To test the involvement of the 20-OH group of CPT as a key structural parameter in the enzyme–DNA–CPT ternary complex, several analogues of CPT were prepared in which the 20-OH substituent was modified. As shown in FIGURE 10, this included the 20-chloro and bromo derivatives of camptothecin as well as 20-aminoCPT, all of which were prepared by known methods.[56] It may be noted that the modified derivatives are all mixtures of isomers at position 20, which is known to affect their activity as topoisomerase I inhibitors; specifically (20R)-CPT has been reported[57] not to inhibit topoisomerase I function.

As shown in TABLE 3, all three of the CPT analogues were capable of stabilizing the covalent binary complex formed from a DNA duplex having a single, preferred topoisomerae I cleavage site. None was as potent as CPT itself, but the potencies of inhibition were good, especially considering the presence of the 20R isomers in each of the analogues. Significantly, the 20-amino analogue of CPT was no more potent than the 20-haloCPT derivatives in this assay, implying that the ability of 20-aminoCPT to act as an H-bond donor did not enhance its potency of stabilization of the covalent binary complex.

Also shown in TABLE 3 are the off-rates of the individual analogues from the ternary complex following treatment with NaCl. Interestingly, both 20-chloroCPT and 20-bromoCPT had off-rates from the enzyme–DNA–inhibitor ternary complex very close to that of CPT itself, implying a similarity of function, and also produced a pattern of DNA cleavage sites very similar to that of CPT when added to an incubation mixture containing the enzyme and a DNA restriction fragment having several topoisomerase I cleavage sites. In contrast, 20-aminoCPT had an off-rate from the ternary complex too fast to be measured. Thus, the presence of a 20-OH group does not seem to be required for the formation of topoisomerase I–DNA–inhibitor complexes of the type formed by CPT itself. Finally, it may be noted that 20-chloroCPT and 20-bromoCPT inhibited the growth of a yeast strain that lacked the homologous topoisomerase I, but that harbored a plasmid from which the human enzyme was expressed. Although both of the halo derivatives were less potent than CPT itself (IC_{50} values of 2.1 and 6.7 μM for 20-chloroCPT and 20-bromoCPT, respectively, versus 0.2 μM for CPT), both of the halo derivatives were substantially more cytotoxic than 20-amino CPT (IC_{50} 47 μM).[56]

These findings argue that the 20-OH group of CPT is not essential for formation of a ternary complex with topoisomerase I and DNA, and they diminish the likelihood that the 20-OH group participates as an H-bond donor in the formed ternary complex.

CONCLUSION

The use of camptothecin analogues as probes of topoisomerase I function has permitted structural distinctions to be made between the enzyme-DNA covalent binary complexes leading to DNA products having altered structures. They have also permitted an evaluation of the participation of the 20-OH of CPT as an H-bond donor to topoisomerase I residues within the enzyme–DNA–CPT ternary complex.

REFERENCES

1. BEEN, M.D. & J.J. CHAMPOUX. 1981. DNA breakage and closure by rat liver type 1 topoisomerase: separation of the half-reactions by using a single-stranded DNA substrate. Proc. Natl. Acad. Sci. USA **78:** 2883–2887.
2. HALLIGAN, B.D., J.L. DAVIS, K.A. EDWARDS & L.F. LIU. 1982. Intra- and intermolecular strands transfer by HeLa DNA topoisomerase I. J. Biol. Chem. **257:** 3995–4000.
3. BULLOCK, P., W. FORRESTER & M. BOTCHAN. 1984. DNA sequence studies of simian virus 40 chromosomal excision and integration in rat cells. J. Mol. Biol. **174:** 55–84.
4. BULLOCK, P., J.J. CHAMPOUX & M. BOTCHAN. 1985. Association of crossover points with topoisomerase I cleavage sites: a model for nonhomologous recombination. Science. **230:** 954–958.
5. MCCOUBREY, W.K. & J.J. CHAMPOUX. 1986. The role of single-strand breaks in the catenation reaction catalyzed by the rat type I topoisomerase. J. Biol. Chem. **261:** 5130–5137.

6. CHAMPOUX, J.J. & P.A. BULLOCK. 1988. Possible role for the eucaryotic type I topoisomerase with DNA. *In* Illegitimate Recombination in Genetic Recombination. R. Kucherlapati & K.R. Smith, Eds.: 655–666. American Society for Microbiology. Washington, DC.
7. LANDY, A. 1989. Dynamic, structural, and regulatory aspects of lambda site-specific recombination. Annu. Rev. Biochem. **58**: 913–949.
8. LIU, L.F. 1989. DNA topoisomerase poisons as antitumor drugs. Annu. Rev. Biochem. **58**: 351–375.
9. IKEDA, H. 1990. *In* DNA Topology and Its Biological Effects. N.R. Cozzarelli & J.C. Wang, Eds.: 341–359. Cold Spring Harbor Laboratory Press. Cold Spring Harbor, NY.
10. SHUMAN, S. 1991. Recombination mediated by vaccinia virus DNA topoisomerase I in *Escherichia coli* is sequence specific. Proc. Natl. Acad. Sci. USA **88**: 10104–10108.
11. SVEJSTRUP, J.Q., K. CHRISTIANSEN, I.I. GROMOVA, *et al.* 1991. New technique for uncoupling the cleavage and religation reactions of eukaryotic topoisomerase I. The mode of action of camptothecin at a specific recognition site. J. Mol. Biol. **222**: 669–678.
12. SHUMAN, S. 1992. DNA strand transfer reactions catalyzed by vaccinia topoisomerase I. J. Biol. Chem. **267**: 8620–8627.
13. DEGRASSI, F., R. DESALVIA & L. BERGHELLA. 1993. The production of chromosomal alteration by beta-lapachone, an activator of topoisomerase I. Mutat. Res. **288**: 263–267.
14. SEKIGUCHI, J., N.C. SEEMAN & S. SHUMAN. 1996. Resolution of Holliday junctions by eukaryotic DNA topoisomerase I. Proc. Natl. Acad. Sci. USA **93**: 785–789.
15. CASTANO, I.B., S. HEATH-PAGLIUSO, B.U. SADOFF, *et al.* 1996. A novel family of TRF (DNA topoisomerase I-related function) genes required for proper nuclear segregation. Nucleic Acids Res. **24**: 2404–2410.
16. ROSSI, F., E. LABOURIER, T. FORNÉ *et al.* 1996. Specific phosphorylation of SR proteins by mammalian DNA topoisomerase I. Nature **381**: 80–82.
17. TAZI, J., F. ROSSI, E. LABOURIER, *et al.* 1997. DNA topoisomerase I: Customs officer at the border between DNA and RNA worlds? J. Mol. Med. **75**: 786–800.
18. LABOURIER, E., F. ROSSI, I. GALLOUZI, *et al.* 1998. Interaction between the N-terminal domain of human DNA topoisomerase I and the arginine-serine domain of its substrate determines phosphorylation of SF2/ASF splicing factor. Nucleic Acids Res. **26**:2955–2962.
19. ROSSI, F., E. LABOURIER, I. GALLOUZI, *et al.* 1998. The C-terminal domain but not the tyrosine 723 of human DNA topoisomerase I active site contributes to kinase activity. Nucleic Acids. Res. **26**: 2963–2970.
20. WANG, J.C. 1987. DNA topoisomerases: nature∠s solution to the topological ramifications of the double-helix structure of DNA. Harvey Lect. **81**: 93–110.
21. OSHEROFF, N. 1989. Biochemical basis for the interactions of type I and type II topoisomerases with DNA. Pharmacol. Ther. **41**: 223–241.
22. CHEN, A.Y. & L.F. LIU. 1994. DNA topoisomerases: Essential enzymes and lethal targets. Annu. Rev. Pharmacol. Toxicol. **34**: 191–218.
23. GUPTA, M., A. FUJIMORE & Y. POMMIER. 1995. Eukaryotic DNA topoisomerases I. Biochim. Biophys. Acta **1262**: 1–4.
24. HSIANG, Y.-H., R. HERTZBERG, S.M. HECHT & L.F. LIU. 1985. Camptothecin induces protein-linked DNA breaks via mammalian DNA topoisomerase I. J. Biol. Chem. **260**: 14873–14878.
25. THOMSEN, B., S. MOLLERUP, B.J. BONVEN, *et al.* 1987. Sequence specificity of DNA topoisomerase I in the presence and absence of camptothecin. EMBO J. **6**: 1817–1823.
26. ANDOH, T., K. ISHII, Y. SUZUKI, *et al.* 1987. Characterization of a mammalian mutant with a camptothecin-resistant DNA topoisomerase I. Proc. Natl. Acad. Sci. USA **84**: 5565–5569.
27. HSIANG, Y.-H. & L.F. LIU. 1988. Identification of mammalian DNA topoisomerase I as an intracellular target. Cancer Res. **48**: 1722–1726.
28. GUPTA, R.S., R. GUPTA, B. ENG, *et al.* 1988. Camptothecin-resistant mutants of Chinese hamster ovary cells containing a resistant form of topoisomerase I. Cancer Res. **48**: 6404–6410.

29. KJELDSEN, E., B. BONVEN, T. ANDOH, et al. 1988. Characterization of a camptothecin-resistant human DNA topoisomerase I. J. Biol. Chem. **263:** 3912–3916.
30. MATSUZAKI, T., T. YOKOKURA, M. MUTAI & T. TSUROU. 1988. Inhibition of spontaneous and experimental metastasis by a new derivative of camptothecin, CPT-11, in mice. Cancer Chemother. Pharmacol. **21:** 308–312.
31. HERTZBERG, R.P., M.J. CARANFA & S.M. HECHT. 1989. On the mechanism of topoisomerase I inhibition by camptothecin: evidence for binding to an enzyme-DNA complex. Biochemistry **28:** 4629–4638.
32. HERTZBERG, R.P., M.J. CARANFA, K.G. HOLDEN, et al. 1989. Modification of the hydroxy lactone ring of camptothecin: inhibition of mammalian topoisomerase I and biological activity. J. Med. Chem. **32:** 715–720.
33. JAXEL, C., K.W. KOHN, M.C. WANI, et al. 1989. Structure-activity study of the actions of camptothecin-derivatives on mammalian topoisomerase I. Evidence for a specific receptor-site and a relation to antitumor activity. Cancer Res. **49:** 1465–1469.
34. HSIANG, Y.H., L.F. LIU, M.E. WALL, et al. 1989. DNA topoisomerase I-mediated DNA cleavage and cytotoxicity of camptothecin analogues. Cancer Res. **49:** 4385–4389.
35. KINGSBURY, W.D., J.C. BOEHM, D.R. JAKAS, et al. 1991. Synthesis of water-soluble (aminoalkyl)camptothecin analogues: Inhibition of topoisomerase I antitumor activity. J. Med. Chem. **34:** 98–107.
36. CHAMPOUX, J.J. 1981. DNA is linked to the rat liver DNA nicking-closing enzyme by a phosphodiester bond to tyrosine. J. Biol. Chem. **256:** 4805–4809.
37. STIVERS, J.T., S. SHUMAN & A.S. MILDVAN. 1994. Vaccinia DNA topoisomerase I: kinetic evidence for general acid-base catalysis and a conformational step. Biochemistry **33:** 15449–15458.
38. CHRISTIANSEN, K. & O. WESTERGAARD. 1992. Involvement of eukaryotic topoisomerase I in illegitimate recombination: generation of deletions and insertions. In DNA Repair Mechanisms, Alfred Benzon Symposium 35. V.A. Bohr, K. Wassermann & K.H. Kraemer, Eds.: 361–371. Munksgaard. Copenhagen.
39. CHRISTIANSEN, K., A.B.D. SVEJSTRUP, A.H. ANDERSON & O. WESTERGAARD. 1993. Eukaryotic topoisomerase I-mediated cleavage requires bipartite DNA interaction. Cleavage DNA substrates containing strand interruptions implicates a role for topoisomerase I in illegitimate recombination. J. Biol. Chem. **268:** 9690–9701.
40. HENNINGFELD, K.A., T. ARSLAN & S.M. HECHT. 1996. Alteration of DNA primary structure by DNA topoisomerase I. Isolation of the covalent topoisomerase I-DNA binary complex in enzymatically competent form. J. Am. Chem. Soc. **118:** 11701–11714.
41. CHRISTIANSEN, K., B.R. KNUDSEN & O. WESTERGAARD. 1994. The covalent eukaryotic topoisomerase I–DNA intermediate catalyzes pH-dependent hydrolysis and alcoholysis. J. Biol. Chem. **269:** 11367–11373.
42. ARSLAN, T., A.T. ABRAHAM & S.M. HECHT. 1998. Structurally altered substrates for DNA topoisomerase I. Effects of inclusion of a single 3'-deoxynucleotide within the scissile strand. Nucleosides & Nucleotides **17:** 515–530.
43. ARSLAN, T., A.T. ABRAHAM & S.M. HECHT. 1998. DNA duplexes containing 3'-deoxynucleotides as substrates for DNA topoisomerase I cleavage and ligation. J. Biol. Chem. **273:** 12383–12390.
44. HENNINGFELD, K.A. & S.M. HECHT. 1995. Topoisomerase I-mediated illegitimate recombination with duplex DNA substrates containing branches, nicks and gaps. Biochemistry **34:** 6120–6129.
45. WANG, X. 1999. Analysis of topoisomerase I-mediated reorganization of DNA structure. Ph.D. thesis, University of Virginia, Charlottesville, Virginia.
46. SCHIMKE, R. T., S. W. SHERWOOD, A. B. HILL & R. N. JOHNSTON. 1986. Overreplication and recombination of DNA in higher eukaryotes: Potential consequences and biological implications. Proc. Natl. Acad. Sci. U.S.A. **83:** 2157–2161.
47. MEUTH, M. 1989. In Mobile DNA. D. E. BERG & M. M. HOWE, Eds.: 833 ff. American Society for Microbiology. Washington, DC.
48. SOLOMON, E., J. BORROW & A. D. GODDARD. 1991. Chromosome aberrations and cancer. Science. **254:** 1153–1160.

49. LIU, L. F. 1990. Anticancer drugs that convert DNA topoisomerases into DNA damaging agents. *In* DNA Topology and Its Biological Effects. Cold Spring Harbor Laboratory: 371–389. Cold Spring Harbor, NY.
50. HSIANG, Y., M.G. LIHOUR & L.F. LIU. 1989. Arrest of replication forks by drug-stabilized topoisomerase I-DNA cleavable complexes as a mechanism of cell killing by camptothecin. Cancer Res. **49:** 5077–5082.
51. WANG, X., L.-K. WANG, W.D. KINGSBURY, *et al.* 1998. Differential effects of camptothecin derivatives on topoisomerase I-mediated DNA structure modification. Biochemistry **37:** 9399–9408.
52. WANG, X., G.F. SHORT, III, W.D. KINGSBURY, *et al.* 1998. Effects of camptothecin analogues on DNA transformations mediated by calf thymus and human DNA topoisomerases I. Chem. Res. Toxicol. **11:** 1352–1360.
53. REDINBO, M.R., L. STEWART, P. KUHN, *et al.* 1998. Crystal structures of human topoisomerase I in covalent and noncovalent complexes with DNA. Science **279:** 1504–1513.
54. STEWART, L., M.R. REDINBO, X. QIU, *et al.* 1998. A model for the mechanism of human topoisomerase I. Science **279:** 1534–1541.
55. FAN, Y., J.N. WEINSTEIN, K.W. KOHN, *et al.* 1998. Molecular modeling studies of the DNA-topoisomerase I ternary cleavable complex with camptothecin. J. Med. Chem. **41:** 2216–2226.
56. WANG, X., X. ZHOU & S.M. HECHT. 1999. Role of the 20-hydroxyl group in camptothecin binding by the topoisomerase I-DNA binary complex. Biochemistry **38:** 4374–4381.
57. JAXEL, C., K.W. KOHN, M.C. WANI, *et al.* 1989. Structure-activity study of the actions of camptothecin derivatives on mammalian topoisomerase I: evidence for a specific receptor site and a relation to antitumor activity. Cancer Res. **49:** 1465–1469.

Preclinical and Clinical Trials of Topoisomerase Inhibitors

NAGAHIRO SAIJO[a]

National Cancer Center Hospital, Tsukiji 5-1-1, Chuo-ku, Tokyo 104-0045, Japan

ABSTRACT: CPT-11, developed by Yakult Honsha, has achieved the position of standard chemotherapy for colorectal cancer in the United States and in Western countries because CPT-11+5FU+LV showed survival benefit compared with 5FU-LV in two randomized controlled trials. CPT-11 has been distributed to almost all countries. In Japan, combination therapy of CDDP+CPT-11 was significantly superior to CDDP-VP-16 in the treatment of extensive disease small cell lung cancer. This combination is also active against non-small cell lung cancer. Daiich Pharmaceutical Co. developed a more active nonmasked form of camptothecin derivative, DX-8915f. The phase I study of a new camptothecin inhibitor, DX-8915f, has just been completed. The new topoisomerase I inhibitors of indolocarbazol derivatives, NB-506 and J107088, developed by Banyu Co., have strong antitumor activity and a wide therapeutic ratio. The phase I trial of J107088 is currently ongoing in the United States and Japan. These do not show any cross-resistance to MDR drugs.

INTRODUCTION

DNA topoisomerase I has been demonstrated to be involved in various genetic processes such as DNA replication, transcription, and recombination.[1] Camptothecin (CPT) isolated from the Chinese tree *Camptotheca acuminata* in 1966 has a novel structure and mechanism of action.[2] The clinical development of CPT was discontinued because of its intolerable adverse effects, although it showed a broad antitumor spectrum.[3]

CPT-11 substituted with ethyl and carbonyloxy piperidinopiperidine into CPT was semisynthesized to increase its solubility and to decrease the toxicity.[4] Based on data of the phase II study, CPT-11 was approved against non-small cell lung cancer, small cell lung cancer, and uterine cervical cancer in 1994 in Japan.[5] It is distributed to almost all countries based on the results of randomized and nonrandomized clinical trials.

A new camptothecin derivative, DX-8951f, was developed by the Daiichi Pharmaceutical Co. In addition, topoisomerase I inhibitors with the structural formula of indolocarbazole have been introduced in Japan. Recent progress in preclinical and clinical studies of topoisomerase inhibitors are reviewed.

[a]Voice: 03-3542-2511(2320); fax: 03-3542-6520.
nsaijo@gan2.res.ncc.go.jp

CPT-11 IN THE TREATMENT OF COLORETAL CANCER

First-line chemotherapy for patients with advanced coloretal cancer has been a 5-FU–containing regimen combined with folinic acid (LV). The response rate of this regimen is only about 25% if it is given as first-line chemotherapy. The initial responders become refractory to 5-FU + LV after a couple of courses of the same chemotherapy. The prognosis of patients with refractory colon cancer is extremely poor. It is believed that the best supportive care is standard treatment for 5-FU–refractory patients. In the United States, CPT-11 was given as a 90-minute infusion of 125 mg/m^2 weekly for 4 weeks followed by 2 weeks of rest. The overall response rate among the 304 patients was 12.8%. Stable disease was experienced in 148 patients (49%). Overall, the onset of response was rapid, and the duration of response was 6 months (ranging from 2.6–15.1 months) and median survival was 9 months (0.3–36 months).

Based on these data, investigators from 11 European countries designed a prospective, multicenter, randomized trial comparing CPT-11 with the best supportive care in advanced colorectal cancer with prior 5-FU–based therapy.[6] A 2:1 randomization schedule was used in favor of CPT-11. Patients were not stratified before randomization. An imbalance was noted between the two study groups with regard to performance status. This imbalance favored the CPT-11 arm.

A significant difference in overall survival was noted in favor of CPT-11. As adverse events, neutropenia (22%) and diarrhea (22%) were more common in the CPT-11 arm, and asthenia was more frequent in the best supportive care arm. QOL analyses favored the CPT-11 arm. From this evidence, it can be concluded that CPT-11 significantly prolongs survival, improves QOL, and controls tumor-related symptoms and that best supportive care is no longer considered acceptable in patients with 5-FU refractory colorectal cancer.

Cutsem *et al.*[7] reported the results of another randomized, controlled, pan European trial. Patients were randomized to either CPT-11 ($n = 127$) or what the investigators considered to be best care, such as a high dose infusional 5-FU–based regimen ($n = 129$). All patients had documented disease progression while on 5-FU or within 3 months of the last 5-FU infusion. At 12 months, 45% of patients in the CPT-11 arm were alive compared to only 32% of patients in the 5-FU arm. The median progression-free survival time with CPT-11 was 4.2 months compared to 2.9 months for infusional 5-FU. QOL also favored the CPT-11 arm. Patients receiving CPT-11 experienced a greater incidence of grade III or IV neutropenia, vomiting, and diarrhea, whereas those treated with 5-FU were more likely to experience grade III/IV mucositis, rash, and non-neutropenic fever. In both groups the quality of life was well maintained despite frequent side effects.

These two randomized controlled trials have clearly established a strong role for CPT-11 in second-line therapy.

These data strongly suggest that CPT-11 could be used as first-line therapy against advanced colorectal cancer. The combination of CPT-11 and 5-FU/folinic acid is also of great interest. Randomized controlled trials were scheduled to evaluate the efficacy of CPT-11 as first-line chemotherapy against advanced colorectal cancer. The study was a prospective, open-label, phase III trial to evaluate the efficacy of CPT-11/5-FU/LV when compared with 5-FU/LV alone. There were two study arms. In the first trial, weekly CPT-11/5-FU and daily × 5-FU/LV (Mayo regimen) were compared.[8] A CPT-11 only arm was included in order to assess the activity and reliability of CPT-11 in a multicenter trial. The primary endpoint was progression-free survival. Secondary endpoints were time to treatment failure, response rate, overall survival, safety, and QOL. A total of 683 patients were randomized and more than 200 patients in each arm received the scheduled chemotherapy. The compliance of chemotherapy was approximately 80%. Progression-free survival was significantly greater in the CPT-11/5-FU/LV arm, with CPT-11 alone showing nearly the same result as did 5-FU/LV. Time to treatment failure was better in CPT-11/5-FU/LV (5.0 months) than with LV/FU (3.8 months) and CPT-11 alone (3.1 months). Response rate was better in CPT-11/5-FU/LV (33%) than in 5-FU/LV (18%). Overall survival at 12 months was not statistically different between the two main arms of this trial. There was a trend towards increased survival at 18 months with CPT-11/5-FU/LV. Grade 3/4 diarrhea was associated with a CPT-11–containing regimen more frequently than with 5-FU/LV. On the other hand, the incidence of grade 4 neutropenia, neutropenic fever, and mucositis was statisticallly significantly higher in the 5-FU/LV arm. It was concluded that a weekly CPT-11/5-FU/LV regimen could be a new standard regimen in first-line therapy of patients with metastatic colon cancer.

Another multinational trial chaired by Douillard et al.[9] compared an infusional 5-FU/LV regimen with a regimen containing 5-FU/LV plus CPT-11.[9] Only chemotherapy-naive patients were included; however, adjuvant chemotherapy was allowed if it had ended at least 6 months before randomization. A total of 187 patients were randomized to FU/LV alone and 198 patients to 5-FU/LV + CPT-11. Most patients received a biweekly schedule. The control arm schedule included a loading dose of LV 200 mg/m^2 followed by a bolus of 5-FU 400 mg/m^2. This was repeated on days 1 and 2 every 2 weeks. The investigational arm was administered exactly the same 5-FU/LV regimen; in addition, CPT-11 180 mg/m^2 was given 1 day before 5-FU/LV. The response rate was highly statistically significantly better in the CPT-11 arm with seven complete responders. The median duration of response, period of disease stabilization, median time to disease progression, and overall survival favored combined chemotherapy. QOL score and performance status were maintained in good condition in the CPT-11 arm. The addition of CPT-11 to 5-FU/LV was associated with more hematologic toxicity including one treatment-related death. More non-hematologic toxicities such as diarrhea, asthenia, and alopecia were also experienced in the combined chemotherapy group; however, these toxicities were easily managed and not cumulative.

Accordingly, two randomized controlled trials demonstrated that combined CPT-11 and 5-FU/LV was better than 5-FU/LV alone with regard to survival, time to progression, response rate, and QOL. This regimen will be used as a reference arm for a clinical trial in advanced colorectal cancer.

CPT-11 IN THE TREATMENT OF NON-SMALL CELL LUNG CANCER

A multi-institutional phase II study conducted against 69 stage IIIB and IV non-small cell lung cancer demonstrated a high response rate (48%) and median survival of 44 weeks with tolerable toxicity.[10]

Yakult Honsha Co., Ltd and Daiich Pharmaceutical Co., Ltd. organized two study groups against advanced non-small cell lung cancer. West and East Japan groups have conducted three- and two-armed prospective randomized controlled trials, respectively.

Trial of the CPT-11 Lung Cancer Study Group West[11]

Eligibility criteria of the trial are age 18–75, stage IIIB and IV tumor with no symptomatic brain metastases, ECOG PS 0-2, and no prior chemotherapy. From July 1995 to January 1998, 398 patients were randomly assigned to receive arm A (CDDP 80 mg/m^2 on day 1 and CPT-11 60 mg/m^2 on days 1, 8, and 15), arm B (CDDP 80 mg/m^2 on day 1 and VDS 3 mg/m^2 on days 1, 8, and 15), or arm C (CPT-11 alone 100 mg/m^2 on days 1, 8, and 15). Among 398 patients, 378 were evaluable for response, toxicity, and survival. They consisted of 77% male and 23% female patients, with stage IIIB (37%) and stage IV (63%). The majority of patients (93%) were PS0. Objective responses were observed in 55 (43%), 38 (31%), and 26 patients (21%) in arms A, B, and C, respectively. Grade 4 neutropenia occurred at 36.2%, 53.2%, and 7.9% in arms A, B, and C, respectively. Grade 3 or worse diarrhea was observed at 12.6%, 4.0%, and 15.0% in arms A, B, and C, respectively. Overall survivals were 51.7, 47.4, and 47.1 weeks and 1-year survivals were 48.5%, 39.5%, and 43.5% in arms A, B, and C, respectively. In stage IV disease, survival was statistically significantly different between arm A (53.9 weeks) and B (37.9 weeks).

Trial of the CPT-11 Lung Cancer Study Group East[12]

This group conducted two armed randomized controlled trials comparing CPT-11 and CDDP (arm A) with CDDP and VDS (arm B) against inoperable stage IIIB and stage IV non-small cell lung cancer. The doses of anticancer drugs were the same as those for the West group. The response rates for arms A and B were 29% and 22%, and median survival was 45.4 and 49.6 weeks, respectively. It was concluded that regimen A was as active as regimen B.

Trial of the Japanese Clinical Oncology Group (JCOG) against Extensive Disease Small Cell Lung Cancer (ED-SCLC)[13]

Combination chemotherapy with etoposide (VP-16) and CDDP is considered to be a standard regimen for the treatment of small cell lung cancer (SCLC). Phase II study of CPT 11 (60 mg/m^2) and CDDP (60 mg/m^2) produced an 86% response rate and 13.2 months of median survival in ED-SCLC.[9] JCOG conducted a randomized multicenter phase III study of CPT-11 plus cisplatin and etoposide plus cisplatin. The initial sample size was 230 (115 cases in each arm). Enrollment in this study was terminated in December 1998 in accordance with recommendations of an interim analysis because of the statistically significant difference in survival.

Between November 1995 and November 1998, 154 patients were randomized, 77 into each arm to this study. The study arms consisted of 60 mg/m^2 of CPT-11 on days 1.8 and 15 and 60 mg/m^2 of cisplatin on day 1 every 4 weeks for four courses. The standard arm consisted of 100 mg/m^2 of etoposide on days 1, 2, and 3, and 80 mg/m^2 of cisplatin on day 1 every 3 weeks for four courses. The CR rate was 2% in the CP arm and 13% in the EP arm, and the overall response rate was 89% in the CP arm and 67% in the EP arm ($p = 0.013$). Median survival and the 1-year survival rate were 420 days and 60% in the CP arm and 300 days and 40% in the EP arm, respectively. The CP arm showed significantly better survival compared with standard treatment in the EP arm ($p = 0.0047$ by the log-rank test). JCOG grade 3/4 leukopenia occurred in 27% of the patients in the CP arm and 52% in the EP arm ($p = 0.003$), grade 3/4 neutropenia developed in 66% in the CP arm and 92% in the EP arm ($p = 0.0002$), and grade 3/4 thrombocytopenia was found in 5% in the CP arm and 19% in the EP arm ($p = 0.01$). Grade 3/4 diarrhea was seen in 16% in the CP arm and in none of the patients in the EP arm ($p = 0.0001$). The other nonhematological toxicities did not differ between the two arms. There were four treatment-related deaths, three in the CP arm and one in the EP arm; two of them were caused by infection accompanied by neutropenia and the others by bleeding from the metastatic site and pneumonitis, respectively. In conclusion, four cycles of CPT-11 plus cisplatin every 4 weeks yielded significant improvement in survival over standard etoposide plus cisplatin, with less myelosuppression, in patients with extensive-disease small-cell lung cancer.

Combined Modality against Stage III Non-Small Cell Lung Cancer

CPT-11 combined with CDDP is one of the most active regimens in advanced non-small cell lung cancer (NSCLC). Thoracic radiotherapy (TRT) combined with weekly CPT-11 was promising and feasible for locally advanced NSCLC.[14] A 2-cycle, phase II study of CPT-11/CDDP as induction chemotherapy followed by weekly CPT-11 with concomitant TRT was conducted in JCOG.[15] Eligible patients had unresectable stage III NSCLC, performance status (PS) 0 or 1, and no prior therapy. Patients were treated with the following regimen: CDDP 80 mg/m^2 on days 1 and 29 with CPT-11 60 mg/m^2 on days 1, 8, 15, 29, 36, and 43, and 30 mg/m^2 on days 57, 64, 71, 78, 85, and 92. TRT was initiated on day 57 at 2 Gy/day (total 60 Gy). From February 1998 to January 1999, 68 patients were enrolled in the study. Toxicities of grade 3/4 during induction CT were primarily: neutropenia, 41%/31%; and diarrhea, 14%/5%. Grade 3/4 toxicities during concomitant TRT and CPT-11 consisted of: neutropenia, 10%/6%; esophagitis, 4%/0%; and hypoxia, 4%/2%. No treatment-related deaths occurred. Response rate was 63.6% (CR 5.9%, PR 57.4%); median survival time has not yet been reached. Estimated 1-year survival was 71.7%. These results indicate that treatment strategy consisting of induction CT followed by TRT combined with CPT-11 is feasible even in a cooperative group setting and that CPT-11 may be a promising radiation sensitizer for locally advanced NSCLC.

NEW CAMPTOTHECIN DERIVATIVE, DX-8951F

Preclinical Activity

In an investigation to develop water-soluble and non-pro-drug CPT derivatives with strong antitumor activity, Daiichi Pharmaceutical Co. succeeded in obtaining DX-8951f, a hexacyclic compound having an amino group and a fluorine atom at positions 1 and 5, respectively. DX-8951f is more potent than SN-38 or topotecan in its topoisomerase I inhibitory activity and cytotoxicity.[16] In experiments to determine the anticancer spectrum of DX-8951f, cytotoxicity was evaluated *in vitro* against 32 malignant cell lines. DX-8951f showed stronger antitumor activity than did other CPT derivatives such as SN-38, topotecan, or camptothecin. The pattern of activity of DX-8951f was similar to that of SN-38 and other topoisomerase I inhibitors. Topotecan reportedly is subjected to p glycoprotein-mediated resistance. On the other hand, DX-8951f was obviously less affected by p glycoprotein even compared with SN-38. *In vivo* it shows a favorable toxicity profile and lack of esterase-dependent activation and metabolism. These characteristics contribute to a high therapeutic index and to low intersubject variability in pharmacokinetics and toxicity. The antitumor activity is not modulated by multidrug resistance gene and is observed in a concentration- and time-dependent manner. The antitumor activity of three doses of DX-8951f administered i.v. at 4-day intervals against human gastric adenocarcinoma SC-6 xenografts was greater than that of CPT-11 or topotecan. Maximum body weight reduction and number of toxic deaths indicate that the toxicity of DX-8951f may be less than that of CPT-11 or topotecan at an effective dose level. Preclinical studies indicate that DX-8951f may be a hopeful drug for clinical trial.

Mechanisms of Resistance to DX-8951f[17]

To elucidate the mechanisms of its cytotoxicity, a DX-8951f-resistant cell line, SBC-3/DXCL1, from human small cell lung cancer cells (SBC-3) was established by stepwise exposure to DX-8951f. SBC-3/DXCL1 cells were approximately 400 times more resistant to DX-8951f than were parent cells. SBC-3/DXCL1 cells showed a high degree of cross-resistance to other topo I inhibitors such as CPT-11, SN-38, and camptothecin, but not to non-topo I targeting agents such as cisplatin, adriamycin, etoposide, and vincristine. The mechanisms of resistance of SBC-3/DXCL1 cells to DX-8951f were examined. Intracellular accumulation of DX-8951f by SBC-3 and SBC-3/DXCL1 cells did not differ significantly. Although the topo I activity of nuclear extracts obtained from SBC-3/DXCL1 cells was the same as that of the parent cells, topo I of SBC-3/DXCL1 cells was resistant to the inhibitory effects of DX-8951f and SN-38. Immunoblotting using anti-topo I antibody demonstrated similar protein levels of topo I in SBC-3 and SBC-3/DXCL1 cells. The active topo I protein of SBC-3/DXCL1 was eluted by a high concentration of NaCl (0.4 N) compared with that of SBC-3 (0.3 N). DX-8951f stabilized the DNA-topo I cleavable complex from SBC-3 cells, as measured by topo I-mediated cleavage assay. In SBC-3/DXCL1 cells, DX-8951f also stabilized the DNA-topo I complex, but with a 10-fold lower efficiency. These results suggest that a qualitative change in topo I contributes, at least partially, to the resistance to DX-8951f ion SBC-3/DXCL1 cells. Therefore, SBC-3/DXCL1 cells may have a unique mechanism of resistance to topo I-directed antitumor drugs.

Clinical Trial of DX-8951f[18–22]

In clinical trials of DX-8951f, Daiichi Pharmaceutical Co. took a strategy of global development, meaning that toxicity and efficacy criteria, definition of dose-limiting toxicity and maximum tolerated dose, inclusion and exclusion criteria, and supportive care are standardized in all protocols. Eight protocols were started simultaneously in Japan, USA, and Europe. Clinical data from three regions were shared and utilized for further clinical trials. Totally, six schedules were used as shown in TABLE I. All phase I trials have been completed. Dose-limiting toxicity was myelosuppression such as neutropenia and thrombocytepenia. The nadir of neutropenia was experienced on days 12–15 and recovery was observed on day 22. Main gastrointestinal toxicity was nausea and vomiting, which were easily controlled by antiemetics. Human pharmacokinetic study was consistent with a two- or three-compartment model. Elimination t1/2 was more than 8 hours. T1/2, Vss, and Cl were dose independent. C_{max} and AUC linearly correlated with the dose of DX-8951f. Based on the phase I study, the recommended schedules for the phase II study are weekly 30-minute infusions daily × 5 days q 3 weeks and weekly 30-minute infusions.

SUMMARY

After the successful development of CPT-11, many topoisomerase I inhibitors were introduced not only in preclinical experiments but also in clinical trials. Although topoisomerase I inhibitors are cytotoxic drugs, the molecular target is very clear in this class of drugs. It should be stressed that CPT-11–containing regimens have achieved a position of global standard chemotherapy against colorectal cancer. Recently, deposit form camptothecins have also been developed. The role of topoisomerase I inhibitors will be greatly expanded in the near future.

ACKNOWLEDGMENTS

The authors gratefully acknowledge the following collaborators: (1) **National Cancer Center Hospital:** Tetsuo Kodama, Tomohide Tamura, Yuichiro Ohe, Hideo Kunito, Ikuo Sekine, Noboru Yamamoto, Yoshiko Akiyama, Hitoshi Kusaba, Hirokazu Watanabe, Masahiro Sawada, Akira Inoue, Tatsu Shimoyama, Katsuyuki Hotta, and Hruyasu Murakami. (2) **National Cancer Center Hospital East:** Yutaka Nishiwaki, Ryutaro Kakinuma, Taketoshi Matsumoto, Kaoru Kubota, Hironobu Ohmatsu, Koichi Goto, Yasutsuna Sasaki, and Hironobu Minami. (3) **National Cancer Center Research Institute:** Kazuto Nishio, and Fumihiko Kanzawa. (4) **Japanese Clinical Oncology Group:** Kiyoshi Mori, Koshiro Watanabe, Kazumasa Noda, Akira Yokoyama, Takahiko Sugiura, Shinichiro Nakamura, Masaaki Kawahara, Masahiro Fukuoka, Kaoru Matsui, and Shunich Negoro.

REFERENCES

1. WANG, J.C. 1985. DNA topoisomerases. Annu. Rev. Biochem. **54:** 665–697.
2. WALL, M.E., M.C. WANI, C. E. COOK, *et al.* 1969. Plant antitumor agents. I. The isolation and structure of camptothecin, a novel alkaloidal leukemia and tumor inhibitor from *Camptotheca acuminata.* J. Am. Chem. Soc. **88:** 3888–3890.
3. MUGGIA, F.M., P.J. CREAVEN, H.H. HANSEN, *et al.* 1972. Phase I clinical trial of weekly and daily treatment with camptothecin sodium (NSC-100880). Cancer Chemother. Rep. **56:** 515–521.
4. SAWADA, S., T. YOKOKURA & T. MIYASAKA. 1996. Synthesis of CPT-11 (irinotecan hydrochloride trihydrate). *In* The Camptothecins from Discovery to the Patient. P. Pantazis, B.C. Giovanella & M.L. Rothenberg, Eds. Ann. N.Y. Acad. Sci. **803:** 13–28.

5. SAIJO, N. 1996. Clinical trials of irinotecan hydrochloride (CPT, campto injection, topotecan injection) in Japan. *In* The Camptothecins from Discovery to the Patient. P. Pantazis, B.C. Giovanella & M.L. Rothenberg, Eds. Ann. N.Y. Acad Sci. **803:** 292–305.
6. CUNNINGHAM, D., S. PYRHONEN, R.D. JAMES, *et al.* 1998. A phase III multicenter randomized study of CPT-11 versus supportive care alone in patients with 5-FU resistant metastatic colorectal cancer. Proc. ASCO **17:** 1.
7. CUSTEM, E.V., E. BAJETTA, N. NIEDERLE, *et al.* 1998. A phase III multicenter randomized trial comparing CPT-11 to infusional 5-FU regimen in patients with advanced colorectal cancer after 5-FU failure. Proc. ASCO **17:** 984.
8. SALTZ, L.B., P.K. LOCKER, N. PIOTTA, *et al.* 1999. Weekly irinotecan, leucovorin, and fluorouracil is superior to daily x 5 LV/5-FU in patients with previously untreated metastatic colorectal cancer. Proc. ASCO **18:** 898.
9. DOUILLARD, J.Y., D. AINNINGHAM, A.D. ROTH, *et al.* 1999. A randomized phase III trial comparing irinotecan + 5-FU/folinic acid to the same schedule of FU/FA in patients with metastatic colorectal cancer as front line chemotherapy. Proc. ASCO **18:** 899.
10. MASUDA, N., M. FUKUOKA, A. FUJITA, *et al.* & the CPT-11 lung cancer study group. 1998. A phase II trial of combination of CPT-11 and cisplatin for advanced non-small cell lung cancer. Br. J. Cancer **78:** 251–256.
11. MASUDA, N., M. FUKUOKA, S. NEGORO, *et al.* & the CPT-11 lung cancer study group West. 1999. Randomized trial comparing cisplatin and irinotecan versus cisplatin and vindesine versus irinotecan alone in advanced non-small cell lung cancer, a multicenter phase III study. Proc. ASCO **18:** 1774.
12. NIHO, S., K. NAGAO, Y. NISHIWAKI, *et al.* & the CPT-11 lung cancer study group. 1999. Randomized multicenter Phase III trial of irinotecan and cisplatin versus cisplatin and vindesine in patients with advanced non-small cell lung cancer. Proc. ASCO **18:** 1897.
13. NODA, K., Y. NISHIWAKI, M. KAWAHARA, *et al.* for the members of JCOG. 2000. Randomized phase III study of CPT-11 and cisplatin versus etoposide and cisplatin in ED-SCLC. Proc. ASCO 19.
14. TAKEDA, K., S. NEGORO, S. KUDOH, *et al.* 1999. Phase I/II study of weekly irinotecan and concurrent radiation therapy for locally advanced non-small cell lung cancer. Br. J. Cancer **79:** 1462–1467.
15. YAMAMOTO, N., M. FUKUOKA, S. NEGORO, *et al.* for the members of JCOG. 2000. Induction chemotherapy with CTP-11 and cisplatin followed by thoracic irradiation combined with weekly CPT-11 against stage III NSCLC. Proc. ASCO 19.
16. MITSUI, I., E. KUMAZAWA, Y. HIROTA, *et al.* 1995. A new water-soluble comptothecin derivative, DX-8951f, exhibits potent antitumor activity against human tumors *in vitro* and *in vivo*. Jpn. J. Cancer Res. **86:** 776–782.
17. NOMOTO, T., K. NISHIO, T. ISHIDA, *et al.* 1998. Characterization of a human small-cell lung cancer cell line resistant to a new soluble camptothecin derivative, DX-8951f. Jpn. J. Cancer Res. **89:** 1179–1186.
18. JOHNSON, T., C. GEYER, R. JAGAR, *et al.* 1998. Phase I and PK study of DX-8951f, a novel hexacyclic camptothecin analog, on a 30 min infusion daily for 5 day every 3 week schedule. Proc. ASCO **17:** 756.
19. ROYCE, M., P.M. HOFF, R. BRITO, *et al.* 1999. Phase I trial of DX-8951f, a novel camptothecin analogue, administered by 24-hr continuous infusion. Proc. ASCO **17:** 757.
20. DAVIDSON, K., E. IZBICKA, T. LAURENCE, *et al.* 1999. Anti cancer activity of DX-8951f, a water soluble camptothecin analog, against human tumor specimens taken directly from adult or pediatric patients. Proc. ASCO **17:** 758.
21. MINAMI, H., Y. SASAKI, Y. SHIGEOKA, *et al.* 1999. Phase I study and pharmacology of DX-8951f, a new camptothecin derivative, administered over 30 min every 3 weeks. Proc. 1999 AACR-NCI-EORTC Int. Conf. 326.
22. KAMIYA, Y., N. YAMAMOTO, Y. YAMADA, *et al.* 1999. Phase I and PK study of DX8951f., a novel camptothecin analog given as 30 min infusion daily for 5 days. Proc. 1999 AACR-NCI- EORTC Int. Conf. 327.

Homocamptothecins: E-Ring Modified CPT Analogues

OLIVIER LAVERGNE,[a,c] DANIELE DEMARQUAY,[a] PHILIP G. KASPRZYK,[b] AND DENNIS C.H. BIGG[a]

[a]*Institut Henri Beaufour, Les Ulis, France*

[b]*Biomeasure Inc., Milford, Massachusetts 01757, USA*

ABSTRACT: Homocamptothecins (hCPT) are modified camptothecins (CPT) with a seven-membered β-hydroxylactone instead of the naturally occurring six-membered α-hydroxylactone. This E-ring modification fully conserves the ability to stabilize topo I-DNA single-strand breaks and stimulates high levels of DNA cleavage. A key feature is the irreversibility of E-ring opening, which should give reduced toxicity. Substituted hCPTs have been selected for their high antiproliferative activity on a panel of tumor cell lines, including those with cross resistance, and were found to be active at very low doses in a variety of human tumor xenografts when administered orally. BN 80915, a difluoro-hCPT, has entered clinical trials.

INTRODUCTION

This project was initiated in the mid-1990s, when topotecan and irinotecan were first granted approval for clinical use, one decade after topoisomerase (topo)-I had been established as the molecular target of camptothecin (CPT) and three decades after isolation of the natural product. It was clear at the time that all biologically active CPT analogues were indeed susbtituted CPTs[1] and that if the CPT skeleton was to be kept, the opportunity for novelty would be low, with only four substitution sites allowed (TABLE 1). Altering the skeleton of CPT therefore appeared as the only way to innovate. Because of its high chemical reactivity, the most attractive site was the lactone, and tampering with this ring was a stimulating idea that could give some clue as to its role in stabilizing the topo I–DNA complex. Modifying the lactone was especially challenging because all prior attempts failed to yield biologically active compounds, and strong prejudice existed against any structural change to the E-ring of CPT.

CPT has an intriguing mechanism of action, because it neither interacts with topo-I alone[2] nor does it bind to DNA.[3,4] Its biological activity comes from its capacity to stabilize the "cleavable complex," a transient molecular species in which a tyrosine residue of topo I binds covalently to DNA via its phosphodiester backbone and generates a single-strand break. It is the interaction between three components, CPT, topo I, and DNA, that eventually leads to irreversible chromatin damage and

---

[c]Address for correspondence: Institut Henri Beaufour, 5 avenue du Canada, 91966 Les Ulis, France. Fax: (33) 1 69 07 38 02.

olivier.lavergne@beaufour-ipsen.com

TABLE 1. Structures of CPT analogues

Compound	Code name	R^1	R^2	R^3	R^4
Camptothecin	CPT	H	H	H	H
Topotecan	TPT	H	–OH	–CH$_2$N(CH$_3$)$_2$	H
Irinotecan	CPT-11	H	piperidino-piperidine carbonyloxy	H	–CH$_2$CH$_3$
	SN-38	H	–OH	H	–CH$_2$CH$_3$
Lurtotecan	GG-211	–OCH$_2$CH$_2$O–		H	–CH$_2$-(4-methylpiperazin-1-yl)
Rubitecan	9-NC	H	H	–NO$_2$	H
	9-AC	H	H	–NH$_2$	H
Exatecan	DX-8951	F	–CH$_3$	–CH$_2$CH(NH$_2$)– (fused)	

triggers cell death.[5] This mechanism accounts for the good correlation between the number of stabilized cleavable complexes and the antiproliferative properties of CPT analogues,[6] although the ternary complex has so far eluded isolation in crystalline form and its structure remains speculative.[7,8] In particular, it is still unknown if a covalent bond involving the E-ring carboxyl group of CPT and a nucleophilic site within the topo I–DNA complex (FIG. 1) exists.

Lactones are cyclic carboxylic esters and, as such, are a rather stable molecule, about as sensitive to hydrolysis as ethyl acetate, for example. It is the adjacent hydoxyl group or, more precisely, the inductive effect from the electronegative oxygen that renders the carboxyl group of CPT highly reactive. The idea was therefore to remove this electronic influence with as little structural alteration as possible, by inserting a methylene spacer between the carboxylic and alcoholic functions of the E-ring. The alcohol moiety was seen as a particularly necessary structural feature to stabilize the cleavable complex, because neither deshydroxy-CPT nor the nonnatural enantiomer of CPT is biologically active.

SEMISYNTHESIS

Various syntheses of CPT were adaptable to our purposes, but they often consisted of lengthy multistep sequences. It therefore appeared more convenient to start from CPT itself, or any readily available derivative, with the heterocyclic backbone

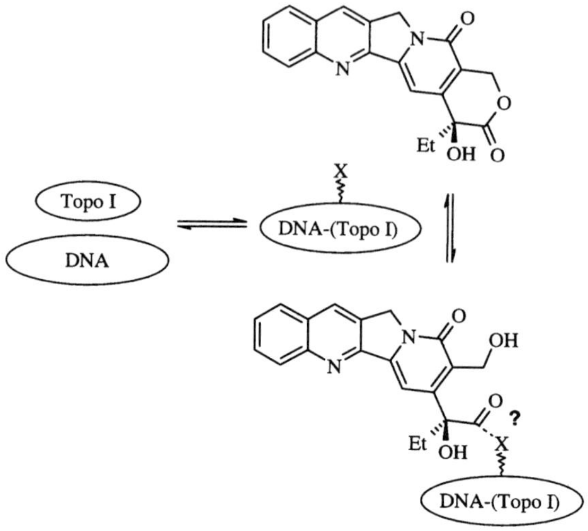

FIGURE 1. Camptothecin (CPT) mode of action via hypothetical covalent interaction.

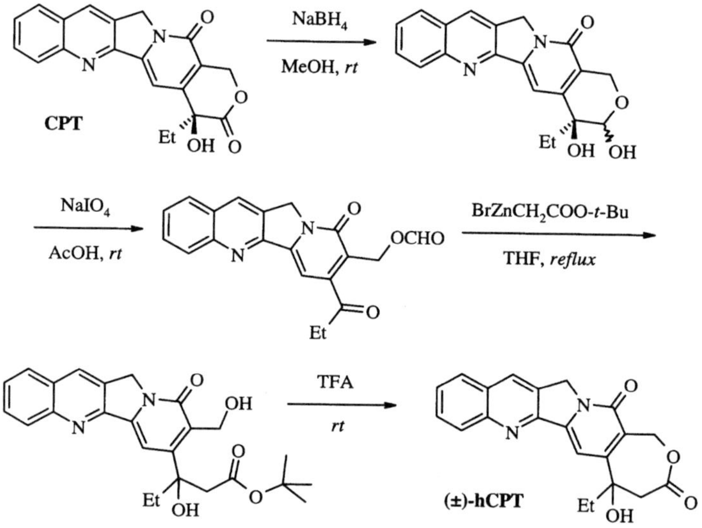

FIGURE 2. Semisynthetic preparation of homocamptothecin (hCPT).

as well as the necessary functionality already in place. A four-step method, shown in FIGURE 2, was rapidly established to validate the project. [9]Formyloxy-mappicine-ketone, obtained from CPT in two easy synthetic steps, was submitted to a Reformastsky type reaction, a classical method for the preparation β-hydroxyesters, and a subsequent acid treatment gave the desired product. This novel CPT analogue bears a seven-membered β-hydroxylactone ring instead of the naturally occuring six-membered α-hydroxylactone. Since a one-carbon ring expansion is chemically termed a homologation, the name "homocamptothecin" (hCPT) was coined to designate this new compound. The semisynthetic procedure turned out to be amenable to the preparation of multigram quantities of racemic hCPT, from which the two enantiomerically pure forms were obtained via a chemical resolution of the ring-open carboxylate conterpart.[10]

PHARMACOLOGY OF hCPT

The first pharmacological results were surprisingly good. Be it in isolated enzyme or in cell culture, homologation of the CPT lactone did *not* result in a dramatic drop of biological activity, as previously seen with other modifications of the E-ring. In a relaxation assay of supercoiled DNA with purified calf thymus topo I, hCPT was as potent as CPT, whereas in terms of antiproliferative activity on the L1210 murine leukemia cell line, hCPT was about 10-fold better.[9] This was very encouraging and called for more testing. Confirmation of the preliminary results was obtained when using human topo I instead of the bovine enzyme. This greater potency hCPT could be due to a number of factors: both drugs stimulated cleavage by topo I at T/G sites, but hCPT, in addition, induced cleavage at specific sites containing the sequence AAC/G.[11] Furthermore, higher levels of protein-linked DNA were found in P388 murine leukemia cells treated with hCPT than in those treated with CPT, as detected by a KCl/SDS coprecipitation method, and an immonoblot assay on fractions obtained from a CsCl gradient of P388 cell lysates enabled identification of higher levels of endogenous topo I trapped onto DNA in hCPT-treated cells.[11] Similarly, hCPT showed superior antiproliferative activity on a panel of human tumor cell lines. Finally, the two drugs were compared *in vivo* on intraperitoneally implanted L1210 murine leukemia cells and on subcutaneous HT29 xenografts. The results were again more than convincing, with hCPT showing greater efficacy than CPT, along with activity over a broader range of doses.[12] The startling contrast with the previously reported modifications of the lactone was high; instead of losing or abolishing biological activity, hCPT quantitatively outperformed the benchmark CPT in a variety of tests.

NOT JUST ANOTHER CPT

Many CPT derivatives are more potent than the parent natural product, but as just mentioned, they are substituted CPT with the intact six-membered lactone and its attendant disadvantages. The new seven-membered lactone, on the other hand, brings unique chemical properties that make hCPT qualitatively different from CPT. The insertion of a methylene spacer between the carboxyl and alcohol functions has two important consequences. First, removal of the electronic influence of the hydroxyl group considerably reduces the rate of hydrolytic opening, so that therapeutically useful plasma levels may be sustained more readily. Second, enlargement to a seven-membered ring renders the ring opening reaction *irreversible*, even under mildly acidic conditions. These two features explain the differences between the two compounds in their hydrolytic profiles obtained on incubation in human plasma at 37°C

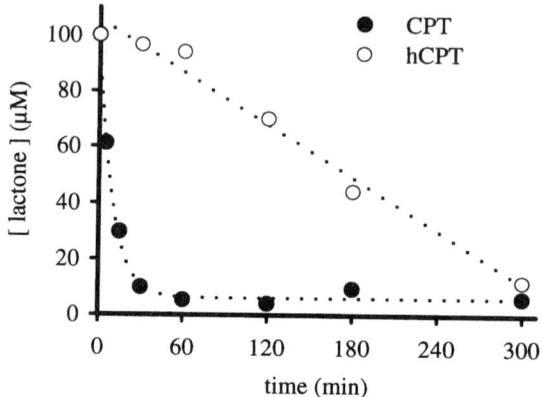

FIGURE 3. Hydrolytic profiles of CPT and hCPT.

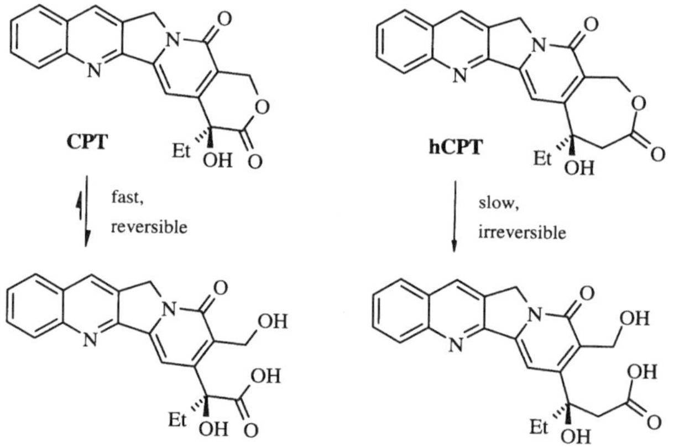

FIGURE 4. Hydrolysis of CPT and hCPT.

(FIG. 3). The slow and irreversible ring opening of hCPT translates into a linear decay, in contrast to the rapid hydrolysis to a pH-dependent equilibrium corresponding to an exponential decay for CPT. The unique solution behavior of hCPT (FIG. 4), unseen in any classical six-membered CPT analogue, may afford new, improved drugs with better efficacy because of the higher lactone AUC values. In addition, the irreversible character of this hydrolysis should reduce the propensity to induce hemorrhagic cystitis, by preventing the accumulation of biologically active material in the urinary tract. It should be remembered that the clinical development of CPT-sodium was halted by severe and unpredictable toxicity, particularly hemorrhagic cystitis, and that patients currently enrolled in clinical trials with 9-nitrocamptothecin have to absorb close to 3 liters of fluid daily to minimize this type of adverse event.

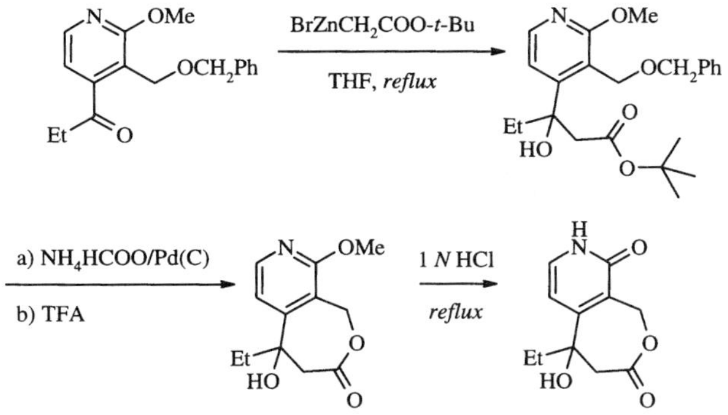

FIGURE 5. Preparation of the DE-moiety.

TOTAL SYNTHESIS

Because hCPT was found to be such a promising template, it became clear that the scope of the semisynthetic route would be too narrow to provide sufficient substituent diversity, and a totally synthetic approach had to be devised for the preparation of new hCPT analogues. An original strategy based on the coupling of a pyridone with a quinoline and elegantly employed by Daniel Comins for a short synthesis of CPT[13] was modified to enable the preparation of hCPT analogues. In this process an AB-quinoline was coupled to a DE-moiety, and subsequent cyclization formed the C ring of the pentacyclic template. Because of its convergent character and the ready access to the required substituted AB-quinolines,[14] this method seemed amenable to an analogue generation program. The only lengthy multistep sequence was restricted to the preparation of the DE-moiety, consisting of a pyridone fused to a seven-membered β-hydroxylactone (FIG. 5), which was a common precursor for all envisaged analogues. Its preparation came logically from our previous semisynthesic experience, since the β-hydroxycarboxylic moiety could be obtained by a Reformatsky reaction on a 4-propionylpyridine with an adjacent protected hydroxymethyl group. The resulting process was rapidly scaled-up to provide multigram quantities, initially in racemic form[10] and subsequently in enantiomerically pure form.[15]

A wide array of options was available for the quinoline synthons, starting from relatively simple precursors to more elaborate patterns to provide, for example, better water solubility or enhanced lipophilicity. The first synthetic hCPT made was an ethylenedioxy analogue, shown in FIGURE 6, which was our leading molecule in terms of activity for only a short period of time because more potent derivatives kept coming out of the chemistry laboratory.[16] Obviously certain criteria had to be applied to weed out the less promising compounds while keeping the hCPT analogues endowed with higher anticancer potential. These selection criteria were: potent and selective topo I inhibition, high antiproliferative activities on a panel of human tumor cell lines (including multidrug-resistant cell lines), elevated plasma stability, and good oral bioavailability.

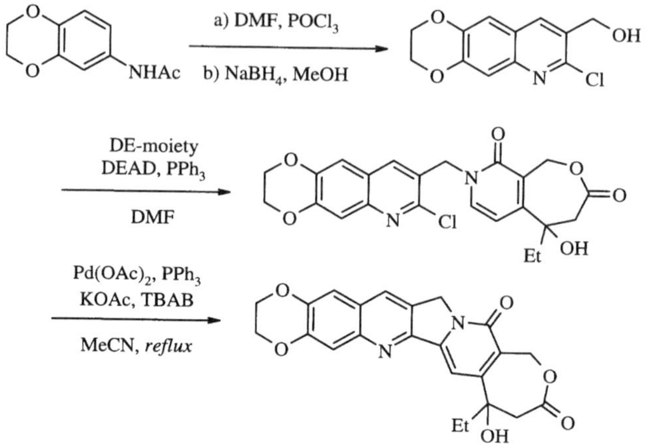

FIGURE 6. Synthesis of an ethylenedioxy-hCPT.

FLUORINATED hCPTS

Starting from simple quinolines, readily available from the corresponding anilines, a first series of halogen- and alkoxyl-substituted hCPTs was obtained. Although tested as racemic mixtures, these compounds were found to be as active as native CPT, as shown in TABLE 2, and three of them displayed elevated topo I inhibition in this assay, with less than 40% relaxed DNA. The A427 human lung carcinoma[17] cell line (perhaps due to its mutant *p53* tumor suppressor gene) provided the means to discriminate compounds, giving IC_{50} values that were spread over several log units of concentration. Some compounds showed very high potency, such as methylenedioxy-hCPT and some fluorinated hCPTs. Surprisingly, the most active compounds in terms of antiproliferative activity were fluorinated hCPTs, not ethylenedioxy or methylenedioxy compounds as in the CPT series. The previously reported SAR in the CPT series was therefore not completely transposable to the hCPTs, perhaps because of subtle differences in the interactions with the cleavable complexes revealed by changes in specificity in drug-induced DNA cleavages by topo I. Another interesting result from this first set of data was that unlike topotecan and, to a lesser extent, SN-38 (the biologically active metabolite of the prodrug CPT-11), halogenated hCPTs performed well on cell lines overexpressing P-glucoprotein (PgP) and MRP multidrug-resistant associated proteins. These were important, and clinically relevant, selection criteria in view of the cross-resistance that often develops with different chemotherapies.

To further explore the benefit of fluoro substituents, a second series of compounds was prepared in enantiopure form.[15] As shown in TABLE 3, the position of the fluorine substituent in the A-ring was found to have a pronounced influence on biological activity. Considering the four monofluorinated analogues, lower levels of relaxed DNA were observed when R^3 is a fluorine, than with fluorine at R^1 or R^2, whereas R^4 appeared to be the least favorable position. The DNA cleavage values

TABLE 2. Biological activities of racemic substituted hCPTs

Compound	Substituents		Activity	
	A	B	Topo I[a]	A427[b]
hCPT	H	H	60	12
	Cl	H	57	0.36
	F	H	47	7.7
	OMe	F	26	0.0083
	Me	F	18	0.00081
	Me	Cl	59	0.031
	F	Cl	61	0.023
	F	F	56	0.10
	-OCH$_2$CH$_2$O-		50	
	-OCH$_2$O-		58	0.62
CPT	-	-	64	24

[a]Percent relaxed DNA obtained with 100 μM of test compound in the calf thymus topo I mediated relaxation of supercoiled pUC19 plasmid DNA assay.

[b]Mean values (nM) from three determinations of 50% inhibitory concentrations by WST assay on A427 cell line.

obtained for unsubstituted hCPT were comparable to those of compounds fluorinated at R^1 or R^2, and ortho as well as meta difluorinated compounds were very efficient in inhibiting supercoiled DNA relaxation. The antiproliferative activities of these fluoro-hCPTs on HT29 human colon adenocarcinoma were in agreement with their inhibition of the relaxation of supercoiled DNA mediated by topo I. Within this series of compounds, those bearing a fluorine atom at R^3 were highly active topo I poisons and up to 10-fold more potent than CPT in terms of cytotoxicity on the HT29 cell line. The difluoro derivative BN 80915 ($R^2 = R^3 = F$) has been selected for further development as a highly active hCPT-based topo I poison, providing an optimal balance between potency and stability.

PRE-CLINICAL STUDY OF BN 80915

BN 80915 outperformed current clinical topo I poisons in terms of activity, and for each drug, the hydrolytic profiles in human plasma were in agreement with the chemical reactivity of their respective lactone, that is, a slow linear decay for BN 80915 instead of exponentially delaying curves for TPT and SN-38. A reduction in

TABLE 3. Biological activities of enantiomerically pure fluorinated hCPTs

	Substituents				Activity	
Compound	R^1	R^2	R^3	R^4	Topo I[a]	HT29[b]
hCPT	H	H	H	H	49	30
	F				39	20
		F			58	27
			F		28	11
				F	86	190
	F		F		33	10
		F	F		25	8.4
	H	H	H	H	49	30
CPT	-	-	-	-	85	80

[a]Percent relaxed DNA obtained with 10 μM of test compound in the calf thymus topo I-mediated relaxation of supercoiled pUC19 plasmid DNA assay.
[b]Mean values (nM) from three determination of 50% inhibitory concentrations by WST assay on HT29 cell line.

adverse effects may therefore be expected from BN 80915 due to the irreversible ring opening of its lactone. When tested on multidrug-resistant tumor cell lines that overexpress PgP and MRP proteins, BN 80915 exerted higher cytotoxicity than did TPT and SN-38 relative to the parent, nonresistant, strains.

Further benchmarking of BN 80915 was performed on human colon cancer samples obtained from surgical resection and cultured under organotypical conditions.[18] Measurement of cell proliferation in these *ex vivo* tumor tissue cultures by tritiated thymidine autoradiography showed BN 80915 to be significantly more active in inhibiting human cancer cell proliferation than TPT or SN-38.

The drugs were compared *in vivo* in athymic mice xenografted with various tumorigenic cell lines of human origin. With DU145 human prostate cancer cells, for example, tumor-like colonies growing to 2,000 mm³ were obtained in about 40 days in untreated mice. When the mice were treated with 100 mg/kg of CPT-11 administered i.p. on a once-a-week schedule repeated three times, significant inhibition of tumor growth was recorded to about 800 mm³ at day 40. BN 80915 was administered orally following the same schedule, but at a dose of 1 mg/kg. As shown in FIGURE 7, pronounced tumor regressions were obtained in the BN 80915-treated group. An average tumor of about 250 mm³ at day 40 shows the high potential of the hCPT-based compound as an anticancer drug.

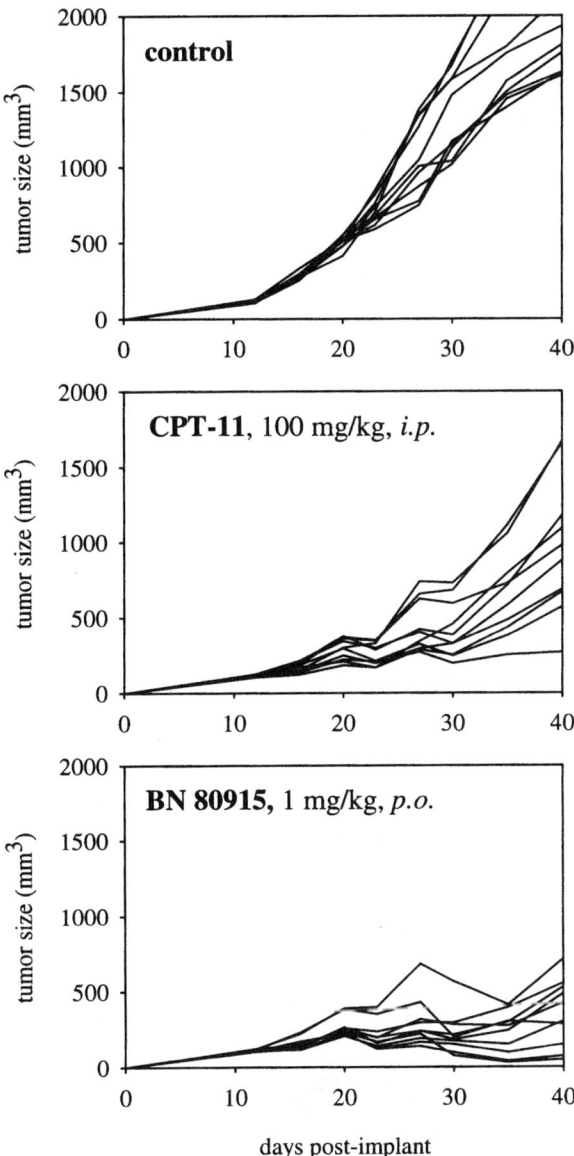

FIGURE 7. Responses of DU145 nonandrogen-dependent human prostate tumor xenografts to CPT-11 and BN 80915. Mice bearing subcutaneous tumors were treated on days 11, 18, and 25 postimplant with vehicle (*upper panel*), CPT-11 (*center panel*), and BN 80915 (*lower panel*). Each curve represents the growth of an individual tumor.

CONCLUSION

Topotecan and irinotecan are already successfully used in the clinic and provide better therapeutic options to treat cancer patients. It is hoped that the signs of higher efficacy and reduced side-effect potential seen with BN 80915 will be beneficial to patients. To that end, oral and i.v. formulations of BN 80915 are currently undergoing clinical evaluation in Europe.

REFERENCES

1. LAVERGNE, O. & D.C.H. BIGG. 1998. The other camptothecins: recent advances with camptothecin analogues other than irinotecan and topotecan. Bull. Cancer Spec. No. **1:** 51–58.
2. HERTZBERG, R.P., M.J. CARANFA & S.M. HECHT. 1989. On the mechanism of topoisomerase I inhibition by camptothecin: evidence for binding to an enzyme-DNA complex. Biochemistry **28:** 4629–4638.
3. LI, L.H., T.J. FRASER, E.J. OLIN & B.K. BHUYAN. 1972. Action of camptothecin on mammalian cells in culture. Cancer Res. **32:** 2643–2650.
4. FUKADA, M. 1985. Action of camptothecin and its derivatives on deoxyribonucleic acid. Biochem. Pharmacol. **34:** 1225–1230.
5. HOLM, C., J.M. COVEY, D. KERRIGAN & Y. POMMIER. 1989. Differential requirement of DNA replication for the cytotoxicity of DNA topoisomerase I and II inhibitors in Chinese hamster DC3F cells. Cancer Res. **49:** 6365–6368.
6. JAXEL, C., K.W. KOHN, M.C. WANI, *et al.* 1989. Structure-activity study of the actions of camptothecin derivatives on mammalian topoisomerase I: evidence for a specific receptor site and a relation to antitumor activity. Cancer Res. **49:** 1465–1469.
7. REDINBO, M.R., L. STEWART, P. KUHN, *et al.* 1998. Crystal structures of human topoisomerase I in covalent and noncovalent complexes with DNA. Science **279:** 1504qP1513.
8. FAN, Y., J.N. WEINSTEIN, K.W. KOHN, *et al.* 1998. Molecular modeling studies of the DNA-topoisomerase I ternary cleavable complex with camptothecin. J. Med. Chem. **41:** 2216–2226.
9. LAVERGNE, O., L. LESUEUR-GINOT, F. PLA RODAS & D.C.H. BIGG. 1997. BN 80245: an E-ring modified camptothecin with potent antiproliferative and topoisomerase I inhibitory activities. Bioorg. Med. Chem. Lett. **7:** 2235–2238.
10. LAVERGNE, O., L. LESUEUR-GINOT, F. PLA RODAS, *et al.* 1998. Homocamptothecins: synthesis and antitumor activity of novel E-ring-modified camptothecin analogues. J. Med. Chem. **41:** 5410–5419.
11. BAILLY, C., A. LANSIAUX, L. DASSONNEVILLE, *et al.* 1999. Homocamptothecin, an E-ring modified camptothecin analogue, generates new topoisomerase I-mediated DNA breaks. Biochemistry **38:** 15556–15556.
12. LESUEUR-GINOT, L., D. DEMARQUAY, R. KISS, *et al.* 1999. Homocamptothecin, an E-ring modified camptothecin with enhanced lactone stability, retains topoisomerase I-targeted activity and antitumor properties. Cancer Res. **59:** 2939–2943.
13. COMINS, D.L., M.F. BAEVSKY & H. HONG. 1992. A 10-step, asymmetric synthesis of (S)-camptothecin. J. Am. Chem. Soc. **114:** 10971–10972.
14. METH-COHN, O., B. NARINE & B. TARNOWSKI. 1981. A versatile new synthesis of quinolines and related fused pyridines. Part 5. The synthesis of 2-chloroquinoline-3-carbaldehydes. J. Chem. Soc. Perkin Trans. I 1520–1530.
15. LAVERGNE, O., D. DEMARQUAY, C. BAILLY, *et al.* 2000. Preparation and *in vitro* activity of enantiomerically pure, fluorinated homocamptothecins as potent topoisomerase I poisons. J. Med. Chem. **43:** 2285–2289.
16. LAVERGNE, O., J. HARNETT, A. ROLLAND, *et al.* 1999. BN 80927: a novel homocamptothecin with inhibitory activities on both topoisomerase I and topoisomerase II. Bioorg. Med. Chem Lett. **9:** 2599–2602.

17. GIARD, D.J., S.A. AARONSON, G.J. TODARO, *et al.* 1973. *In vitro* cultivation of human tumors: establishment of cell lines derived from a series of solid tumors. J. Natl. Cancer Inst. **51:** 1417–1423.
18. PHILIPPART, P., L. HARPER, C. CHABOTEAUX, *et al.* 2000. Homocamptothecin, an E-ring-modified camptothecin, exerts more potent antiproliferative activity than other topoisomerase I inhibitors in human colon cancers obtained from surgery and maintained *in vitro* under histotypical culture conditions. Clin. Cancer Res. **6:** 1557–1562.

The Cascade Radical Annulation Approach to New Analogues of Camptothecins

Combinatorial Synthesis of Silatecans and Homosilatecans

DENNIS P. CURRAN,[a] HUBERT JOSIEN, DAVID BOM, ANA E. GABARDA, AND WU DU

Department of Chemistry and Center for Combinatorial Chemistry, University of Pittsburgh, Pittsburgh, Pennsylvania 15260, USA

ABSTRACT: An overview of the cascade radical annulation approach to the camptothecin family of antitumor drugs is presented. This combinatorial synthetic approach involves two key steps: (1) *N*-propargylation of a lactone/pyridone D/E ring fragment and (2) cascade radical annulation of an A-ring isonitrile to form rings B and C. The synthesis is probably the most flexible and general route to the camptothecin class of molecules. The parallel synthesis of several libraries of silatecan and homosilatecan libraries is summarized. One of the first-generation silatecans, DB-67, is emerging as a serious candidate for cancer chemotherapy.

INTRODUCTION

Thanks to rapid recent advances in the laboratory and the clinic, the members of the camptothecin family of antitumor agents are increasingly recognized as key members in the existing arsenal of useful chemotherapeutic agents.[1,2] The structures of the parent and several of the most important members of the camptothecin family are shown in FIGURE 1. Although camptothecin itself is no longer a candidate for clinical use, its congeners, topotecan and irinotecan, have recently been approved for use in the clinic in several countries.

The analogues shown in FIGURE 1 can be used to exemplify the current level of understanding of the structure–activity relationship in the camptothecin family. The A and B rings are very tolerant of substitution and modification in camptothecin, and over the years A/B modification has been an enduring theme in producing camptothecin analogues with improved activities or other desirable properties. On the other hand, modification of the C, D, or E ring has usually reduced, often even abolished, activity. A major exception to this generalization is the recently reported "homocamptothecin," which bears an expanded E-ring lactone.[3] The homocamptothecin series of compounds is especially important because the opening of the lactone

---

[a]Address for correspondence: Dennis P. Curran, Ph.D., Department of Chemistry and Center for Combinatorial Chemistry, University of Pittsburgh, Pittsburgh, PA 15260. Voice: 412-624-8240; fax: 412-624-9861.
curran@pitt.edu

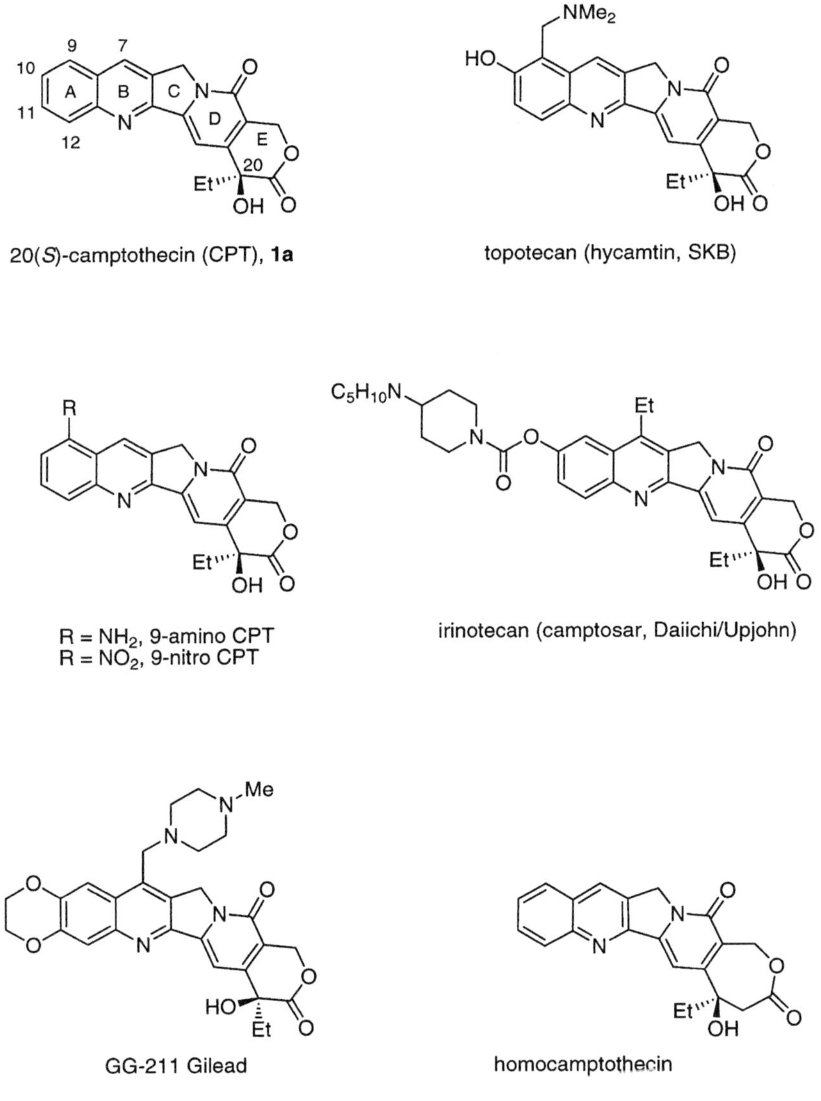

20(S)-camptothecin (CPT), **1a**

topotecan (hycamtin, SKB)

R = NH$_2$, 9-amino CPT
R = NO$_2$, 9-nitro CPT

irinotecan (camptosar, Daiichi/Upjohn)

GG-211 Gilead

homocamptothecin

FIGURE 1. Camptothecin and important congeners.

ring of camptothecins is a source of dynamic instability in the body.[4] Ring expansion is the first modification of the E-ring lactone that favorably addresses the dynamic instability problem while retaining activity. The broad structure–activity trends are currently accommodated by two different but related models for camptothecin binding to the topo I/DNA cleavable complex.[5–8]

The medicinal studies of the camptothecin family of antitumor agents have been driven by synthetic chemistry, and approaches to camptothecin analogues have advanced several times over the course of the past three decades. Many early analogues, including topotecan and irinotecan, were prepared from camptothecin itself by semi-synthesis. During the late 1970s, an approach to the camptothecin ring system based on the classical Friedlander condensation was established by several groups, and this has been used to make many of the known totally synthetic analogues of camptothecin.[9] Important new routes to the camptothecins have appeared over the last few years. These often focus on the parent but can be sufficiently general to provide new analogues by total synthesis.[10–19] Especially noteworthy is the route of Comins, variants of which have been used to make both GG-211 and homocamptothecin.

THE "CASCADE RADICAL ANNULATION" APPROACH TO CAMPTOTHECINS

In 1992, we introduced a fundamentally new route to the camptothecin class of molecules that involved a cascade radical reaction of isonitriles discovered earlier in our lab.[20,21] This "first-generation" route did not prove very practical for analogue synthesis, and a revamped "second-generation" route was introduced in 1995.[22] This synthesis transformed the "cascade radical route" to camptothecins into a method of major practical value. The two central steps in the radical cascade route are shown in FIGURE 2. Propargylation[23] of the enantiopure pyridone lactone 2 (step 1) fol-

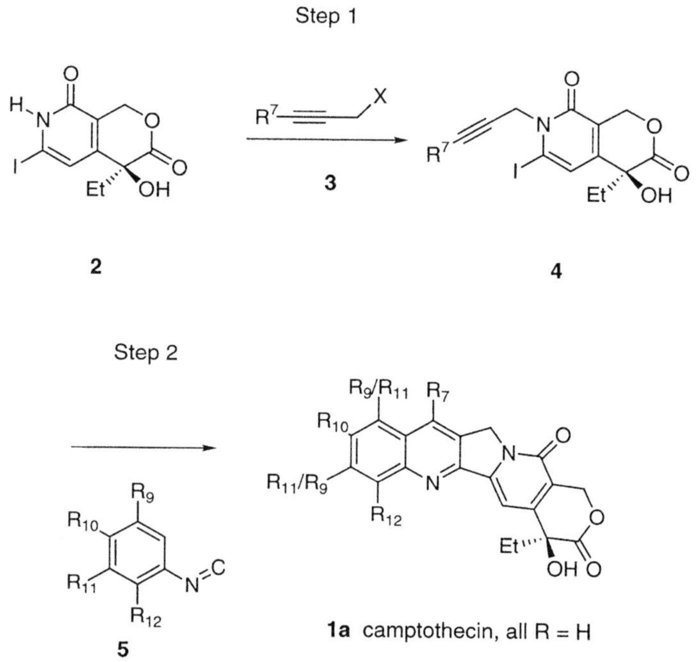

FIGURE 2. The cascade radical strategy is a combinatorial approach to the camptothecin class.

lowed by radical annulation with phenyl isonitrile or a substituted phenyl isonitrile (step 2) directly provides camptothecin (if all R = H) or an analogue. This cascade radical annulation step is the centerpiece of the synthesis. The route has high convergence and is suited to prepare most known types of camptothecins.

The radical cascade route is proving more general than the Friedlander and other routes to make camptothecin analogues. There are both strategic and tactical reasons for this. From the strategy standpoint, the radical cascade route is a true combinatorial approach that divides the molecule into three pieces (**2**, **3**, and **5**). Importantly, the B-ring carbon (C7) and its substituent (R^7) in **4** are divided from the A-ring and its substituents in **5**. This greatly simplifies the synthesis of the starting materials in

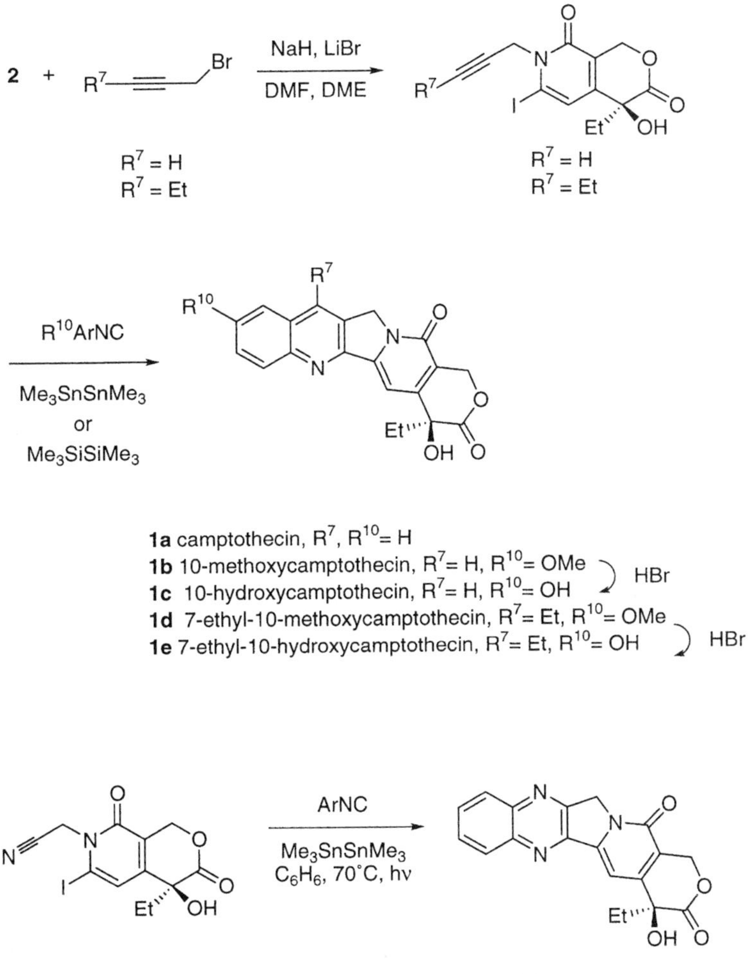

FIGURE 3. Synthesis of camptothecin and representative relatives.

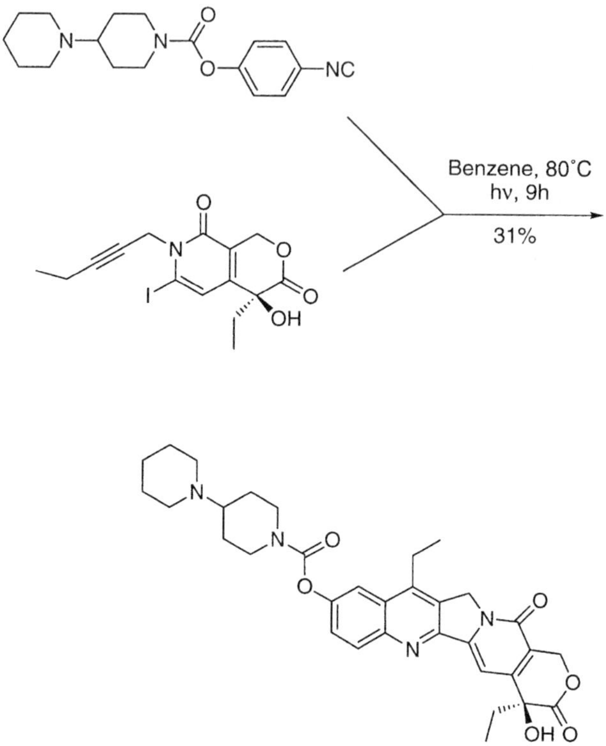

FIGURE 4. Direct synthesis of irinotecan.

addition to making the synthesis more modular. Additional advantages accrue because the radical cascade forms two rings in one step. From the tactical standpoint, the conditions for the radical reaction are much milder than those for the Friedlander condensation (more functional groups survive the key reaction), and the radical reaction is much more general (more components participate in the reaction).

The syntheses of a few representative camptothecin analogues by the cascade radical annulation route are summarized in FIGURE 3. Syntheses of 20(S)-camptothecin **1a**, 10-hydroxycamptothecin **1c** (a natural product and the standard precursor from which topotecan is made in one step), 10-hydroxy-7-ethyl camptothecin **1e** (SN-38), and 7-azacamptothecin **1f** (an active analogue never before made in nonracemic form[24,25]) are highlighted. These simple products are exemplary of the >30 known camptothecin derivatives that we have made over the last five years. Considerably more complex products have been made, including the FDA-approved irinotecan and lurtotecan (GG211). This work resoundingly demonstrates the generality and the versatility of the radical cascade route, and a full paper describing much of it has appeared.[26]

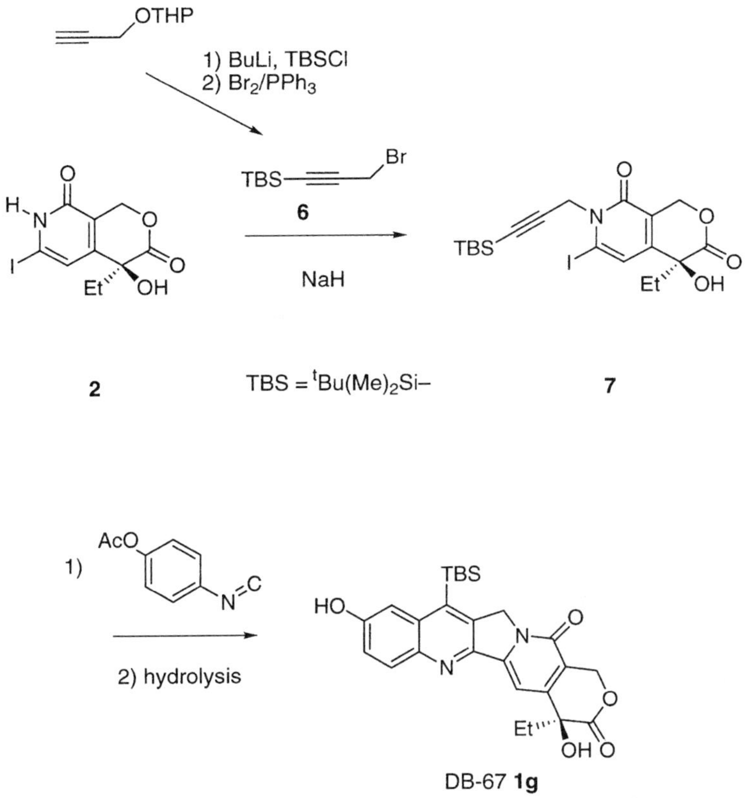

FIGURE 5. Synthesis of DB-67.

The direct synthesis of irinotecan **1d** is summarized in FIGURE 4. This is of special value because it does not pass through the active metabolite SN38 (**1e**). Thus, the method offers significant safety advantages since the synthesis of the (less toxic) prodrug does not pass through the (more toxic) drug.

In addition to making most of the important known camptothecin analogues, we have used the radical cascade route to make more than 200 new analogues of camptothecin. We chose compounds that would not be readily available by semi-synthesis or by the Friedlander approach. Early in this work, we made an important discovery: the introduction of a silyl group on the 7-position of camptothecin is highly beneficial. This has led to a new class of camptothecin derivatives that we have named "silatecans." A recent publication reveals the structure and preliminary cell and enzymes assays of about 25 silatecans.[27] More information about these compounds is found in the chapter by Professor Thomas Burke in this volume.

Among the several preclinical leads discovered, the most promising is 10-hydroxy-7-*t*-butyldimethylsilylcamptothecin.[28] This was synthesized by David Bom and currently goes by its notebook code: DB-67. The synthesis of DB-67 (**1g**) is representative of the other silatecans and is shown in FIGURE 5. The THP ether of pro-

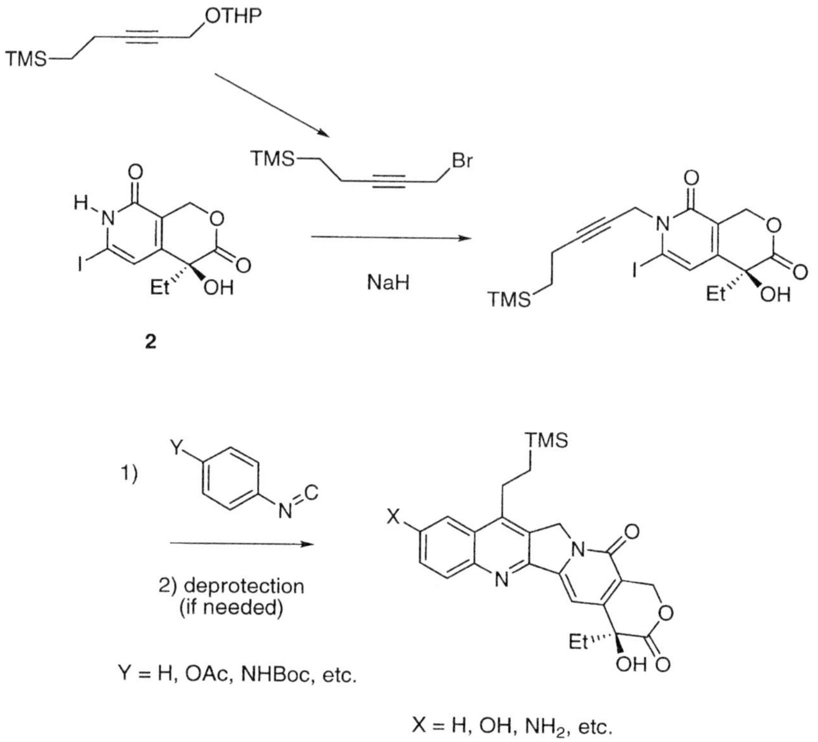

FIGURE 6. Synthesis of alkylene spaced silatecans.

pargyl alcohol is silylated and then brominated to provide the requisite propargylating agent **6**. This is then used to *N*-propargylate pyridone lactone **2** to give radical precursor **7**. Reaction of **7** with readily available *p*-acetoxyphenyl isonitrile followed by deacylation provides DB-67 (**1g**). DB-67 has been made on >10 gram scale, and the material is now being used for formulation, toxicology, and other preclinical studies. Over 100 g of the key precursor **2** have been prepared in enantiomerically pure form. Thus, the cascade annulation route not only provides large numbers of derivatives due to its combinatorial nature, but it also provides large quantities of derivatives.

Silatecans can also be made with an alkyl spacer in between the ring and the silyl group by simply preparing the requisite propargyl bromide and using it to alkylate the key lactone pyridone precursor **2**. Examples of several that have been made are shown in FIGURE 6.

Analogue work on the original silatecan class of molecules has been suspended, and, with the selection of DB-67 by the NCI RAID (Rapid Access to Intervention Development) program,[29] work on this class of compounds has focused on preclinical development. On the synthesis front, the clear yet different advantages shown by the silatecans and homocamptothecin suggested that a combination of the two features might be valuable, so we set out to make a new class of molecules called

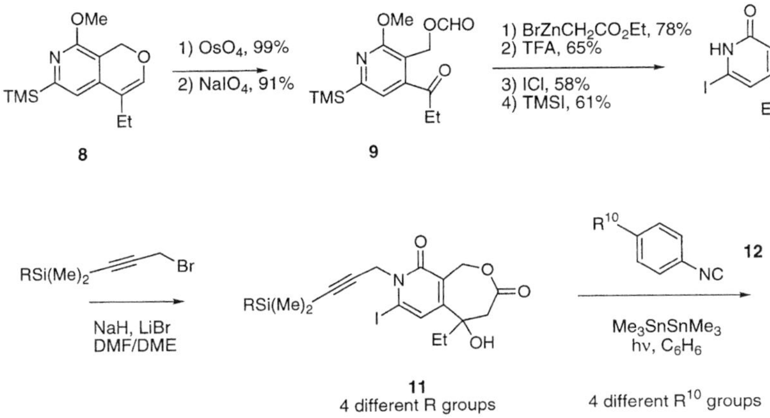

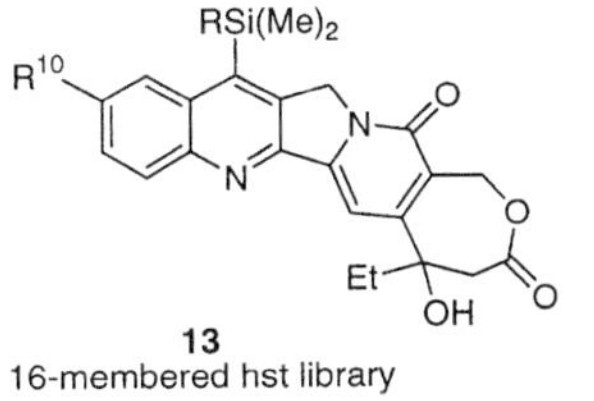

R^{10} \ R	Et	Pr	i-Pr	i-Bu
CH_3O	36%	35%	41%	37%
CH_3	49%	27%	31%	32%
F	28%	24%	27%	27%
CF_3	31%	44%	37%	37%

FIGURE 7. Combinatorial synthesis of homosilatecans.

homosilatecans (hst). First, a synthesis of the racemic DE radical ring precursor **10** was developed (FIG. 7), and four new "homosilatecan" analogues were prepared. Three of the new homosilatecans were markedly superior to homocamptothecin in terms of human blood stability and lipophilicity.[30] Next, a library of 16 new homosilatecans **13** was made, and these are now being evaluated.

The synthesis of the first homosilatecan library is summarized in FIGURE 7. The key ring expanded lactone-pyridone **10** was prepared on gram scale in racemic form. Next, small quantities (about 50–100 mg) were separately propargylated under standard conditions to make four new precursors **11**. These compounds bear different silyl groups (R) at the terminus of the propargyl group. The 16-compound library was then made by synthesizing all possible combinations of the four lactone pyridones **11** with four isonitriles **12**. This initial library was prepared by hand and purified by flash chromatography, but the preparation, purification, and analysis in subsequent libraries have been expedited by using facilities in the University of Pittsburgh's Center for Combinatorial Chemistry.

In the more recent libraries, the reagent and reactants are mixed in small vials. These are placed collectively in front of a sunlamp and simultaneously irradiated for two hours. The vials are then transferred to a Hewlett-Packard solution-phase synthesizer, which works the reactions up by solid-phase extraction and evaporation. This workup removes the tin, excess isonitrile, and other impurities, and provides new homosilatecans in reasonable purities (70–90%). However, these purities are not sufficient for testing, so the library is then purified on a Gilson serial HPLC with a robot liquid handler. This convenient instrument provides start-to-finish automated purification with no intervention. Finally, the tubes containing the product were concentrated on a vacuum centrifuge to give 5–10 mg of each pure silatecan, which was characterized by automated LC/MS. We are just completing the synthesis of a 115-member library of new homosilatecan derivatives, and this is described in a poster in this volume.

CONCLUSIONS

The cascade radical annulation approach to the camptothecin family of antitumor agents has important ramifications from the standpoint of both synthetic and medicinal chemistry. From the synthesis vantage point, the work shows the power of cascade radical reactions to quickly make complex molecules under exceedingly mild conditions. From the standpoint of combinatorial synthetic strategy, it also shows the importance of building rings in diversity-generating steps, as opposed to the more common strategy of appending diversity elements onto existing rings. From the standpoint of medicinal chemistry, the synthesis is an enabling technology. It allows the evaluation of a wide variety of analogues that would be difficult or impossible to make by other routes.

ACKNOWLEDGMENTS

We thank the National Institutes of Health for funding this work. Support on instrumentation for the Center for Combinatorial Chemistry from Hewlett-Packard, Parke-Davis, Merck, and the University of Pittsburgh is also gratefully acknowledged. We also warmly thank our biological collaborators, Dr. Yves Pommier, Dr. T.-C. Chou, and especially Professor Thomas Burke, and their respective co-workers.

REFERENCES

1. POTMESIL, H. & H. PINEDO, Eds. 1995. Camptothecins: New Anticancer Agents. CRC Press. Boca Raton, FL.
2. PANTAZIS, P. & B.C. GIOVANELLA, Eds. 1996. The Camptothecins: From Discovery to Patient. Ann. N.Y. Acad. Sci. **803**: 335pp.
3. LAVERGNE, O., L. LESUEUR-GINOT, F. PLA RODAS & D.C.H. BIGG. 1997. BN80245: an E-ring modified camptothecin with potent antiproliferative and topoisomerase I inhibitory activities. Bioorg. Med. Chem. Lett. **7**: 2235–2238.
4. BURKE, T.G., A.E. STAUBUS, A.K. MISHRA & H. MALAK. Liposomal stabilization of camptothecins lactone ring. J. Am. Chem. Soc. **114**: 8318–8319.
5. LIMA, C.D., J.C. WANG & A. MONDRAGON. 1994. 3-Dimensional structure of the 67K N-terminal fragment of *E. coli* DNA topoisomerase-I. Nature **367**: 138–146.
6. FAN, Y.W., K.W. KOHN, L. SHI & Y. POMMIER. 1998. Molecular modeling studies of the DNA-topoisomerase I ternary cleavable complex with camptothecin. J. Med. Chem. **41**: 2216–2226.

7. REDINBO, M.R., L. STEWART, P. KUHN, et al. 1998. Crystal structures of human topoisomerase I in covalent and noncovalent complexes with DNA. Science **279:** 1504–1513.
8. STEWART, L., M.R. REDINBO, X.Y. QIU, et al. 1998. A model for the mechanism of human topoisomerase I. Science **279:** 1534–1541.
9. SCHULTZ, A.G. 1973. Camptothecin. Chem. Rev. **73:** 385–405.
10. COMINS, D.L., M.F. BAEVSKY & H. HONG. 1992. A 10-step, asymmetric synthesis of (S)-camptothecin. J. Am. Chem. Soc. **114:** 10971–10972.
11. WANG, S., C.A. COBURN, W.G. BORNMANN & S.J. DANISHEFSKY. 1993. Concise total syntheses of D,L-camptothecin and related anticancer drugs. J. Org. Chem. **58:** 611–617.
12. COMINS, D.L., H. HONG & G. JIANHUA. 1994. Asymmetric synthesis of camptothecin alkaloids: a nine-step synthesis of (S)-camptothecin. Tetrahedron Lett. **35:** 5331–5334.
13. COMINS, D.L., H. HONG, J.K. SAHA & J.H. GAO. 1994. A six-step synthesis of (+/−)-camptothecin. J. Org. Chem. **59:** 5120–5121.
14. RAO, A.V.R., J.S. YADAV & V. MURALIKRISHNA. 1994. Regioselective synthesis of camptothecin. Tetrahedron Lett. **35:** 3613–3616.
15. FANG, F.G., S.P. XIE & M.W. LOWERY. 1994. Catalytic enantioselective synthesis of 20(S)-camptothecin: a practical application of the sharpless asymmetric dihydroxylation reaction. J. Org. Chem. **59:** 6142–6143.
16. COMINS, D.L. & J.K. SAHA. 1995. Asymmetric synthesis of a key camptothecin intermediate from 2-fluoropyridine. Tetrahedron Lett. **36:** 7995–7998.
17. FORTUNAK, J.M.D., A.R. MASTROCOLA, M. MELLINGER, et al. 1996. Novel syntheses of camptothecin alkaloids. 1. Intramolecular [4+2] cycloadditions of N-arylimidates and 4H-3,1-benzoxazin-4-ones as 2-aza-1,3-dienes. Tetrahedron Lett. **37:** 5679–5682.
18. FORTUNAK, J.M.D., J. KITTERINGHAM, A.R. MASTROCOLA, et al. 1996. Novel syntheses of camptothecin alkaloids. 2. Concise synthesis of (S)-camptothecins. Tetrahedron Lett. **37:** 5683–5686.
19. CIUFOLINI, M.A. & F. ROSCHANGAR. 1996. Total synthesis of (+)-camptothecin. Angew. Chem. Int. Ed. **35:** 1692–1694.
20. CURRAN, D.P. & H. LIU. 1992. New 4+1 radical annulations—a formal total synthesis of (+/−)-camptothecin. J. Am. Chem. Soc. **114:** 5863–5864.
21. CURRAN, D.P., H. LIU, H. JOSIEN & S.B. KO. 1996. Tandem radical reactions of isonitriles with 2-pyridonyl and other aryl radicals: scope and limitations, and a first generation synthesis of (+/−)-camptothecin. Tetrahedron **52:** 11385–11404.
22. CURRAN, D.P., S.B. KO & H. JOSIEN. 1995. Cascade radical reactions of isonitriles: a second-generation synthesis of 20(S)-camptothecin, topotecan, irinotecan, and GI-147211C. Angew. Chem. Int. Ed. **34:** 2683–2684.
23. LIU, H., S.B. KO, H. JOSIEN & D.P. CURRAN. 1995. Selective N-functionalization of 6-substituted-2-pyridones. Tetrahedron Lett. **36:** 8917–8920.
24. SAWADA, S., S. MATSUOKA, K. NOKATA, et al. 1991. Synthesis and antitumor activity of 20(S)-camptothecin derivatives: A-ring modified and 7,10-disubstituted camptothecins. Chem. Pharm. Bull. **39:** 3183.
25. SAWADA, S., S. OKAJIMA, R. AIYAMA, et al. 1991. Synthesis and antitumor activity of 20(S)-camptothecin derivatives: carbamate-linked, water-soluble derivatives of 7-ethyl-10- hydroxycamptothecin. Chem. Pharm. Bull. **39:** 1446.
26. CURRAN, D.P., D. BOM & H. JOSIEN. 1998. A general synthetic approach to the 20(S)-camptothecin family of antitumor agents by a regiocontrolled cascade radical cyclization of arylisonitriles. Chem. Eur. J. **7:** 67–81.
27. JOSIEN, H., D. BOM, D.P. CURRAN, et al. 1997. 7-Silylcamptothecins (silatecans): a new family of camptothecin antitumor agents. Bioorg. Med. Chem. Lett. **7:** 3189–3295.
28. POLLACK, I.F., M. ERFF, D. BOM, et al. 1999. Potent topoisomerase I inhibition by novel silatecans eliminates glioma proliferation in vitro and in vivo. Cancer Res. **59:** 4898–4905.
29. http://dtp.nci.nih.gov/
30. BOM, D., D.P. CURRAN, A.J. CHAVAN, et al. 1999. Novel A,B,E-ring-modified camptothecins display high lipophilicity and markedly improved human blood stabilities. J. Med. Chem. **42:** 3018–3022.

Structure–Activity Relationship of Alkyl Camptothecin Esters

ZHISONG CAO,[a] PANAYOTIS PANTAZIS, JOHN MENDOZA, JANET EARLY, ANTHONY KOZIELSKI, NICK HARRIS, DANA VARDEMAN, JOACHIM LIEHR, JOHN S. STEHLIN, AND BEPPINO GIOVANELLA[a]

The Stehlin Foundation for Cancer Research and St. Joseph Hospital Cancer Laboratory, Houston, Texas 77003, USA

ABSTRACT: The cytotoxicity of camptothecin (CPT) esters 1–6 was measured. Like parental camptothecin, esters 2 and 3, but not 1, 4, 5, and 6, inhibited proliferation of human leukemia cells in culture and induced programmed cell death as assessed by flow cytometry studies. Exhibition of similar levels of antiproliferative activities of CPT 2 and 3 required different incubation time periods in cell cultures, with CPT and 3 requiring the shortest and longest periods, respectively. Both 2 and 3 were inactive against cells resistant to the semisynthetic CPT derivative 9-nitrocamptothecin and unable to stabilize DNA-topoisomerase I (Topo I) "cleavable complexes" in a cell-free system, suggesting that Topo I activity was required but insufficient for the mechanism of action of 2 and 3. Mouse liver homogenate converted esters to parental CPT, but the conversion rates were different with different esters. Of four tested esters in this experiment, ester 2 had the fastest conversion rate. *In vivo* studies showed that ester 2 had an exceptional lack of toxicity in nude mice, even at enormous doses, and demonstrated extensive activity against human breast and colon tumors grown as xenografts in immunodeficient nude mice, whereas no antitumor activity was observed for the other esters. In conclusion, ester 2 is a prodrug of the antitumor compound CPT, and it can be administered at very high doses in mice with no appearance of toxicity. This study provides a basis for further evaluation of CPT ester 2 as an investigational anticancer agent.

INTRODUCTION

Camptothecin (CPT) is a naturally occurring alkaloid. The structure of this compound was established by Wall *et al*. in 1966.[1] Camptothecin functions as an inhibitor of topoisomerase I, an enzyme that plays an important role in DNA replication.[2] Although camptothecin has potent antitumor activity, it has a serious problem with toxicity. The clinical use of this compound as an anticancer agent is thus limited. In order to overcome this problem, researchers have made extensive efforts to modify the camptothecin molecule. Over the years, many new CPT derivatives have been prepared.[3–20] Whereas until now the derivatives made have not met the criterion that

---

[a]Address for correspondence: Zhisong Cao, Ph.D., or Beppino Giovanella, The Stehlin Foundation for Cancer Research, 1918 Chenevert Street, Houston, TX 77003. Voice: 713-756-5750; fax: 713-756-5783.
zcao@pipeline.com

the inherent antitumor activity of CPT be maintained while the toxicity is reduced, they have offered important information about critical structural features necessary for activity.

Clinical trials and structure–activity studies have shown that the intact α-hydroxy lactone of the CPT molecule is required for maximum activity.[21] The sodium salts of the open form of CPT lactone have severe toxicity and much lower activity than the intact lactone itself. For example,[7] one antitumor assay with the carboxylate sodium salt of CPT against P388 rodent leukemia cells showed that this open form of the compound has only one-tenth of the potency of the lactone molecule. This confirmed the importance of the intact lactone ring E for both passive diffusion of the drug into cancer cells as well as interaction with its cellular target, topoisomerase I. It is now well established that the physiological plasma pH 7.4 and human blood components variably affect conversion of the lactone to the carboxylate form of each CPT derivative, with the water-insoluble compounds being more susceptible to this conversion. More information about structural and functional properties of various CPT derivatives and their stabilization in the bloodstream can be found in literature.[22–24]

In our laboratory, CPT has shown a spectacular level of activity against a wide spectrum of human tumors grown as xenografts in nude mice, but very little activity in clinical trials with cancer patients.[25–27] This difference in antitumor activity has been associated with the finding that the hydrolysis of CPT lactone to carboxylate is much faster in human plasma.[24,26] Thus, to extend the biological life span of the active drug by protecting the lactone moiety of the molecule is critical to the drug's development. Our hypothesis is that modification of the CPT molecule at position 20 by attaching a water-insoluble ester side chain will stabilize the intact lactone ring; and, if so, the potency of the drug will be increased, and the toxicity will be decreased. The first water-insoluble alkyl ester, camptothecin 20(S)-acetate, was prepared by Wall *et al.* in 1966[1] and then prepared in our laboratory with a modified procedure.[28] This ester was tested against the L1210 system and was inactive.[29]

Previously, we reported the synthesis of six alkyl camptothecin esters.[28,30] In this report, we describe biological studies that indicate a relationship between the antitumor activity and the length of the ester side chain for these alkyl CPT esters.

MATERIALS AND METHODS

Drugs

All CPT esters used in the biological studies described in this report were prepared according to our previous reports.[28,30]

Determination of Drug-Induced Antiproliferative Activity and Toxicity in Cultured Cells

To assess the antiproliferative activity of the various CPT esters, identical cell cultures received equimolar concentrations of these esters, and the cell number per milliliter was counted. Stocks consisted of fine suspensions of esters in polyethylene glycol (PEG-400; Aldrich). Control cultures received only the carrier. The cell num-

TABLE 1. Growth inhibition of U-937 cells treated with CPT esters

Treatment	Growth percent (at 120 hr)
Untreated cells	100
+CPT	0
+CPT-acetate 1	92 ± 4
+Ester 2	31 ± 2
+Ester 3	44 ± 2
+Ester 4	96 ± 5
+Ester 5	92 ± 5
+Ester 6	94 ± 4

ber was counted at 24, 72, and 120 hours of treatment. Control compounds included the parental compound CPT as a positive control and the CPT ester 1 (CPT-acetate) as a negative control. The targeted cells included the HL-60 and U-937 cell lines, which have shown differential sensitivity to CPT congeners. The results for growth inhibition of U-937 cells treated with CPT esters are shown in TABLE 1.

Flow cytometry analysis was used to identify the cell cycle phase targeted by the esters and quantify the extent of ester-induced cell death (apoptosis). The virtues of flow cytometry over other methods to study drug-induced cell cycle perturbations and apoptosis have been reviewed.[22,31] Cell cycle perturbations and apoptotic fractions were determined with an Epics-Elite laser flow cytometer (Coulter Corp., Hialeah, FL) and analyzed with the Multicycle program (Phoenix Flow Systems, San Diego, CA). Flow cytometry methodology has routinely been used at our laboratory to study anticancer drugs including various CPT congeners.[22,23,31]

Preparation of Liver Homogenate

A 6-month-old, super Swiss female mouse was sacrificed, and the liver was surgically removed and placed in a Dounce homogenizer standing in ice. Approximately four volumes of ice-cold 0.5 M KCl were added, and the liver was homogenized with 20 strokes of a tight-fitting pestle. The homogenate was centrifuged at 15000×g for 15 min at 4°C, and the supernatant was transferred to a glass container standing on ice. This supernatant, hereafter called liver homogenate, was used for incubation of the 2 ester.

Incubation of Ester in Liver Homogenate

The homogenate was transferred from 4°C to a 37°C waterbath and incubated for 10 min. Subsequently, ester in DMSO (10 mg/ml) was added to the homogenate and mixed well. The final concentrations of ester and DMSO in the incubated mixture were 10 µg/ml and 0.1%, respectively. An aliquot was removed (0-time aliquot), and incubation continued at 37°C. Aliquots were subsequently removed at 6 hr, 24 hr, and 48 hr of the incubation period. Each aliquot removed was immediately mixed with four volumes of ice-cold acidified ethanol, and stored at −20°C. When all samples were collected, they were centrifuged at 15,000×g for 10 min to remove the precipi-

TABLE 2. Determination of percent conversion of esters 2–4 in mouse liver homogenate

Time (hr)	Ester 2		Ester 3		Ester 4		Ester 5	
	% 2	% CPT	% 3	% CPT	% 4	% CPT	% 5	% CPT
0	88	0	79	0	88	0	93	0
6	48	52	50	50	55	26	73	15
24	20	68	45	54	54	27	72	17
48	10	79	34	57	51	35	70	16

tated protein. The clarified supernatant was then analyzed for ester and CPT contents by HPLC using fluorescence spectroscopy. The results are shown in TABLE 2.

Incubation of Ester 2 in PBS

Ester 2 was finely suspended in PBS. The final concentration of 2 in PBS was 1000 ng/ml. The suspension was incubated at 37°C. A 100-µl portion of PBS suspension was removed at time points of 0, 6, 24, and 48 hr and analyzed by HPLC.

HPLC Procedure for the Determination of Percent Conversion of Esters

A 100-µl portion of solution was taken from the top homogeneous layer of the above-centrifuged mixture, injected through a 2-ml loop onto a C-8 Microsorb column, and chromatographed with 45% methanol in water—10 mM ammonium formate (pH 2.0) as mobile phase. The components of the drug were detected by a fluorescence detector at 347/418 nm. The peaks were integrated, and the percent conversion for each ester was determined. CPT has a characteristic retention time of 3.5 min, and esters have retention times in the range of 12.0 to 14.0 min.

General Procedure for Measurements of in Vivo Toxicity and Antitumor Activity

All the animal experiments were performed on nude Swiss mice of the National Institutes of Health high-fertility strain. They were bred and raised in our laboratory under strict pathogen-free conditions.[32] The tumors used for the anticancer activity determination were human xenografts originally obtained from human biopsies and then carried in our laboratory by serial transplantation from nude mouse to nude mouse. For the in vivo toxicity and antitumor activity determination, a tumor xenograft growing in a nude mouse, approximately 1 cm^3 in size, was excised sterilely, minced finely with iridectomy scissors, and suspended in RPMI tissue culture medium at the ratio 1:10 vol/vol. One-half of 1 ml of this suspension, containing about 50 mg tumor mince wet-weight, was inoculated subcutaneously on the upper half of the dorsal thorax of the mouse. Groups of six animals were used. The drug (ester) was finely suspended in cottonseed oil and was then injected into the stomach cavity of the mouse through the anterior abdominal wall by using a 26-gauge needle. The weekly schedule previously established for 9-nitrocamptothecin injection was once a day, five days on, and two days off. This schedule was employed throughout all the animal experiments. Treatment was initiated when the tumor had an exponential growth and reached a volume of about 200 mm^3, that is, when it had become well-vascularized. Tumors growing in animals were checked and measured with a caliper once a week.

RESULTS AND DISCUSSION

The structural drawings of alkyl CPT esters 1–6 are shown in FIGURE 1. CPT ester 1, camptothecin acetate, was reported by Wall et al. in 1966 and was prepared with acetic anhydride as the acylating agent.[1] This compound was recently prepared in our laboratory with trichloroethane as an acylating agent.[28] The detailed syntheses of esters 2–6 are described in our previous article.[30]

The relative antiproliferative activity of the esters in cell cultures was investigated. The antiproliferative activity of the CPT esters was assayed in cultures of human HL-60 and U-937 leukemia cells. The negative controls, that is, 100% cell growth, included untreated cultures and cultures treated with an inactive ester 1, camptothecin 20(S)-acetate. The parental compound CPT served as the positive control, that

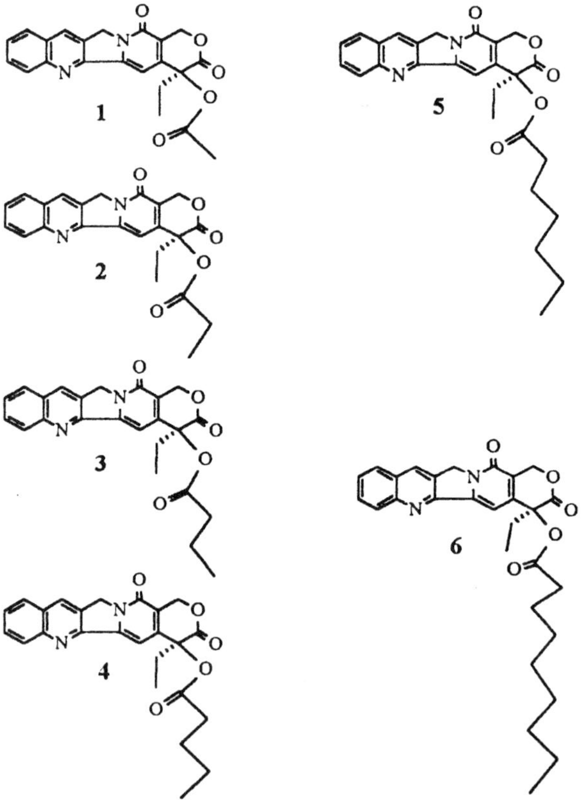

FIGURE 1. Structures of esters 1–6.

is, 100% growth inhibition agent. The study compared the effectiveness of equimolar ester concentrations over various periods of treatment. The results indicated that concentrations lower than 0.2 µM were completely ineffective for some of the esters, whereas CPT concentrations higher than 0.2 µM had killed all the cells very rapidly at 120 hr. TABLE 1 summarizes the results of growth inhibition of U-937 cells treated with 0.2 µM of esters for 120 hr. CPT completely inhibited growth and induced cell death as monitored by microscopy, whereas esters 1, 4, 5, and 6 were virtually unable to exhibit any growth inhibitory effect. In contrast, esters 2 and 3 dramatically inhibited cell growth, although not as effectively as CPT. It was also apparent that 2 was more potent than 3. A similar pattern of responses was observed for HL-60 cells treated with the various esters and CPT (results not shown), but the extent of growth inhibition differed from that observed for U-937 cells, suggesting a cell type–dependent drug effectiveness (also see results of flow cytometry below). Because of these observations, we extended our studies to investigate the patterns of cell cycle perturbations induced by these esters. It has been demonstrated that CPT-treated cancer cells are initially arrested in late S-phase, and subsequently die by apoptosis, whereas CPT-treated normal and normal-like cells are arrested in the boundary of late-S/G_2 and do not undergo apoptotic death. Further, after a critical period of S-phase arrest, the cancer cells die even after CPT is removed from the culture, whereas removal of CPT from cultures of S/G_2-arrested normal cells allows these cells to re-enter cycling.[23,33] The differential response of normal and cancer cells to CPT is not understood yet, but it is very likely associated with differentially regulated cyclins. However, this differential effect of CPT on normal and cancer cells has not been reported for other anticancer drugs except thymidine.[34]

Drug-induced cell cycle perturbations and apoptosis were monitored and quantitated by flow cytometry, a method that we have routinely used to study effectiveness of various anticancer drugs including CPT congeners.[22,23,35] FIGURE 2 shows the results (histograms) of a flow cytometry study of the drug-treated HL-60 cells. In pilot experiments, it was found that CPT concentrations above 0.02 µM were highly toxic for HL-60 but not for U-937 cells. Therefore, the control compound CPT was used at 0.02 µM and 0.2 µM in the studies of HL-60 and U-937 cells, respectively. Untreated HL-60 cells showed no difference in the histograms at 24 hr, 72 hr, and 120 hr, while the apoptotic fraction remained at low levels of 2–5% (histograms A,H,O). On the other hand, 0.02 µM CPT induced perturbations in the cell cycle fractions and increased apoptotic death, which became more extensive as the treatment period was prolonged (B,I,P). CPT-acetate 1 induced small cell cycle perturbations (C,J,Q), which had no significant inhibitory effect on the cell growth. Further, ester 2 had no effect on the cell cycle at 24 hr (D), but dramatic perturbations were observed at 72 hr of treatment (K), which were followed by the appearance of a significant apoptotic fraction of 15% in the cultures as the treatment was extended to 120 hr (R). Further, significant cell cycle perturbations were observed at 120 hr of treatment with 3 (S), but not at shorter periods of treatment (E,L). These results suggested that the 2 activity appears faster than the 3 activity. Finally, esters 4 (F,M,T), 5 (G,N,U), and 6 (histograms not shown) were completely ineffective in inducing detectable perturbations in the cell cycle at any time within the 120-hr treatment. Since U-937 cells are less sensitive than HL-60 cells to CPT, we also compared by flow cytometry the sensitivity of the U-937 cells to the CPT esters including the negative control, CPT-ac-

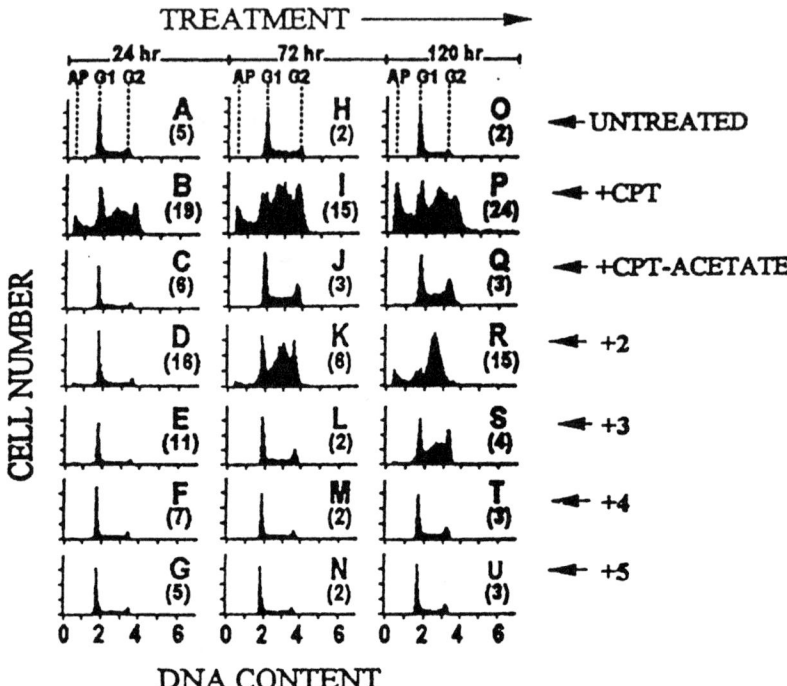

FIGURE 2. Histograms of U-937 cells treated with CPT esters. *Top*: Treatment with CPT, CPT-acetate, and esters 2–5 for 120 hours (5 days). *Bottom*: Extended treatment with CPT-acetate and esters 2–4 for 240 hours (10 days).

etate 1. All drugs were used at a final concentration of 0.2 µM. The resulting histograms are shown in FIGURE 3. Growth of the untreated cells had virtually ceased, and the cells were mostly arrested at G_1 at 120 hr as the culture reached confluence (A,H,O). Similar results were observed in the cell cultures treated with CPT-acetate 1 (C,J,Q), esters 4 (F,M,T), 5 (G,N,U), and 6 (histograms not shown). A low grade of induction of perturbations was detected in 3-treated cells (E,L,S), whereas ester 2 induced extensive perturbations and apoptosis (D,K,R). It should be noted that the side chains of the alkyl esters 2 and 3 contain 2 and 3 carbon atoms, respectively, whereas more carbon atoms are contained in the side chains of esters 4, 5 and 6 (see FIG. 1). Therefore, it appears that the 2- and 3-carbon side chains delay the exhibition of biological activity, whereas chains with 1 carbon (CPT-acetate 1), or 4 carbons (4), or more (5 and 6) completely hinder the activity. Finally, the U-937 cells were more susceptible than HL-60 cells to ester 2 treatment for the same period (compare FIG. 2, K to FIG. 3, K and FIG. 2, R to FIG. 3, R). This higher sensitivity of U-937 cells to ester 2 was observed reproducibly, and it is rather unlikely to be due to the small difference in generation times of the cells (21 hr for U-937 cells and 24 hr for HL-60 cells), but other possibilities exist including differences in ester-metabolizing enzymes, cell cycle- and apoptosis-regulating enzymes and factors, and so forth.

The delayed responses of both the leukemia HL-60 and U-937 cells to 2 and particularly 3 (see FIGS. 2 and 3) suggested that longer treatment with these esters was required for exhibition of increased biological activity. Again, this possibility was investigated by flow cytometry analysis of U-937 cells (FIG. 3, AA to OO) treated with 2 (histograms DD, II, NN,), 3 (EE, JJ, OO) and 4 (CC, HH, MM) compared to control cells in untreated cultures (AA, FF, KK) and cultures treated with CPT-acetate 1 (BB, GG, LL) for a period up to 10 days. Untreated cells or cells treated with 1 and 4 were arrested at G_1 by day 6 because of confluence (AA,BB,CC), then started to die by apoptosis as they remained in culture for 8 (FF, GG, HH) and 10 (KK, LL, MM) days. In contrast, esters 2 and 3 resulted in increased depletion of the G_1 population at days 6 (DD, EE), 8 (II, JJ) and 10 (NN,OO) because the cells traversing the S phase were arrested there, then died by apoptosis. At day 10, no live cells were detected in the 2-treated culture (NN), whereas some cells were still alive in the 3-treated culture (OO). These results confirmed our previous observations (FIGS. 2 and 3) that ester 3 exhibited more delayed biological activity than ester 2. In addition, the delayed exhibition of CPT activity by 2 suggested that ester 2 could be a prodrug requiring metabolic conversion to the parental compound CPT. This metabolic conversion was confirmed by the action of a mouse liver enzyme(s), presumably an esterase, that de-esterified esters by cleaving the side ester bond (TABLE 2). The results of TABLE 2 show that ester 2 (which has a shorter C_2-ester chain) has the fastest conversion rate and ester 5 (which has a longer C_5-ester chain) has the lowest conversion rate, implying that the conversion rate of esters to the parental CPT is related with the length of side alkyl ester chain. In order to confirm that the conversion of esters to CPT in mouse liver homogenate is catalyzed by enzymes (or esterases) and does not occurr by simple hydrolysis, a portion of powders of ester 2 was suspended in PBS and incubated at 37°C for 48 hours. No conversion was observed by HPLC analysis.

In one study we found that ester 2 concentrations that induced apoptosis in U-937 cells were completely ineffective in inducing apoptosis in 9NC-resistant U-937 cells that contained either normal levels of topoisomerase I unable to bind 9NC[36] or very low levels of this enzyme.[37] In another study, 10 μM 2 failed to sustain DNA degradation induced by the nuclear enzyme topoisomerase I in a cell-free system, whereas complete DNA degradation was observed in presence of 0.1 μM CPT (results not shown). Together these results and the results described earlier in this report indicated to us that intact topoisomerase I was required for exhibition of the 2 activity, and confirmed that 2 was devoid of the "topoisomerase I-poisoning" activity known to be exhibited by the parental CPT.[23,31,38] In other words, topoisomerase-I is insufficient for showing 2 activity. An enzymatic metabolism for releasing the active parental CPT has to be involved. The interaction between CPT esters and a metabolic enzyme, presumably an esterase, requires a strict spatial fitness. A shorter or a longer side ester chain is not spatially suitable for the interaction. Only those esters with a 2- or 3-carbon side chain showed the delayed activity.

Overall, the results from TABLE 1 together with the observations obtained from cell cultures indicate that, of these tested esters, ester 2 is active, ester 3 is slightly active, and the other esters are not active. Thus, the *in vitro* assays showed a cell antiproliferative order of 2>3>1~4-6.

The results obtained from *in vivo* assays correlated well with the *in vitro* observations. For example, esters 2–5 were tested against human CLO breast carcinomas

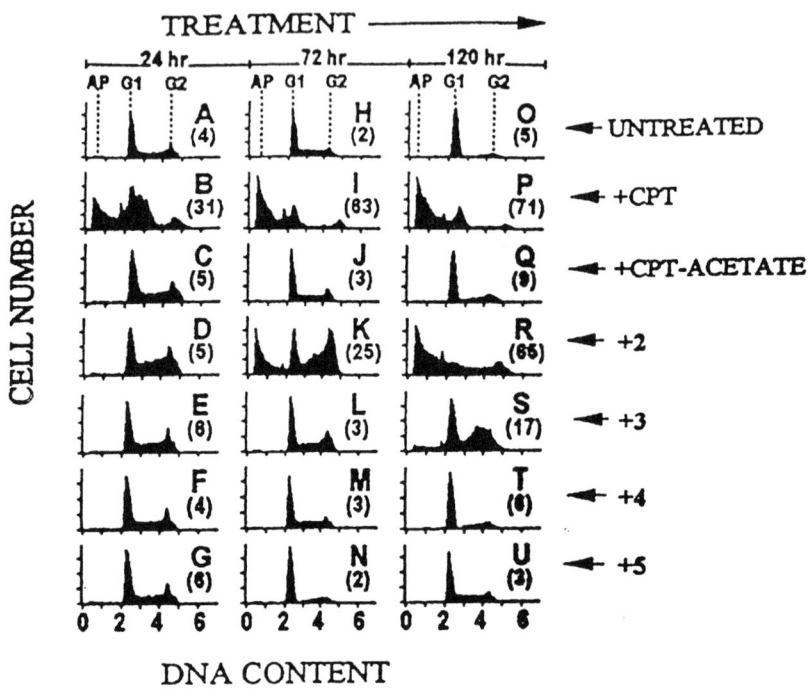
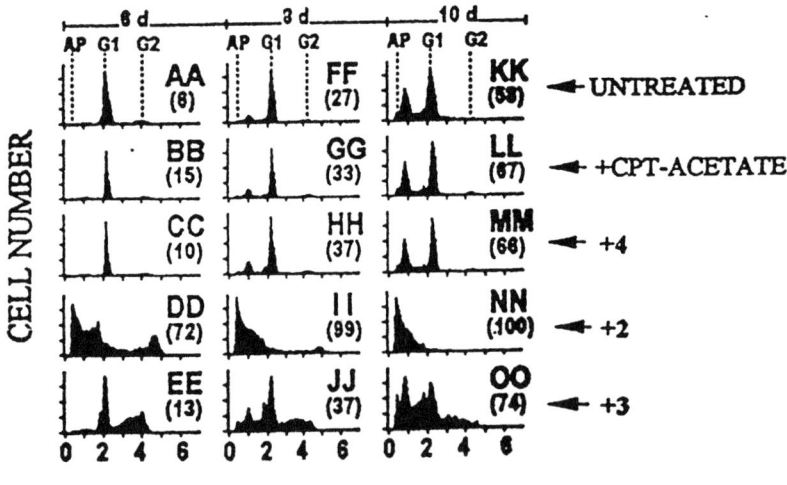

FIGURE 3. Histograms of the treatment of HL-60 cells with CPT esters. G1 = G0 + G1; G2 = G2 + M; AP = apoptosis. The numbers in parentheses indicate percentage of apoptotic cells in the cell culture.

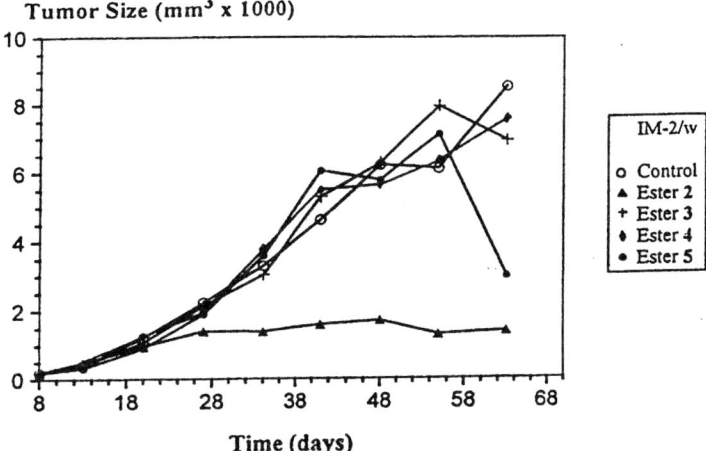

FIGURE 4. Antitumor activity of esters 2–5 against human breast carcinoma with a dose of 4 mg/kg. Animals were treated 13 times and sacrificed at day 69. The treatments were stopped at day 51.

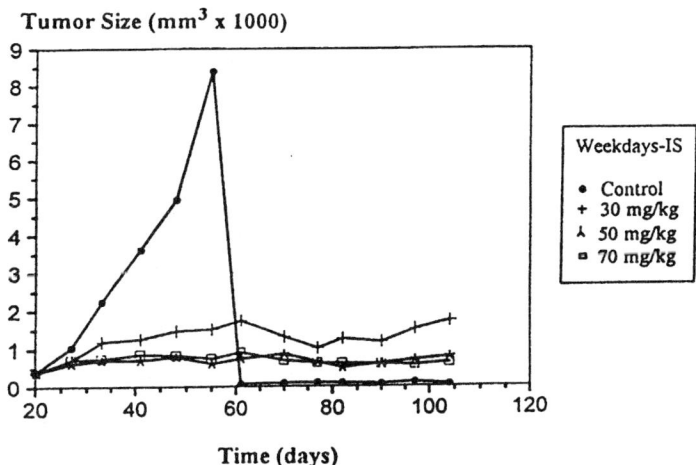

FIGURE 5. Antitumor activity against human colon carcinoma with different doses. Animals were treated in groups of 5. Control mice (4 out of 5) were sacrificed on day 56 because of large tumors.

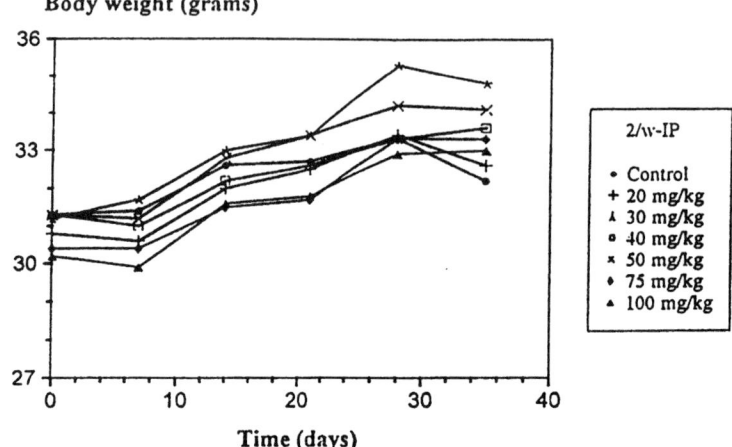

FIGURE 6. Toxicity of prodrug 2 in nude mice at different doses.

in nude mice grown as xenografts with a twice-weekly dose of 4 mg/kg. The experimental results are shown in FIGURE 4. It is clear from FIGURE 4 that only the group of mice treated with ester 2 showed the tumor growth inhibition. Esters 3–5 failed to show any antitumor activity at this dose level. The antitumor ability of ester 2 was also tested against several tumors of diverse tissue origin grown as xenografts in nude mice treated with various nontoxic doses. The effect of ester 2 on the size and growth inhibition of a human colon tumor is shown in FIGURE 5. Mice in the control group were dead at day 56. All doses of ester 2 applied in this experiment induced tumor growth inhibition. It is possible that diverse types of tumors exhibit various esterase activities, and therefore, regression of these tumors will require different 2 doses. In other words, variability in esterase activity may be an important determinant of conversion of 2 to parental CPT and subsequent effectiveness. If this were the case, then strategies would be developed to increase the conversion of ester 2 to CPT lactone near or at a specific tumored tissue.

The *in vivo* toxicity was also measured in terms of body weight. In general, toxicity is readily detected in these animals as loss of body weight. A 10–15% loss of body weight is generally considered to be a sign of toxicity. FIGURES 6 and 7 show the toxicity of ester 2 in nude mice with different doses. The change of body weight of mice is recorded as a function of treatment time. FIGURE 6 does not show any sign of toxicity. Actually, as was found in the control group, body weights of mice treated with all indicated doses of ester 2 were slightly increased. As shown in FIGURE 7, body weight losses in mice were not observed even when the dose reached as high as 200 mg/kg. A slight body weight loss (~10%) was observed when the dose of ester 2 reached 300 mg/kg. Thus, ester 2 showed an exceptional lack of toxicity.

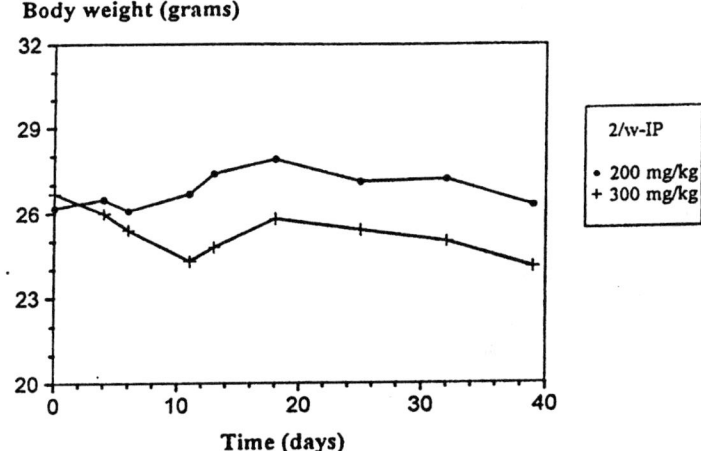

FIGURE 7. Toxicity of prodrug 2 in nude mice at different doses. Survival rate of treated mice in each group was 100% (3 out of 3).

CONCLUSION

The activity of alkyl CPT esters varies depending on the length of their side alkyl ester chain. The results presented in this report strongly indicate that camptothecin-20(S)-propionate 2 and other CPT lactone esters can be developed into highly effective and nontoxic prodrugs for anticancer treatment.

ACKNOWLEDGMENT

The authors wish to thank Y-H. Hsiang for assays measuring stabilization of topoisomerase I-DNA complexes and the Stehlin Foundation and the Friends of the Stehlin Foundation for financial support.

REFERENCES

1. WALL, M.E., M.C. WANI, C.E. COOK, et al. 1996. Plant antitumor agents. I. The isolation and structure of camptothecin, a novel alkaloidal leukemia and tumor inhibitor from *Camptotheca acuminata*. J. Am. Chem. Soc. **88:** 3888–3890.
2. OSHEROFF, N. 1989. Biochemical basis for the interactions of type I and type II topoisomerases with DNA. Pharmacol. Ther. **41:** 223–241.
3. PLATTNER, J.J., R.D. GLESS, G.K. COOPER & H. RAPPORT. 1974. Synthesis of some DE and CDE ring analogues of camptothecin. J. Org. Chem. **39:** 303–311.
4. DANISHEFSKY, S. & S.J. ETHEREDGE. 1974. Synthesis and biological evaluation of DE-AB-camptothecin. J. Org. Chem. **39:** 3430–3432.

5. BRISTOL J.A., D.L. COMINS, R.W. DAVENPORT, et al. 1975. Analogs of camptothecin. J. Med. Chem. **18:** 535–537.
6. SUGASAAWA, T., T. TOYODA, N. UCHIDA & K. YAMAGUCHI. 1976. Experiments on the synthesis of *dl*-camptothecin. 4. Synthesis and antileukemic activity of *dl*-camptothecin analogs. J. Med. Chem. **19:** 675–679.
7. WANI, M.C., P.E. RONMAN, L.T. LINDLEY & M.E. WALL. 1980. Plant antitumor agents. 18. Synthesis and biological activity of camptothecin analogs. J. Med. Chem. **23:** 554–560.
8. WANI, M.C., A.W. NICKOLAS & M.E. WALL. 1986. Plant antitumor agents. 23. Synthesis and antileukemic activity of camptothecin analogs. J. Med. Chem. **29:** 2358–2363.
9. WANI, M.C., A.W. NICKOLAS, G. MANIKUMAR & M.E. WALL. 1987. Plant antitumor agents. 25. Total synthesis and antileukemic activity of ring A substituted camptothecin analogs. Structure–activity correlations. J. Med. Chem. **30:** 1774–1779.
10. NICKOLAS, A.W., M.C. WANI, G. MANIKUMAR, et al. 1990. Plant Antitumor Agent. 29. Synthesis and biological activity of ring D and ring E modified analogues of camptothecin. J. Med. Chem. **33:** 972–978.
11. KINGSBURG, W.D., J.C. BOEHM, D.R. JAKAS, et al. 1991. Synthesis of water soluble (aminoalkyl)camptothecin analogues: inhibition of topoisomerase I and antitumor activity. J. Med. Chem. **34:** 98–107.
12. EJIMA, A., H. TERASAWA, M. SUGIMORI, et al. 1992. Antitumor agents. V. Synthesis and antileukemic activity of E-ring modified (RS)-camptothecin. Chem. Pharm. Bull. **40:** 683–688.
13. YAEGASHI, T., S. SAWADA, H. NAGATA, et al. 1994. Synthesis and antitumor activity of 20 (S)-camptothecin derivatives. A-ring-substituted 7-ethylcamptothecins and their E-ring-modified water soluble derivatives. Chem. Pharm. Bull. **42:** 2518–2525.
14. PEEL, M.R. & D.D. STEINBACK. 1994. The synthesis and evaluation of flexible analogs of the topoisomerase I inhibitor, camptothecin. Bioorg. Med. Chem. Lett. **4:** 2753–2758.
15. WANG, H.K., S.Y. LIU, K.W. HWANG, et al. 1995. Antitumor agents. 160. The synthesis of 5-substituted camptothecins as potential inhibitor of DNA topoisomerase I. Bioorg. Med. Chem. Lett. **5:** 77–82.
16. LUZZIO, M.J., J.M. BESTERMAN, D.L. EMERSON, et al. 1995. Synthesis and antitumor activity of novel water soluble derivatives of camptothecin as specific inhibitors of topoisomerase I. J. Med. Chem. **38:** 395–401.
17. SYDER, L., W. SHEN, W.G. BORNMANN & S.I. DANISHEFSKY. 1994. Synthesis of 18-noranhydrocamptothecin analogs which retain topoisomerase I inhibitory function. J. Org. Chem. **59:** 7033–7037.
18. FANG, F., S. XIE & M.W. LOWERY. 1994. Catalytic enantioselective synthesis of 20 (S)-camptothecin: a practical application of the sharpless asymmetric dihydroxylation reaction. J. Org. Chem. **59:** 6142–6143.
19. COMINS, D.L., H. HAO & J. GAO. 1994. Asymmetric synthesis of camptothecin alkaloids: a nine step synthesis of (S)-camptothecin. Tetrahedron Lett. **35:** 5331–5334.
20. RAMA RAO, A.V., J.S. YADAV & M. VALLURI. 1994. Regioselective synthesis of camptothecin. Tetrahedron Lett. **35:** 3613–3616.
21. CARRIGAN, S.W., P.C. FOX, M.E. WALL, et al. 1997. Comparative molecular field analysis and molecular modeling studies of 20-(S)-camptothecin analogs as inhibitors of DNA topoisomerase I and anticancer/antitumor agents. J. Comput. Aided Mol. Design **11:** 71–78.
22. PANTAZIS, P., D. VARDEMAN, J. MENDOZA, et al. 1995. Sensitivity of camptothecin-resistant human leukemia cells and tumors to anticancer drugs with diverse mechanisms of action. Leuk. Res. **19:** 43–55.
23. PANTAZIS, P. 1995. Preclinical studies of water-insoluble camptothecin congeners: cytotoxicity, development of resistance, and combination treatments. Clin. Cancer Res. **1:** 1235–1244.
24. BURKE, T.G. 1993. Chemistry of the camptothecins in the bloodstream: drug stabilization and optimization of activity. Ann. N.Y. Acad. Sci. **803:** 29–31.

25. GIOVANELLA, B.C., H.R. HINZ, A.J. KOZIELSKI, *et al.* 1991. Complete growth inhibition of human cancer xenografts in nude mice by treatment with 20 (S) camptothecin. Cancer Res. **51:** 3052–3055.
26. NATELSON, E., B.C. GIOVANELLA, C.F. VERSCHRAEGEN, *et al.* 1996. Phase I clinical and pharmacological studies of 20-(S)-camptothecin and 20-(S)-9-Cao Z nitrocamptothecin as anticancer agents. Ann. N.Y. Acad. Sci. **803:** 224–230.
27. GIOVANELLA, B.C. Unpublished results.
28. CAO, Z. 1997. An alternative preparation of camptothecin 20(S)-acetate. Synth. Commun. **27:** 2013–2019.
29. WALL, M.E. & M.C. WANI. 1984. Antineoplastic structure–activity relationships of camptothecin and related analogs. Natural products and drug development. Alfred Benzon Symposium **20:** 253–265. Copenhagen.
30. CAO, Z., N. HARRIS, A. KOZIELSKI, *et al.* 1998. Alkyl esters of camptothecin and 9-nitrocamptothecin: synthesis, in vitro pharmacokinetics, toxicity, and antitumor activity. J. Med. Chem. **41:** 31–37.
31. PANTAZIS, P. 1995. The water-insoluble camptothecin analogues: promising drugs for the effective treatment of hematological malignancies (review). Leuk. Res. **19:** 775–778.
32. GIOVANELLA, B.C. & J.S. STEHLIN. 1973. Heterotransplantation of human malignant tumors in "nude" thymusless mice. I. Breeding and maintenance of "nude" mice. J. Natl. Cancer Inst. **51:** 615–617.
33. PANTAZIS, P., J.A. EARLY, J.T. MENDOZA, *et al.* 1994. Cytotoxic efficacy of 9-nitrocamptothecin in the treatment of human malignant melanoma cells *in vitro*. Cancer Res. **54:** 771–776.
34. LEE, S.S., B.C. GIOVANELLA & J.S. STEHLIN. 1977. Selective lethal effect on thymidine on human and mouse tumor cells. J. Cell. Physiol. **92:** 401–405.
35. NATELSON, S., P. PANTAZIS & E.A. NATELSON. 1994. L-Homoserine hydroxamic acid as an antitumor agent. Chim. Clin. Acta **229:** 133–145.
36. RUBIN, E., P. PANTAZIS, A. BHARTI, *et al.* Identification of a mutant human topoisomerase I with intact catalytic activity and resistance to 9-nitrocamptothecin. J. Biol. Chem. **269:** 2433–2439.
37. PANTAZIS, P., J.T. MENDOZA, A. DEJESUS, *et al.* 1994. Partial characterization of human leukemia U-937 cell sublines to 9-nitrocamptothecin. Eur. J. Haematol. **43:** 135–144.
38. WALL, M.E. & M.C. WANI. 1996. Camptothecin: discovery to clinic (review). Ann. N.Y. Acad. Sci. **803:** 1–12.

Conjugation of Camptothecins to Poly-(L-Glutamic Acid)

JACK W. SINGER,[a,d] PETER DE VRIES,[a] RAMA BHATT,[a] JOHN TULINSKY,[a] PETER KLEIN,[a] CHUN LI,[b] LUKA MILAS,[c] ROBERT A. LEWIS,[a] AND SIDNEY WALLACE[b]

[a]*Cell Therapeutics Inc., Seattle, Washington 98119, USA*

[b]*Division of Diagnostic Imaging and* [c]*Division of Radiation Oncology, M.D. Anderson Cancer Center, University of Texas, Houston, Texas, USA*

ABSTRACT: Conjugation of water-insoluble cancer chemotherapeutic drugs to macromolecular polymers can lead to improved pharmaceutical properties and improved therapeutic ratios due to accumulation of the polymer–drug conjugate in tumor tissue through the enhanced permeability and retention (EPR) to macromolecules associated with tumor vasculature. Pharmaceutical shortcomings of certain active camptothecins including difficulty in formulation and instability of the active lactone form due to interactions with human albumin might be improved by conjugation to polymers. In this report, conjugations of camptothecin (CPT), 10-hydroxy-CPT, and 9-amino-CPT to poly-(L-glutamic acid) (PG) are described; coupling was accomplished either through the 20(S)-hydroxyl or 9 and 10 substituents with and without the use of a glycine linker. Studies using a PG paclitaxel conjugate (PG-TXL), which is currently in Phase I testing, demonstrated that PG enhanced aqueous solubility, prolonged plasma residence time, and greatly increased the distribution of paclitaxel to tumor tissue in a murine model. In this report, we describe the use of similar conjugation technology for CPT derivatives and demonstrate that these difficult to formulate compounds can be rendered water soluble, that their maximum tolerated doses are increased, and that they retain substantial anti-tumor activity in syngeneic and xenogeneic tumor models. Preliminary data suggest that PG with molecular weights between 37 and 50 kDa with CPT loading between 14% and 37% with or without glycine linkers display enhanced efficacy compared with nonconjugated camptothecins administered at their maximum tolerated dose.

INTRODUCTION

Conjugation of cytotoxic chemotherapeutic drugs to polymeric macromolecules can yield more favorable pharmacokinetic profiles, reduced toxicity, and enhanced efficacy.[1–4] We have been evaluating the ability of covalently linked polymers of L-glutamic acid (PG) to improve the pharmaceutical properties and therapeutic indices of several classes of oncologic agents including taxanes and camptothecins. The advantages for PG over other currently available polymers are its biodegradability,

---

[d]Address for correspondence: Jack W. Singer, Cell Therapeutics Inc., 201 Elliott Avenue West, Seattle, WA 98119.
jsinger@ctiseattle.com

its multiple available conjugation sites for drugs, and its ability to solubilize extremely hydrophobic molecules.

Although camptothecin (CPT) and its derivatives, generically termed "camptothecins" are important anticancer agents (reviewed in Refs. 5, 6), their full clinical potential has yet to be realized because of a lack of aqueous solubility of the most active compounds and the instability of the pharmacologically critical lactone ring in the presence of human albumin. At physiological pH, in the absence of human albumin, approximately 20% of CPT is present in the lactone form.[7–9] The 150-fold preferential binding of the carboxylate form to human serum albumin (binding constant: 6×10^7 M^{-1})[10] shifts the equilibrium to the inactive carboxylate form.[7,9,11,12] 9-amino-CPT and CPT are rapidly and almost completely converted to their respective carboxylate forms upon contact with human albumin. In an initial attempt to improve solubility, the sodium salt of CPT was developed and evaluated by a Phase I/II clinical program. Unfortunately, the sodium salt of CPT was relatively inactive compared to the parent drug[13] and proved to be both toxic and weakly active in patients.[4,14–16] Instability in human plasma also contributed to a low therapeutic index for 9-amino-CPT despite robust activities in animal models.

Aqueous solubility and plasma stability have been advanced by two camptothecin derivatives that have been developed and commercialized. Irinotecan is a water-soluble, inactive prodrug for the highly insoluble and active compound SN-38. The ratio of the area-under-the-curve (AUC) values for irinotecan:SN-38 is approximately 50:1 and depends on an enzymatic conversion step that can vary among patients.[17] The ethyl substitution at the C-7 position decreases the interaction of the open chain carboxylate form of SN-38 with human serum albumin, thereby increasing persistence of the lactone form.[18] A second water-soluble camptothecin derivative, topotecan, although a less potent topoisomerase 1 inhibitor than CPT *in vitro*, is more stable as the result of weaker interactions of its carboxylate form with human albumin, and it is clinically active.[18,19] Lactone instability in human plasma appears to be the predominant reason for the difficulty in clinically developing CPT or 9-amino-CPT. In an attempt to enhance the lactone AUC, 72-hour infusions of 9-amino-CPT were evaluated. Less than 10% of 9-amino-CPT was in the lactone form at steady state when dosed by 72-hour infusion,[20–24] and the clinical activity in Phase II studies was marginal.[25–28] 9-Nitro-CPT is currently in advanced development as an oral prodrug for 9-amino-CPT.[29] In initial studies, comparing steady-state AUCs, about 13% of 9-nitro-CPT was in the lactone form.[11]

An alternative approach to overcome the pharmaceutical and pharmacokinetic shortcomings of camptothecins is to covalently bind them to neutral polymers such as polyethylene glycol (PEG)[30–32] or to charged polymers exemplified by PG. Using these approaches, the water solubility of the most active camptothecins can be adequately enhanced so as to allow parenteral administration in aqueous medium. Conjugation through the 20(S)-hydroxyl group may also protect the lactone from interactions with human albumin. In addition to the differential effects of electroneutrality versus charge, another difference between PEG and PG is the presence of multiple conjugation sites on the γ-carboxylic acids of PG, in contrast to the two sites on PEG. Although theoretically each γ-carboxylic acid of PG could be covalently coupled to a molecule of interest, with highly hydrophobic molecules such as taxanes or camptothecins, only about 1 in 8 sites can be occupied before aqueous solubility is significantly diminished. The ability to conjugate large numbers of molecules of active drug on each PG decreases the total mass of polymer needed to administer a given dose compared to the analogous PEG conjugates.

We are currently proceeding with the clinical development of our first PG–hydrophobic drug conjugate, PG–paclitaxel (PG-TXL), in which each paclitaxel molecule is linked at the 2'-OH group by an ester linkage to a γ-carboxylic acid of a glutamic acid in PG.[33–35] Preclinical studies demonstrated that PG-TXL (37% paclitaxel by weight) linked to a 31- to 50-kDa PG backbone is readily soluble in aqueous media, is inactive *in vitro* because coupling to a paclitaxel site is required for tubulin binding, has a prolonged plasma residence time compared to free paclitaxel, and has increased distribution to tumor tissue.[36] The latter effect is characteristic of polymeric drug conjugates of >20 kDa[37] that take advantage of the biological properties of enhanced permeability of tumor vessels and retention for macromolecules due to lack of lymphatic drainage (EPR). Systemically administered macromolecules are preferentially distributed to the tumor,[2,38] to be either hydrolyzed extracellularly or taken up by pinocytosis with degradation and release of the active drug by lysosomal enzymes.[39] We found that increasing the loading of PG-TXL from 25% to 37% substantially improved efficacy without altering toxicity and that 50% loading by weight was essentially equivalent to 37% loading for efficacy (unpublished data). With paclitaxel, approximately 10% of the potential conjugation sites were occupied when PG was loaded at 37%. At this level of loading, the material is stable in circulation and resistant to release of free paclitaxel by plasma esterases. Studies in mice and rats demonstrated that PG-TXL has a higher maximum tolerated dose (MTD) and enhanced efficacy compared with paclitaxel in Cremophor and ethanol.[33,34] Unlike free paclitaxel, PG-TXL was active in multidrug-resistant tumors that overexpressed *mdr1* (unpublished data).

On the basis of our experience with PG-TXL, we have begun a program to identify an optimal PG-CPT conjugate structure on the basis of *in vivo* activity, and then to optimize this conjugate for clinical development.

MATERIALS AND METHODS

On the basis of the experience with PG-TXL, several camptothecins were chosen to be evaluated as PG conjugates on the basis of their relative topoisomerase I inhibitory activities and efficacies in murine tumor models. A lack of efficacy in human clinical trials was not considered relevant since conjugation to a polymer might be expected to yield a compound with different pharmacokinetics, toxicity profile, biodistribution, and stability profiles than the free parent drug. TABLE 1 indicates the relative topoisomerase I inhibitory activities of several camptothecins and their relative stabilities in the lactone forms in human plasma. We chose to evaluate CPT,[13] SN-38,[5] 9-amino-CPT,[28] and 10-hydroxy-CPT.[6,40,41]

The initial PG conjugates of camptothecins were synthesized so that the γ-carboxylic acid of PG was covalently linked to the 20(S)-hydroxyl substituent of the camptothecins through an ester bond with and without a glycine linker (FIG. 1). Additionally, conjugates of 9-amino-CPT and 10-hydroxy-CPT were prepared using amide or ester linkages at the 9- and 10-position substituents, respectively. The effect of conjugation using a glycine linker attached to the amino group of 9-amino-CPT

TABLE 1. Anti-topoisomerase 1 activity and human plasma stability of selected camptothecin derivatives

Compound	Percent inhibition of double-stranded DNA relaxation at 10 μM[41]	Stability in human plasma (percent lactone at steady state)[44]
CPT	52	0.5%
10-hydroxy-CPT	73	4%
SN-38	73	38%
9-amino-CPT	91	<10%

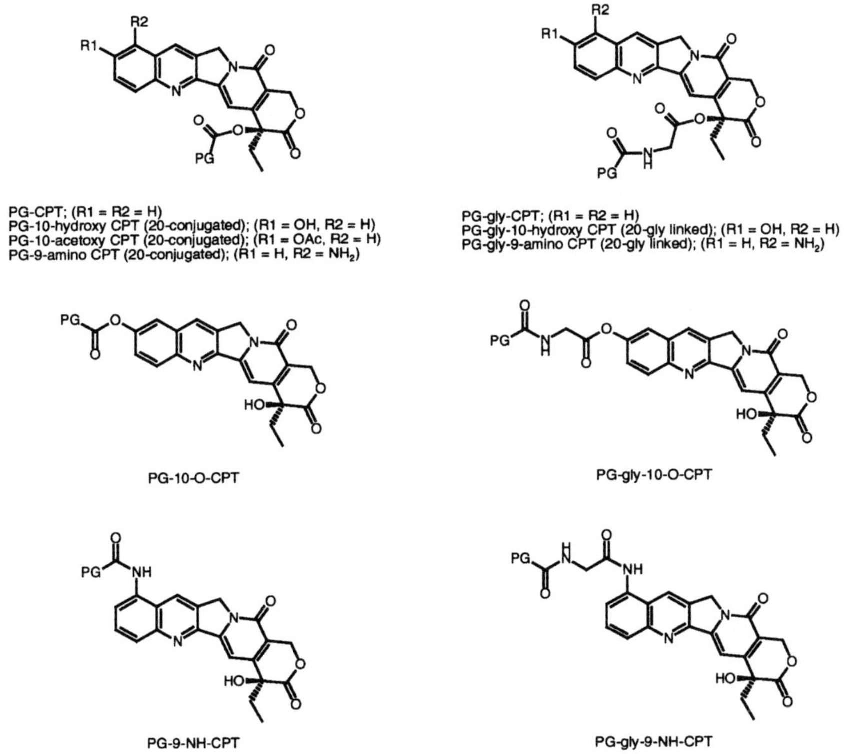

PG-CPT; (R1 = R2 = H)
PG-10-hydroxy CPT (20-conjugated); (R1 = OH, R2 = H)
PG-10-acetoxy CPT (20-conjugated); (R1 = OAc, R2 = H)
PG-9-amino CPT (20-conjugated); (R1 = H, R2 = NH$_2$)

PG-gly-CPT; (R1 = R2 = H)
PG-gly-10-hydroxy CPT (20-gly linked); (R1 = OH, R2 = H)
PG-gly-9-amino CPT (20-gly linked); (R1 = H, R2 = NH$_2$)

PG-10-O-CPT

PG-gly-10-O-CPT

PG-9-NH-CPT

PG-gly-9-NH-CPT

FIGURE 1. Structures of camptothecin conjugates.

or the 10-hydroxyl group of 10-hydroxy-CPT was also examined (FIG. 1). In the following sections, the synthesis and characteristics of these conjugates are described, as are preliminary studies in tumor-bearing mice. To optimize the therapeutic ratio of PG–camptothecins, we are exploring the use of short linker molecules, varying the molecular weight of the PG backbone, and changing the number of molecules of the camptothecins loaded on each PG molecule.

RESULTS

Conjugation of 20(S)-CPT

Because all of the active camptothecins possess the 20(S)-hydroxyl functionality as a lactone ring substituent, we took advantage of this group in our conjugation chemistry. Direct conjugation of CPT to PG through the 20(S)-hydroxyl group was accomplished using chloromethylpyridinium iodide (CMPI) as coupling reagent with 4-dimethylaminopyridine (DMAP) as the organic base.

To evaluate the efficacy of our conjugation chemistry, we undertook to verify that covalent conjugation had occurred and that weight loading of the drug on the polymer was of the expected magnitude. To determine how much of the CPT in PG-CPT (directly conjugated) was covalently bound to PG, the conjugate was treated with 2% methanol in dichloromethane and sonicated for 3 hours. Thin-layer chromatography (TLC) analysis of the organic extract failed to detect unreacted CPT. Analysis of the ^{1}H NMR spectrum of the conjugate confirmed that CPT was covalently bound to PG (see TABLE 2). To determine the amount of drug loaded on the polymer, we subjected a portion of the directly conjugated PG-CPT to basic hydrolysis to release the conjugated CPT, which also opens the lactone ring to the free carboxylate salt. Following acidification to reclose the carboxylate to the lactone, CPT was obtained that was identical to an authentic sample by comparisons of both TLC behavior and ^{1}H NMR spectra. The weight of the released CPT was calculated to be 14% weight loading of CPT on the polymer. Comparison of the UV absorbance at 364 nm of PG-CPT with a standard curve obtained from CPT also indicated 14% weight loading.

Additionally, conjugation of CPT to PG through the 20(S)-hydroxyl group was achieved by interposition of a glycine linker. Conjugation of CPT glycinate ester[30] to PG through the glycine free amino group using diisopropylcarbodiimide (DIPC) and DMAP yielded glycine-linked PG-CPT (PG-gly-CPT).

Conjugation of 10-Hydroxy-CPT

Under conditions of direct conjugation of 10-hydroxy-CPT to PG using CMPI and DMAP, PG-10-O-CPT was isolated as the exclusive product. This assertion is based on the results of an analogous coupling of 10-hydroxy-CPT with Boc-L-glutamic acid α-*tert*-butyl ester under the same reaction conditions. The ^{1}H NMR spectrum of the latter product displayed characteristic shifts of signals due to 10-hydroxy-CPT aromatic protons, whereas signals due to lactone ethyl protons were not shifted.

Conjugation of 10-hydroxy-CPT to PG through the 10-hydroxyl group was also accomplished by interposition of a glycine linker. To achieve the needed selectivity in the site of conjugation, a method to differentiate the 10- and 20-hydroxyl groups on 10-hydroxy-CPT was required. Treatment of 10-hydroxy-CPT with the symmetrical anhydride of Boc-glycine and pyridine yielded solely the corresponding 10-(*N*-Boc)-glycinate ester. Treatment of the latter with trifluoroacetic acid (TFA) effected cleavage of the *N*-Boc protecting group. The resulting 10-glycinate ester of 10-hydroxy-CPT was conjugated with PG using DIPC and DMAP to give PG-gly-10-O-CPT. Exclusive coupling to the α-amino group of the glycine was inferred on the basis of an analogous coupling of the 10-glycinate ester of 10-hydroxy-CPT with

TABLE 2. Loading, NMR spectra, and MTD of PG-camptothecins

CPT	Percent CPT in conjugate (w+/w+)	Aqueous solubility	Diagnostic signals in 300 MHz ^{1}H NMR spectra (DMSO-d6)	Murine single-dose MTD (i.p.) (mg eq. CPT/kg)
PG-CPT (20-O-conjugated)	14	11 mg/ml	δ 12.1 (broad singlet, PG γ-COO$\underline{H}$), 7.4–8.5 (multiple broad signals, Ar-$\underline{H}$), 5.6 (broad singlet, lactone -C$\underline{H}_2$-), 0.9 (broad signal, CPT C$\underline{H}_2$C$\underline{H}_3$)	60–80 mg eq. CPT/kg
PG-Gly-CPT (20-O-conjugated)	37	25 mg/ml	δ 12.1 (broad singlet, PG γ-COO$\underline{H}$), 7.4-8.5 (multiple broad signals, Ar-$\underline{H}$), 5.6 (broad singlet, lactone -C$\underline{H}_2$-), 0.9 (broad signal, CPT C$\underline{H}_2$C$\underline{H}_3$)	60–80 mg eq. CPT/kg
PG-10-acetoxy-CPT (20-O-conjugated)	13	10 mg/ml	δ 12.1 (broad singlet, PG γ-COO$\underline{H}$), 7.2–8.6 (multiple broad signals, Ar-$\underline{H}$); 5.4 (singlet, lactone –C$\underline{H}_2$-); 5.2 (singlet, C5-$\underline{H}_2$); 0.9 (broad triplet, CPT C$\underline{H}_2$C$\underline{H}_3$)	10–20 mg eq. CPT/kg
PG-10-O-CPT	13	10 mg/ml	δ 12.1 (broad singlet, PG γ-COO$\underline{H}$), 7.2–8.6 (multiple broad signals, Ar-$\underline{H}$); 5.4 (singlet, lactone –C$\underline{H}_2$-); 5.2 (singlet, C5-$\underline{H}_2$); 0.9 (broad triplet, CPT C$\underline{H}_2$C$\underline{H}_3$)	50 mg eq. CPT/kg
PG-gly-10-O-CPT	20	>10 mg/ml	δ 12.1 (broad singlet, PG γ-COO$\underline{H}$), 7.2–8.8 (multiple broad signals, Ar-$\underline{H}$); 5.4 (singlet, lactone –C$\underline{H}_2$-); 5.2 (singlet, C5-$\underline{H}_2$); 0.9 (broad signal, CPT C$\underline{H}_2$C$\underline{H}_3$)	10–50 mg eq. CPT/kg
PG-10-hydroxy-CPT (20-O-gly-linked)	19	>10 mg/ml	δ 12.1 (broad singlet, PG γ-COO$\underline{H}$), 7.0–8.5 (multiple broad signals, Ar-$\underline{H}$); 5.4 (singlet, lactone –C$\underline{H}_2$-); 5.2 (singlet, C5-$\underline{H}_2$); 0.9 (broad signal, CPT C$\underline{H}_2$C$\underline{H}_3$)	>50 mg eq. CPT/kg
PG-9-amino-CPT (20-O-conjugated)	NA	>10 mg/ml	δ 12.1 (broad singlet, PG γ-COO$\underline{H}$), 8.8 (broad singlet, C7-$\underline{H}$), 7.2–8.0 (multiple broad signals, Ar-$\underline{H}$), 5.4 (broad singlet, lactone -C$\underline{H}_2$-), 0.9 (broad signal, CPT C$\underline{H}_2$C$\underline{H}_3$).	>25 mg eq. CPT/kg
PG-9-NH-CPT	14	7 mg/ml	δ 12.1 (broad singlet, PG γ-COO$\underline{H}$), 8.8 (broad singlet, C7-$\underline{H}$), 7.2–8.0 (multiple broad signals, Ar-$\underline{H}$), 5.4 (broad singlet, lactone -C$\underline{H}_2$-), 0.9 (broad signal, CPT C$\underline{H}_2$C$\underline{H}_3$).	>25 mg eq. CPT/kg

Boc-L-glutamic acid α-*tert*-butyl ester under the same reaction conditions. The ^{1}H NMR spectrum of this reaction product displayed characteristic shifts of signals due to 10-hydroxy-CPT aromatic protons, whereas signals due to lactone ethyl group protons were not shifted.

Conjugation of 10-hydroxy-CPT to PG through the 20(S)-hydroxyl group involved interposition of a glycine linker. Treatment of 10-hydroxy-CPT with di-*tert*-butyl dicarbonate and pyridine provided exclusively the corresponding 10-O-Boc derivative. The latter was 20-O-acylated with Boc-glycine using DIPC and DMAP. Removal of both Boc-protecting groups with TFA followed by conjugation with PG provided PG-gly-10-hydroxy-CPT (20-O-gly linked).

Conjugation of the 10-hydroxy-CPT derivative, 10-acetoxy-CPT,[42] to PG was accomplished using CMPI and DMAP to provide PG-10-acetoxy-CPT (20-O-conjugated).

Conjugation of 9-Amino-CPT

As with 10-hydroxy-CPT, coupling of 9-amino-CPT to PG under conditions of direct conjugation (CMPI and DMAP) took place on the aromatic A-ring heteroatom substituent, in this case producing PG-9-NH-CPT as the exclusive product. This outcome was inferred on the basis of results of an analogous coupling of 9-amino-CPT with Boc-L-glutamic acid α-*tert*-butyl ester that afforded a product whose ^{1}H NMR spectrum displayed characteristic shifts of signals due to the 9-amino-CPT aromatic protons, whereas signals due to lactone ethyl protons were not shifted.

Conjugation of 9-amino-CPT to PG through the 20-hydroxyl group was achieved by interposition of a glycine linker. Conjugation of the glycinate ester of 9-amino-CPT [43] to PG through the α-amino group of glycine using DIPC and DMAP provided PG-gly-9-NH-CPT.

IN VIVO BIOLOGICAL ACTIVITIES

CPT Conjugates

The MTD and relative efficacy of direct and glycine-conjugated PG-CPT were initially tested using single intraperitoneal (i.p.) injections in C57BL/6 mice carrying subcutaneous B16 melanomas. Although B16 melanoma is only weakly responsive to CPT, this model was used to screen various compounds for preliminary efficacy assessment due to its reproducibility and utility in rapidly assessing anti-tumor activity. Tumors were produced in the muscle of the right interscapular region by injecting 1×10^5 murine melanoma cells (B-16-F0; ATCC CRL-6322) in a volume of 0.2 ml PBS supplemented with 2% FBS. Native camptothecins were dissolved in a mixture of 8.3% Cremophor/8.3% ethanol in 0.75% saline. Test compounds and vehicle control were administered in 0.5 ml, 7 or 8 days after tumor cell implantation, when the tumors had grown to between 5 and 10 mm^3. CPT conjugates were dissolved in a 0.1 M Na$_2$HPO$_4$ solution by sonication at 45°C for 45–60 minutes. All injections were given i.p. Each treatment group consisted of 10 mice randomly allocated to each group on the basis of tumor size. Tumor volume was calculated according to the formula (length × width × height)/2. Mice with tumors equal to or greater than 2000 mm³ were euthanized by cervical dislocation. Tumor efficacy of test compounds was determined by calculating the tumor growth delay (TGD), which was defined as the mean difference in days for the tumors in the treatment group minus the mean time for the tumors in the control group to reach a fixed volume. An unpaired Student's *t*-test was done to determine statistical differences. The compounds were tested in additional syngeneic and xenogeneic tumor models after the MTD and efficacy were determined in the B16 model.

For directly coupled CPT, PG-CPT, the maximum loading achieved was approximately 14% (weight of CPT/total weight of conjugate). A glycine linker (PG-gly-CPT) allowed loading of up to 37% and enhanced aqueous solubility (TABLE 2). The single dose maximum tolerated dose (MTD) by i.p. injection was similar for PG-CPT and PG-gly-CPT in the C57BL/6 (80 mg equivalent [eq.] CPT/kg). In comparison the MTD for free CPT was 12 mg eq. CPT/kg, when formulated in Cremophor/ethanol.

Syngeneic Tumor Models

PG-CPT and PG-gly-CPT coupled to 33-kDa PG both produced equivalent tumor growth delays in the B16 model (4.3 and 3.4 days, respectively; $p < 0.0001$ for both compared to controls; FIG. 2). When 50-kDa PG was used as the carrier for PG-gly-CPT, enhanced efficacy was observed, compared with the 33-kDa PG with a TGD of 5.2 days at 80 mg eq. CPT/kg ($p < 0.01$ compared to PG-gly-CPT using 33-kDa PG; FIG. 2). This observation is consistent with the expected lower renal clearance

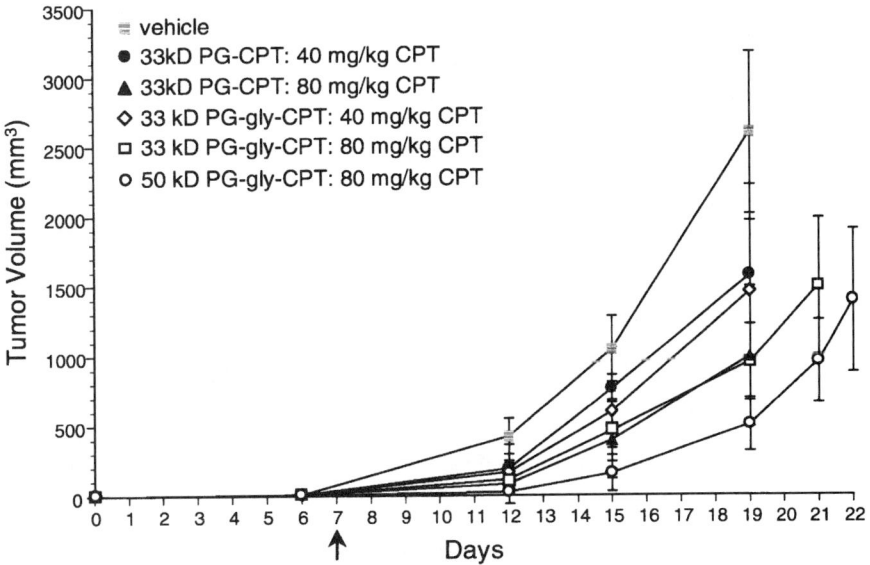

FIGURE 2. Antitumor activity of single-dose PG-CPT and PG-gly-CPT on B16 melanoma in C57BL/6 mice. PG-CPT contained 14% CPT by weight and PG-gly-CPT contained 37% CPT by weight. The doses in the figure legend are based on CPT equivalents.

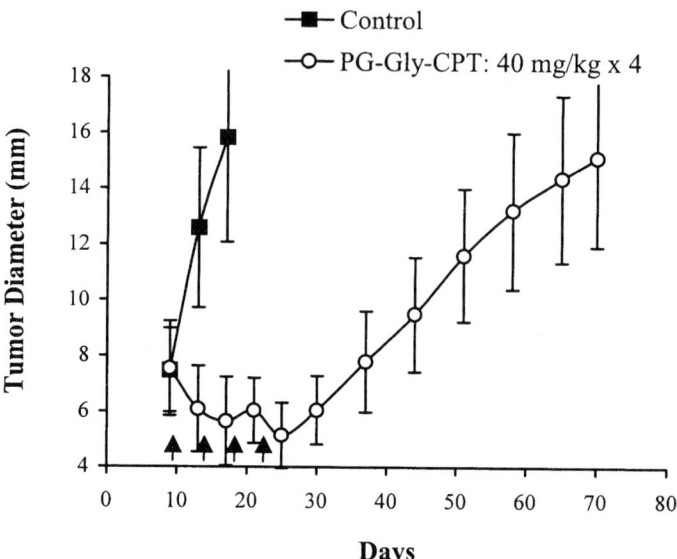

FIGURE 3. Antitumor activity of PG-gly-CPT on H322 human lung cancer inoculated s.c. in nude mice. The drug was injected i.v. on days 9, 13, 17, and 21 at an equivalent CPT dose of 40 mg eq. CPT/kg when tumors measured 7–8 mm in diameter. The TGD compared to control was 40 days. Data are presented as means ($n = 10$) ± SE.

rate for a higher molecular weight conjugate. In preliminary single-dose studies, PG-CPT at 40 mg eq. CPT/kg and PG-gly-CPT at 80 mg eq. CPT/kg, a dose somewhat above the MTD in this experiment, had major anti-tumor activity in mice bearing the MCA-4 breast cancer or the OCa-1 ovarian cancer (data not shown).

Human Tumor Xenografts

Female nude mice with 7–8 mm in diameter H322 human lung cancer xenografts had PG-gly-CPT injected i.v. on days 9, 13, 17, and 21 at a CPT equivalent dose of 40 mg/kg. The TGD was 40 days (FIG. 3).

Female nude mice with 7–8 mm diameter subcutaneous H460 human non-small cell lung cancer xenografts were treated with PG-gly-CPT on days 1, 5, 9, and 13 at a dose of 40 mg eq. CPT/kg per injection. The tested dose of 40 mg eq. CPT/kg i.v. every 4th day × 4 modestly exceeded the MTD. Although there were no deaths, weight loss was approximately 20% of the starting weight, and TGD was 43 days for the PG-gly-CPT-treated mice (FIG. 4A). In a second experiment, directly conjugated PG-CPT was tested on the same schedule but administered i.p., and it also produced substantial growth delay (FIG. 4B). For the direct conjugate, this dose produced no overt toxicity.

PG-gly-CPT was also tested on female nude mice inoculated subcutaneously with 1.5×10^6 H1299 human lung cancer cells. Due to excessive weight loss at 40 mg eq., CPT/kg in the prior experiment in nude mice, the dose was lowered to 30 mg eq. CPT/kg every 4th day × 4. This dose was well tolerated and a TGD of 32 days was observed (FIG. 5).

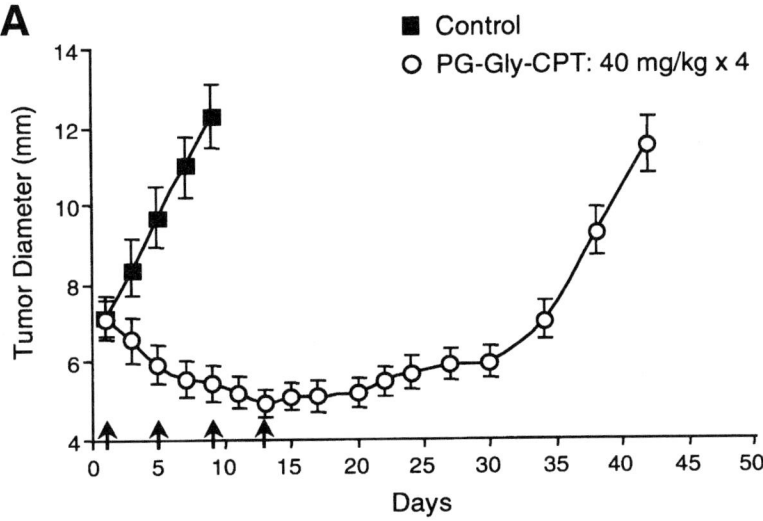

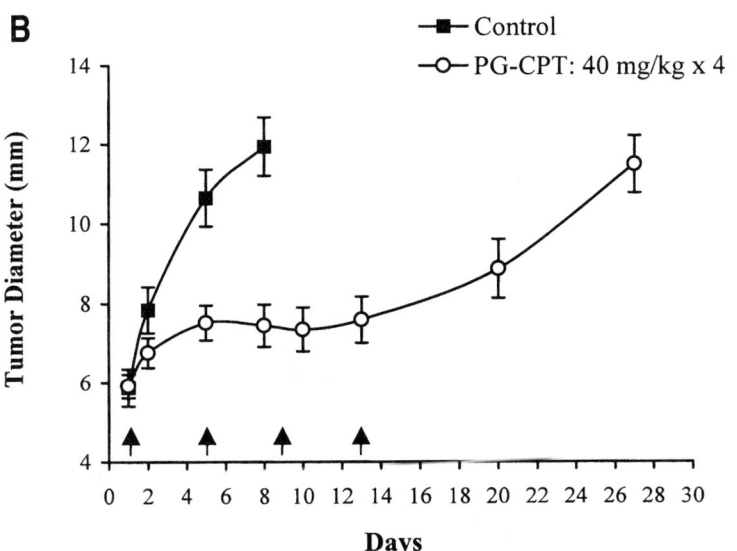

FIGURE 4. Antitumor activity of PG-gly-CPT on H460 human lung cancer inoculated s.c. in nude mice (**Panel A**). The drug was injected i.v. on days 1, 5, 9, and 13 at an equivalent CPT dose of 40 mg eq. CPT/kg when tumors measured 8 mm in diameter. Weight loss of 20% of starting weight occurred, suggesting this dose was somewhat over the MTD. The TGD was 43 days. In a second experiment, directly conjugated PG-CPT was tested by i.p. administration on H460 using an otherwise identical dose and schedule (**Panel B**). No toxicity was observed. The TGD was 34 days. Data are presented as means ($n = 10$) ± SE.

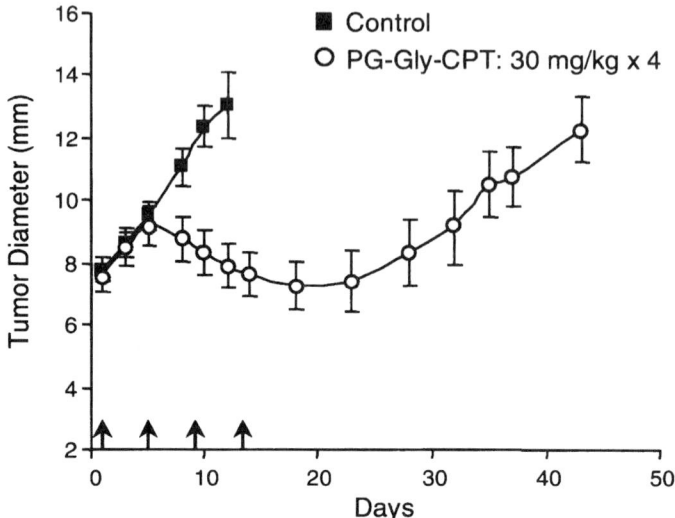

FIGURE 5. Antitumor activity in mice bearing subcutaneous H1299 human lung tumors. Female nude mice were inoculated s.c. with 1.5×10^6 H1299 human lung cancer cells. In view of the weight loss observed at 40 mg eq. CPT/kg, PG-gly-CPT was injected on days 1, 5, 9, and 13 at equivalent CPT dose of 30 mg eq. CPT/kg. A TGD of 32 days was observed. Data are presented as means ($n = 10$) ± SE.

10-Hydroxy-CPT Conjugates

10-hydroxy-CPT conjugates have undergone preliminary studies in the B16 model. The most active conjugate in these studies is the material directly conjugated or glycine conjugated through the 20-hydroxyl group. In initial experiments, the directly (20-O)-coupled material (PG-10-acetoxy-CPT; 20-O-conjugated) appeared more active at 50 mg eq. CPT/kg than a 20-O-glycine-linked conjugate; however, this dose was below the MTD for both compounds (FIG. 6). At 50 mg eq. CPT/kg, 20-O-hydroxy-CPT produced a TGD of 5.3 days ($p < 0.01$ compared to control). It is of interest that the MTD for PG-10-O-CPT (conjugated through the 10-hydroxyl group) is between 10 and 50 mg eq. CPT/kg. However, even at the highly toxic dose of 50 mg eq. CPT/kg, it was not as effective as the 20-hydroxy directly coupled, 10-acetoxy- or the 20-O-glycine-conjugated 10-hydroxy-CPT.

9-Amino-CPT Conjugates

The testing of these conjugates is currently in progress. Preliminary studies indicate that PG-9-NH-CPT and PG-9-amino-CPT (20-O-conjugated) are active in the B16 melanoma model and have MTDs in excess of 25 mg eq. CPT/kg.

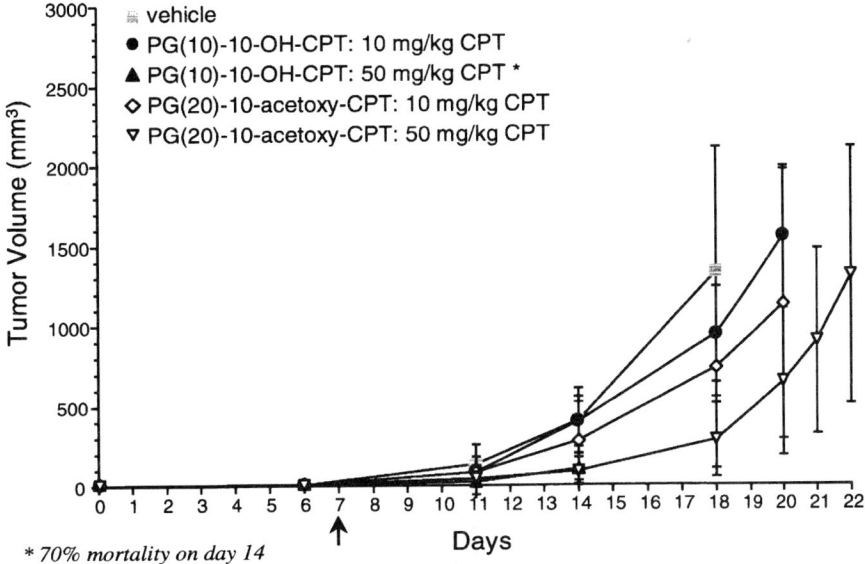

FIGURE 6. Antitumor activity of single-dose PG-10-hydroxy-CPT linked to PG either through the 10-hydroxy group (PG-10-O-CPT) or through the 20(S)-hydroxyl group (PG-10-acetoxy-CPT; 20-O-conjugated)) on B16 melanoma in C57BL/6 mice. The MTD for PG-10-acetoxy-CPT was ≥ 50 mg eq. CPT/kg whereas that for the PG-10-0-CPT was between 10 and 50 mg eq. CPT/kg.

DISCUSSION AND CONCLUSIONS

These studies indicate that it is feasible to covalently link camptothecins to PG, either directly or with a glycine linker to form a water-soluble and biologically active macromolecular conjugate. As observed for PG–taxane conjugates, the MTD for these conjugates is several-fold higher than that for the free camptothecins. Although pharmacokinetic data are not yet available for PG-camptothecins, studies of a similar conjugate with paclitaxel revealed a prolonged plasma half-life and improved distribution to tumor tissue compared to paclitaxel administered in Cremophor and ethanol.[36] It is anticipated from studies of PG-TXL that PG-camptothecin conjugates will be stable in plasma and not subject to esterolysis by plasma enzymes. For camptothecins such as CPT, 10-hydroxy-CPT, and 9-amino-CPT, which are highly bound to human albumin in the carboxylate form, a major advantage of conjugation is likely to be stabilization of the lactone, particularly since effective conjugates can be made through an ester linkage to the 20(S)-hydroxyl group. We anticipate that with optimization of a PG–camptothecin conjugate, based on varying the loading, the domain of chemical linkage between the camptothecin and PG, and the PG molecular weight, a PG-camptothecin may become an attractive candidate for clinical development. Such a compound may address some of the pharmaceutical shortcomings of this important class of drugs.

REFERENCES

1. CASSIDY, J., D.R. NEWELL, S.R. WEDGE & J. CUMMING. 1993. Pharmacokinetics of high molecular weight agents. Pharmacokinetics Cancer Chemo. **17:** 315–339.
2. MATSUMURA, Y. & H. MAEDA. 1986. A new concept for macromolecular therapeutics in cancer chemotherapy: mechanism of tumoritropic accumulation of proteins and the antitumor agent smancs. Cancer Res. **46:** 6387–6392.
3. VASEY, P.A., S.B. KAYE, R. MORRISON, et al. 1999. Phase I clinical and pharmacokinetic study of PK1 [N-(2- hydroxypropyl)methacrylamide copolymer doxorubicin]: first member of a new class of chemotherapeutic agents—drug–polymer conjugates. Cancer Research Campaign Phase I/II Committee [see comments]. Clin. Cancer Res. **5:** 83–94.
4. MUGGIA, F.M., P.J. CREAVEN, H.H. HANSEN, et al. 1972. Phase I clinical trial of weekly and daily treatment with camptothecin (NSC-100880): correlation with preclinical studies. Cancer Chemother. Rep. **56:** 515–521.
5. ROTHENBERG, M.L. 1997. Topoisomerase I inhibitors: review and update. Ann. Oncol. **9:** 837–855.
6. MUGGIA, F.M. & I. DIMERY. 1996. Camptothecin and its analogs. In The Camptothecins: From Discovery to the Patient. P. Pantazis, B.C. Giovanella & M.L. Rothenberg, Eds. Ann. N.Y. Acad. Sci. **803:** 213–223.
7. MI, Z. & T.G. BURKE. 1994. Marked interspecies variations concerning the interactions of camptothecin with serum albumins: a frequency-domain fluorescence spectroscopic study. Biochemistry **33:** 12540–12545.
8. MI, Z. & T.G. BURKE. 1994. Differential interactions of camptothecin lactone and carboxylate forms with human blood components. Biochemistry **33:** 10325–10336.
9. CHOURPA, I., J.M. MILLOT, G.D. SOCKALINGUM, et al. 1998. Kinetics of lactone hydrolysis in antitumor drugs of camptothecin series as studied by fluorescence spectroscopy. Biochim. Biophys. Acta **1379:** 353–366.
10. CREAVEN, P.J., L.M. ALLEN & F.M. MUGGIA. 1972. Plasma camptothecin (NSC-100880) levels during a 5-day course of treatment: relation to dose and toxicity. Cancer Chemother. Rep. **56:** 573–578.
11. NATELSON, E.A., B.C. GIOVANELLA, C.F. VERSCHRAEGEN, et al. 1996. Phase I clinical and pharmacological studies of 20-(s)-camptothecin and 20-(s)-9-nitrocamptothecin as anticancer agents. Ann. N.Y. Acad. Sci. **803:** 224–230.
12. BURKE, T.G. & Z. MI. 1993. Preferential binding of the carboxylate form of camptothecin by human serum albumin. Anal. Biochem. **212:** 285–287.
13. GIOVANELLA, B.C., H. HINZ, A.J. KOZIELSKI, et al. 1991. Complete growth inhibition of human cancer xenografts in nude mice by treatment with 20-(S)-camptothecin. Cancer Res. **51:** 3052–3055.
14. GOTTLIEB, J.A. & J.K. LUCE. 1972. Treatment of malignant melanoma with camptothecin (NSC-1008800). Cancer Chemother. Rep. **56:** 103–105.
15. GOTTLIEB, J.A., A.M. GUARINO, J.B. CALL, et al. 1970. Preliminary pharmacologic and clinical evaluation of camptothecin sodium (NSC-100880). Cancer Chemother. Rep. **54:** 461–470.
16. MOERTEL, C.G., A.J. SCHUTT, R.J. REITEMEIER & R.G. HAHN. 1972. Phase II study of camptothecin (NSC-100880) in the treatment of advanced gastrointestinal cancer. Cancer Chemother. Rep. **56:** 95–101.
17. Product monograph for Camptosar brand of irinotecan.
18. BURKE, T.G. & Z. MI. 1994. The structure basis of camptothecin interactions with human serum albumin: impact on drug stability. J. Med. Chem. **37:** 40–46.
19. MI, Z., H. MALAK & T.G. BURKE. 1995. Reduced albumin binding promotes the stability and activity of topotecan in human blood. Biochemistry **34:** 13722–13728.
20. LANGEVIN, A.M., D.T. CASTO, P.J. THOMAS, et al. 1998. Phase I trial of 9-aminocamptothecin in children with refractory solid tumors: a pediatric oncology group study. J. Clin. Oncol. **16:** 2494–2429.
21. TAKIMOTO, C., M.T. MARINO, M.D. LIANG, et al. 1997. Pharmacodynamics and pharmacokinetics of a 72-hour infusion of 9-aminocamptothecin in adult cancer patients. J. Clin. Oncol. **15:** 1492–1501.

22. EDER, J.P. JR., J.G. SUPKO, T. LYNCH, et al. 1998. Phase I trial of the colloidal dispersion formulation of 9-amino-20(s)-camptothecin administered as a 72-hour continuous intravenous infusion. Clin. Cancer Res. **4:** 317–324.
23. SIU, L.L., A.M. OZA, E.A. EISENHAUER, et al. 1998. Phase I and pharmacologic study of 9-aminocamptothecin colloidal dispersion formulation given as a 24-hour continuous infusion weekly times four every 5 weeks. J. Clin. Oncol. **16:** 1120–1130.
24. DAHUT, W., N. HAROLD, C. TAKIMOTO, et al. 1996. Phase I and pharmacologic study of 9-aminocamptothecin given by 72-hour infusion in adult cancer patients. J. Clin. Oncol. **14:** 1236–1244.
25. PAZDUR, R., E. DIAZ-CANTON, W.P. BALLARD, et al. 1997. Phase II trial of 9-aminocamptothecin administered as a 72-hour continuous infusion in metastatic colorectal carcinoma. J. Clin. Oncol. **15:** 2905–2909.
26. PAZDUR, R., D.C. MEDGYESY, R.J. WINN, et al. 1998. Phase II trial of 9-aminocamptothecin (NSC 603071) administered as a 120-hr continuous infusion weekly for three weeks in metastatic colorectal carcinoma. Invest. New Drugs **16:** 341–346.
27. VOKES, E.E., R.H. ANASARI, G.A. MASTERS, et al. 1998. A phase II study of 9-aminocamptothecin in avanced non-small-cell lung cancer. Ann. Oncol. **9:** 1085–1090.
28. POTMESIL, M., S.G. ARBUCK, C. TAKIMOTO, et al. 1996. 9-Aminocamptothecin and beyond: preclinical and clinical studies. *In* The Camptothecins: From Discovery to the Patient. P. Pantazis, B.C. Giovanella & M.L. Rothenberg, Eds. Ann. N.Y. Acad. Sci. **803:** 231–246.
29. HINZ, H., N.J. HARRIS, E.A. NATELSON & B.C. GIOVANELLA. 1994. Pharmacokinetics of the in vivo and in vitro conversion of 9-nitro-20(S)-camptothecin to 9-amino-20(S)-camptothecin in humans, dogs and mice. Cancer Res. **54:** 3096–3100.
30. GREENWALD, R.B., A. PENDRI, C.D. CONOVER, et al. 1998. Camptothecin-20-PEG ester transport forms: the effect of spacer groups on antitumor activity. Bioorg. Med. Chem. **6:** 551–562.
31. CONOVER, C.D., A. PENDRI, C. LEE, et al. 1997. Camptothecin delivery systems: the antitumor activity of a camptothecin-20-O-polyethylene glycol ester transport form. Anticancer Res. **17:** 3361–3368.
32. CONOVER, C.D., R.B. GREENWALD, A. PENDRI, et al. 1998. Camptothecin delivery systems: enhanced efficacy and tumor accumulation of camptothecin following its conjugation to polyethylene glycol via a glycine linker. Cancer Chemother. Pharmacol. **42:** 407–414.
33. LI, C., D.F. YU, R.A. NEWMAN, et al. 1998. Complete regression of well-established tumors using a novel water-soluble poly(L-glutamic acid)–paclitaxel conjugate. Cancer Res. **58:** 2404–2409.
34. LI, C., J.E. PRICE, L. MILAS, et al. 1999. Antitumor activity of poly(L-glutamic acid)-paclitaxel on syngeneic and xenografted tumors [In Process Citation]. Clin. Cancer Res. **5:** 891–897.
35. LI, C., R.A. NEWMAN & S. WALLACE. 1999. Reformulating paclitaxel. Sci. Med. **6:** 32–41.
36. LI, C., R.A. NEWMAN, Q. WU, et al. 2000. Biodistribution of paclitaxel and poly(L-glutamic acid)-paclitaxel conjugate in mice with ovarian OCa-1 tumor. Cancer Chemother. Pharmacol. In press.
37. SEYMOUR, L.W. & R. DUNCAN. 1987. Effect of molecular weight (MW) of *n*-(2-hydroxypropyl)methacrylamide copolymers on body distribution and rate of excretion after subcutaneous, intraperitoneal, and intravenous administration to rats. J. Biomed. Materials Res. **21:** 1359–1361.
38. PIMM, M.V., A.C. PERKINS, J. STROHALM, et al. 1996. Gamma scintigraphy of the biodistribution of ^{123}I-labelled *n*-(2-hydroxypropyl)methacrylamide copolymer-doxorubicin conjugates in mice with transplanted melanoma and mammary carcinoma. J. Drug Targeting **3:** 375–383.
39. MCCORMICK-THOMSON, L.A. & R. DUNCAN. 1989. Poly(amino acid) copolymers as a potential soluble durg delivery system. 1. pinocytic uptake and lysosomal degradation measured in vitro. J. Bioact. Compat. Polym. **4:** 242–251.

40. CREASEY, W.A., M. RICHARDS, D. GIL & K.C. TSOU. 1983. Action of (s)-10-hydroxycamptothecin on P388 leukemia and distribution of the drug in mice. Cancer Treat. Rep. **67:** 179–182.
41. JAXEL, C., K.W. KOHN, M.C. WANI, *et al.* 1989. Structure–activity study of the actions of camptothecin derivatives on mammalian topoisomerase I: evidence for a specific receptor site and a relation to antitumor activity. Cancer Res. **49:** 1465–1469.
42. MIYASAKA, T., S. SAWADA, K. NOKATA & M. MUTAI. 1985. Photochemical Process for Preparing Camptothecin Derivatives. US Patent. 4,545,880.
43. WALL, M.E., M.C. WANI, A.W. NICHOLAS, *et al.* 1993. Plant antitumor agents. 30. Synthesis and structure activity of novel camptothecin analogs. J. Med. Chem. **36:** 2689–2700.
44. BURKE, T.G. & Z. MI. 1993. Ethyl substitution at the 7 position extends the half-life of 10-hydroxycamptothecin in the presence of human serum albumin. J. Med. Chem. **36:** 2580–2582.

9-Nitrocamptothecin Liposome Aerosol Treatment of Human Cancer Subcutaneous Xenografts and Pulmonary Cancer Metastases in Mice

VERNON KNIGHT,[a,f] EUGENIE S. KLEINERMAN,[c,d] J. CLIFFORD WALDREP,[a] BEPPINO C. GIOVANELLA,[e] BRIAN E. GILBERT,[b] AND NADEZHDA V. KOSHKINA[a]

[a]*Molecular Physiology and Biophysics, and* [b]*Molecular Virology and Microbiology, Baylor College of Medicine, Houston, Texas 77030, USA*

[c]*Cancer Biology and* [d]*Pediatrics, University of Texas M.D. Anderson Cancer Center, Houston, Texas, USA*

[e]*Stehlin Foundation for Cancer Research at St. Joseph's Hospital, Houston, Texas, USA*

ABSTRACT: The purpose of this study was to test the anticancer properties of the water-insoluble derivative of camptothecin, 9-nitrocamptothecin (9NC), administered in a liposome formulation (L-9NC) in aerosol to mice with subcutaneous xenografts of three human cancers and in mice with murine melanoma and human osteosarcoma pulmonary metastases. The drug was formulated with dilauroylphosphatidylcholine and nebulized in particle sizes of 1.2–1.6 µm mass median aerodynamic diameter and a geometric standard deviation of 2.0. The aerosol was generated with the nebulizer flowing at 10 l/min and delivered to mice in sealed plastic cages or in a nose-only exposure chamber. Aerosol was administered for 15 min to 2 hr daily, delivering deposited doses in the respiratory tract of 8.1–306.7 µg of 9NC/ kg. With subcutaneous tumors, growth was greatly inhibited or tumors were undetectable after several weeks of treatment. We also showed that oral dosage with L-9NC had no detectable effect on cancer growth, and thus the benefit from aerosol treatment was due to pulmonary deposition and not the larger fraction of drug deposited in the nose of mice during aerosol treatment which is promptly swallowed. Intramuscular L-9NC in slightly larger doses than given in the aerosol had detectable anticancer activity, but it was significantly less than in mice receiving the drug by aerosol. With metastatic pulmonary cancers, treated animals showed highly significantly less cancer growth than control animals. L-9NC aerosol showed a major therapeutic benefit in the treatment of subcutaneous human cancer xenografts in nude mice, suggesting that cancers at systemic sites might be responsive to this treatment. In addition, the strong anticancer effect of L-9NC aerosol on pulmonary metastases offers a therapeutic approach for treatment of pulmonary cancers. Thus, L-9NC aerosol may have applicability in the treatment of cancers throughout the body.

[f]Address for correspondence: Department of Molecular Physiology and Biophysics, Baylor College of Medicine, One Baylor Plaza, Houston, TX 77030. Voice: 713-798-5725; fax: 713-798-3125.

INTRODUCTION

The 9-nitrocamptothecin (9NC) derivative used in the following studies has demonstrated potent antitumor effects against human ovarian and malignant melanoma in the human xenograft–nude mouse model when administered intramuscularly in the dose range of 1–4 mg/kg per day.[1–3] The same workers also found that intragastric injection of cotton seed oil suspensions of 9NC, at 1.0 mg/kg per day, 5 days per week for several weeks was also effective against several human cancer xenografts.[4,5]

Previous work in this laboratory has shown that certain drugs delivered to the respiratory tract in a liposome formulation may have advantages over other methods of treatment. The inhalation route is noninvasive and yields high lung concentrations of drug that are reached immediately. Toxicity is often less than by other routes, and these characteristics of aerosol treatment have been demonstrated in the treatment of pulmonary as well as systemic disease.[6–11]

In this report we describe the beneficial effect of a liposome aerosol containing 9NC (L-9NC) on subcutaneous xenografts of human breast, colon, and lung cancer in nude mice[12]; on pulmonary metastases of murine melanoma in C57BL/6 mice; and on pulmonary metastases of a human osteosarcoma xenografts in nude mice.[13,14]

MATERIALS AND METHODS

Chemicals

9NC was purchased from ChemWerth (Woodbridge, CT). Dilauroylphosphatidylcholine (DLPC) was purchased from Avanti Polar Lipids (Alabaster, AL). Tertiary butanol was obtained from Fisher Scientific, dimethylsulfoxide from Sigma, and pyrogen-free, sterile water for irrigation was from Baxter Healthcare Corporation (Deerfield, IL).

Human Cancer Subcutaneous Xenografts

Swiss immunodeficient nude mice of the NIH-1 high-fertility strain, bred and housed at the Stehlin Foundation for Research, Houston, Texas, were used. Tumors were implanted at the Stehlin Institute, and the mice were transferred to Baylor College of Medicine for experimental treatments. Human breast cancer (CLO), human colon cancer (SQU), and human lung cancer (SPA) were used in the study.

Cells and Pulmonary Tumor Metastases in Animal Models

B16F10 murine melanoma cells were purchased from ATCC (Rockville, MD) and maintained in tissue culture using DMEM supplemented with 10% fetal calf serum (FCS). Medium supplements were obtained from Gibco (Grand Island, NY). To induce pulmonary metastases, B16F10 cells were injected intravenously, 1×10^5 cells in 0.2 ml of medium via tail vein in female C57BL/6 mice (Harlan Sprague-Dawley). Lung metastases could be visually detected within a week after cell inoculation.

SAOS-LM6 (LM6) cell line was derived from SAOS-2 human osteosarcoma cells by repeating cycling of tumor cells in nude mice.[13] LM6 cells were maintained *in vitro* using EMEM medium supplemented with 10% FCS. LM6 cells, 1×10^6 in 0.2 ml, were injected into the tail vein of male nu/nu mice. Following intravenous injection, visible, macroscopic pulmonary metastases were present by 8 weeks.

Liposome Preparation and Aerosol Dosage of 9NC in Liposome Aerosol

The procedure for L-9NC preparation is described elsewhere.[12,15] The ratio of DLPC to 9NC was 50:1 (wt:wt). Lyophilized powder was reconstituted with water for irrigation (Baxter Laboratories) to a concentration of 0.2 or 0.5 mg of 9NC/ml. Empty liposomes composed of DLPC were prepared as described before[12] without adding 9NC to the formulation; the concentration of lipid after adding water for aerosol administration was 10 or 25 mg/ml.

Dosages in mice were based on a 30-g mouse with a minute volume of 30 ml (1 l/min per kg of body weight)[16] and an average of 30% deposition of the inhaled aerosol.[3] The deposited doses in this study were calculated as shown by the following example: 8.5 µg of 9NC/l in the aerosol $\times$ 0.03 l/min (mouse minute volume) $\times$ 0.3 (fraction of inhaled aerosol deposited) $\times$ 30 min (treatment time)/0.03 kg (weight of mouse) = 76.7 µg/kg. The deposited dose of DLPC in the lungs was about 50-fold higher. Dosage calculations were based on measurements of 9NC in aerosol recovered on the Andersen/ACFM nonviable ambient particle sizing sampler (Andersen Instruments, Atlanta, GA).

Treatment with Aerosol L-9NC

Treatment of mice with subcutaneous tumors was started when the subcutaneous nodules were readily palpable, a period of two or three weeks. The size of nodules was measured at regular intervals with calipers, usually in three dimensions.

In the melanoma model, aerosol treatment was started the next day after B16 cells were injected intravenously into C57BL/6 mice. Mice were divided into groups and treated five times per week for 16–21 days. Aerosol was administered to groups of mice in sealed cages. Drug suspension (10 ml) containing 0.5 mg of 9NC and 25 mg of DLPC/ml was added to an AeroTech II nebulizer (CIS-USA, Bedford, MA). The nebulizer was operated at a flow rate of 10 liters of air per min. If the mice were treated for an hour or more per day, they received half of the treatment in the morning and the other half in the afternoon.

In the osteosarcoma model, at week 9 after injection of LM6 cells when visible metastatic tumor nodules on the surface of the lungs (macroscopic metastases) were expected to be present,[13] mice were divided into groups and aerosol treatment was given for 30 min for 5 days/week for 8 or 10 weeks as described above for the B16 model. Mice were sacrificed at the end of treatment. Lungs were removed, and the tumor nodules were counted and measured. Microscopic disease was assessed by sectioning the lungs and staining with hematoxylin and eosin.

Statistics

Comparisons of lung weights and various tumor indices were made with the two-tailed Student's *t* test or the two-tailed Mann-Whitney rank sum test. For statistical analysis, "too numerous to count" (i.e., >200) was assigned a value of 200, and tumor foci diameters less than 0.5 mm were assigned a value of 0.25 mm. For experiment #1 in TABLE 2, a mean tumor diameter of 4 mm (range: 0–8 mm) was used in the calculation of tumor areas for the untreated group.

RESULTS

Measurement of the Size and Electron Microscopic Appearance of L-9NC Liposomes

Samples were obtained from the reservoir of the nebulizer at start and at 17 and 30 min later. Because liquid in the reservoir of the nebulizer is continuously recycled through the nebulizer, shear effects can be conveniently assessed on reservoir samples. Material from the nebulizer was examined in the Submicron Particle Sizer Model 370 (NICOMP), Particle Sizing Systems, Santa Barbara, CA. Data were collected until the percent error was <1.5. The liposomes at 0-time were about 2500 nm in diameter, whereas at 17 and 30 min the size had reduced to about 300 nm in diameter. Electron microscopy performed on material recovered from aerosol showed multilamellar particles resembling liposomes with a majority of diameters of about 100 nm.[12]

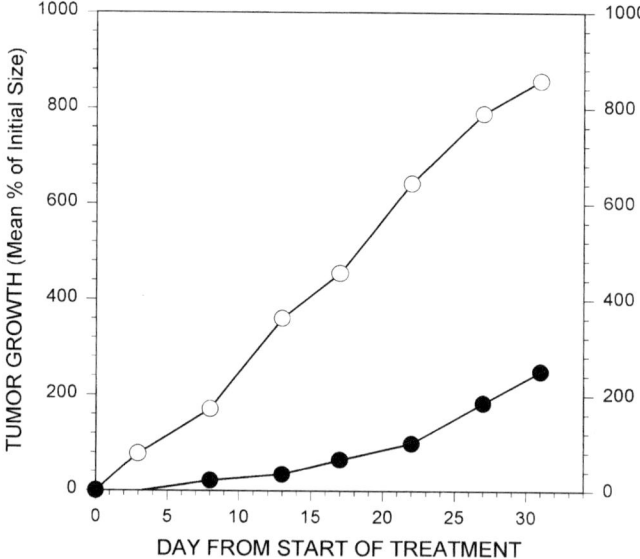

FIGURE 1. Treatment of human breast cancer (CLO) xenografts in nude mice with 9-NC-DLPC liposome aerosol. Aerosol was administered 15 min daily, five consecutive days weekly in a period of 0–31 days. The calculated dose was 8.1 µg of 9-NC/kg per day. Values are means ± SD. The mean (± SD) size of tumors at start of treatment was 90.7 ± 97.2 mm². (○ untreated, $n = 5$; ● 9-NC-DLPC liposomes, $n = 6$.) Adapted from a figure published in *Cancer Chemotherapy and Pharmacology* (Knight et al.[12]).

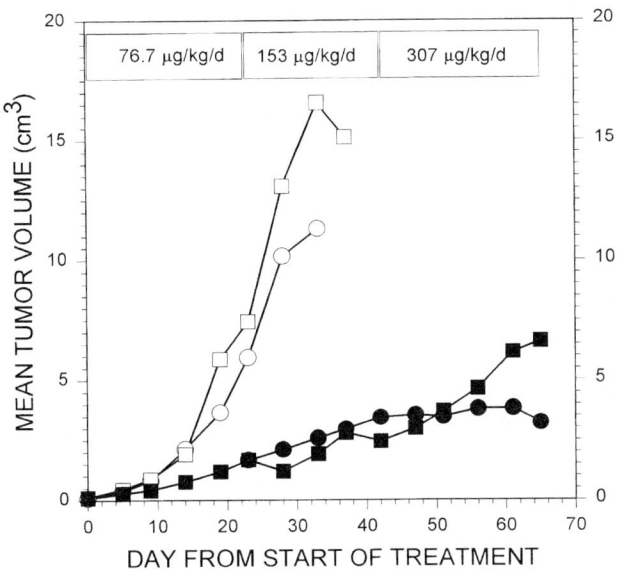

FIGURE 2. Treatment of human colon cancer (SQU) xenografts in nude mice with 9-NC-DLPC liposome aerosol. The following dosing schedules were used: 76.7 µg/kg 9-NC per day for 5 consecutive days per week from day 0 to day 62 (constant dose): or 76.7 µg/kg 9-NC per day for 5 consecutive days per week from day 0 to day 23, 153.4 µg/kg per day twice daily for 5 consecutive days per week from day 24 to 42 and 307.7 µg/kg per day twice daily for 5 consecutive days per week from day 43 to day 65 (increasing dose). Values are means ± SD. Symbols: ○ untreated, $n = 10$; □ DLPC-only liposomes, $n = 10$; ■ 9-NC-DLPC liposomes, constant dose, $n = 8$; ● 9-NC-DLPC liposomes, increasing dose, $n = 7$. Adapted from a figure published in *Cancer Chemotherapy and Pharmacology* (Knight et al.[12]).

Effect of L-9NC on Subcutaneous Xenografts of Human Cancer in Nude Mice

FIGURE 1 shows a major reduction in growth of human breast tumor (CLO) in nude mice treated for only 15 minutes daily (8.1 µg 9NC/kg), five days per week over a period of 31 days compared to controls. FIGURE 2 shows reduced growth of human colon cancer cells (SQU) with a fixed dose of 76.7 µg/kg, five days per week over a period of 62 days in one group of treated mice and an escalating dosage over this period of 76.7, 153.4, and 306.7 µg/kg in the other. Control animals received no treatment or DLPC only. Despite different doses, the two treated groups showed nearly identical reduced growth of cancer, and the DLPC controls were nearly identical to the untreated controls. FIGURE 3 shows the effect of escalating dosage of L-9NC on growth of human lung cancer (SPA) with significantly reduced growth in the treated animals. Of note is the finding that oral dosage with L-9NC in an amount slightly greater than given by aerosol had no effect on growth of the cancer. FIGURE 4 shows an effect of intramuscular L-9NC that is intermediate and significantly different from both L-9NC aerosol-treated animals and no treatment.

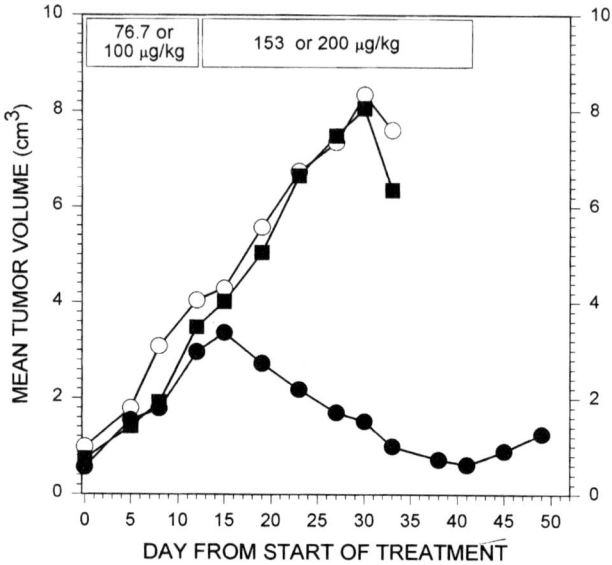

FIGURE 3. Treatment of human lung cancer (SPA) xenografts in nude mice with 9-NC-DLPC liposome aerosol or oral administration. The aerosol dosage was 76.7 µg/kg 9-NC per day for five consecutive days per week from day 0 to day 12. The dose was increased to 153.4 µg/kg per day twice daily for five days per week from day 13 to day 41. The oral 9-NC-DLPC liposomes in aqueous suspension were administered at 100 and 200 µg/kg 9-NC per day following the same regimen as aerosol treatments. Values are means ± SD. (○ untreated, $n = 11$; ■ oral 9-NC-DLPC liposomes, $n = 11$; ● aerosol 9-NC-DLPC liposomes, $n = 11$). Adapted from a figure published in *Cancer Chemotherapy and Pharmacology* (Knight *et al.*[12]).

Effect of L-9NC Aerosol on Experimental B16 Murine Melanoma Pulmonary Metastases

The lungs of mice treated for five weeks with aerosol L-9NC had markedly less B16 melanoma lung metastases than untreated control mice. The summarized data of the lung weights from three experiments performed with this animal model are presented in FIGURE 5.

In Experiment 1 (TABLE 1), 10 mice received no treatment and 12 mice received 153 µg of 9-NC/kg during a 1-hr aerosol exposure, 5 days a week over a 21-day period. The total dosage of 9-NC received during the treatment was 2.3 mg/kg. Statistical analysis gave p values (Student's t test, two-tailed) for treated versus control animals as follows: lung weights, $p = 0.0005$; number of tumor foci, $p = 0.001$; and number of mice with foci larger than 1 mm, $p = 0.001$. In a second experiment (FIG. 5), 12 mice were treated with L-9-NC aerosol, and 10 mice served as untreated controls. Animals were treated 2 hr per day (306 µg of 9-NC/kg), 5 times weekly for 16 days. Total deposited dose of 9-NC during this treatment was 3.7 mg/kg. Lung weights were used in this experiment to approximate tumor content of lungs, because a linear regression analysis of lung weights in Experiment 1 demonstrated a significant correlation with the number of tumors ($r = 0.76$, $p < 0.0001$; Pearson cor-

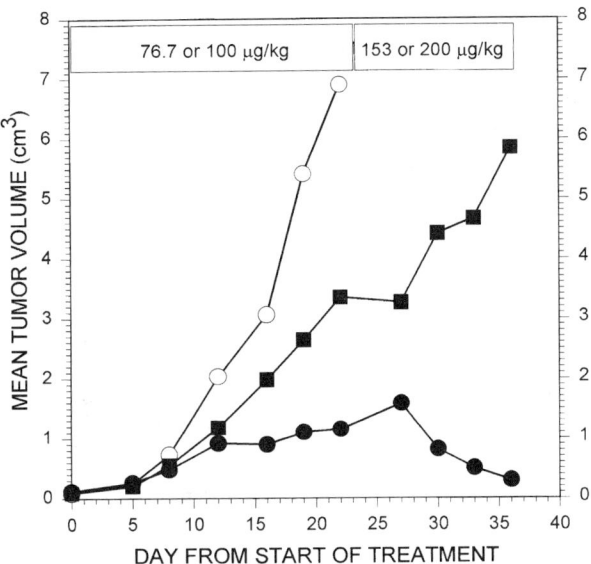

FIGURE 4. Treatment of nude mice with human lung cancer (SPA) xenografts with 9-NC-DLPC liposomes administered by aerosol using a nose-only exposure device or by intramuscular injection. Values are means ± SD. (○ untreated, $n = 8$; ● aerosol, 76.7 µg/kg 9-NC per day, 5 days per week from day 0 to day 23, then the dosage doubled from day 24 to day 36, $n = 8$; ■ intramuscular injections into the hind legs, 100 µg/kg 9NC per day, then 200 µg/kg per day on the same schedule as aerosol treatment, $n = 8$). Adapted from a figure published in *Cancer Chemotherapy and Pharmacology* (Knight et al.[12]).

relation, two-tailed). Lung weights were more than four times greater in the untreated animals than in the L-9NC-treated group (FIG. 1, $p < 0.001$; Student's t test, two-tailed).

In Experiment 3 (FIG. 5), lung weights of both untreated mice and mice given empty liposomes showed similar increases. The difference between the untreated and DLPC-treated groups was not statistically significant ($p = 0.331$; Student's t test, two-tailed). FIGURE 6 shows lungs from untreated and DLPC-only treated mice from Experiment 3 compared to L-9NC-treated mice in Experiment 2. The top and middle rows, untreated and DLPC-only treated, respectively, show enlarged lungs with many large tumors compared to smaller lungs with many fine pigmented tumors in mice treated with L-9NC aerosol (bottom row).

Effect of L-9NC Aerosol on Human LM6 Osteosarcoma Pulmonary Metastases

L-9NC aerosol treatment was also effective against LM-6 osteosarcoma metastases in the lungs. As shown in TABLE 2, Experiment 1, 10 of 11 control mice had large visible tumors in the lungs after 8 weeks of treatment 16 weeks after tumor injection. Lung sections also revealed multiple microscopic foci in the 10 animals with tumors. The remaining animal had no visible or microscopic disease detected. By contrast, none of the 11 animals treated for 8 weeks with L-9NC aerosol (treatment

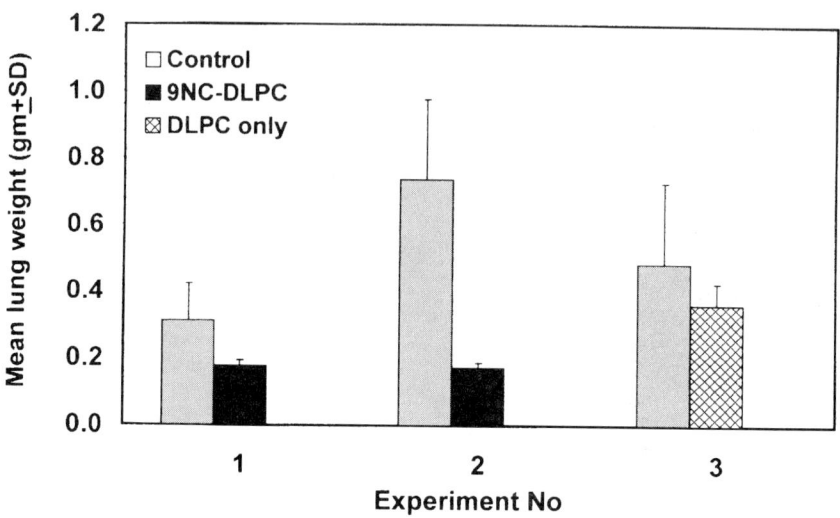

FIGURE 5. Effect of 9-NC liposome aerosol treatment on B16 murine melanoma experimental pulmonary metastases in C57BL/6 mice. Shown are mean lung weights of experimental groups. Mice were injected with 100,000 cells in 0.2 ml via tail vein. Treatment was started day after injection, 5 days per week. Dose was 153 µg/kg of 9-NC/day given during a 1-hr exposure from the Aerotech II nebulizer. Exp. 1: Treatment period, 21 days; untreated vs. treated, $p = 0.0005$. Exp. 2: Treatment period, 16 days; untreated vs. treated, $p < 0.0001$. Exp. 3: Treatment period, 21 days; control vs. DLPC only, $p = 0.331$.

received on weeks 9–16; total deposited dose of 9NC during this period was 3.1 mg/kg) had visible disease in their lungs ($p < 0.0001$; Student's t test, two-tailed). Microscopic tumor foci only were seen in 4 of the 11 mice, indicating disease regression or growth inhibition. Both the mean number of tumor foci and mean tumor area were significantly reduced in the 9-NC-treated group compared to untreated animals ($p < 0.0003$ and $p < 0.0002$, respectively; Mann-Whitney rank sum test, two-tailed).

In Experiment 2 when the treatment was extended to 10 weeks and the total of administered drug was 3.8 mg/kg, similar results were seen. The number of visible lung metastases was significantly less in treated mice than in untreated and DLPC-only treated mice ($p = 0.0001$; Student's t test, two-tailed). The number of mice with visible lung metastases in the untreated and DLPC-treated groups was not statistically different ($p = 0.635$; Student's t test, two-tailed). Statistical analysis of microscopic lung metastases revealed that in the L-9NC-treated group the mean number of tumors was much smaller than in untreated or DLPC-only treated groups ($p < 0.0008$ and $p = 0.005$, respectively; Mann-Whitney rank sum test, two-tailed). This difference was reflected in a significant reduction in mean tumor area in the L-9NC-treated group compared to the untreated and DLPC-only groups ($p = 0.002$ and $p = 0.013$, respectively; Mann-Whitney rank sum test, two-tailed). Despite a tendency for mean number of tumors and mean tumor areas to be lower in the DLPC-treated group in comparison with the untreated group, the differences were not statistically significant ($p = 0.115$ and $p = 0.149$, respectively; Mann-Whitney rank sum test, two-tailed).

TABLE 1. Effect of 9-nitrocamptothecin liposome aerosol treatment on murine B16 melanoma lung metastases (Experiment 1)[a]

Mouse No.	Lung weight (mg)	Tumors on lung surface[b]		
		No. of tumors	Size of largest tumor, diameter (mm)	Percent of total of largest tumors
Untreated				
1	372	183	2.5	50
2	504	149	2.5	50
3	212	68	1.25	50
4	334	83	2.5	50
5	486	85	4.0	50
6	194	85	1.0	50
7	223	54	2.0	50
8	255	39	2.0	50
9	286	64	2.5	50
10	253	38	2.0	50
Mean ± SD	311 ± 111	85 ± 47	2.2 ± 0.8	50 ± 0
L-9NC treated				
1	163	31	1.0	20
2	183	40	0.75	22
3	158	53	0.5	17
4	169	39	0.5	20
5	199	27	0.5	37
6	151	34	0.5	15
7	169	42	0.5	17
8	189	23	0.5	22
9	187	32	0.5	19
10	207	27	0.5	33
11	170	16	0.5	25
12	179	25	0.5	12
Mean ± SD	177 ± 17	32 ± 10	0.6 ± 0.2	22 ± 7

[a]B16 melanoma cells (1×10^5/0.2 ml injection) were given intravenously. Treatment was started the next day. Mice were treated for 1 hr, 5 times weekly for 3 weeks; lungs were weighed, and tumor nodules counted and measured.

[b]Tumors on lung surface were counted, and diameters were measured. The size and percentage occurrence of the largest tumors were recorded.

DISCUSSION

We report here the use of liposome aerosol therapy consisting of the anticancer drug 9-nitrocamptothecin and the neutral lipid DLPC formulated into liposomes in the treatment of B16 murine melanoma and human osteosarcoma lung metastases and on various human cancer xenograft models in mice. L-9NC aerosol therapy was effective in inhibiting the growth of both tumors and, in some cases, with near elimination of tumor cells from the lungs.

TABLE 2. 9-Nitrocamptothecin liposome aerosol treatment of human osteosarcoma lung metastases in a nude mouse model[a]

Treatment	Visible lung metastases	Microscopic lung metastases		
		Median No. [Range]	Mean No. ±SD	Mean tumor area (mm^2 ± SD)
Experiment 1 Untreated ($n = 11$)	10/11	16 [0–39]	18.5 ± 12.5	252 ± 170
9-NC ($n = 11$)	0/11	0 [0–4]	0.9 ± 1.6	0.05 ± 0.08
Experiment 2 Untreated ($n = 11$)	9/11	15 [0 – >200]	60.7 ± 80.3	294 ± 615
DLPC Only ($n = 11$)	7/11	2 [0–15]	4.6 ± 5.5	1.2 ± 1.4
9-NC ($n = 11$)	1/11	0 [0–1]	0.1 ± 0.3	0.2 ± 0.6

[a]SAOS-LM6 human osteosarcoma cells (1×10^6 per 0.2 ml injection) were given intravenously and allowed to grow for 8 weeks. Beginning week 9, mice were treated 5 times weekly for 8 weeks (Exp. 1) or 10 weeks (Exp. 2) with L-9NC aerosol (76.7 µg/kg/30 min treatment). At the end of 16 weeks (Exp. 1) or 18 weeks (Exp. 2) mice were sacrificed, lungs were removed, and tumor nodules were counted and measured. n = number of mice/group.
[b]Number of nude mice with lung metastases/number of mice injected with cells.

Aerosol treatment of B16 melanoma pulmonary metastases demonstrated a strong inhibition of tumor growth after 16–21 days of treatment. Treatment for 8–10 weeks was required to achieve a significant reduction of the LM-6 osteosarcoma tumor nodules. The dosages used in this study were 3 to 20 times lower than the dosages of 9-NC that were previously found to be effective when given by the intramuscular, intravenous, or intragastric routes in mice.[15,17] A possible explanation for the apparently greater therapeutic efficacy of aerosol treatment may stem from the immediate deposition of high concentrations of 9-NC throughout the respiratory tract. Pharmacokinetic studies done with the parent compound, camptothecin, showed a rapid increase in drug concentration in the lungs during aerosol treatment, with smaller but substantial amounts deposited in the liver, kidney, and spleen.[18] Drug was shown to disappear from lungs soon after treatment was stopped, with a somewhat slower disappearance from other sites. It may be that this method preserves more of the active lactone form of 9NC on the lung surfaces where there is little albumin[19] to bind and inactivate the drug. The speed of the first-pass transport of 9-NC to subcutaneous xenograft tumors following aerosol liposomal therapy has been previously reported[18] and may also be important in producing the antitumor effects seen in these present aerosol studies.

It is of interest to note the differences in the handling of inhaled aerosols by mice and men.[16] The minute ventilation per unit of body weight in mice is 1.0 ml/g, compared to 0.1 ml/g in humans, a 10-fold difference. Mice deposit approximately 30% of inhaled particles in the respiratory tract, which includes the nose, trachea, and

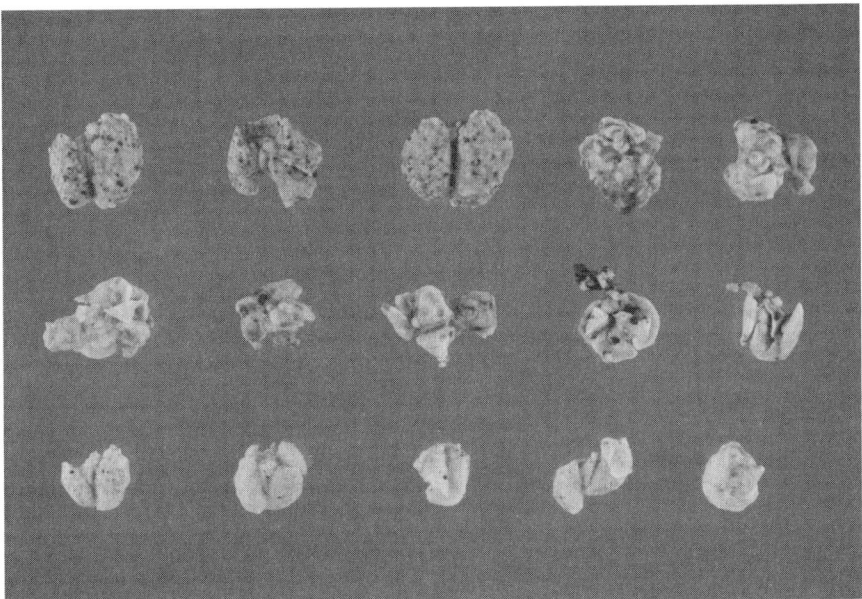

FIGURE 6. Photographs of lungs with B16 melanoma pulmonary metastases. *Top row*: lungs from untreated mice. The first three lungs and the last two lungs in the row are from mice untreated for 16 days (Exp. 2) and 21 days (Exp. 3), respectively. *Middle row*: lungs from mice that received DLPC-only aerosol treatment for 21 days (Exp. 3). *Bottom row*: lungs from mice that received L-9NC aerosol therapy for 16 days (Exp. 2).

lungs; whereas humans deposit about 70% of the inhaled particles throughout the respiratory tract with nose breathing. Pulmonary deposition in mice accounts for only 10% of the inhaled volume,[20] while humans with mouth breathing will deposit 20% of inhaled particle in the lung parenchyma (Weibel generations 17–23 constitute the alveolated portion of the human lung, K. Keyhani and P. Scherer, University of Pennsylvania, unpublished). The net effect of these differences is that, overall, mice will deposit approximately twofold more particles in the lung periphery per unit of body weight than humans. Because the maximum tolerated oral dose of 9NC in humans is 1.0 to 1.5 mg/m^2 per day (26 to 39 μg/kg in an adult),[21] it should be easily possible to administer therapeutic doses of 9NC to humans by liposome aerosol. Although our studies indicated that camptothecin, the parent component of 9NC, is rapidly cleared from the pulmonary tissue after aerosol treatment of mice,[18] DLPC remains in the lungs for many hours in humans[22,23] and rats[24] studied with ^{99m}Tc-labeled DLPC.

In previous studies with subcutaneous xenografts,[13] we found that the oral dosage of L-9NC in amounts greater than those given by aerosol had no detectable anticancer effect. This suggests that direct delivery of the drug to the tumor in the lungs by aerosol administration may be the main basis for the activity of this agent. Aerosol L-9NC therapy may also be effective against metastatic disease outside the lungs. Aerosol liposomal camptothecin treatment resulted in appreciable concentrations of drug in tumors and in brains of treated animals.[18] We anticipate a similar pharmacokinetic pattern for L-9NC.

It is current practice to administer aerosol to patients through a mouth-only breathing mask, which substantially avoids nasal and pharyngeal deposition of drug. This provides a deposition of the particles from approximately 20% of the inhaled volume in the lung parenchyma; moreover less than 5% of inhaled particles will deposit elsewhere in the respiratory tract. Therefore, mouth breathing can target particles to the lungs with great efficiency and is an effective way to administer liposomal aerosol chemotherapy for the treatment of pulmonary metastases. Mouth-only breathing masks avoid particle deposition in the nasopharynx, which are promptly swallowed and, therefore, constitute oral medication rather than aerosol medication.

In summary, these studies have demonstrated that L-9NC aerosol therapy is effective in the treatment of melanoma and osteosarcoma pulmonary metastases in mice. Because drugs in the camptothecin family are presently being used in the treatment of primary lung cancer, aerosol L-9NC therapy may offer an additional therapeutic approach for this disease. A number of other anticancer drugs can also be delivered in the liposomal formulation by aerosol. Thus, the aerosol route could provide a broad base for this type of cancer chemotherapy. Previous studies showing the activity of aerosol L-9NC against various subcutaneous tumor xenografts in nude mice[13] indicate that this approach may be useful in the treatment of metastatic disease outside the lungs as well. Inhalation therapy has the advantage of being a noninvasive route for administration of medications. It can also be given at home under supervision, thus reducing clinic visits and the cost of therapy and thus yielding greater patient freedom. A Phase I clinical trial using aerosol L-9NC in patients with advanced pulmonary malignancies is now under way.[25]

ACKNOWLEDGMENTS

This research was supported by the Clayton Foundation for Research, Houston, Texas and National Institutes of Health Grant CA 42992 (ESK) and Core Grant CA-16672.

REFERENCES

1. GIOVANELLA, B.C., E. NATELSON, N. HARRIS, et al. 1996. Protocols for the treatment of human tumor xenografts with camptothecins. Ann. N.Y. Acad. Sci. **803:** 181–187.
2. GIOVANELLA, B.C., S.O. YIM, J.S. STEHLIN & L.J. WILLIAMS. 1972. Development of invasive tumors in the "nude" mouse after injection of cultured human melanoma cells. J. Natl. Cancer Inst. **48:** 1531–1533.
3. HINZ, H.R., N.J. HARRIS, E.A. NATELSON & B.C. GIOVANELLA. 1994. Pharmacokinetics of the *in vivo* and *in vitro* conversion of 9-nitro-20(S)-camptothecin to 9-amino-20(S)-camptothecin in humans, dogs, and mice. Cancer Res. **54:** 3096–3100.
4. PANTAZIS, P., A.J. KOZIELSKI, D.M. VARDEMAN, et al. 1993. Efficacy of camptothecin congeners in the treatment of human breast carcinoma xenografts. Oncol. Res. **5:** 273–281.
5. PANTAZIS, P., J.T. MENDOZA, A. DEJESUS, et al. 1994. Partial characterization of human leukemia U-937 cell sublines resistant to 9-nitrocamptothecin. Eur. J. Haematol. **53:** 135–144.

6. GILBERT, B.E., M.B. BLACK, J.C. WALDREP, et al. 1997. Cyclosporin A liposome aerosol: lack of acute toxicity in rats with a high incidence of underlying pneumonitis. Inhal. Toxicol. **9:** 717–730.
7. GILBERT, B.E., C. KNIGHT, F.G. ALVAREZ, et al. 1997. Tolerance of volunteers to cyclosporine A-dilauroylphosphatidylcholine liposome aerosol. Am. J. Respir. Crit. Care Med. **156:** 1789–1793.
8. GILBERT, B.E. & V. KNIGHT. 1996. Pulmonary delivery of antiviral drugs in liposome aerosols. Sem. Ped. Infect. Dis. **7:** 148–154.
9. GILBERT, B.E. & R.T. PROFFITT. 1996. Aerosolized AmBisome treatment of pulmonary *Cryptococcus neoformans* infection in mice. J. Aerosol Med. **9:** 263–276.
10. GILBERT, B.E., P.R. WYDE, G. LOPEZ-BERESTEIN & S.Z. WILSON. 1994. Aerosolized amphotericin B-liposomes for treatment of systemic *Candida* infections in mice. Antimicrob. Agents Chemother. **38:** 356–359.
11. GILBERT, B.E., P.R. WYDE & S.Z. WILSON. 1992. Aerosolized liposomal amphotericin B for treatment of pulmonary and systemic *Cryptococcus neoformans* infections in mice. Antimicrob. Agents Chemother. **36:** 1466–1471.
12. KNIGHT, V., N.V. KOSHKINA, J.C. WALDREP, et al. 1999. Anti-cancer effect of 9-nitrocamptothecin liposome aerosol on human cancer xenografts in nude mice. Cancer Chemother. Pharmacol. **44:** 177–186.
13. JIA, S-F., L.L.WORTH & E.S. KLEINERMAN. 1999. A nude mouse model of human osteosarcoma lung metastases for evaluating new therapeutic strategies. Clin. Exp. Metastasis **17(6):** 501–506.
14. KOSHKINA, N.V., E.S. KLEINERMAN, C. WALDREP, et al. 2000. 9-Nitrocamptothecin liposome aerosol treatment of melanoma and osteosarcoma lung metastases in mice. Clin. Cancer Res. **6(7):** 2876–2880.
15. GIOVANELLA, B.C., E. NATELSON, N. HARRIS, et al. 1996. Protocols for the treatment of human tumor xenografts with camptothecins. Ann. N.Y. Acad. Sci. **803:** 181–186.
16. PHALEN, R.F. 1984. Inhalation Studies: Foundations and Techniques. CRC Press, Inc. Boca Raton, FL.
17. THOMPSON, J., C.F. STEWART & P.J. HOUGHTON. 1998. Animal models for studying the action of topoisomerase I targeted drugs. Biochim. Biophys. Acta **1400:** 301–311.
18. KOSHKINA, N.V., B.E. GILBERT, J.C. WALDREP, et al. 1999 Distribution of camptothecin after delivery as a liposome aerosol or following intramuscular injection in mice. Cancer Chemother. Pharmacol. **44:** 187–192.
19. PATTON, J.C. 1996. Mechanisms of macromolecule absorption by the lungs. Adv. Drug Deliv. Rev. **19:** 3–36.
20. THOMAS, R.L. 1969. Deposition and initial translocation of inhaled particles in small laboratory animals. Health Phys. **16:** 417–428.
21. VERSCHRAEGEN, C.F., E.A. NATELSON, B.C. GIOVANELLA, et al. 1998. A phase I clinical and pharmacological study of oral 9-nitrocamptothecin, a novel water-insoluble topoisomerase I inhibitor. Anti-cancer Drugs **9:** 36–44.
22. FARR, S.J., I.W. KELLAWAY, D.R. PARRY-JONES & S.G. WOOLFREY. 1985. ^{99m}Technetium as a marker of liposomal deposition and clearance in the human lung. Int. J. Pharmaceut. **26:** 303–316.
23. VIDGREN, M., J.C. WALDREP, J. ARPPE, et al. 1995. A study of ^{99m}technetium-labelled beclomethasone dipropionate dilauroylphosphatidylcholine liposome aerosol in normal volunteers. Int. J. Pharmacol. **115:** 209–216.
24. MORIMOTO, Y. & Y. ADACHI. 1982. Pulmonary uptake of liposomal phosphatidylcholine upon intrathecal administration to rats. Chem. Pharm. Bull. **30:** 2248–2251.
25. VERSCHRAEGEN, C., B.E. GILBERT, A. HUARINGA, et al. 2000. Feasibility, phase I, and pharmacological study of aerosolized liposomal 9-nitro-20(s)-camptothecin (L9NC) in patients with advanced malignancies in the lungs. Proc. Am. Assoc. Clin. Oncol. In press.

Modified Lactone/Carboxylate Salt Equilibria *in Vivo* by Liposomal Delivery of 9-Nitro-Camptothecin

DIANA S-L. CHOW,[a,c] LING GONG,[a] MICHAEL D. WOLFE,[a] AND BEPPINO C. GIOVANELLA[b]

[a]*College of Pharmacy, University of Houston, Texas Medical Center, Houston, Texas 77030, USA*

[b]*Stehlin Foundation for Cancer Research, Houston, Texas 77002, USA*

ABSTRACT: The lactone stability of camptothecins is critical for their anticancer activity. A stable liposomal 9-nitro-camptothecin formulation was developed to circumvent the drawbacks of low aqueous solubility and lactone instability and to provide sustained release of the agent in blood circulation. The potential merits of the formulation were demonstrated by its profoundly improved lactone stability *in vivo*, favorable pharmacokinetic and biodistribution characteristics in rats, and enhanced preclinical efficacy in tumor-bearing athymic mice.

INTRODUCTION

Camptothecins, topoisomerase I inhibitors, represent the most important and the newest class of anticancer drugs other than taxanes[1] introduced into clinical practice since the approval of Cisplatin. Camptothecin (CPT) is a water-insoluble, natural alkaloid extracted from the Chinese trees *Camptotheca acuminata* and *Mappia foetida* in the late 1960s.[2] The clinical application of CPT was hampered initially because of its severe side effects, including hemorrhagic cystitis, gastrointestinal toxicities, and myelosuppression revealed in early clinical trials using the sodium salt of CPT. Nevertheless, intensive interest and research efforts resurged in the early 1980s, after the antitumor mechanism of the agent was elucidated as novel inhibition of topoisomerase I.[3] The agent thus offers tissue selectivity for chemotherapy, because the enzyme level is higher in malignancy than in normal tissues.

CPT and its analogues have a broad spectrum of antitumor activity against human colon, ovarian, lung, and breast cancers in the preclinical athymic mouse model.[4–8] Chemically, the analogues share the common features of a planar aromatic five-ring system with a lactone moiety in the E-ring and an S-configuration at C-20, with dif-

[c]Address for correspondence: Diana S-L. Chow, College of Pharmacy, University of Houston, 1441 Moursund St., Texas Medical Center, Houston, TX 77030. Voice: (713)-795-8308; fax: (713)-795-8305.
dchow@uh.edu

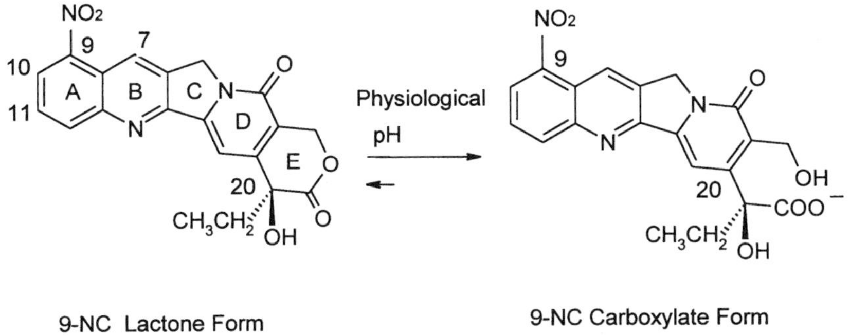

FIGURE 1. Chemical structures of 9-nitrocamptothecin (9-NC) and its carboxylate salt.

ferent substituents at C-7, C-9, C-10, and C-11. The lactone moiety is unstable and rapidly hydrolyzes to its carboxylate form at physiological pH (FIG. 1). The carboxylate form is significantly less potent in activity than its lactone form. Therefore, research efforts are still currently active, using formulation[9,10] or synthetic[11,12] approaches to protect the lactone moiety from opening *in vivo* for the maximal activity of camptothecins.

At present, two water-soluble analogues of CPT, topotecan (Hycamtin®) and irinotecan (Campto®), were approved by the FDA as a second-line therapy for metastatic ovarian cancer and colorectal cancer, respectively. However, the response rates of clinical anticancer activity of these two products were modest, 12–50% depending on the type of cancer being treated.[13] The treatment efficacy is schedule-dependent, because the cytotoxic activity of topoisomerase I inhibitors is cell-cycle specific to the S-phase.[13] Nevertheless, the optimal treatment dose and schedule in the clinic are still unknown and are yet to be defined by ongoing clinical investigations.[2,13,14] It is recognized to be essential to maintain a low lactone plasma level, below the toxic threshold, over an extended period of time to achieve optimal therapeutic effects.[15,16] In preclinical studies, it was observed that lower 9-nitro-camptothecin (9-NC) or 9-amino-camptothecin (9-AC) concentrations applied for long periods of treatment were more effective in inducing apoptosis than higher concentrations for short periods.[6]

Regardless of the commercial availability of water-soluble topotecan and irinotecan, newer analogues, including water insoluble derivatives of 9-AC and 9-NC and water-soluble derivatives of lurtotecan (GG211, G1147211, GW211) and DX8951, are presently at different stages of clinical development. Current clinical trials are directed to better characterize the clinical anticancer spectra; to establish the optimal dose, schedule, and route of administration; and to define their uses in combination with other chemotherapeutic agents and as radiation sensitizers or antiviral agents. These studies are also intended to determine whether the new analogues will have improved toxicity and efficacy profiles over the approved agents.[2,13]

There has been increased interest in the lipophilic analogues, CPT, 9-AC, and 9-NC.[17] The cytotoxic potency of camptothecins in clinical trials varied widely with a descending order of SN 38 (the active metabolite of irinotecan) > CPT > 9-NC >

9-AC > topotecan >> irinotecan.[17] CPT and 9-NC have been identified to have superior antitumor activity *in vitro* and in preclinical *in vivo* models.[5-8] The delivery of these lipophilic analogues, however, is a challenging task. The lactone stability has been a concern for camptothecins, and it is even more so with the lipophilic analogues, because their lactone moiety was less stable than those of SN 38, irinotecan, and topotecan.[13] In addition, the oral capsule forms of CPT and 9-NC used in clinical trials yielded low and erratic bioavailabilities,[2] which is consistent with the dissolution rate-limiting, incomplete absorption characteristics known to be associated with highly lipophilic agents.

Therefore, the objectives of this project were (a) to develop a stable liposomal 9-NC formulation (lipo-9NC) intended to circumvent the drawbacks of low aqueous solubility and lactone instability and to provide sustained release of the agent in blood circulation and (b) to demonstrate the potential merits of the formulation with its improved lactone stability *in vivo*, favorable pharmacokinetics and biodistribution in Sprague-Dawley rats, and enhanced preclinical efficacy in tumor-bearing athymic mice.

MATERIALS AND METHODS

Lipo-9NC Formulation

The lipo-9NC formulation, consisting of phospholipid ($t_g > 37°C$), cholesterol, and short-chain PEG fatty acid, was prepared using rehydration of dried lipid film followed by sonication. The preparation was characterized by entrapment efficiency, vesicle size, and *in vitro* release in the presence of rat plasma and human plasma.

In Vitro *Release Characteristics*

The *in vitro* release profiles of 9-NC from the formulation, as in contact with human and rat plasma at 37°C, respectively, were characterized using the dialysis method.[18] Briefly, the formulation was mixed with plasma (1:2, vol/vol) and dialyzed against normal saline (in a volume 150 times that of the mixture) through semipermeable dialysis tubing with a MWCO of 12–14,000. Aliquots (0.3 ml) of release medium were withdrawn at determined time intervals up to 6 hours, and the medium was replenished with the same volume of fresh saline. The concentration of lactone 9-NC was determined by direct injection of the sample onto the HPLC column. The concentration of total 9-NC was assayed after acidifying the sample to pH 2 with an equal volume of 0.85% H_3PO_4 solution before the HPLC assay.

The initial release rate was determined from the slope of the initial linear portion of the release profile, and the extent of release up to 6 hours was evaluated.

Pharmacokinetics

The lipo-9NC formulation or free 9-NC was administered intravenously (i.v.) via jugular vein cannula to Sprague-Dawley rats ($n = 4$ for each group) at a single dose of 2.5 mg/kg. The free 9-NC was solubilized in a co-solvent system of DMSO:PEG400:ethanol:normal saline (3:3:2:2 by volume) and administered either alone or in combination with the sham liposome. The plasma samples were collected at determined time intervals up to 6 hours and stored at −20°C until assay. The lactone and total 9-NC were extracted from the plasma samples at physiological pH and acidic pH (pH = 2), respectively, using solid-phase extraction. The extraction eluents were evaporated to dryness and reconstituted in the mobile phase before the HPLC assay.

The plasma concentration profiles for both lactone and total 9-NC were constructed. The parameters of half-life ($t_{1/2}$), overall exposure (AUC), clearance (CL), and volume distribution at steady state (V_{ss}) were derived from the profiles using a noncompartmental model of WinNonlin®.

Biodistribution

The lipo-9NC or free 9-NC (2.5 mg/kg) was injected into rats via the tail vein. At each time point, 0.5, 1, 2, 4, and 6 hours post-dose, four rats were sacrificed for harvesting liver, lung, spleen, heart, and kidneys. The organs were stored at −20°C until assay.

Each thawed sample was divided into two parts and homogenized, followed by the solid-phase extraction of the supernatant at the physiological and acidic pH for the quantification of lactone and total 9-NC, respectively. The extracts were evaporated to dryness and reconstituted in the mobile phase before the HPLC assay.

Bar graphs were constructed for both lactone and total 9-NC in each treatment group, and the AUC values were calculated from the profiles for each organ.

HPLC Assay

The samples were eluted from the reversed-phase C_8 HPLC column with the mobile phase consisting of acetonitrile/0.1% acetic acid (32:68, vol/vol), pH = 5.1, at 1 ml/min, and quantified by a spectrophotometric detector at 370 nm. CPT was used as the internal standard.

Antitumor Efficacy

The antitumor efficacy of 9-NC with i.v.[18] and intramuscular (i.m.)[19] administrations of lipo-9NC was evaluated in an athymic mouse model bearing human colon carcinoma SC1008, SC1162, or breast carcinoma Clouser tumors. Three studies were performed, with doses of 1.5 and 2.5 mg/kg for i.v. and 0.25, 0.5, 0.75, and 1.0 mg/kg for i.m. administrations. The control groups received either no treatment or sham liposome vehicle. The reference group was the free 9-NC in the co-solvent system or in NCI emulsion. The dose was administered twice weekly for various durations, 3–8 weeks.

Tumor size and animal survival were evaluated for efficacy. The body weights were recorded to monitor the toxicity.

Statistics

Student's t test was performed to compare the parameters between the lipo-9NC and free 9-NC groups. The level of significance was $p < 0.05$.

TABLE 1. *In vitro* release of 9-NC from lipo-9NC and free 9-NC formulations as incubated with human or rat plasma at 37°C

Parameter	Total 9-NC**	
	Lipo-9NC	Free 9-NC
Human plasma		
Initial release rate (%/hr)	11.8 ± 1.1*	39.7 ± 4.0
Percent released at 6 hr	42.5 ± 12.5*	80.3 ± 7.2
Rat Plasma		
Initial release rate (%/hr)	8.8 ± 0.9*	51.7 ± 5.2
Percent released at 6 hr	32.8 ± 9.8*	96.9 ± 1.9

*$p < 0.05$, as lipo-9NC compared with free 9NC.
** Mean ± SD, $n = 3$.

RESULTS AND DISCUSSION

Lipo-9NC Formulation Characteristics[18]

A stable liposomal preparation with a low lipid-to-drug ratio was capable of encapsulating 95% of the 9-NC, which is known to crystallize easily during the preparation of liposomes. The mean vesicle size was 900 nm. The formulation yielded sustained *in vitro* release of 9-NC in the presence of rat or human plasma. The initial release rates were 11.8 and 8.8% per hour in human and rat plasma, respectively, three- to sixfold slower than those of free 9-NC. The extent of release was only 42.5 and 32.8% by 6 hours in human and rat plasma, respectively (TABLE 1). It was noted that among the released 9-NC molecules, 40–50% were in lactone form. The lactone protecting effect of lipo-9NC *in vivo* was further demonstrated in the following pharmacokinetic and biodistribution data.

Pharmacokinetics[20,21]

The intravenous administration of free 9-NC or sham liposome together with free 9-NC resulted in a rapid decline of 9-NC in plasma. No 9-NC was detectable 2 hours post dose. However, the liposomal encapsulation yielded a sustained level of 9-NC for more than 6 hours (FIG. 2). The pharmacokinetic parameters were calculated on the basis of the plasma profiles. The liposomal encapsulation resulted in more than a 10-fold increase in the biological half-life ($t_{1/2}$) and more than a fourfold increase in overall exposure (AUC) of total 9-NC, due to the significant decrease in the plasma clearance (CL). The sham liposomes did not modify the pharmacokinetics of free 9-NC (TABLE 2).

In addition, the lactone-protecting effect *in vivo* was clearly demonstrated. The lactone 9-NC constituted 50% of circulating total 9-NC from the lipo-9NC delivery, but only 27% with the treatment of free 9-NC, based on the AUC measurements (TABLE 2). Lipo-9NC resulted in sustained levels of lactone 9-NC in blood circulation because of the significant protection of the lactone ring of 9-NC from hydrolysis *in vivo*.

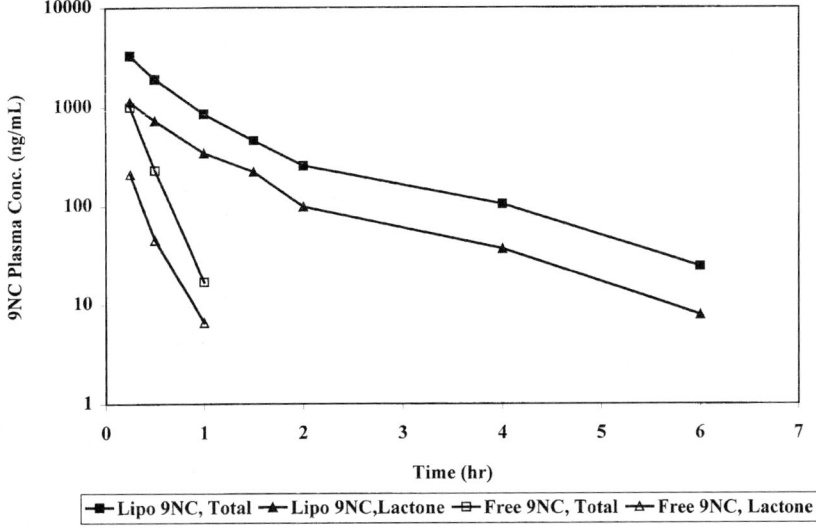

FIGURE 2. Pharmacokinetic profiles of lactone and total 9-NC following a single i.v. dose (2.5 mg/kg) of lipo-9NC or free 9-NC in rats.

TABLE 2. Summary of pharmacokinetic parameters of 9-NC following single i.v. dose (2.5 mg/kg) of lipo-9NC or free 9-NC in rats

	Total 9-NC		Lactone 9-NC	
Parameter**	Lipo-9NC	Free 9-NC	Lipo-9NC	Free 9-NC
$t_{1/2}$ (hr)	1.11 ± 0.19*	0.12 ± 0.03	1.00 ± 0.31*	0.15 ± 0.04
$AUC_{0 \to \infty}$ (ng · hr/ml)	3399.5 ± 201.3*	760.0 ± 205.1	1241.6 ± 105.3*	171.6 ± 50.0
CL (ml/hr)	117.0 ± 7.1*	567.8 ± 147.4	320.1 ± 26.6*	2536.2 ± 716.8
Vss (ml)	113.2 ± 11.2	100.1 ± 32.3	317.9 ± 40.2	490.1 ± 236.8

* $p < 0.05$, as lipo-9NC compared with free 9-NC, Student's t-test.
** Mean ± SD, $n = 4$.

Biodistribution[21,22]

The concentration profiles of total and lactone 9-NC in five major organs were significantly altered after the liposomal encapsulation (FIGS. 3A and B). After the administration of free 9-NC, the drug was eliminated rapidly from all of the organs and was not detectable by 2 hours post dose. The administration of lipo-9NC, however, yielded sustained levels of both lactone and total 9-NC in liver, lung, and spleen (TABLE 3) up to 6 hours. Moreover, more than 50% of the 9-NC retained in the lung and spleen were in lactone form, demonstrating a significant lactone-protecting ef-

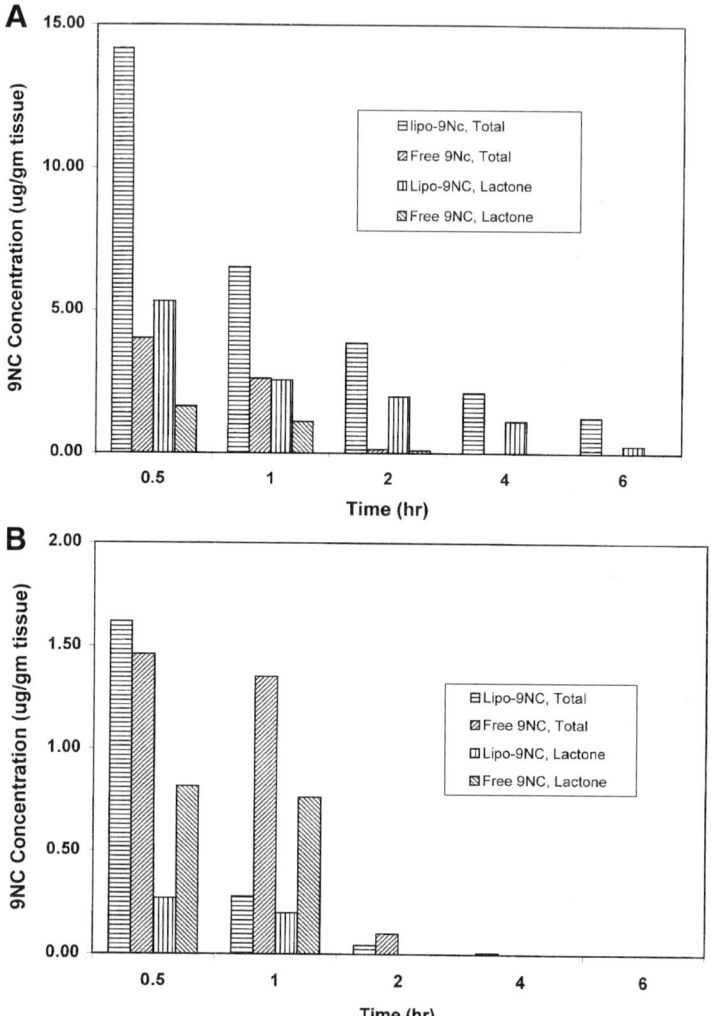

FIGURE 3. Concentrations of lactone and total 9-NC in (**A**) lung and (**B**) kidneys following a single i.v. dose (2.5 mg/kg) of lipo-9NC or free 9-NC in rats.

fect of liposomal encapsulation *in vivo*. The organ exposures of liver, lung, and spleen to lactone 9-NC after lipo-9NC treatment were increased 8, 6, and 4 times, respectively, as compared with those after the treatment of free 9-NC (TABLE 3). These favorable biodistribution characteristics of lipo-9NC offer potential merits in treating patients with cancers in these organs. In heart[18] and kidneys, however, different patterns of tissue distribution were observed (FIG. 3B). The concentrations of 9-NC from lipo-9NC were lower than or comparable to those from free 9-NC in the first hour, but significantly lower afterwards. The organ exposures to lactone 9-NC after lipo-9NC treatment in heart and kidneys, although these are highly perfused

TABLE 3. AUC_{0-6} (ng · hr/g tissue) of total and lactone 9-NC in rat organs following single i.v. dose (2.5 mg/kg) of lipo-9NC or free 9-NC

Organ	AUC_{0-6} (ng · hr/g tissue)[a]			
	Total 9-NC		Lactone 9-NC	
	Lipo-9NC	Free 9-NC	Lipo-9NC	Free 9-NC
Liver	433.8 ± 108.5*	70.3 ± 36.7	88.5 ± 28.1*	—
Lung	23237.1 ± 1341.5*	4153.1 ± 2313.1	10042.4 ± 722.8*	1790.5 ± 1095.9
Spleen	2075.9 ± 183.7*	745.1 ± 141.8	1119.9 ± 88.5*	290.5 ± 144.9
Heart	806.7 ± 231.1	1337.4 ± 759.7	280.2 ± 60.9*	515.1 ± 74.6
Kidneys	1080.8 ± 669.5	1693.1 ± 799.0	222.8 ± 138.2*	899.0 ± 470.0

[a]Mean ± SD, $n = 4$ rats.
*$p < 0.05$, as compared with total 9-NC or lactone 9-NC following free 9-NC injection, Student's t test.

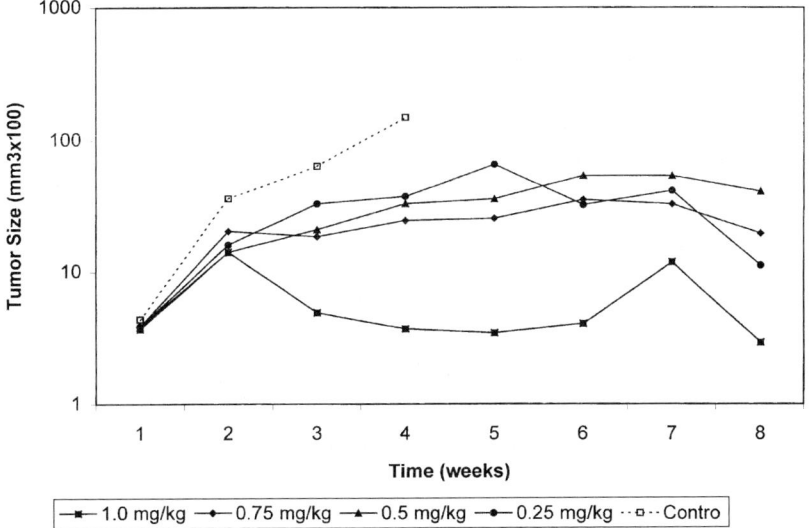

FIGURE 4. Antitumor activity of intramuscular lipo-9NC (twice weekly doses of 0.25–1.0 mg/kg) in breast carcinoma (Clouser)-bearing athymic mice.

organs, were decreased two and four times, respectively, as compared with those after the treatment of free 9-NC (TABLE 3). This observation may tender another potential merit of decreasing drug toxicity in kidneys.

Antitumor Efficacy[19,20,23,24]

The preclinical antitumor activity has been significantly enhanced by the lipo-9NC in the athymic mouse model bearing human colon carcinoma or breast carcino-

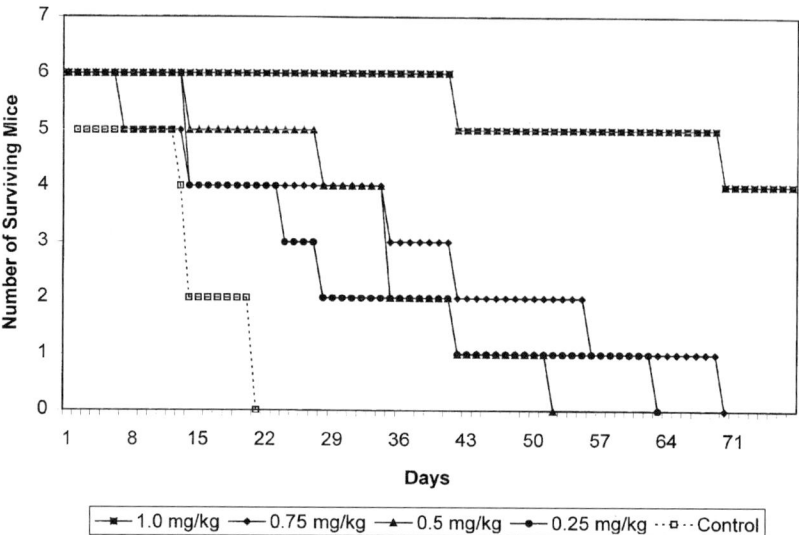

FIGURE 5. Survival profiles of breast carcinoma (Clouser)-bearing athymic mice treated with intramuscular lipo-9NC (twice weekly doses of 0.25–1.0 mg/kg).

ma. The tumor sizes of colon carcinoma in the control mice had increased five times by the end of the study. Intravenous lipo-9NC treatment suppressed the tumor growth entirely at a 2.5 mg/kg dose.[18] The tumor size in lipo-9NC groups did not change appreciably for 42 days and exerted inhibition of tumor growth four times more than with free 9-NC from NCI. At the lipo-9NC dose of 1.5 mg/kg, the tumor growth was significantly suppressed, comparable to the effect of liposomal CPT (lipo-CPT).[18]

Intramuscular administration of lipo-9NC resulted in enhanced efficacy at low doses. The tumors started to shrink after two injections and animals remained tumor free even two weeks after the last injection at a dose of 1 mg/kg. The tumor growth was suppressed entirely, 55%, and 18% at doses of 0.75, 0.5, and 0.25 mg/kg, respectively (FIG. 4). The medium survival days were significantly prolonged from two weeks to 4–6 weeks with 0.25–0.75 mg/kg doses and to longer than 10 weeks with a 1 mg/kg dose (FIG. 5). No toxicity was apparent at the test dose range, when body weight was monitored (FIG. 6).

CONCLUSION

The lipo-9NC formulation exhibited a 100-fold increase in solubilization of 9-NC, from the aqueous solubility of 0.025 mg/ml to 2.5 mg/ml. The lactone moiety *in vitro*, when in contact with rat plasma and human plasma, as well as *in vivo* was profoundly protected. The circulation retentions of the lactone form of 9-NC were prolonged 3–10 times with substantially higher levels. Moreover, the delivery system changed the inherent biodistribution pattern of 9-NC. Sustained exposure to the

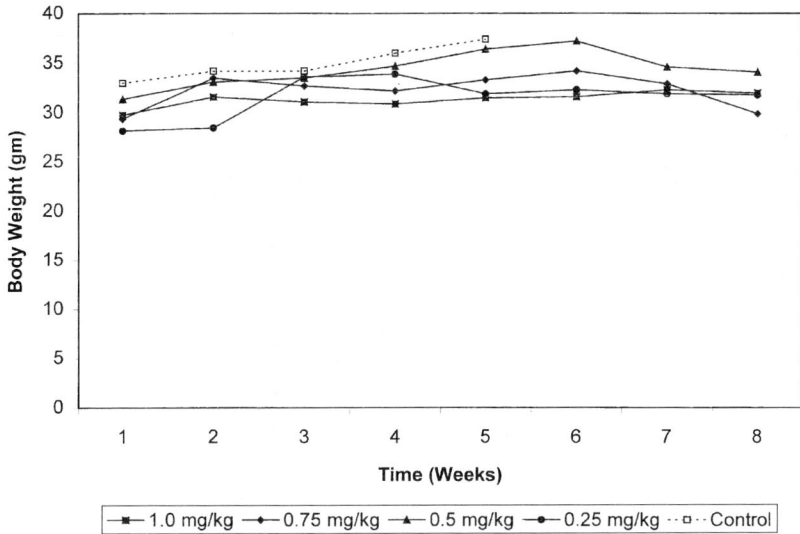

FIGURE 6. Body weights of breast carcinoma (Clouser)-bearing athymic mice treated with intramuscular lipo-9NC (twice weekly doses of 0.25–1.0 mg/kg).

lactone form of 9-NC was achieved in lung, liver, and spleen with lipo-9NC in the rat model. The favorable distribution offers the potential merit of passive targeting. Most encouragingly, the preclinical efficacy in the tumor-bearing athymic mouse model with human colon or breast carcinoma was enhanced by the intravenous or intramuscular administration of lipo-9NC.

REFERENCES

1. WALL, M.E. 1998. Camptothecin and taxol: discovery to clinic. Med. Res. Rev. **18:** 299–314.
2. HERBEN, V.M.M., W.W.B. HUININK, J.H.M. SCHELLENS & J.H. BEIJNEN. 1998. Clinical pharmacokinetics of camptothecin topoisomerase I inhibitors. Pharm. World Sci. **20:** 161–172.
3. HSIANG, Y.H., R. HERTZBERG, S. HECHT & L.F. LIU. 1985. Camptothecin induces protein-linked DNA breaks via mammalian DNA topoisomerase I. J. Biol. Chem. **260:** 14873–14878.
4. GIOVANELLA, B.C., J.S. STEHLIN, M.E. WALL, et al. 1989. DNA topoisomerase I-targeted chemotherapy of human colon cancer in xenografts. Science **246:** 1046–1048.
5. GIOVANELLA, B.C., H.R. HINZ, A.J. KOZIELSKI, et al. 1991. Complete growth inhibition of human cancer xenografts in nude mice by treatment with 20-(S)-camptothecin. Cancer Res. **51:** 3052–3055.
6. PANTAZIS, P., J.A. EARLY, A.J. KOZIELSKI, et al. 1993. Regression of human breast carcinoma tumors in immuno-deficient mice treated with 9-nitrocamptothecin: differential response of nontumorigenic and tumorigenic human breast cells *in vitro*. Cancer Res. **53:** 1577–1582.
7. PANTAZIS, P., J.A. EARLY, J.T. MENDOZA, et al. 1994. Cytotoxic efficacy of 9-nitrocamptothecin in the treatment of human malignant melanoma cells *in vitro*. Cancer Res. **54:** 771–776.

8. HINZ, H.R., N.J. HARRIS, E.A. NATELSON & B.C. GIOVANELLA. 1994. Pharmacokinetics of the *in vivo* and *in vitro* conversion of 9-nitro-20-(S)-camptothecin to 9-amino-20-(S)-camptothecin in humans, dogs, and mice. Cancer Res. **54:** 3096–3100.
9. CONOVER, C.D., R.B. GREENWALD, A. PENDRI, *et al.* 1998. Camptothecin delivery systems: enhanced efficacy and tumor accumulation of camptothecin following its conjugation to polyethylene glycol via a glycine linker. Cancer Chemother. Pharmacol. **42:** 407–414.
10. SADZUKA, Y., S. HIROTSU & S. HIROTA. 1999. Effective irinotecan (CPT-11) containing liposomes: intraliposomal conversion to the active metabolite SN-38. Jpn. J. Cancer Res. **90:** 226–232.
11. HAN, Z., Z. CAO, D. CHATTERJEE, *et al.* 1999. Propionate and butyrate esters of camptothecin and 9-nitrocamptothecin as antileukemia prodrugs *in vitro*. Eur. J. Haematol. **62:** 246–255.
12. LESUEUR-GINOT, L., D. DEMARQUAY, R. KISS, *et al.* 1999. Homocamptothecin, an E-ring modified camptothecin with enhanced lactone stability, retains topoisomerase I-targeted activity and antitumor properties. Cancer Res. **59:** 2939–2943.
13. TAKIMOTO, C.H., J. WRIGHT & S.G. ARBUCK. 1998. Clinical application of the camptothecins, Biochim. Biophys. Acta **1400:** 107–119.
14. O'REILLY, S. 1999. Topotecan: what dose, what schedule, what route? Clin. Cancer Res. **5:** 3–5.
15. POTMESIL, M. 1994. Camptothecins: from bench research to hospital wards. Cancer Res. **54:**1431.
16. GERRITS, C.J.H., M.J.A. DE JONGE, J.H.M. SCHELLENS, *et al.* 1997. Topoisomerase I inhibitors: the relevance of prolonged exposure for present clinical development. Br. J. Cancer **76:** 952–962.
17. TANIZAWA, A., A. FUJIMORI, Y. FUJIMORI & Y. POMMIER. 1994. Comparison of topoisomerase I inhibition, DNA damage and cytotoxicity of camptothecin derivatives presently in clinical trials. J. Natl. Cancer Inst. **86:** 836–842.
18. GONG, L. 1998. Development of 9-nitrocamptothecin liposomal formulation: preformulation, pharmacokinetics, biodistribution and antitumor activity in rats and mice. Ph.D. dissertation, University of Houston, Houston, TX.
19. CHOW, D.S-L., M.D. WOLFE & B.C. GIOVANELLA. 2000. Intramuscular (i.m.) delivery of liposomal 9-nitrocamptothecin (9NC) in a tumor bearing athymic mouse model. Proc. Am. Assoc. Cancer Res. **41:** 324, Abstract #2055.
20. GONG, L., B.C. GIOVANELLA & D.S-L. CHOW. 1998. Improved lactone stability of 9-nitro-camptothecin *in vitro* and *in vivo* by liposomal formulation. Proc. Am. Assoc. Cancer Res. **39:** 430, Abstract #2926.
21. GONG, L. & D.S-L. CHOW. 1998. Pharmacokinetics and biodistribution of liposomal 9-nitrocamptothecin (9NC) and free 9NC in rats. Presented at the 12th National Meeting of the American Association of Pharmaceutical Scientists, Pharm. Res. (Suppl.): Abstract #3027.
22. GONG, L., B.C. GIOVANELLA & D.S-L. CHOW. 1999. Sustained organ exposure to 9-nitro-camptothecin (9NC) lactone form by liposomal delivery. Proc. Am. Assoc. Cancer Res. **40:** 417, Abstract #2756.
23. CHOW, D.S-L., G. CHEN, L. GONG & B.C. GIOVANELLA. 1997. Pharmacokinetics and *in vivo* anti-tumor activity of liposomal encapsulated camptothecin and its analogue. Proc. Am. Assoc. Cancer Res. **38:** 258, Abstract #1733.
24. CHOW, D.S-L., G. CHEN, L. GONG & B.C. GIOVANELLA. 1997. Liposomal camptothecin and 9-nitrocamptothecin: formulation, pharmacokinetics and pre-clinical anti-tumor activity. Proceedings of the 24th International Symposium on Controlled Release of Bioactive Materials, Stockholm, Sweden, pp. 919–920, Abstract #6520.

New Analogues of Camptothecins
Activity and Resistance

EPIE BOVEN,[a] ANNEMARIE H. VAN HATTUM, ILSE HOOGSTEEN, HENNIE M.M. SCHLÜPER, AND H.M. PINEDO

Department of Medical Oncology, Vrije Universiteit Medical Centre, Amsterdam, The Netherlands

INTRODUCTION

Semisynthetic analogues of camptothecin have been developed with the aim of better efficacy and reduced toxicity when compared to topotecan and CPT-11. Among them are DX-8951f [(1S,9S)-1-amino-9-ethyl-5-fluoro-2,3-dihydro-9-hydroxy-4-methyl-1H,12H-benzo[de]pyrano[3′,4′:6,7]indolizino[1,2-b]quinoline-10,13(9H,15H)-dione methanesulfonate dihydrate][1] and BNP1350 (7-[(2-trimethylsilyl)ethyl]-20(S)camptothecin),[2] which are currently in phase I–II clinical trials. DX-8951f is a water-soluble derivative, while BNP1350 is a highly lipophilic compound. Preclinical activity data indicate that both drugs have the potential for a greater therapeutic index than camptothecins in clinical use. We have studied DX-8951f and BNP1350 for their efficacy in a variety of human tumor xenografts. In addition, we analyzed possible mechanisms of resistance in drug-selected variants of the human ovarian cancer cell line A2780.

MATERIALS AND METHODS

Drugs

DX-8951f (Daiichi Pharmaceutical Co., Tokyo, Japan), BNP1350 (BioNumerik Pharmaceuticals Inc., San Antonio, TX), SN-38 (Daiichi), camptothecin (Sigma, St. Louis, MO), all dissolved in DMSO, and topotecan (SmithKline Beecham Pharmaceuticals, King of Prussia, PA), as clinically formulated, were further diluted in tissue culture medium for the *in vitro* antiproliferative assay. For *in vivo* use, DX-8951f was dissolved in water, and for BNP1350 the vehicle BNP-PF4 (BioNumerik) was used.

Cell Lines and Antiproliferative Assay

A2780 human ovarian cancer cells and resistant variants 2780DX8 (grown in 8 nM DX-8951f), 2780K4 (grown in 4 nM BNP1350), 2780K32 (grown in 32 nM

---

[a]Address for correspondence: Epie Boven, M.D., Ph.D., Department of Medical Oncology, Vrije Universiteit Medical Centre, De Boelelaan 1117, 1081 HV Amsterdam, The Netherlands. Voice: 31-20-4444336; fax: 31-20-4444355.
e.boven@azvu.nl

BNP1350), and ADDP (cisplatin-resistant)[3] were cultured in supplemented Dulbecco's modified Eagle's medium (Gibco, Breda, NL). Drug activity experiments were carried out with the MTT assay and a 96-hour drug exposure time. All concentrations were tested in four replicate wells, and each experiment was performed at least three times. The results were expressed as the IC_{50}, which is the concentration of the drug inducing a 50% inhibition of growth of treated cells when compared to control cell growth. The resistance factor (RF) was calculated by dividing the IC_{50}-resistant variant: IC_{50} wild-type cells.[4]

Human Tumor Xenografts and Treatment

Tumors derived from colon cancer and ovarian cancer were grown s.c. in both flanks of nude mice (Harlan, Horst, NL). Treatment was given at maximum tolerated doses in various schedules depending on the drug. Treatment was started at the time that tumors had a mean volume of 100–150 mm^3, and groups consisted of 5–6 mice each. Drug efficacy was expressed as the percentage of growth inhibition.[5]

Resistance Features

Topoisomerase I nuclear protein was measured by Western blot using a polyclonal antibody from scleroderma patient serum (TopoGEN, Columbus, OH), and topoisomerase I catalytic activity was determined with the DNA relaxation assay.[4] The presence of breast cancer resistance protein (BCRP)[6] was detected on cytospin preparations with monoclonal antibody BXP-34 (Prof. R.J. Scheper, Vrije Universiteit Medical Centre, Amsterdam, NL).

RESULTS AND DISCUSSION

Antitumor Activity

DX-8951f was given at a dose of 17.5 mg/kg i.p. weekly ×2, and growth inhibition >50% was obtained in three of five human tumor xenografts, all three derived from ovarian cancer. Efficacy of the weekly schedule was more pronounced than the equitoxic schedule 1.5 mg/kg i.p. daily ×5. BNP1350 was given 1.0 mg/kg i.p. daily ×5 and induced a growth inhibition >50% in six of seven human tumor xenografts derived from both colon cancer and ovarian cancer. BNP1350 1.5 mg/kg daily ×5 given by oral route proved to be as effective as the i.p. schedule; oral bioavailability was presumably 67%.

Drug Resistance Studies

DX-8951f-induced resistance in 2780DX8 cells showed a RF of 9.3. SN-38 and topotecan were highly cross-resistant, while the activity of camptothecin and BNP1350 was not clearly affected. Topoisomerase I protein and activity were not reduced in 2780DX8 cells, but cells demonstrated pronounced BCRP expression. Cells were also highly resistant against mitoxantrone, suggesting the presence of BCRP as the mechanism of resistance.[6,7] BNP1350-induced resistance in 2780K4 and 2780K32 cells showed RFs of 41 and 90, respectively. All topoisomerase I inhibitors were cross-resistant. Topoisomerase I protein was unchanged, but activity was reduced in BNP1350-selected variants. In addition, in 2780K32 cells resistance was more pronounced against SN-38, topotecan, and DX-8951f, which may likely be attributed to the moderate expression of BCRP in these cells. Cisplatin-resistant ADDP cells with a RF of 14 were also resistant against all topoisomerase I inhibitors having RFs in the same order of magnitude. In this cell line, topoisomerase I protein and activity were not changed. It thus appears that increased DNA repair enzymes will also affect sensitivity to camptothecins.

CONCLUSIONS

Both DX-8951f and BNP1350 have antitumor activity in preclinical *in vivo* tumor systems. BNP1350 may be a suitable candidate for oral treatment of cancer. In order to determine schedule dependency of DX-8951f in ovarian cancer patients, a clinical phase II trial has recently been initiated studying the daily ×5 every 3 weeks schedule and the weekly ×3 every 4 weeks schedule. The efficacy of both drugs is decreased when topoisomerase I activity is reduced or when DNA damage repair is increased. DX-8951f is a drug that is affected by the presence of BCRP, but to a lesser extent than SN-38 and topotecan.

REFERENCES

1. MITSUI, I., E. KUMAZAWA, Y. HIROTA, *et al.* 1995. A new water-soluble camptothecin derivative, DX-8951f, exhibits potent antitumor activity against human tumors *in vitro* and *in vivo*. Jpn. J. Cancer Res. **86:** 776–782.
2. HAUSHEER, F., K. HARIDAS, M. ZHAO, *et al.* 1998. Karenitecins (PART II): a novel class of orally active highly lipophilic topoisomerase inhibitors. Proc. Am. Assoc. Cancer Res. **39:** 420–421.
3. SCANLON, K.J., T. FUNATO, B. PEZESHKI, *et al.* 1990. Potentiation of azidothymidine cytotoxicity in cisplatin-resistant human ovarian carcinoma cells. Cancer Comm. **2:** 339–343.
4. JANSEN, W.J.M., T.M. HULSCHER., J. VAN ARK-OTTE, *et al.* 1998. CPT-11 sensitivity in relation to the expression of p170-glycoprotein and multidrug resistance-associated protein. Br. J. Cancer **77:** 359–365.
5. JANSEN, W.J.M., G.M. KOLFSCHOTEN, C.A.M. ERKELENS, *et al.* 1997. Anti-tumor activity of CPT-11 in experimental human ovarian cancer and soft-tissue sarcoma. Int. J. Cancer **73:** 891–896.
6. BRANGI, M., T. LITMAN, M. CIOTTI, *et al.* 1999. Camptothecin resistance: role of the ATP-binding cassette (ABC), mitoxantrone-resistance half-transporter (MXR), and potential for glucuronidation in MXR-expressing cells. Cancer Res. **59:** 5938–5946.
7. MALIEPAARD, M., M.A. VAN GASTELEN, L.A. DE JONG, *et al.* 1999. Overexpression of the *BCRP/MXR/ABCP* gene in a topotecan-selected ovarian tumor cell line. Cancer Res. **59:** 4559–4563.

Intraperitoneal Topoisomerase-I Inhibitors

Preliminary Findings with 9-Aminocamptothecin

FRANCO MUGGIA, LEONARD LIEBES, MILAN POTMESIL,[a] ANNE HAMILTON, HOWARD HOCHSTER, GILA HORNREICH, JOAN SORICH, ANDREA DOWNEY, AND HEATHER WASSERSTROM

Department of Medicine-Division of Oncology, Department of Radiology, and the Comprehensive Kaplan Cancer Center, New York University School of Medicine, New York, New York 10016, USA

ABSTRACT: The i.p. administration of topoisomerase I (Topo I) inhibitors has a pharmacologic advantage over intravenous application, including preservation of the biologically active lactone form. In our ongoing study, patients have received 9-amino-20(S)-camptothecin (9-AC) i.p. on days 1, 3, 5, 8, 10, and 12, repeated every 4 weeks. The daily dose has been escalated to level IV of 1.5 mg/m^2 (9.0 mg/m^2 per course), median of 3 cycles, range 1–4, with a reversible Grade 3 neutropenia in one patient. Responses included one CR (resolution of a pleural effusion), two patients without progressive disease (PD), two not evaluable, and two patients too early for evaluation. The area under the curve (AUC)ip/AUCpl ratio (pharmacologic advantage) ranged from 7.6 to 16.5 on average, and, using nonlinear modeling, the pharmacologic decay data were fit to one- or two-compartmental models. Overall, a 9-AC i.p. application is well tolerated and anticipated to be an active regimen against i.p. malignancies, particularly those known to be sensitive to systemic Topo-I inhibitors.

INTRODUCTION

Several general principles, defining the suitability of a systemically active chemotherapeutic agent for intraperitoneal (i.p.) locoregional treatment, have been established[1–5]: (1) A substantial difference exists between i.p. drug levels over time, expressed as area under the curve (AUCip), and the AUCpl in plasma, representing systemic blood flow supplying susceptible normal tissues and extraperitoneal tumors. AUCip/AUCpl is referred to as the "pharmacologic advantage" of the i.p. route specific for a particular drug and schedule. Depending on the rate of drug clearance from the i.p. cavity and systemic drug metabolism, pharmacologic advantage varies among drug classes. (2) Drug "penetrance" into tumor cells and tumor metastatic nodules: on the basis of preclinical findings, camptothecins have a 10-fold increase in intracellular partitioning compared to extracellular drug concentrations.[6] (3) Tolerance of peritoneal surfaces to the direct local effect of a drug. (4) Efflux from the peritoneal cavity via surface capillaries into blood circulation including the

---

[a]Address for correspondence: Milan Potmesil, M.D., New York University School of Medicine, Department of Radiology, 550 First Avenue, New York, NY 10016. Voice: 212-263-6486; fax: 212-263-8104.

milan.potmesil@med.nyu.edu

portal venous system, compared to the drug efflux via lymphatics: this is generally higher for compounds with a molecular weight of <1,000 daltons. Activity against liver tumors may be enhanced should the drug clearance be predominantly by the portal-vein route.[5] Such portal clearance is applicable to the disposition of camptothecins, fluoropyrimidines, or platins.

Optimal conditions for i.p. therapeutic protocols are met through careful assessment of the size and extent of i.p. tumor involvement and the absence of i.p. adhesions preventing fluid distribution throughout the cavity. Such an optimal situation may be achieved by surgical or systemic (chemical) debulking and by considering i.p. therapy at the first reassessment.[3,7,8] Few if any benefits of the i.p. treatment can be expected in patients with bulky intra-abdominal disease, in patients subjected to repeated surgery, and/or in the presence of extensive intra-abdominal adhesions preventing adequate drug distribution. Negative reports of treatment can often show suboptimal conditions among patients selected for i.p. regimens including bulky disease, or the selection of drugs that may not be suitable for i.p. administration. The role of i.p. therapy has been somewhat defined for patients with ovarian cancer, whereas for gastrointestinal cancers and other malignancies further study is needed.

CLINICAL EXPERIENCE WITH INTRAPERITONEAL CHEMOTHERAPY

Epithelial ovarian cancer is a major cause of morbidity and mortality among women in the United States. The standard approach to the treatment of stages III and IV has been surgical reduction of tumors, followed by an i.v. platinum- and taxane-based regimen. Although two-thirds of patients respond to this combination chemotherapy, the majority are documented to have residual disease or will eventually experience relapse within the peritoneal cavity. In responding patients, residual disease may be documented at a planned surgical reassessment, a procedure that can be combined with i.p. consolidation. Alternatively, recurrences are documented at a median time of 1.5 years by laparoscopy, CT scan, a serum marker (CA-125), or by physical examination. Locoregional therapy has been extensively explored in these patients. In earlier studies, i.p. carboplatin yielded mixed results,[9-11] possibly reflecting a suboptimal selection of patients. A later study, using i.p. consolidation either with FUDR (floxuridine, 2'-deoxy-5-fluorouridine) or with mitoxantrone, reported encouraging prolongation of disease-free and overall survival for the former.[12] Cisplatin has shown both local penetration into cancer nodules and good systemic distribution. Therefore, the drug alone or in combination has often been used as i.p. consolidation of the disease for patients at a high risk of recurrences in spite of their favorable response to the first-line treatment.[8] The most conclusive results, rekindling interest in i.p. therapy, have recently been reported in two Phase-III studies.[13,14] The trials, comparing initial treatment of a small-volume residual advanced ovarian cancer with either intravenous (i.v.) or i.p. cisplatin, have found that the i.p. route of drug administration was less toxic and significantly improved progression-free survival of patients. The i.p. treatment repertoire has been recently enhanced by the use of paclitaxel.[15] This drug has an excellent pharmacological advantage when administered i.p., and this role, together with i.p. cisplatin, is being explored in a Phase-III study of the Gynecologic Oncology Group (GOG).[16]

The i.p. instillation of FUDR has been further investigated either alone or in combination with i.p. platins, leucovorin, or with systemic hydroxyurea (reviewed in Muggia et al.[8]). As noted earlier, a randomized Phase-II SWOG study of patients with ovarian cancer selected i.p. FUDR alone over i.p. mitoxantrone in prolonging the relapse-free survival.[12] In addition to these studies, i.p. FUDR was combined with i.p. cisplatin in patients with gastric cancer. Following neoadjuvant chemotherapy and gastric resection, patients on this protocol were consolidated with i.p. FUDR treatment, resulting in a median four-year actuarial survival, a marked improvement over historical controls.[17] Overall, results of trials studying the treatment with i.p. FUDR, either alone or in combination with leukovorin or cisplatin, show good tolerance of the modality by patients with minimal residual disease that is confined to the peritoneal cavity and encouraging potential for disease-free survival.[18,19]

This experience in patients with ovarian or gastrointestinal cancer raises the prospect of effective consolidation with suitable new compounds to be used in patients with residual i.p. disease. Camptothecins, DNA topoisomerase-I (Topo-I) inhibitors, have a potential advantage for i.p. administration, that is, good local tolerance and sustained stability of their biologically active lactone form in the acidic medium used for i.p. administration. The tolerance has been confirmed by two trials of i.p. topotecan combined with systemic chemotherapy.[20,21] We are reporting preliminary observations made with the i.p. administration of another Topo-I inhibitor, 9-amino-20(S)-camptothecin (9-AC).

DEVELOPMENT OF 9-AMINO-20(S)-CAMPTOTHECIN

9-AC, a semisynthetic analogue of camptothecin, was developed, and its biochemistry, pharmacology, preclinical antitumor effectiveness, and toxicities studied in Topo I–directed molecular screens and tissue-culture cell lines[22,23] by an academic consortium in collaboration with the National Cancer Institute (NCI)/Division of Cancer Treatment (DCT) and Pharmacia & Upjohn. 9-AC has shown activity against inherently resistant human cancers such as colon cancer and melanoma growing as xenografts in immunodeficient mice.[24–28] The *in vivo* studies also revealed essential information on the optimal pharmacokinetics and pharmacodynamics of 9-AC, and established the principles of clinical scheduling. It was shown in the mouse that a gradual release of biologically active 9-AC lactone from a subcutaneous 9-AC depot induces a low plasma level of the lactone with the terminal half-life in excess of 17 hours, and this was accompanied by excellent antitumor activity.[26,27,29]

In 1989, 9-AC was selected by the NCI/DCT for further evaluation. Clinical trials have suggested that the frequency and duration of i.v. administration may determine the antitumor effectiveness of the drug.[30–37] We have previously studied 9-AC in a Phase-I trial (CTEP T92-0163, NYU 92-37) using 21-day and 14-day i.v. continuous infusions (CI),[38,39] paralleling our experience with a low-dose 21-day CI of topotecan.[40] Among 17 evaluable patients with ovarian cancer treated on the 21-day CI schedule with 9-AC, there were two complete remission (CR) and three partial remissions. Dose-limiting toxicities included leukopenia and thrombocytopenia, whereas nonhematologic toxicities were mild. The maximally tolerated dose (MTD) for the CD-formulated 9-AC, delivered over 21 days, is 0.5–0.6 mg/m^2 per day (10.5–12.6 mg/m^2 per course).[6,7] A Phase-I trial of oral 9-AC has been reported,[41] providing an alternative to prolonged i.v. administration of 9-AC. Considering our experience with i.v. 9-AC administration,[26,27,29] we have selected a protracted schedule for the i.p. study.

INTRAPERITONEAL ADMINISTRATION OF 9-AMINO-20(S)-CAMPTOTHECIN IN A PHASE-I STUDY

9-AC has several favorable attributes expected in a compound that is effective by the i.p. route: (1) clearance of a substantial portion of i.p. 9-AC before reaching the systemic circulation due to the bile excretion and disposition in feces[42,43] (contributing in turn to a markedly higher AUCip over AUCpl); (2) preclinical evidence for good i.p. tolerance; (3) preservation of biologically active lactone in an acidic pH[44]; and (4) enhanced accumulation of the lactone in tumor cells.[6]

This study seeks to determine the type and extent of toxicities of 9-AC administered every 28 days i.p. in a cycle of six applications delivered over a 12-day period. CD-formulated 9-AC for injections (IDEC Pharmaceuticals, Inc.) was dissolved in special diluent (20% dextrose U.S.P., 0.9% NaCl U.S.P., and sterile water for injection, QSAD), and the volume adjusted by saline (0.9% NaCL U.S.P. and sterile water

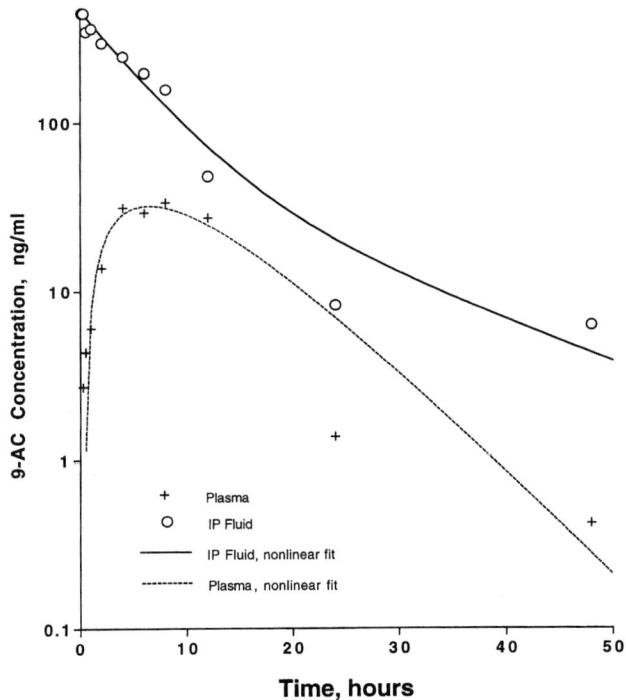

FIGURE 1. Comparison of pharmacokinetic decay of 9-AC in i.p. fluid (o) and plasma (+). The nonlinear model fits for i.p. fluid (———) and plasma (- - -) are also shown.

TABLE 1. Studied dose levels

Dose level	mg/m²/application (number of i.p. applications/course^a^)	mg/m²/course	Number of patients entered
I	0.208 (6)	1.25	1
II	0.42 (6)	2.5 (100%)	1
III	1.0 (6)	6.0 (140%)	3
IV	1.5 (6)	9.0 (50%)	2
V	2.25 (6)	13.5 (50%)	
VI	3.0 (6)	18.0 (34%)	
VII	4.0 (6)	24.0 (34%)	
VIII	5.0 (6)	30.0 (25%)	

^{a}Starting Monday, the i.p. drug applications are planned for day 1, 3, 5, 8, 10 and 12 of a treatment course. Each application is diluted in 1.0 l/m² of special diluent/saline and delivered i.p. by gravity.

EXAMPLE: A female patient with a BSA of 1.5 m² will receive, at level III, six applications of 1.5 l of special diluent/saline with 1.5 mg of 9-AC each. The total dose/course of 9.0 mg is delivered in 6 applications over 12 days in 9 l of special diluent/saline.

for injection, QSAD, pH 6.8) to 1 l/m².[45] All 9-AC concentrations in this trial are calculated on body surface-area (BSA) basis expressed in m², and the volume of fluid given i.p. is adjusted to 1 l/m², thus the concentration is constant per dose level. The fractionation employed over 12 days is practical and avoids possible fluid build-up in spite of prolonged treatment cycles. Additional objectives of the trial include pharmacological studies and, when feasible, documentation of antitumor activity.

Eligibility is directed towards patients with predominantly small i.p. tumor metastases <1.0 cm in diameter, and includes ovarian cancer with epithelial histology, other gynecological tumors, breast, gastric, colorectal, appendiceal, or pancreatic cancer and cancer of unknown primary source, as well as other epithelial malignancies with predominantly i.p. manifestations. Patients with ovarian cancer have to receive standard therapy before entry into this trial. Except for colorectal cancer treated systemically, also eligible are postoperative patients with other cancers of the digestive system who are considered to have a high probability of a local recurrence.

The pretreatment intervention consists of insertion of a Tenckhoff catheter or an implantable peritoneal device, usually placed at the time of surgery. The catheter is placed in the abdominal cavity under laparoscopic control or by laparotomy, with precautions as dictated by good clinical practice.[46] Laparoscopy is planned if deemed important for the patient's management.

To date, seven patients have been treated on the protocol, with a median age of 54 years (range 27–74 years), consisting of four men and three women: four with colon, two with epithelial ovarian, and one with gastric carcinoma. Five patients had previous chemotherapy. Trial patients received a median of three treatment cycles (range 1–4), and level IV of the escalation schema has been reached (see TABLE 1), with reversible grade 3 neutropenia in one patient. Local toxicity was classified as Grade 1 and 2 of the abdominal pain score[47] in one patient each. A reversible irritation around the Huber needle inserted into the device has been noted, which required

TABLE 2. Summary of 9-AC pharmacokinetic parameter estimates

No. of patients	Dose (mg/m^2)	AUC-i.p. (ng/ml) × hr	$t_{1/2}$-i.p. hours	C_{max}-i.p. (ng/ml)	AUC-pl (ng/ml) × hr	$t_{1/2}$-p.l. hours	C_{max}-p.l. (ng/ml)	AUC i.p./pl ratio
$n=1$	0.208	473	5.2	112	28.7 ± 27.1	4.5 ± 1.8	4 ± 2.1	16.5
$n=2$	0.42	933 ± 126	3.2 ± 1.3	243 ± 163	71.2 ± 51.6	8.9 ± 4.0	7 ± 4.1	13.1
$n=3$	1	3846 ± 105	7.9 ± 3.6	486 ± 104	504 ± 77	16.5 ± 11.2	25.4 ± 8.6	7.6

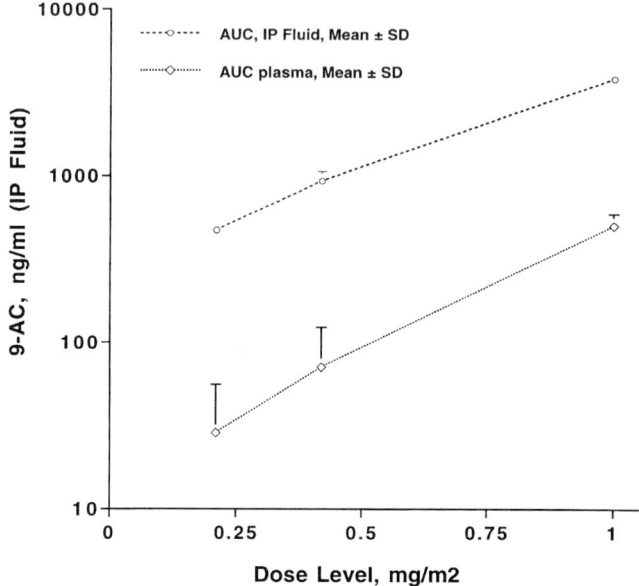

FIGURE 2. Comparison of the dose proportionally for the 9-AC AUC determination for i.p. fluid (- - -) and plasma (———).

antibiotics on one occasion. Responses included one CR (resolution of a pleural effusion), two patients without progressive disease during the treatment, two not evaluable, and two patients who are too early in the treatment for evaluation.

Aliquots of i.p. fluid and blood plasma were obtained during the first cycle of treatment from six patients. Blood was handled and processed using the method established for clinical studies of 9-AC pharmacokinetics.[48,49] Handling of i.p. fluid samples followed the technique established for plasma collection. Blood and i.p. fluid was sampled before i.p. drug installation, and at 5, 15, and 30 min and 1, 2, 4, 6, 8, 12, 24, and 48 hours for the first and fifth or sixth i.p. drug application. Plasma or i.p. fluid in the amount of 2 ml was obtained from heparinized aliquots, 9-AC lactone was separated using solid-phase separation under neutral conditions or from acidified aliquots. The method allows sample storage up to two month before reversed-phase HPLC analysis. An acidic pH 2.55 isocratic HPLC mobile phase is used to enhance 9-AC fluorescence, and this step enhances the fluorescence 50-fold compared to the original method. The detection method determines the total 9-AC (lactone plus inactive hydrolyzed form) and the lactone form separately.[47,48] TABLE 2 summarizes the results of pharmacokinetic studies. There is a 10.9-fold increase of 9-AC AUC in peritoneal fluid compared to plasma AUC (FIG. 1), with i.p. AUC and C_{max} showing dose dependency in both i.p. fluid and plasma (FIG. 2). Drug elimination half-life in i.p. fluid is significantly shorter (5.9 hr) than in plasma (12 hr). Reasonably high concentrations of 9-AC lactone have been achieved in the i.p. environment.

ACKNOWLEDGMENTS

This work was supported in part by the Lynne Cohen Foundation, UO1 CA 76642, GCRC MO1 RR 00096, and the Cancer Center Core Grant CA 16087.

REFERENCES

1. DEDRICK, R.L., C.E. MYERS, P.M. BUNGAY, et al. 1978. Pharmacokinetic rationale for peritoneal drug administration in the treatment of ovarian cancer. Cancer Treat. Rep. **62:** 1–12.
2. DEDRICK, R.L. & M.F. FLESSNER. 1997. Pharmacokinetic problems in peritoneal drug administration: tissue penetration and surface exposure. J. Natl. Cancer Inst. **89:** 480–487.
3. HOWELL, S.B. 1993. Regional chemotherapy. In Cancer Medicine. J.F. Holland et al., Eds.: XV–4: 640–652. Lea and Febiger. Philadelphia/London.
4. SUGARBAKER, P.H. 1996. Peritoneal carcinomatosis: natural history and rational therapeutic intervention using intraperitoneal chemotherapy. In Peritoneal Carcinomatosis: Drugs and Diseases. Cancer Treatment and Research. P.H. Sugarbaker, Eds. Kluger Academic Publishers. Boston.
5. ALEXANDER, H.R., D.L. BARTLETT, D.L. FRAKER, et al. 1996. Regional treatment strategies for unresectable primary and metastatic cancer confined to the liver. In Cancer. Principles and Practice of Oncology. V.T. DeVita, Jr., S. Hellman, S.A. Rosenberg, Eds. **10:** 1–19. J.B. Lippincott. Philadelphia, PA.
6. POTMESIL, M., L. LIEBES, J. DRYGAS, et al. 1996. Camptothecins with lipophilic moiety as potential tools in regional chemotherapy. Program/Proceedings of the American Society of Clinical Oncology. 32nd Annual Meeting, Abstr. 1600, p. 500, Philadelphia, PA.
7. MARKMAN, M. 1986. Intraperitoneal antineoplastic agents for tumors principally confined to the peritoneal cavity. Cancer Treat. Rep. **13:** 219–242.
8. MUGGIA, F.M., T. SAFRA, S. JEFFERS, et al. 1999. Intraperitoneal therapy with fluoropyrimidines in the treatment of ovarian and gastrointestinal cancers. In Current Clinical Oncology. Regional Chemotherapy: Clinical Research and Practice. M. Markman, Ed. Chapt. 13: 213–223. Humana Press. Totowa, NJ.
9. TEN-BOKKEL-HUININK, W.W., D.J. VAN WARMERDAM, A.C. DUBBLEMAN, et al. 1994. Intraperitoneal-administered carboplatin in patients with ovarian cancer: influence of a dwell time on toxicity and response. Ann. Oncol. **5:** 133–139.
10. GUASTALLA, J.P., C. LHOMME, P. KERBRAT, et al. 1994. Phase II trial of intraperitoneal carboplatin in ovarian carcinoma patients with macroscopic disease at second laparotomy: a multicentre study of French Federation Nationale des Centres Lutte Contre le Cancer. Ann. Oncol. **5:** 127–132.
11. SPEYER, J.L., U. BELLER, N. COLOMBO, et al. 1990. Intraperitoneal carboplatin: favorable results in women with minimal residual ovarian cancer after cisplatin therapy. J. Clin. Oncol. **8:** 1335–1341.
12. MUGGIA, F.M., P.Y. LIU, D.S. ALBERTS, et al. 1996. Intraperitoneal mitoxantrone or floxuridine: effects on time-to-failure and survival of patients with minimal residual ovarian cancer after second-look laparotomy—a randomized Phase II study by the Southwest Oncology Group. Gynecol. Oncol. **61:** 395–402.
13. ALBERTS, D.S., P.Y. LIU, E.V. HANNIGAN, et al. 1996. Intraperitoneal cisplatin plus intravenous cyclophosphamide versus intravenous cisplatin plus intravenous cyclophosphamide for stage III ovarian cancer. N. Engl. J. Med. **335:** 1950–1955.
14. MARKMAN, M. 1999. Intraperitoneal therapy of ovarian cancer. Oncology **1:** 18–21.
15. MCGUIRE, W.P., W.J. HOSKINS, M.F. BRADY, et al. 1996. Cyclophosphamide and cisplatin compared with paclitaxel and cisplatin in patients with stage III and IV ovarian cancer. N. Engl. J. Med. **334:** 1–6.
16. MARKMAN, M., E. ROWINSKY, T. HAKES, et al. 1992. Phase I trial of intraperitoneal taxol: a Gynecologic Oncology Group study. J. Clin. Oncol. **10:** 1485–1491.

17. CROOKES, P., C.G. LEICHMAN, L. LEICHMAN, et al. 1997. Systemic chemotherapy for gastric carcinoma followed by postoperative intraperitoneal therapy. Cancer, Special Section, **79:** 1767–1775.
18. MUGGIA, F.M., S. JEFFERS, L. MUDERSPACH, et al. 1997. Phase I/II study of intraperitoneal floxuridine and platinums (cisplatin and/or carboplatin). Gynecol. Oncol. **66:** 290–294.
19. MUGGIA, F.M., A. TULPULE, A., RETZIOA, et al. 1994. Intraperitoneal 5-fluoro-2′-deoxyuridine with escalating doses of leucovorin: pharmacology and clinical tolerance. Invest. New Drugs **12:** 197–206.
20. HOFSTRA, L.S., A.M. BOS, E.G. DE VRIES, et al. 2000. Intraperitoneal topotecan with standard iv paclitaxel in ovarian cancer is feasible. Program/Proceedomgs of the American Society of Clinical Oncololgy, 36th Annual Meeting, Abstr. 1548, p. 391a, New Orleans, LA.
21. MUGGIA, F.M. & H. HOCHSTER. 1997. Phase I topotecan and cisplatin intraperitoneal therapy for solid tumors of the peritoneum. Protocol NYU 97-40.
22. JAXEL, C., K.W. KOHN, M.C. WANI, et al. 1989. Structure activity study of the actions of camptothecin derivatives on mammalian topoisomerase I. Evidence for a specific receptor site and for a relation to antitumor activity. Cancer Res. **49:** 1465–1469.
23. HSIANG, Y.-H., L.F. LIU, M.E. WALL, et al. 1989. DNA topoisomerase I-mediated DNA cleavage and cytotoxicity of camptothecin analogs. Cancer Res. **49:** 4385–4389.
24. GIOVANELLA, B.C., J.S. STEHLIN, M.E. WALL, et al. 1989. DNA topoisomerase I-targeted chemotherapy of human colon cancer in xenografts. Science **246:** 1046–1048.
25. GIOVANELLA, B.C., H.R. HINZ, A.J. KOZIELSKI, et al. 1991. Complete growth inhibition of human cancer xenografts in nude mice by treatment with 20-(S)-camptothecin. Cancer Res. **51:** 3052–3055.
26. POTMESIL, M., B.C. GIOVANELLA, L.F. LIU, et al. 1991. Preclinical studies of DNA topoisomerase I-targeted 9-amino and 10,11-methylenedioxy camptothecins. In DNA Topoisomerases in Cancer. M. Potmesil & K.W. Kohn, Eds.: 299–311. Oxford University Press. New York.
27. POTMESIL, M., B.C. GIOVANELLA, M.E. WALL, et al. 1993. Preclinical and clinical development of DNA topoisomerase I inhibitors in the United States. In Molecular Biology of DNA Topoisomerases and Its Application to Chemotherapy. T. Andoh, H. Ikeda & M. Oguro, Eds. Chapt. 29: 301– 311. CRC Press. Tokyo.
28. POTMESIL, M., D. VARDEMAN, A.J. KOZIELSKI, et al. 1995. Growth inhibition of human cancer metastases by camptothecins in newly developed xenograft models. Cancer Res. **55:** 5637–5641.
29. SUPKO, J.G., J. PLOWMAN, D.J. DYKES, et al. 1992. Relationship between the schedule dependence of 9-amino-20(S)-camptothecin (AC; NSC 603071) antitumor activity in mice and its plasma pharmacokinetics. Proc. Am. Assoc. Cancer Res. **33:** 432, Abstr. 2578.
30. POTMESIL, M. 1994. Camptothecins: from bench research to hospital wards. Cancer Res. **54:** 1431–1439.
31. Clinical Brochure 9-Amino-20(S)-camptothecin, NSC 603071, Investigational New Drug. 1992. Division of Cancer Treatment, National Cancer Institute, Bethesda, MA.
32. EDER, J.P. JR., J.G. SUPKO, T. LYNCH, et al. 1998. Phase I trial of colloidal dispersion formulation of 9-amino-20(S)-camptothecin administered as a 72-hour intravenous infusion. Clin. Cancer Res. **4:** 317–324.
33. SIU, L.L., A.M. OZA, E.A. EISENHAUER, et al. 1998. Phase I and pharmacologic study of 9-aminocamptothecin colloidal dispersion formulation given as a 24-hour continuous infusion weekly times four every 5 weeks. J. Clin. Oncol. **16:** 1122–1130.
34. RUBIN, E., V. WOOD, A. BHARTI, et al. 1995. A phase I and pharmacokinetic study of a new camptothecin derivative, 9-aminocamptothecin. Clin. Cancer Res. **1:** 269–276.
35. DAHUT, W., N. HAROLD, C. TAKIMOTO, et al. 1996. Phase I and pharmacologic study of 9-aminocamptothecin given by 72-hr infusion in adult cancer patients. J. Clin. Oncol. **14:** 1236–1244.
36. TAKIMOTO, C.H., W. DAHUT, M.T. MARINO, et al. 1997. Pharmacokinetics and pharmacodynamics of a 72-hr infusion of 9-aminocamptothecin in adult patients. J. Clin. Oncol. **15:** 1492–1501.

37. POTMESIL, M., S.G. ARBUCK, C.H. TAKIMOTO, et al. 1996. 9-Aminocamptothecin and beyond: preclinical and clinical studies. In The Camptothecins: From Discovery to the Patient. P. Pantazis, B.C. Giovanella, M.L. Rothenberg, Eds. Ann. N.Y. Acad. Sci. **803**: 321–247.
38. HOCHSTER, H., M. POTMESIL, L. LIEBES, et al. 1996. A Phase I study of 9-amino-camptothecin (9-AC) by prolonged infusion of 21 days. In 9th NCI-EORTC Symposium on New Drugs in Cancer Therapy. Abstract book, abstract #461, p. 130, Amsterdam, The Netherlands.
39. HOCHSTER, H., L. LIEBES, J. SPEYER, et al. 1997. Phase I and pharmacodynamic study of prolonged infusion of 9-amino-camptothecin (9-AC) in two formulations. Program/Proceedings of the American Society of Clinical Oncology, 33rd Annual Meeting, Abstr. 1507 p. 476, Denver, CO.
40. HOCHSTER, H., L. LIEBES, J. SPEYER, et al. 1994. Phase I trial of low dose continuous topotecan infusion in patients with cancer: an active and well-tolerated regimen. J. Clin. Oncol. **12**: 553–559.
41. DE JONGE, M.J.A., C.J.A. PUNT, H. GELDERBLOM, et al. 1999. Phase I and pharmacologic study of oral (PEG-1000) 9-aminocamptothecin in adult patients with solid tumors. J. Clin. Oncol. **17**: 2219–2226.
42. SMITH, P.L., J.G. LIEHR, A.E. AHMED, et al. 1992. Pharmacokinetics of tritium labeled camptothecin in nude mice. Proc. Am. Assoc. Cancer Res. **33**: 432, abstract 2579.
43. POTMESIL, M., L. LIEBES, J. DRYGAS, et al. 1996. Novel camptothecins with lipophilic moieties. Proc. Am. Assoc. Cancer Res. **37**: 432, abstract 2951.
44. GABR, A., A. KUIN, M. AALDERS, et al. 1997. Cellular pharmacokinetics and cytotoxicity of camptothecin and topotecan at normal and acidic pH. Cancer Res. **57**: 4811–4816.
45. MUGGIA F.M., H. HOCHSTER, E. NEWMAN, et al. 1997. A Phase I study of intraperitoneal administration of 9-amino-20(S)-camptothecin to patients with cancer predominantly confined to the peritoneal cavity. CTEP Protocol T97-0123, NYU 97-53.
46. ASH, S.R. 1996. Peritoneal access devices for intraperitoneal chemotherapy. In Peritoneal Carcinomatosis: Principles of Management. P.H. Sugarbaker, Cancer Treatment and Research Series. E.J. Freireich, Ed. Chapt. 25: 387–413. Kluver Academic Publishers.
47. TAKIMOTO, C.H., R.W. KLECKER, W.L. DAHUT, et al. 1994. Analysis of the active lactone form of 9-aminocamptothecin in plasma using solid-phase extraction and high-performance liquid chromatography. J. Chromatogr. **655**: 97–104.
48. SUPKO, J.G. & L. MALSPEIS. 1992. Liquid chromatography analysis of 9-amino-camptothecin in plasma monitored by fluorescence induced upon postcolumn acidification. J. Liq. Chromatogr. Clin. Anal. **15**: 3261–3272.

Transport of Topoisomerase I Inhibitors by the Breast Cancer Resistance Protein

Potential Clinical Implications

JAN H.M. SCHELLENS,[a,c,d] MARC MALIEPAARD,[a] RIK J. SCHEPER,[b] GEORGE L. SCHEFFER,[b] JOHAN W. JONKER,[a] JOHAN W. SMIT,[a] JOS H. BEIJNEN,[a,c] AND ALFRED H. SCHINKEL[a]

[a]*The Netherlands Cancer Institute, Department of Medical Oncology and Experimental Therapy, Amsterdam, The Netherlands*

[b]*Free University, Department of Pathology, Amsterdam, The Netherlands*

[c]*Division of Drug Toxicology, Faculty of Pharmacy, Utrecht University, Utrecht, The Netherlands*

ABSTRACT: The multidrug resistance protein BCRP (breast cancer resistance protein) is a member of the ATP-binding cassette family of drug transporters. Overexpression of BCRP caused by exposure of cells to mitoxantrone (MX) or doxorubicin/verapamil resulted in a resistance pattern that is different from what is generally seen in the case of P-glycoprotein and MRP1 overexpression. Recently, the BCRP gene has been described in ovarian, breast, colon, and gastric cancer and fibrosarcoma cell lines. Our human tumor cells T8 and MX3, derived from the ovarian cancer cell line IGROV1 by stepwise increased exposure to topotecan and MX, are resistant to topotecan, CPT11, SN38, and 9-aminocamptothecin as well as MX. Increased energy-dependent efflux of affected drugs was noted. BCRP is a very efficient transporter of topotecan. Our recent studies, using the monoclonal antibody (mAb) BXP34, revealed that BCRP is located in the plasma membrane of the T8 and MX3 cell lines. Preliminary results of staining of human tumor cells showed low or absent levels of BCRP in a panel of solid tumors and acute myeloid leukemia cells.

INTRODUCTION

The clinical pharmacology of a great number of anticancer drugs is largely affected by the presence of drug transporters in a wide variety of normal tissues. It concerns in particular anticancer drugs of natural source or origin, such as the anthracyclin antitumor antibiotics, the taxane drugs paclitaxel and docetaxel, and the vinca alkaloids. These drugs are substrates for the membrane-bound drug efflux pump P-glycoprotein (P-gp).[1,2] An increasing number of transporters have recently been characterized molecularly, biochemically, and pharmacologically. The most intensively studied drug transporter is the multidrug resistance (mdr) protein P-gp.

---

[d]Address for correspondence: J.H.M. Schellens, Department of Medical Oncology, The Netherlands Cancer Institute, Plesmanlaan 121, 1066 CX Amsterdam, The Netherlands. Voice: +31 20 512 2569; fax + 31 20 512 2572.
jhm@nki.nl

P-gp is an ATP-binding cassette protein of 170 kDa that is expressed in a wide variety of normal tissues such as the epithelial layer of the gastrointestinal tract, the bile canaliculi in the liver, the blood–brain barrier, the testes, the placenta, and excretory organs such as the suprarenal gland.[3–6] Recent studies revealed that P-gp has protective and excretory functions. It protects the brain against a range of harmful toxins, that after uptake into the body circulate in the blood compartment by making the blood–brain barrier pharmacologically impermeable. Also in the placenta P-gp has a protective function for the fetus, which can be exerted because of its localization at the apical site of the syncytiotrophoblast. In the liver it contributes to the excretion of drugs into the bile canaliculi, such as paclitaxel and doxorubicin. In the gastrointestinal tract P-gp modulates the uptake, and possibly also the biotransformation, of substrate drugs through a concerted action with the drug-metabolizing enzyme system cytochrome P450 (CYP) in the intestinal epithelial layer. Previous studies in genetically modified mdr (P-gp) knockout mice revealed that the oral bioavailability of substrate drugs, such as paclitaxel, is highly increased compared with the very low (<10%) bioavailability in P-gp proficient wild-type mice.[7] Effective blockade of P-gp in wild-type mice by oral application of cyclosporin A or PSC833 resulted in a highly significant increase of systemic exposure of the orally administered model substrate paclitaxel compared with oral administration of paclitaxel alone.[8,9] A proof-of-principle study in patients using the oral combination of paclitaxel and cyclosporin A has confirmed these laboratory observations.[10,11] The apparent bioavailability of paclitaxel in patients when given alone was 5%, which increased to at least 40% when given orally in combination with cyclosporin A. The safety of the oral route was very good. This has been the starting point for additional clinical studies, some of which are presently still ongoing. The aim is to improve the oral pharmacokinetics of the substrate drugs paclitaxel and docetaxel by blockade of P-gp in the gut wall by co-administration of a P-gp blocker, such as cyclosporin A or GF120918 (GG918). The ultimate goal is to develop an oral treatment strategy for these taxane drugs in order to improve patient convenience, make therapy more practical, and enable development of chronic treatment schedules.

P-gp has also been widely associated with clinical drug resistance in preclinical models. Overexpression of P-gp results in a significantly increased drug efflux and therefore decreased intracellular accumulation of substrate anticancer drugs. Based on the well-established relationships between drug exposure and cell survival, this P-gp overexpression results in decreased tumor cell kill. Blockade of P-gp by co-incubation of an effective blocker can restore tumor cell sensitivity by increased drug accumulation. Also, in artificial tumor models *in vivo,* comparable relationships have been described. Overexpression of P-gp can result in tumor resistance, and blockade of P-gp can restore tumor sensitivity to affected substrate drugs. Clinical implications of P-gp expression in tumor tissue are less clear. Previous studies in patients with solid tumors and hematologic malignancies failed to show that coadministration of a P-gp blocker resulted in increased anticancer drug efficacy. However, the study design of some of these studies had significant limitations.[12–14] It is to be hoped that currently ongoing studies, which employ more effective and selective P-gp blockers, will be more conclusive.

In addition to P-gp, other ABC transporters have been characterized such as the multidrug-related protein family MRP. Up to now, MRPs 1–7 have been cloned, and normal tissue distribution has at least partly been established. The function of the

MRPs is not yet as well established as that of P-gp, but assessment of physiologic function as well as implications of overexpression, as have been found in some tumor tissues, are the subjects of extensive ongoing investigations. The canalicular organic anion transporter MRP2, which is involved in hepatic transport of bilirubin glucuronide, is also involved in biliary excretion of CPT11 and its active metabolite SN38.[15]

Recently, another ABC transporter has been identified. It concerns the 72-kDa (half)-transporter protein BCRP.[16-19] Studies using mRNA established that BCRP is expressed in normal tissue such as the placenta, liver, and small and large intestine; but the exact cellular localization is currently unknown, because monoclonal antibodies are not yet available. In addition, the physiologic function of BCRP is still unknown. Our studies are directed toward determining the implications of overexpression of BCRP in tumor cell line models, to describe the expression of BCRP in normal and tumor tissues, and to establish the potential clinical implications of BCRP expression for the pharmacokinetic behavior of substrate drugs. In this study we describe human tumor cell lines that overexpress BCRP and the development of antibodies (mAbs) against BCRP and speculate on clinical implications of BCRP expression.

MATERIALS AND METHODS

Development of Cell Lines

Two cell lines were developed and denoted T8 and MX3. Both cell lines were derived from the human epithelial ovarian cancer cell line IGROV1. The T8 cell line was developed by intermittent exposure of IGROV1 to increasing concentrations of the camptothecin-derived topoisomerase I inhibitor topotecan, and the MX3 cell line was developed by continuous exposure of IGROV1 cells to increasing concentrations of MX. Topotecan exposure was increased up to 950 nM, after which single cells were selected. These cells were exposed once weekly to topotecan for 1 hour. MX concentrations were increased up to 340 nM, after which single cells were selected. These cells were exposed in culture to MX for 1 hour every week. Details of the development of T8 and MX3 have previously been described.[20]

Cross Resistance Pattern

Selected drugs were tested for cross-resistance using the sulforhodamine B (SRB) assay.

Accumulation and Efflux of Topotecan and MX

Accumulation was studied using IGROV1, T8, and MX3 cells under energy proficient and ATP-deprived incubation conditions as previously described.[20] Drug concentrations were determined by validated HPLC assays (topotecan[21]) or flow cytometry (MX).

TABLE 1. Cross-resistance of the topotecan (T8)- and MX (MX3)-derived sublines of the human ovarian cancer cell line IGROV1 to selected drugs

	IC_{50} IGROV1 (nM)	Resistance factor T8	Resistance factor MX3
Topotecan	12.6	52*	14*
9-Aminocamptothecin	2.64	79*	16*
SN38	1.95	176*	44*
Camptothecin	3.15	4.3*	1.9**
MX	30.4	11*	11*
Cisplatin	547	1.4	0.7
5FU	1754	1.8	1.0
Paclitaxel	1.32	1.8	1.5
Doxorubicin	88.2	0.5	0.9

ABBREVIATION: MX = mitoxantrone.
* $p < 0.001$.
** $p = 0.06$.

Development of Monoclonal Antibodies

Female Balb/c mice were injected in the footpad with sonicated BCRP-overexpressing MCF7 MR cells emulsified in Freund's complete adjuvant. Booster injections were given on days 10, 20, 30, and 34 before fusion. Cells of draining lymph nodes were fused with mouse myeloma cells as previously described.[22] The established mAb was denoted BXP34. Subsequently, hybridoma supernatants were tested on cytospin preparations of tumor cell lines.

RESULTS

The T8 and MX3 cell lines showed significant resistance to both topotecan and MX (TABLE 1). Both T8 and MX3 showed a significant cross-resistance to CPT11, its active metabolite SN38, 9-aminocamptothecin, and MX. There was a moderate (T8) to weak (MX3) crossresistance to camptothecin (TABLE 1). There was no cross-resistance to the P-gp substrate drugs paclitaxel and doxorubicin.

Accumulation studies revealed that intracellular concentrations of topotecan and MX under equal incubation conditions were significantly lower in both T8 and MX3. In T8 and MX a four- to fivefold lower accumulation of topotecan and MX was found. The initial rate of efflux was significantly higher in T8 and MX3, accounting for the observed accumulation difference. Under ATP-depleted conditions there were no significant differences anymore in accumulation and efflux of topotecan and MX in T8 and MX3 compared with the parental IGROV1.

The developed mAb, denoted BXP34, was used for staining of the described cell lines. No staining for BCRP was found in cytospins of IGROV1, in contrast to T8 and MX3 which showed intensive staining. BXP34 was found to be specific for BCRP as described previously.[22] Further analysis showed, as expected, clear plasma membrane staining for BCRP.

Preliminary results of staining of tumor tissue revealed no or very low levels of staining on cryosections of a panel of renal cell cancer, breast cancer, and acute myeloid leukemia cells obtained from chemotherapy-naive as well as from chemotherapy-pretreated patients.

DISCUSSION

Incubation of the human ovarian cancer cells IGROV1 with increasing concentrations of topotecan and MX3 resulted in development of resistant sublines T8 and MX3 that remain resistant when exposed to topotecan and MX for 1 hour every week. The mechanism of resistance is increased efflux of topotecan and MX. In particular the initial rate of efflux is significantly higher than in the parental cell line IGROV1. The increased efflux is clearly ATP-dependent, which has been described in detail elsewhere.[20] Additional investigations revealed that P-gp is not overexpressed in T8 and MX3 cells and also that the MRPs do not appear to play a role in the resistance to topotecan and MX in these cells (results not shown). BCRP overexpression was shown in T8 and MX3 by Northern analysis.[20] In addition, our studies showed intensive staining of BCRP in T8 and MX3 and no staining in IGROV1 using the recently developed mAb BXP34, which further supports the possibility that BCRP is involved in the mechanism of resistance. BCRP staining was observed in the plasma membrane, as was expected. BCRP has been cloned previously and identified as a so-called half-transporter that most likely needs dimerization to become functionally active.[16-18]

Cell survival studies showed that T8 and MX3 are cross-resistant to other camptothecin-derived topoisomerase I inhibitors such as CPT11, its active metabolite SN38, and 9-aminocamptothecin. Both cell lines showed, however, a moderate or weak cross-resistance to camptothecin. T8 and MX3 showed clear cross-resistance to MX, but not to the P-gp substrate drugs paclitaxel and doxorubicin. The latter observation is of interest because human breast cancer cells MCF7, which developed BCRP overexpression by exposure to doxorubicin plus verapamil, clearly showed resistance to doxorubicin as well as to MX and topotecan.[16] In addition, a comparable observation was made in mouse cell lines selected for resistance to topotecan, MX, or doxorubicin.[23]

The mAb BXP34 was used to stain other cell lines and cryosections of a panel of tumor tissues. BCRP staining was found positive in the topotecan-selected cell line T8 and in the MX-selected cell lines MX3 and MCF7 MX. In addition, intensive staining was found in the BCRP-transfected MCF7/BCRP cells.[22] On cryosections very low or no staining was found in a panel of primary as well as chemotherapy-treated human solid tumors and leukemia samples. In particular, BCRP was found negative in renal cell cancer, breast cancer, and acute myeloid leukemia.

In vitro, BCRP overexpression clearly plays a significant role in tumor cell resistance, as could be shown in studies by us using T8 ad MX3 cells and by others using MX and doxorubicin/verapamil-derived cell lines and BCRP-transfected cells. Preliminary immunohistochemistry studies using a panel of tumor cells of patients do not give a clear indication that BCRP plays a significant role in clinical resistance to affected substrate drugs. However, additional functional (pharmacologic) studies are necessary to determine the clinical implications of BCRP expression in patients. In these studies the use of an effective blocker of BCRP is an essential tool. Such a blocker, GF120918, has recently been described.[24] This compound was developed as a blocker of P-gp and is still being investigated in the clinic to revert resistance to the P-gp substrate probes doxorubicin and paclitaxel. Our preliminary results reveal that the bioavailability of oral topotecan, which is low and on the order of 30% in patients,[25] can be significantly enhanced by oral coadministration of the BCRP blocker GG918.

Furthermore, additional studies using mAbs should be performed to determine the expression of BCRP in normal human tissue. Previously, expression of BCRP using mRNA data was observed in placenta, small intestine, and colon.[17] This profile suggests BCRP involvement in protection of the fetus and in regulation of uptake of compounds from the GI tract. Studies are in progress at our institute to unravel these potential physiologic functions of BCRP.

ACKNOWLEDGMENT

We are indebted to H. Rosing, R.C.A.M. van Waardenburg, M.A. van Gastelen, and M.C. Ruevekamp-Helmers for excellent support. This work was supported by the Dutch Cancer Society Grants NKI 99-2060 and NKI 2000-2143.

REFERENCES

1. BRADLEY, G., P.F. JURANKA & V. LING. 1988. Mechanism of multidrug resistance. Biochim. Biophys. Acta **948:** 87–128.
2. GOTTESMAN, M.M. & I. PASTAN. 1993. Biochemistry of multidrug resistance mediated by the multidrug transporter. Annu. Rev. Biochem. **62:** 385–427.
3. CORDON-CARDO, C., J.P. O'BRIEN, D. CASALS, et al. 1989. Multidrug-resistance gene (P-glycoprotein) is expressed by endothelial cells at blood–brain barrier sites. Proc. Natl. Acad. Sci USA **86:** 695–698.
4. SUGAWARA, I., I. KATAOKA, Y. MORISHITA, et al. 1988. Tissue distribution of P-glycoprotein encoded by a multidrug-resistant gene as revealed by a monoclonal antibody, MRK16. Cancer Res. **48:** 1926–1929.
5. THIEBAUT, F., T. TSURUO, H. HAMADO, et al. 1987. Cellular localization of the multidrug resistance gene product in normal human tissue. Proc. Natl. Acad. Sci. USA **84:** 7735–7738.
6. SCHINKEL, A.H. 1997. The physiological function of drug-transporting P-glycoproteins. Semin. Cancer Biol. **9:** 161–170.
7. SPARREBOOM, A., J. VAN ASPEREN, U. MAYER, et al. 1997. Limited oral bioavailability and active epithelial excretion of paclitaxel (Taxol) caused by P-glycoprotein in the intestine. Proc. Natl. Acad. Sci. USA **94:** 2031–2035.
8. VAN ASPEREN, J., O. VAN TELLINGEN, A. SPARREBOOM, et al. 1997. Enhanced oral bioavailability of paclitaxel in mice treated with the P-glycoprotein blocker SDZ PSC 833. Br. J. Cancer **76:** 1181–1183.
9. VAN ASPEREN, J., O. VAN TELLINGEN, M.A. VAN DER VALK, et al. 1998. Enhanced oral absorption and decreased elimination of paclitaxel in mice cotreated with cyclosporin A. Clin. Cancer Res. **4:** 2293–2297.
10. MEERUM TERWOGT, J.M., J.H. BEIJNEN, W.W. TEN BOKKEL HUININK, et al. 1998. Coadministration of cyclosporin enables oral therapy with paclitaxel. Lancet **352:** 285.
11. MEERUM TERWOGT, J.M., M.M. MALINGRÉ, J.H. BEIJNEN, et al. 1999. Co-administration of cyclosporin enables oral therapy with paclitaxel. Clin. Cancer Res. **5:** 3379–3384.

12. BRADSHAW, D.M. & R.J. ARCECI. 1998. Clinical relevance of transmembrane drug efflux as a mechanism of multidrug resistance. J. Clin. Oncol. **16(11):** 3674–3690.
13. RAMACHANDRAN, C. & S.J. MELNICK. 1999. Multidrug resistance in human tumors—molecular diagnosis and clinical significance. Mol. Diagn. **4(2):** 81–94.
14. COVELLI, A. 1999. Modulation of multidrug resistance (MDR) in hematological malignancies. Ann. Oncol. **10(Suppl. 6):** 53–39.
15. CHU, X., Y. KATO & Y. SUGIYAMA. 1997. Multiplicity of biliary excretion mechanisms for irinotecan, CPT-11, and its metabolites in rats. Cancer Res. **57:** 1934–1938.
16. DOYLE, L.A., W. YANG, L.V. ABRUZZO, et al. 1998. A multidrug resistance transporter from MCF-7 breast cancer cells. Proc. Natl. Acad. Sci. USA **95:** 15665–15670.
17. ROSS, D.D., W. YANG, L.V. ABRUZZO, et al. 1999. Atypical multidrug resistance: breast cancer resistance protein messenger RNA expression in mitoxantrone-selected cell lines. J. Natl. Cancer Inst. 429–433.
18. MIYAKE, K., L. MICKLEY, T. LITMAN, et al. 1999. Molecular cloning of cDNAs which are highly overexpressed in mitoxantrone-resistant cells: demonstration of homology to ABC transport genes. Cancer Res. **59:** 8–13.
19. ALLIKMETS, R., L.M. SCHRIML, A. HUTCHINSON, et al. 1998. A human placenta-specific ATP-binding cassette gene (ABCP) on chromosome 4q22 that is involved in multidrug resistance. Cancer Res. **58:** 5337–5339.
20. MALIEPAARD, M., M.A. VAN GASTELEN, L.A. DE JONG, et al. 1999. Overexpression of the BCRP/MXR/ABCP gene in a topotecan-selected ovarian tumor cell line. Cancer Res. **59:** 4559–1563.
21. ROSING, H., E. DOYLE, B.E. DAVIES & J.H. Beijnen. 1995. High-performance liquid chromatographic determination of the novel antitumour drug topotecan and topotecan as the total of the lactone plus carboxylate forms in human plasma. J. Chromatogr. B. Biomed. Appl. **668:** 107–115.
22. SCHEFFER, G.L., M. MALIEPAARD, A.C. PIJNENBORG, et al. 2000. Breast cancer resistance protein is localized at the plasma membrane in mitoxantrone- and topotecan-resistant cell lines. Cancer Res. **55:** 4559–4563.
23. ALLEN, J.D., R.F. BRINKHUIS, J. WIJNHOLDS & A.H. SCHINKEL. 1999. The mouse Bcrp1/Mxr/Abcp gene: amplification and overexpression in cell lines selected for resistance to topotecan, mitoxantrone, or doxorubicin. Cancer Res. **59:** 4237–4241.
24. DE BRUIN, M., K. MIYAKE, T. LITMAN, et al. 1999. Reversal of resistance by GF120918 in cell lines expressing the ABC half-transporter, MXR. Cancer Lett. **146:** 117–126.
25. SCHELLENS, J.H.M., G.J. CREEMERS, J.H. BEIJNEN, et al. 1996. Bioavailability and pharmacokinetics of oral topotecan, a new topoisomerase I inhibitor. Br. J. Cancer **73:** 1268–1271.

Pharmacokinetics of Orally Administered Camptothecins

ELORA GUPTA,[a] VIRAL VYAS, FARHEENA AHMED, PATRICK SINKO, THOMAS COOK, AND ERIC RUBIN

UMDNJ-The Cancer Institute of New Jersey, New Brunswick, New Jersey USA

ABSTRACT: Phase I trials of oral camptothecins, including camptothecin (CPT) and irinotecan (CPT-11), have reported substantial interpatient variability in systemic exposure, which could result in suboptimal antitumor activity in some patients or enhanced risk for toxicity in others. This investigation evaluates the contribution of intestinal absorption and first-pass metabolism in the disposition of oral CPT and CPT-11, respectively. The transport of CPT in Caco-2 cell lines (validated model of intestinal drug transport) was concentration dependent and saturable (V_{max}: 34×10^{-5} cm/sec and K_m: 20 μM), and was temperature dependent with an activation energy (E_a) of 11.7 kcal/mole. Cumulatively, this data was indicative of carrier-mediated intestinal transport. In addition, a reduction of transport in the presence of sodium azide plus deoxyglucose suggested ATP dependence. Thus, variable expression and availability of intestinal transporters could contribute to the observed wide variability in the exposure to oral CPT. CPT-11 is hydrolyzed by the ubiquitous enzyme carboxyl esterase to active SN-38, and first-pass metabolism of oral CPT-11 would include both intestinal and hepatic hydrolysis. Incubation of CPT-11 with S9 fractions of human liver and intestinal tissues resulted in variable rates of formation of SN-38. The mean (±SD) specific activities (pmoles/min/mg) were: liver (8.57 ± 10.4, $n = 8$), duodenum (5.06 ± 3.7, $n = 4$), jejunum (6.44 ± 2.8, $n = 5$), ileum (4.81 ± 2.4, $n = 5$), colon (1.93 ± 1.5, $n = 6$), and rectum (0.82, $n = 1$). Interestingly, there was a decrease in SN-38 formation by tumor tissue compared to matched normal liver and colon tissues. Therefore variable first-pass metabolism could contribute to the substantial differences in the systemic exposures to CPT-11 and SN-38 in patients receiving oral CPT-11.

INTRODUCTION

The oral administration of camptothecins is being explored actively for both practical and pharmacological reasons. Ease of administration on an outpatient basis, avoidance of vascular complications, and frequent hospital visits improves quality of life, lowers costs, and enhances patient compliance. Because of the S-phase specificity of these compounds, protracted schedules resulting in sustained exposure to these compounds have been shown to be effective.[1] Thus, steady-state plasma concentrations following continuous oral delivery would ensure therapeutic efficacy of the camptothecins. In addition, the low gastric pH would favor the active lactone ring configuration of the camptothecins.

---

[a]Address for correspondence: Bristol-Myers Squibb, Mail Stop D13-04, PO Box 4000, Princeton, NJ 08543.

In a phase I study of oral camptothecin (CPT), substantial interpatient variability was observed in the rate and extent of systemic availability of the drug.[2] The plasma CPT concentrations observed in this study were associated with toxicity; patients who experienced grade 3 or 4 toxicity had significantly higher plasma CPT steady-state concentrations than patients who did not experience such toxicity ($p = 0.003$). Another important finding of this study was that the extent of decrease of topoisomerase I in peripheral mononuclear blood cells was related to the plasma CPT steady-state concentrations. In a phase I and pharmacokinetic trial of oral irinotecan (CPT-11), substantial interindividual differences in the variability of pharmacokinetic parameters was reported in all dosages.[3] Overall, the variable systemic availability of oral camptothecins results in enhanced toxicity or suboptimal activity and could hinder the viability of this route of administration. It is therefore critical to characterize the mechanistic pathways affecting the oral bioavailability of camptothecins.

Several factors have been attributed to the inconsistent bioavailability of orally administered drugs including intestinal permeability and first-pass metabolism. There is limited information regarding the metabolism of CPT. On the other hand, CPT-11 is a prodrug and is metabolized by the ubiquitous enzyme carboxylesterase to the active metabolite SN-38. Therefore, this investigation focused on the assessment of the mechanism of intestinal absorption of CPT using the human intestinal cell line Caco-2. These cells have been extensively validated as a model for intestinal drug transport, and ease of availability makes them an attractive system for the evaluation of intestinal permeability.[4] For the prodrug CPT-11, which could undergo both hepatic and intestinal first-pass metabolism, we ascertained the *in vitro* activation by human liver and intestine.

MATERIALS AND METHODS

Evaluation of the Intestinal Transport of CPT

Materials

Polycarbonate membrane Snapwell® plates 12 mm in diameter and 0.4 mM in pore size were obtained from Costar (Cambridge, MA), and cell culture media components were purchased from Gibco Life Technologies Inc. (Grand Island, NY). CPT, sodium azide, 2-deoxyglucose, sodium taurocholate, probenecid, and quinine were obtained from Sigma Chemical Co. (St. Louis, MO). Supplies for the HPLC analysis of CPT were obtained from Fisher Scientific Inc. (Fairlawn, NJ).

Transport Studies

Caco-2 cells, obtained from American Type Culture Collection (Rockville, MD), were seeded on Snapwell polycarbonate filter inserts and grown for 28 days before being mounted on side-by-side Ussing type diffusion chambers maintained at 37°C for the permeability studies. The donor (apical) compartment of the chamber contained the drug in MES Ringer's buffer (pH 6.5, containing a maximum of 1.5%

DMSO) and the receptor (basolateral) compartment contained Ringer's buffer (pH 7.4). There was no effect of the DMSO on Caco-2 permeability (data not shown). The fluid in the chambers was circulated using a gas lift mechanism with 5% CO_2 and 95% O_2, and the flow rate was monitored continuously during the experiments. Samples were withdrawn from the receptor chamber at predetermined time intervals and replaced with the same volume of prewarmed Ringer's buffer. Total CPT concentrations in the samples were determined using HPLC.[5] Monolayer integrity was established by unchanged transepithelial electrical resistance (TEER), determined by using EVOM epithelial voltohmeter and EndOhm tissue resistance measurement chamber (World Precision Instruments, Sarasota, FL), at the beginning and at the end of the permeability studies.

Effective permeability (P) was determined by the following equation[6]:

$$P = \frac{V_r}{AC_0} \cdot \frac{dC}{dt}$$

where V_r was the volume of the receptor chamber (5 ml), A was the surface area of the filter (1.13 cm^2), C_0 was the donor CPT concentration and dC/dt was the flux (linear slope of a plot of receptor drug concentration as a function of time). Permeability through the Caco-2 monolayer (P_{mono}) was obtained after correcting for resistance due to the microporous filter (P_f) where P_f was calculated using the same equation as effective permeability.

To determine the existence of carrier mediated and/or passive transport, P_{mono} was determined using increasing drug concentrations. No change in P_{mono} at increasing concentrations would be indicative of drug absorption due to passive transport only. In the event of decreasing flux as a function of concentration (indicative of saturable transport), the Michaelis-Menten kinetic parameters for the saturable transport was determined from a plot of P_{mono} as a function of drug concentration [S], using the following equation.

$$P = \frac{V_{max}[S]}{K_m + [S]} + P_d$$

V_{max} was the maximum flux, K_m was the drug concentration at 50% V_{max} and P_d was the permeability due to nonsaturable passive transport.[7]

Temperature dependence was determined by obtaining the flux of the drug (at K_m) at different temperatures (range 9°C to 37°C). The apparent activation energy (E_a) was determined from the plot of the log P_{mono} as a function of 1/T, where T was the absolute temperature. Based on the Arrhenius equation, the slope of the plot equals E_a/R, where R is the gas constant.

The energy dependence of transport was investigated using donor cell buffer containing 15 mM sodium azide plus 50 mM 2-deoxy-D-glucose, cellular metabolic inhibitors that deplete cellular ATP.

To characterize the intestinal transporter, the permeability of CPT was determined in the presence of several inhibitors. There were: 1 mM probenecid (organic anion transporter), 1 mM quinine (organic cation transporter), and 1 mM taurocholic acid (bile acid transporter). Decrease in CPT receptor concentrations in the presence of an inhibitor would suggest its involvement in the Caco-2 transport of CPT.

TABLE 1. Tissues evaluated for the *in vitro* assessment of hepatic and intestinal metabolism of CPT-11

Region	Tissue type (n)
Liver	Normal (7)
	Tumor (4)
	Matched (4)[a]
Duodenum	Normal (4)
Jejunum	Normal (4)
Ileum	Normal (4)
Colon	Normal (6)
	Tumor (4)
	Matched (4)[a]
Rectum	Normal (1)
	Tumor (1)
	Matched (1)[a]

[a]Matched normal and tumor tissue were obtained from the same patient.

Evaluation of Hepatic and Intestinal Metabolism of CPT-11

Materials

CPT-11 hydrochloride trihydrate solution and SN-38 were gifts from Pharmacia and Upjohn (Kalamazoo, MI). Supplies for performing the incubations were purchased from Sigma (St. Louis, MO). Supplies for the HPLC analysis of CPT were obtained from Fisher Scientific Inc. (Fairlawn, NJ).

In Vitro *Metabolism Studies*

Human intestinal and liver samples (normal and tumor) were obtained through the Tissue Retrieval and Distribution Core Facility of the Cancer Institute (TABLE 1). For matched specimens, a piece of peritumoral tissue (normal) was cut from an area farthest away from the tumor which was distinctly separate from the area of tumor growth. This was accompanied by a sample from the tumor. All samples were placed in cryogenic vials and snap-frozen in liquid nitrogen within 45 min after surgical removal and stored at −80°C. Each tissue sample used in this investigation was accompanied by a pathological assessment which included the tissue type (normal or tumor) and tumor type. None of the patients from whom tumor tissue samples had been obtained were on CPT-11 therapy.

Because carboxyl esterase is present in the microsomal as well as cytosolic fractions, we evaluated tissue metabolic activity using S-9 fractions. The samples were homogenized for 5–10 minutes with 5X buffer (0.154M KCL containing 50 mM Tris-HCL, pH 7.4) and centrifuged at 10,000 × g for 30 minutes at 0°C (Beckman L-80 Ultracentrifuge, Palo Alto, CA). After centrifugation the supernatant (S-9 fraction) was decanted into a prechilled receptacle. The protein concentration was determined by the method of Bradford.[8]

Incubations with CPT-11 were performed in triplicate and initiated by the addition of CPT-11 to the S-9 fractions. The final concentration of CPT-11 in the incubates (100 μg/ml), was similar to the K_m values reported for CPT-11.[9] Aliquots were removed at predetermined time intervals, placed in microcentrifuge tubes containing methanol (to terminate enzymatic reaction), and SN-38 was quantitated by reversed-phase HPLC as described previously.[10] Rates of SN-38 formation were assessed from the initial periods of plots of SN-38 concentration as a function of time, showing linear SN-38 formation. The specific activity was determined as the ratio of the formation rate of SN-38 and the protein concentration.

RESULTS AND DISCUSSION

Evaluation of the Intestinal Transport of CPT

Evidence for Carrier-Mediated Transport of CPT

Permeability through the Caco-2 cell monolayer (P_{mono}) was estimated at increasing CPT concentrations ranging from 1 μM to 100 μM. FIGURE 1 shows the concentration dependence of CPT flux (A) and permeability (B). Decreasing flux with increasing CPT concentrations was indicative of saturable absorption. From the plot of P_{mono} as a function of CPT concentrations, K_m was estimated to occur at 20 μM, V_{max} was 34×10^{-5} cm/sec, and P_d was computed to be 8×10^{-5} cm/sec (hatched line, FIG. 1B). These data suggest that the transport of CPT is carrier mediated and passive diffusion accounts for a minor fraction of the transport.

Temperature Dependence of CPT Transport

The involvement of a carrier-mediated transport of CPT across Caco-2 was further supported by the >6-fold reduction in the P_{mono} of CPT when the temperature was reduced from 37°C to 10.9°C (FIG. 2). The E_a was calculated to be 11.7 kCal/mol. Because the range of E_a values associated with enzymatic reactions or carrier-mediated processes range from 7 to 25 kCal/mol (E_a for passive diffusion <4 kCal/mol),[11] it can be concluded that the transport of CPT across the Caco-2 monolayer is temperature dependent.

Energy Dependence of CPT Transport

The P_{mono} of CPT decreased from 1.132 ± 0.179 cm/sec ($n = 3$) in controls to 0.864 ± 0.284 cm/sec ($n = 3$) in the presence of inhibitors (sodium azide + 2-deoxyglucose), which depletes ATP resources in the Caco-2 cells. Therefore, CPT appears to be transported by an active process across the Caco-2 monolayer.

Effect of Inhibitors on CPT Transport

The organic anion transport inhibitor (probenecid) caused a modest reduction in the intestinal permeability of CPT, whereas inhibitors of organic cation or bile acid transport had no effect (FIG. 3). Lack of substantial inhibition by probenecid, quinine, or taurocholic acid suggests the involvement of a novel transporter or multiple transporters in CPT transport.

Overall, the investigation of transport across Caco-2 monolayers demonstrates that CPT is transported via a carrier-mediated, active process. Variable expression, availability, and activity of transport proteins could lead to inconsistent systemic availability of oral CPT in patients. The investigation also suggests the possibility of the existence of carrier-mediated transport of other camptothecin analogues.

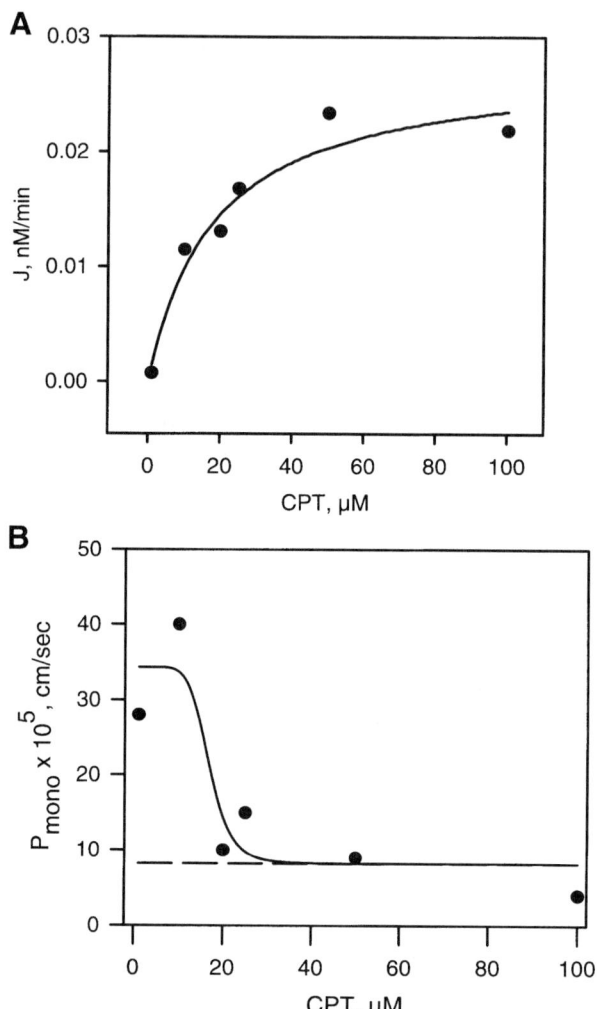

FIGURE 1. Concentration dependency of CPT transport across Caco-2 monolayer. There was evidence of a saturable component in the flux (**A**) and P_{mono} (**B**). *Hatched line* represents transport by passive diffusion (**B**).

Evaluation of Hepatic and Intestinal Metabolism of CPT-11

CPT-11 Hydrolysis by Human Intestinal Tissue

Incubation of CPT-11 with human liver and intestinal samples resulted in the formation of SN-38. We observed substantial interpatient variability in the activities in the liver and the intestine. The mean (±SD) specific activity (pmoles/min per mg), of the tissues were: liver (8.57 ± 10.4, $n = 8$), duodenum (5.06 ± 3.7, $n = 4$), jejunum (6.44 ± 2.8, $n = 5$), ileum (4.81 ± 2.4, $n = 5$), colon (1.93 ± 1.5, $n = 6$), and rectum

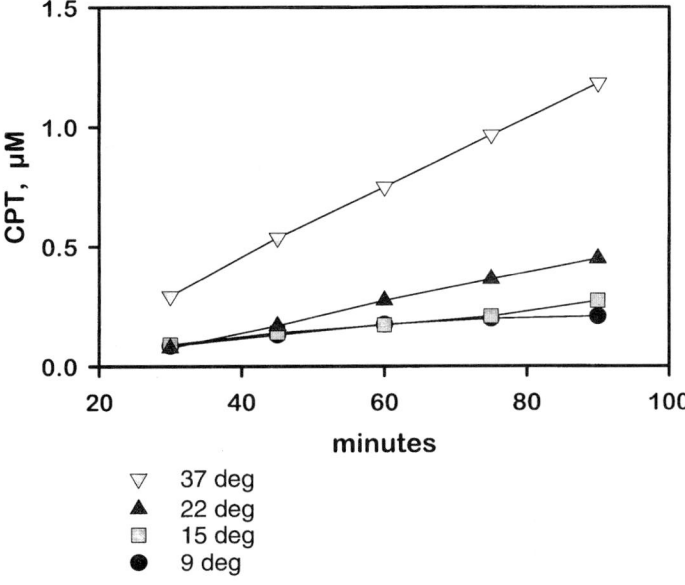

FIGURE 2. Temperature dependence of CPT transport across Caco-2 monolayer. The activation energy was determined to be 11.7 kCal/mole.

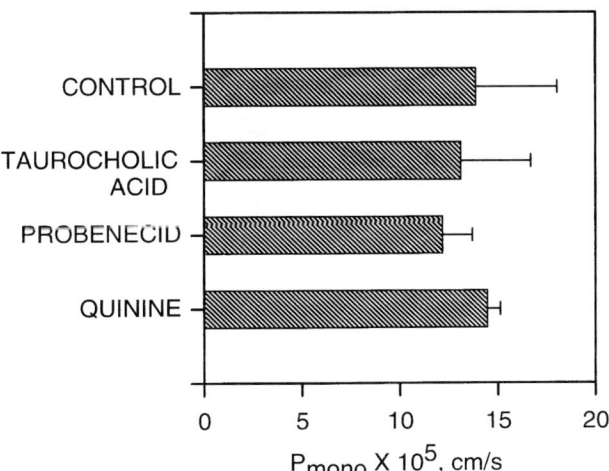

FIGURE 3. Effect of inhibitors on CPT P_{mono}.

(0.82, $n = 1$). In two instances, we were able to obtain tissue samples from hepatic and/or intestinal regions of the same patient. In one patient, the liver tissue exhibited a specific activity of 3.0 pmoles/min per mg while the rectal tissue had a fourfold lower activity of 0.82 pmoles/min per mg. In another patient, the tissue from the duodenum had a specific activity of 8.27 pmoles/min per mg, whereas the tissue for the colon had a substantially lower specific activity of 0.55 pmoles/min per mg. The observation of CPT-11 hydrolysis to SN-38 in all the regions of the intestine is in agreement with reports of the presence of carboxyl esterase activity in proximal and distal small intestine and colon.[12] Overall, a consequence of the variability in specific activities observed in the current investigation could be substantial interpatient differences in the systemic availabilities of CPT-11 and SN-38 following oral CPT-11 administration.

The intestinal activation of CPT-11 observed in the investigation reported here would be an important rationale for the development of oral CPT-11 and would underscore the important contribution of the intestines in the first-pass metabolism of oral CPT-11. In addition, since CPT-11 has been approved for the treatment of patients with refractory colon cancer, it was interesting to note that the colorectal region was active in the metabolism of CPT-11 to SN-38. However, localized activation in intestinal tissue could cause mucosal damage leading to diarrhea, a dose-limiting toxicity of CPT-11 therapy.

Differences in Activity in Matched Normal and Tumor Tissue

We were able to evaluate the carboxylesterase-mediated CPT-11 hydrolysis in matched tissues (normal and tumor) that were obtained from the same patient (FIG. 4). In about 67% of the samples, the tumor tissue had a >25% lower specific activity compared to matched controls. Because of the small sample size, no significant differences in specific activities between the normal and tumor tissues were ob-

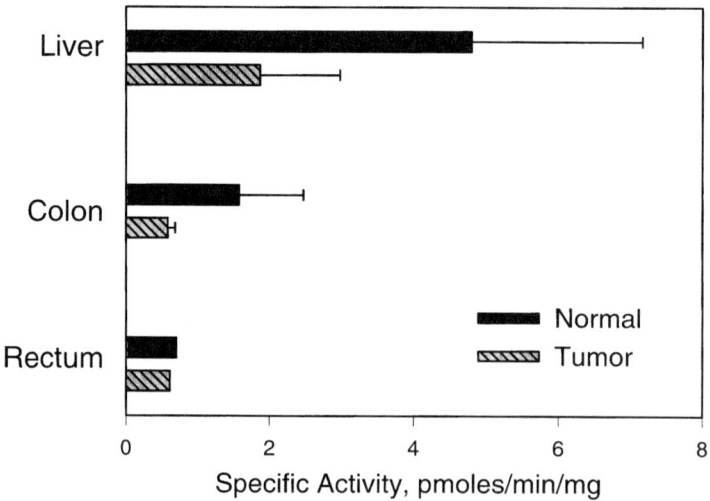

FIGURE 4. Comparison of carboxylesterase activities in matched normal and tumor tissues from liver and colon.

served. Carboxyl esterase expression has been established as one of the cellular sensitivity determinants of CPT-11 cytotoxicity, and reduced carboxyl esterase activity has been implicated as a mechanism of CPT-11 resistance.[13] Reduced SN-38 formation in tumor tissues compared to matched normal tissue could be an important determinant in the assessment of tumor response.

CONCLUSIONS

This investigation explored some of the causes that could contribute to the interpatient variability associated with oral CPT and CPT-11 therapy by in vitro transport studies using Caco-2 cells and in vitro metabolism studies using S9 preparations. The results suggest variable rate and extent of intestinal transport and variable intestinal and hepatic first-pass metabolism as possible causes of the marked differences in the in vivo plasma concentrations of orally administered camptothecins. To enhance the viability of the oral route of administration, two approaches could be implemented. To avoid possible saturation of intestinal transporter(s), a single daily dose could be fractionated and administered multiple times a day. The other approach would be therapeutic drug monitoring in which plasma concentrations of the drug are obtained following the initial dose, and the dosage is individualized to obtain target plasma concentrations in the patients.

REFERENCES

1. GERRITS, C.J.H., M.J.A. DE JONGE, J.H.M. SCHELLENS, et al. 1997. Topoisomerase inhibitors: the relevance of prolonged exposure for present clinical development. B. J. Cancer **67:** 952–962.
2. GUPTA, E., D. TOPPMEYER, R. ZAMEK, et al. 1998. Clinical evaluation of sequential topoisomerase targeting in the treatment of advanced malignancy. Cancer Ther. **1:** 292–301.
3. DRENGLER, R.L., J.G. KUHN, L.J. SCHAAF, et al. 1999. Phase I and pharmacokinetic trial of oral irinotecan administered daily for 5 days every 3 weeks in patients with solid tumors. J. Clin. Oncol. **17:** 685–696.
4. DELIE, F. & W. RUBAS. 1997. A human colonic cell line sharing similarities with enterocytes as a model to examine oral absorption: advantages and limitations of the Caco-2 model. Crit. Rev. Ther. Drug Carrier Syst. **14:** 221–286.
5. AHMED, F., V. VYAS, A. SALEEM, et al. 1998. High-performance liquid chromatographic quantitation of total and lactone 20(S)camptothecin in patients receiving oral 20(S)camptothecin. J. Chromatogr. B **707:** 227–233.
6. YU, H. & P.J. SINKO. 1997. Influence of the microporous substratum and hydrodynamics on resistances to drug transport in cell culture systems: calculation of intrinsic transport parameters. J. Pharm. Sci. **86:** 1448–1457.
7. WALTER, E. & T. KISSEL. 1994. Transepithelial transport and metabolism of thyrotropin-releasing hormone (TRH) in layers of a human intestinal cell line (Caco-2): evidence for an active transport component? Pharm. Res. **11:** 1575–1580.
8. BRADFORD, M. 1976. A rapid and sensitive method for the quantitation of microgram quantities of protein utilizing the principle of protein-dye binding. Anal. Biochem. **72:** 248–254.
9. SLATTER J.G., P. SU, J.P. SAMS, et al. 1998. Bioactivation of the anticancer agent CPT-11 to SN-38 by human hepatic microsomal enzymes and the in vitro assessment of potential drug interactions. Drug Metab. Disp. **25:** 1157–1164.

10. GUPTA, E., T.M. LESTINGI, R. MICK, et al. 1994. Metabolic fate of CPT-11 in humans: correlation of glucuronidation with diarrhea. Cancer Res. **54:** 3723–3725.
11. NG, KA-YUN & R.T. BORCHARDT. 1993. Biotin transport in a human intestinal epithelial cell line (Caco-2). Life Sci. **53:** 1121–1127.
12. SCHWER, H., T. LANGMANN, R. DAIG, et al. 1997. Molecular cloning and characterization of a novel putative carboxylesterase present in human intestine and liver. Biochem. Biophys. Res. Commun. **233:** 117–120.
13. NAGAI, S., M. YAMAUCHI, T. ANDOH, et al. 1995. Establishment and characterization of human gastric and colonic and gastric xenograft lines resistant to CPT-11 (a new derivative of camptothecin). J. Surg. Oncol. **59:** 116–124.

Metabolism of CPT-11

Impact on Activity

LAURENT P. RIVORY[a]

Sydney Cancer Centre, Royal Prince Alfred Hospital, and the University of Sydney, Sydney, Australia

ABSTRACT: Irinotecan (CPT-11) is a semi-synthetic camptothecin with a broad spectrum of clinical activity. It is a prodrug that is cleaved by esterases to the potent topoisomerase I poison, SN-38. In humans, this activation is relatively inefficient, but this may result in a more protracted formation of SN-38 lactone. Some intratumoral activation may also occur, but the significance of this process is uncertain. CPT-11 is metabolized by cytochrome P450 3A to yield a number of comparatively inactive compounds. SN-38 is glucurono-conjugated in the liver, and this metabolite, although inactive, may participate in the enterohepatic cycling of SN-38 after hydrolysis in the intestinal lumen. Overall, the production of SN-38 from CPT-11 is the result of the complex interplay of several metabolic pathways and the source of considerable interpatient variability.

INTRODUCTION

The camptothecins are a major class of anticancer drugs related to 20-(S)camptothecin that act as topoisomerase I poisons. A lack of water solubility plagued the early clinical development of the lead compound, 20-(S)camptothecin. The use of the more soluble carboxylate salt appeared an obvious solution to this problem, but this led to toxicity and an absence of appreciable clinical activity. It is now recognized that the ring-opened carboxylate form has no activity against topoisomerase I and several approaches to overcoming the lack of water solubility of the active lactone form have been investigated. Packaging of camptothecins in liposomes appears feasible, as do alternative forms of administration such as oral, aerosol, and depot formulations. The more conventional, intravenous route of administration is possible with the synthesis of watersoluble camptothecins, such as topotecan and DX-8951, or prodrugs. CPT-11 (also known as irinotecan) belongs to the latter group and was rationally synthesized as a prodrug of a potent but waterinsoluble topoisomerase I poison, SN-38. It was part of a series of 36 carbamate esters of SN-38 produced by Yakult Institute of Microbiological Research. Of these, CPT-11 produced the best activity in murine tumor screens. It is now in use in the clinic and has been proven in the setting of advanced colorectal carcinoma.

---

[a]Medical Oncology, Sydney Cancer Centre, Missenden Road, Camperdown, NSW 2050, Australia. Voice: +61-2-9515 7376; fax: +61-2-9519 1546.
lrivory@canc.rpa.cs.nsw.gov.au

ACTIVATION

As mentioned, CPT-11 is a carbamate ester prodrug of SN-38.[1] Initial work in rodents showed that CPT-11 was rapidly hydrolyzed to SN-38 *in vivo*.[2] In rats, SN-38 and its glucuronide account for 25–50% of the mass balance depending on the dose administered,[3] whereas it is only approximately 12% in patients.[4,5] However, in the rat, the mean residence time of CPT-11 is only 1–2 hours[3] as compared to ~10 hours in patients.[6–9] Assuming the body distribution to be species independent, this indicates a difference in activation rates of approximately 10-fold between rats and patients.

The hydrolysis of CPT-11 to SN-38 has been shown to be mediated by carboxylesterases, which are present in many normal tissues as well as tumor.[2,10–13] A screen of various hepatic carboxylesterases by Satoh *et al.*[14] revealed that the human form was one of the poorest catalysts for this reaction. We confirmed this observation using purified human liver carboxylesterase[11] and showed the steady-state rate of hydrolysis of CPT-11 to be approximately a million times slower than the prototypic carboxylesterase substrate *p*-nitrophenol acetate (*p*NPA). The hydrolysis of CPT-11 by several carboxylesterases has been shown to be deacylation rate-limited.[10,11,15] In this type of reaction, the 4-piperidino-piperidine ester moiety is transferred to the active site serine during the production of SN-38. Regeneration of the active enzyme then requires hydrolysis of the carbamoylated enzyme complex. It is this second step that is extremely slow for human liver carboxylesterase.[11] The fact that the reaction is deacylation rate-limited has broad implications in the study of CPT-11 activation. For one, the determination of the Michaelis-Menten parameters will be entirely dependent on the experimental conditions (i.e., early or steady-state production).[11] Similarly, the identification of potential inhibitors will be experiment-dependent. For example, a potent inhibitor of deacylation would be expected to have little impact on carboxylesterase during a short incubation experiment with CPT-11.

In our studies with purified human liver carboxylesterase,[11] the apparent K_M for the process was 53 μM. This concentration is in excess of the peak concentrations of CPT-11 observed clinically even at the high doses explored in some studies.[7,9] Because of the slow steady-state reaction in this system, we were limited to examining the hydrolysis of CPT-11 in the mixture of lactone and carboxylate found at physiological pH, that is, mostly as the carboxylate. A study of CPT-11 hydrolysis by human liver microsomes over the concentration range of 8.8–146 μM revealed a similar K_M (~50 μM) as seen with the pure enzyme for the carboxylate form.[15] An interesting finding was that the lactone form of CPT-11 was converted to SN-38 at approximately twice the velocity (and with a lower K_M) than that seen with the carboxylate, despite the fact that the two reactions share a common rate-limiting step. Catalytic rate constants are usually expressed as V_{MAX}/K_M and, on that basis, hydrolysis of the lactone form is approximately four times more efficient than for the lactone. Because of the increased lipophilicity of the lactone form and its preferential tissue uptake,[16] it is likely that actual rates of hydrolysis of plasma CPT-11 by hepatic carboxylesterase would be even more in favor of the lactone form. SN-38 lactone accounts for 60–70% of total SN-38 (lactone + carboxylate) found in the plasma of patients,[16–18] which is in contrast to other camptothecins in clinical use.

Although part of this phenomenon may be explained by the stabilizing effects of protein binding on SN-38 lactone,[19] it is possible that the preferential conversion of lactone CPT-11 may be a factor in determining this desired property.

By investigating lower concentrations of CPT-11, Slatter et al.[20] were able to demonstrate the presence of an additional high affinity human liver microsomal esterase capable of hydrolyzing CPT-11. In this case, the K_M was ~2 µM, which makes this saturability of relevance to the comparison of rapid versus slow infusion regimens of CPT-11. Because their experiments were carried out with short incubations, the apparent steady-state K_M may well be even less than the reported value.

During initial phase I studies of CPT-11, the AUC ratio of total SN-38 to CPT-11 was occasionally observed to be highest at the lower CPT-11 doses.[9,21] The wide inter-patient variability in the pharmacokinetics of CPT-11 and SN-38 has made the study of the dose-dependence of CPT-11 pharmacokinetics extremely difficult. Nevertheless, there is emerging data in support of a saturability of SN-38 formation. In general, short infusions (30–90 min) of CPT-11 yield a **molar** ratio of the areas under the curve (AUC) of total SN-38 and CPT-11 of the order of 0.03 to 0.07.[7–9,21,22] In contrast, prolonged infusions (4-, 5-, and 14-day continuous i.v.) yield ratios as high as 0.24.[23] Likewise, in children, the use of protracted daily regimens (daily × 5 for 2 weeks) results in an apparently increased efficiency of conversion of CPT-11 to SN-38[24] in comparison with the high dose every 3-week regimen.[25]

An additional advantage of prolonged infusion protocols is that it provides a steady supply of CPT-11 lactone and this should favor not only formation of SN-38 but also, more specifically, formation of SN-38 lactone, the active species. However, the percentage of the total SN-38 found in its lactone form in recent trials appears to range only from 60–70% with no clear evidence for more pronounced lactonization with prolonged infusion.[16–18]

Recently, it was shown that butyrylcholinesterases are capable of hydrolyzing CPT-11 to SN-38.[26,27] However, the human enzyme is relatively inefficient and has a K_M of approximately 40 µM.[27] Hence, human butyrylcholinesterase is unlikely to be the high affinity esterase described by Slatter et al.[20] and the significance of this enzyme to SN-38 metabolism is unclear.

The original idea behind the synthesis of carbamate esters of SN-38 was to exploit a possible intratumoral activation pathway.[1] *In vitro* studies have shown conflicting results on the correlation between the sensitivity of cell lines and their carboxylesterase activity.[28,29] In general, it would be expected that the exposure of cells *in vitro* to SN-38 would be determined by their own ability to activate CPT-11. This raises the possibility of using ADEPT or GDEPT approaches to increase intratumoral activation of CPT-11. This approach has been investigated with both human and rabbit carboxylesterases.[30–33]

In vivo, however, the exposure of tumor cells to SN-38 will also be dependent on activation by other tissues. In mice, Janssen et al.[29] found that two human colon cancer xenografts had only a fraction of the carboxylesterase activity of organs such as the liver and small intestine. However, they used pNPA as a marker of the esterase activity, and this may not necessarily reflect the distribution of CPT-11 activation. Indeed, other groups have shown that human tumor tissue has comparable, albeit lower rates of CPT-11 conversion than do matched normal samples.[13,34] Importantly, the concentration of CPT-11 used in the study of Guichard et al.[13] was sufficiently low (1 µM) to make such evaluation relevant to the clinical situation. Although tumor conversion was on the whole lower than that in the normal counterparts, the ratio actually exceeded unity in 11 of 28 Duke's C patients.

The presence of CPT-11 converting activity in the intestinal mucosa and liver[2,13,34] is also of potential significance in understanding the pharmacology of orally administered CPT-11. In mice and both adult and pediatric patients, the AUC ratio of SN-38 to CPT-11 is greatly increased by oral administration.[35,36] Part of this difference is likely to be due to first-pass activation during absorption. However, the ratio may be also partly increased as a result of CYP450-mediated oxidation during the first-pass, which would reduce the CPT-11 AUC. The fact that the **absolute** AUCs of SN-38 have been reported to be reduced relative to those observed with intravenous administration of CPT-11 suggests that the situation is more complex than simply the effect of first-pass activation.

The other product of CPT-11 hydrolysis is 4-piperidinopiperidine (4-PP), which is a spontaneous rearrangement of the liberated carbamic acid precursor. This compound also appears capable of inducing apoptosis in cancer cell lines.[37] The typical concentrations required for this effect are high (100–300 mM) and several orders of magnitude in excess of those that can be measured in plasma samples taken from patients treated with CPT-11.[38] However, 4-PP has a very long plasma half-life, and the effects of protracted exposure of both the body and tumors to low concentrations of this compound still remain to be explored.[38]

OXIDATION

CPT-11 undergoes significant oxidative metabolism *in vivo*. In a radiolabeled mass-balance study, it was found that, on average, approximately 15% of a 125 mg/m^2 dose of CPT-11 is excreted as oxidative metabolites.[4] The major product is the aminopentanocarboxylic (APC) derivative of CPT-11, which is a major plasma metabolite in patients.[5,9,39] There is also a less abundant primary amino-piperidine metabolite referred to as NPC.[40] Both are produced by pathways involving the cytochrome P450 3A family[41,42] (FIG. 1). Although it was originally thought that NPC might be produced from APC by an *N*-dealkylation reaction,[39] this does not appear to be the case.[42] Rather, it is more likely that both are produced, among others, from mono- and di-hydroxy intermediates. Several mono-hydroxy metabolites have indeed been observed in plasma, urine, and bile,[39,43,44] but their positioning within the metabolic scheme of CPT-11 is currently unknown. In one study, there was some evidence of a metabolite featuring a mono-hydroxylation on the camptothecin moiety.[43] This is consistent with reports that the rat liver is capable of generating mono-hydroxylated species.[45] Recently, another group and we found that CYP3A5 was capable of producing an additional polar metabolite to those seen with incubations with CYP3A4.[46,47] Renewed attempts to obtain a molecular weight yielded the estimate of 528. However, in our case, the "purified" fraction was eventually identified as corresponding to the photodegradation product PDP-4[48] in terms of retention time, mass/charge, and fragmentation in LC/MS experiments. The retention time was dramatically different from that of the original fraction. Therefore, it is possible that oxidation of CPT-11 by CYP3A5 yields an extremely unstable metabolite with

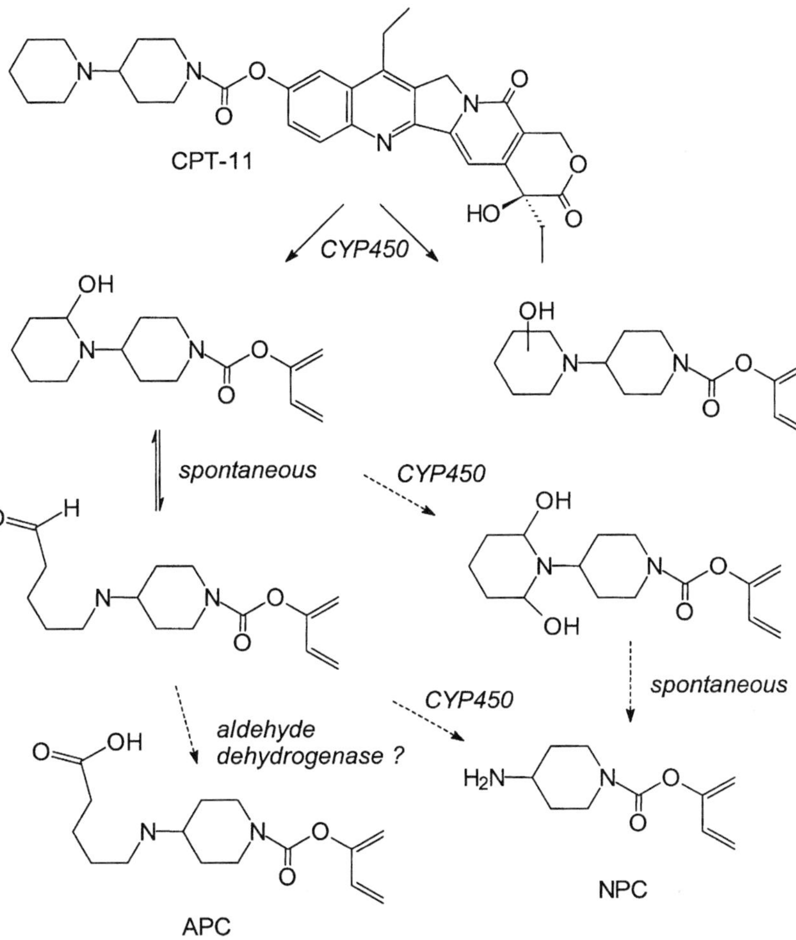

FIGURE 1. Proposed pathway for the CYP450-mediated oxidation of CPT-11. Although only APC and NPC have been characterized to date, there is supporting evidence for the presence of some of the intermediates. The requirement for an additional, non-CYP450 pathway may account for the low rate of production of APC by liver microsomes.

a modification of the lactone ring, which undergoes facile condensation to the PDP-4 mappicine. In a screening of urine and plasma, we did not detect PDP-4 in appreciable quantities,[44] and it is possible that the presence of PDP-4 in the samples analyzed by Lokiec et al.[43] was the result of the photodegradation of CPT-11 itself or, possibly, in view of the foregoing studies, from the conversion of an unstable CYP3A5 product during extensive sample processing. In any case, given that the majority of the mass balance can be explained by the existing known metabolites, the importance of this pathway remains to be clarified.

An intriguing question is whether the oxidative metabolites of CPT-11, which have piperidine ring modifications, have the potential of being activated to SN-38. In the case of APC, it appears that the high polarity of the resulting distal chain is incompatible with hydrolysis by human carboxylesterase,[39] although this may not be the case with the rabbit enzyme.[33] NPC, on the other hand, is significantly converted to SN-38 by both purified carboxylesterase and human liver microsomes.[40]

NPC is a more important CYP450 metabolite *in vitro*, whereas the situation in terms of mass balance is the reverse, with NPC being a minor excretion product.[4,5] Although this may be the result of conversion of NPC to SN-38, an alternative explanation is that the production of the precursor(s) of NPC and APC is CYP450 dependent and that the eventual formation of APC requires a nonmicrosomal system, whereas the corresponding reaction for NPC is also CYP450-mediated. We have investigated the possibility that cytosolic aldehyde reductase is involved in the biosynthesis of APC, but its opposite cofactor requirements to those of CYP450 make this a difficult system to emulate *in vitro*.[46]

Reanalysis of some of the initial phase I plasma specimens indicated that individuals with high plasma SN-38 concentrations generally also had concentrations of both CPT-11 and APC.[9] As mentioned previously, APC is itself not directly activated to SN-38, but the possibility that a lipophilic precursor of APC is preferentially converted to SN-38 remains. Unfortunately, the high multicolinearity of CPT-11, APC, and SN-38 concentrations and the lack of stability of some of the proposed intermediates make this aspect very difficult to explore.

The pharmacokinetics of CPT-11 in patients treated with phenytoin, barbiturates, and steroids (known inducers of CYP3A) show a dramatically increased clearance of CPT-11 but also a greatly reduced exposure to SN-38.[49,50] This would argue against a CYP450-dependent pathway of formation of SN-38. Nevertheless, the effects of these and other drugs (e.g., carbamazepine, valproic acid) used in this population on other enzyme systems may confound this type of analysis.

CONJUGATION

SN-38 is conjugated by UDP-glucuronosyltransferase 1A1[51] (UDPG 1A1), and this inactive metabolite is usually the predominant plasma form of SN-38 *in vivo*.[6,9,43,52,53] Gilbert's disease, which is a mild and often undiagnosed chronic hyperbilirubinemia, is linked to a genetic polymorphism of UDPG 1A1, the predominant isoform involved in the conjugation of bilirubin.[51] Affected individuals usually are homozygous for a variant allele which features an additional TA repeat in the promoter. Genotype/phenotype correlations have been demonstrated with both bilirubin and SN-38 as substrates *in vitro*.[54] Case studies of patients with Gilbert's disease (on the basis of history of unconjugated hyperbilirubinemia) have been reported, and these individuals have greatly reduced glucuronoconjugation of SN-38 as revealed by the AUC ratio of the conjugate to the free SN-38.[55] Importantly, the toxicity of CPT-11 appears to be significantly increased in these patients, in keeping with this reduced ability to deactivate SN-38. The pharmacokinetics of SN-38 have also been shown to be modified according to the UDPG 1A1 genotype in a small pharmacokinetic study.[56] Because of the competition between SN-38 and bilirubin for UDPG 1A1, administration of CPT-11 may cause transient hyperbilirubinemia.[57] Also the pre-treatment plasma concentrations of unconjugated bilirubin appear to correlate with hematologic toxicity and SN-38 pharmacokinetics.[57] It is clear that CPT-11 should be used with the upmost care in patients with reduced capacity to conjugate SN-38.[53,58] The potential exists also for significant drug interactions with other drugs that are extensively glucuronoconjugated, such as valproic acid.[59]

In animal models at least, SN-38 and SN-38 glucuronide appears to participate in significant enterohepatic recirculation with the glucuronide being released by bacterial and mucosal glucuronidase activity.[60] Delayed diarrhea is one of the dose-limiting toxicities of CPT-11, and this has been shown to be greatly reduced in animals treated with inhibitors of β-glucuronidases or broad spectrum antibiotics.[60,61] However, the situation regarding the hydrolysis of SN-38G in man is not as clear, although it is evident that significant SN-38G hydrolytic activity is present in human feces.[4,5]

Glucuronoconjugation of SN-38 has also been reported to be mediated by other isoforms of the UDPG1A family,[62] and overexpression of several of these may contribute to the resistant phenotype of a cell line with greatly increased glucuronoconjugation of SN-38.[63] Surprisingly, in the Ciotti study, UDPGT1A7 was found to conjugate SN-38 much more avidly than did UDPGT1A1.[62] However, the clinical significance of this finding is unclear, because the available evidence listed above suggests that UDPGT1A1 is the principal pathway for conjugation of SN-38 in patients.

CONCLUSIONS

Being a prodrug, CPT-11 has metabolism as one of the principal factors influencing its clinical activity. CPT-11 is inefficiently converted to SN-38 but, paradoxically, this may be a positive factor in determining the clinical activity of this drug because of the "slow-release" effect that results from the large volume of distribution and long mean residence time of CPT-11. Low dose protracted regimens, aside from considerations in terms of anti-tumor activity of schedule-dependent drugs, have an advantage in terms of the efficiency of the conversion to SN-38. The cholinergic toxicity sometimes experienced with CPT-11, although easily managed, is related to CPT-11 itself,[26] and reducing the relative concentrations of the prodrug should translate into an increased therapeutic index as far as nonproliferative toxicity is concerned.

The question of whether tumor activation is relevant remains unanswered. In particular, the properties of tumor esterases are unknown. However, any large difference in deacylation reaction rates or half-saturation constants of normal and tumor tissue esterases could theoretically be used to define optimum regimens of administration of CPT-11.

Although CYP450-mediated metabolism accounts for a small fraction (~15%) of the CPT-11 excretion mass balance, the effects of induction/inhibition of CYP450 appear to be considerable[49,50] and may impact on the therapeutic index of this drug. Studies of new administration regimens should include delineation of metabolism to enable further optimization of treatment with CPT-11.

REFERENCES

1. SAWADA, S., S. OKAJIMA, R. AIYAMA, K. NOKATA, T. FURUTA, T. YOKOKURA, E. SUGINO, K. YAMAGUCHI & T. MIYASAKA. 1991. Synthesis and antitumor activity of 20(S)-camptothecin derivatives: carbamate-linked, water-soluble derivatives of 7-ethyl-10-hydroxycamptothecin. Chem. Pharm. Bull. Tokyo **39:** 1446–1450.
2. KANEDA, N., H. NAGATA, T. FURUTA & T. YOKOKURA. 1990. Metabolism and pharmacokinetics of the camptothecin analogue CPT-11 in the mouse. Cancer Res. **50:** 1715–1720.
3. KANEDA, N. & T. YOKOKURA. 1990. Nonlinear pharmacokinetics of CPT-11 in rats. Cancer Res. **50:** 1721–1725.
4. SCHAAF, L., J. SLATTER, J. SAMS, K. FEENSTRA, M. JOHNSON, P. BOMBARDT, K. CATHCART, M. VERBURG, L. PEARSON, L. COMPTON, et al. 1999. Metabolism and excretion of irinotecan (CPT-11) following IV infusion of [^{14}C]CPT-11 in patients with advanced solid tumor malignancy. Proc. ASCO. **18:** 164a.
5. SPARREBOOM, A., M.J. DE JONGE, P. DE BRUIJN, E. BROUWER, K. NOOTER, W.J. LOOS, R.J. VAN ALPHEN, R. H. MATHIJSSEN, G. STOTER & J. VERWEIJ. 1998. Irinotecan (CPT-11) metabolism and disposition in cancer patients. Clin. Cancer Res. **4:** 2747–2754.
6. CANAL, P., C. GAY, A. DEZEUZE, J.Y. DOUILLARD, R. BUGAT, R. BRUNET, A. ADENIS, P. HERAIT, F. LOKIEC & A. MATHIEU BOUE. 1996. Pharmacokinetics and pharmacodynamics of irinotecan during a phase II clinical trial in colorectal cancer. Pharmacology and Molecular Mechanisms Group of the European Organization for Research and Treatment of Cancer. J. Clin. Oncol. **14:** 2688–2695.
7. CHABOT, G.G., D. ABIGERGES, G. CATIMEL, S. CULINE, M. DE FORNI, J.M. EXTRA, M. MAHJOUBI, P. HERAIT, J.P. ARMAND, R. BUGAT et al. 1995. Population pharmacokinetics and pharmacodynamics of irinotecan (CPT-11) and active metabolite SN-38 during phase I trials. Ann. Oncol. **6:** 141–151.
8. CHABOT, G. . 1997. Clinical pharmacokinetics of irinotecan. Clin. Pharmacokinet. **33:** 245–259.
9. RIVORY, L.P., M.C. HAAZ, P. CANAL, F. LOKIEC, J.P. ARMAND & J. ROBERT. 1997. Pharmacokinetic interrelationships of irinotecan (CPT-11) and its three major plasma metabolites in patients enrolled in phase I/II trials. Clin. Cancer Res. **3:** 1261–1266.
10. TSUJI, T., N. KANEDA, K. KADO, T. YOKOKURA, T. YOSHIMOTO & D. TSURU. 1991. CPT-11 converting enzyme from rat serum: purification and some properties. J. Pharmacobiodyn. **14:** 341–349.
11. RIVORY, L.P., M. . BOWLES, J. ROBERT & S.M. POND. 1996. Conversion of irinotecan (CPT-11) to its active metabolite, 7-ethyl-10-hydroxycamptothecin (SN-38), by human liver carboxylesterase. Biochem. Pharmacol. **52:** 1103–1111.
12. KAWATO, Y., M. AONUMA, Y. HIROTA, H. KUGA & K. SATO. 1991. Intracellular roles of SN-38, a metabolite of the camptothecin derivative CPT-11, in the antitumor effect of CPT-11. Cancer Res. **51:** 4187–4191.
13. GUICHARD, S., C. TERRET, I. HENNEBELLE, I. LOCHON, P. CHEVREAU, E. FRETIGNY, J. SELVES, E. CHATELUT, R. BUGAT & P. CANAL. 1999. CPT-11 converting carboxylesterase and topoisomerase activities in tumour and normal colon and liver tissues. Br. J. Cancer **80:** 364–370.
14. SATOH, T., M. HOSOKAWA, R. ATSUMI, W. SUZUKI, H. HAKUSUI & E. NAGAI. 1994. Metabolic activation of CPT-11, 7-ethyl-10-[4-(1-piperidino)-1- piperidino]carbonyloxycamptothecin, a novel antitumor agent, by carboxylesterase. Biol. Pharm. Bull. **17:** 662–664.
15. HAAZ, M.C., L.P. RIVORY, C. RICHE & J. ROBERT. 1997. The transformation of irinotecan (CPT-11) to its active metabolite SN-38 by human liver microsomes. Differential hydrolysis for the lactone and carboxylate forms. Naunyn Schmiedeberg's Arch. Pharmacol. **356:** 257–262.
16. RIVORY, L.P., E. CHATELUT, P. CANAL, A. MATHIEU BOUE & J. ROBERT. 1994. Kinetics of the in vivo interconversion of the carboxylate and lactone forms of irinotecan (CPT-11) and of its metabolite SN-38 in patients. Cancer Res. **54:** 6330–6333.

17. HERBEN, V., J. SCHELLENS, M. SWART, G. GRUIA, L. VERNILLET, J. BEIJNEN & W. TEN BOKKEL HUININK. 1999. Phase I and pharmacokinetic study of irintotecan administered as a low-dose, continuous intravenous infusion over 14 days in patients with malignant solid tumors. J. Clin. Oncol. **17:** 1897–1905.
18. VAN GROENINGEN, C., W. VAN DER VIJGH, G. GIACCONE, M. KEDDE, H. GALL, M. BART & H. PINEDO. 1997. Phase I clinical and pharmacokinetic study of 5 day CPT-11 hepatic arterial infusion (HAI) chemotherapy. Proc. ASCO. **16:** 219a.
19. BURKE, T.G. & Z. MI. 1994. The structural basis of camptothecin interactions with human serum albumin: impact on drug stability. J. Med. Chem. **37:** 40–46.
20. SLATTER, J.G., P. SU, J.P. SAMS, L.J. SCHAAF & L.C. WIENKERS. 1997. Bioactivation of the anticancer agent CPT-11 to SN-38 by human hepatic microsomal carboxylesterases and the in vitro assessment of potential drug interactions. Drug Metab. Dispos. **25:** 1157–1164.
21. ROTHENBERG, M.L., J.G. KUHN, H.A.D. BURRIS, J. NELSON, J.R. ECKARDT, M. TRISTAN MORALES, S.G. HILSENBECK, G.R. WEISS, L.S. SMITH, G.I. RODRIGUEZ ET AL. 1993. Phase I and pharmacokinetic trial of weekly CPT-11. J. Clin. Oncol. **11:** 2194–2204.
22. ROWINSKY, E.K., L.B. GROCHOW, D.S. ETTINGER, S.E. SARTORIUS, B.G. LUBEJKO, T.L. CHEN, M.K. ROCK & R.C. DONEHOWER. 1994. Phase I and pharmacological study of the novel topoisomerase I inhibitor 7-ethyl-10-[4-(1-piperidino)-1-piperidino]carbonyloxycamptothecin (CPT-11) administered as a ninety-minute infusion every 3 weeks. Cancer Res. **54:** 427–436.
23. TAKIMOTO, C., G. MORRISON, N. HAROLD, M. QUINN, B. MONAHAN, R. BAND, J. COTTRELL, A. GUEMEI, V. LLORENS, H. HEHMAN, et al. 2000. Phase I and pharmacologic study of irinotecan administered as a 96-hour infusion weekly to adult cancer patients. J. Clin. Oncol. **18:** 659–667.
24. FURMAN, W., C. STEWART, C. POQUETTE, C. PRATT, V. SANTANA, W. ZAMBONI, L. BOWMAN, M. MA, F. HOFFER, W. MEYER, et al. 1999. Direct translation of a protracted irinotecan schedule from a xenograft model to a phase I trial in children. J. Clin. Oncol. **17:** 1815–1824.
25. VASSAL, G., A. SANTOS, F. PEIN, D. FRAPPAZ, D. MIGNARD & F. DOZ. 1997. Pharmacokinetics of irinotecan (CPT-11) and its metabolites in children. Proc. AACR. **38:** 505.
26. DODDS, H. & L. RIVORY. 1999. The mechanism for the inhibition of acetylcholinesterases by irinotecan (CPT-11). Mol. Pharmacol. **56:** 1346–1353.
27. MORTON, C.L., R.M. WADKINS, M.K. DANKS & P.M. POTTER. 1999. The anticancer prodrug CPT-11 is a potent inhibitor of acetylcholinesterase but is rapidly catalyzed to SN-38 by butyrylcholinesterase. Cancer Res. **59:** 1458–1463.
28. VAN ARK OTTE, J., M.A. KEDDE, W.J. VAN DER VIJGH, A.M. DINGEMANS, W.J. JANSEN, H.M. PINEDO, E. BOVEN & G. GIACCONE. 1998. Determinants of CPT-11 and SN-38 activities in human lung cancer cells. Br. J. Cancer. **77:** 2171–2176.
29. JANSEN, W.J., B. ZWART, S.T. HULSCHER, G. GIACCONE, H.M. PINEDO & E. BOVEN. 1997. CPT-11 in human colon-cancer cell lines and xenografts: characterization of cellular sensitivity determinants. Int. J. Cancer **70:** 335–340.
30. KOJIMA, A., N.R. HACKETT & R.G. CRYSTAL. 1998. Reversal of CPT-11 resistance of lung cancer cells by adenovirus-mediated gene transfer of the human carboxylesterase cDNA. Cancer Res. **58:** 4368–4374.
31. KOJIMA, A., N.R. HACKETT, A. OHWADA & R.G. CRYSTAL. 1998. In vivo human carboxylesterase cDNA gene transfer to activate the prodrug CPT-11 for local treatment of solid tumors. J. Clin. Invest. **101:** 1789–1796.
32. DANKS, M.K., C.L. MORTON, E.J. KRULL, P.J. CHESHIRE, L.B. RICHMOND, C.W. NAEVE, C.A. PAWLIK, P.J. HOUGHTON & P.M. POTTER. 1999. Comparison of activation of CPT-11 by rabbit and human carboxylesterases for use in enzyme/prodrug therapy. Clin. Cancer Res. **5:** 917–924.
33. GUICHARD, S.M., C.L. MORTON, E.J. KRULL, C.F. STEWART, M.K. DANKS & P.M. POTTER. 1998. Conversion of the CPT-11 metabolite APC to SN-38 by rabbit liver carboxylesterase. Clin. Cancer Res. **4:** 3089–3094.
34. AHMED, F., V. VYAS, A. CORNFIELD, S. GOODIN, T.S. RAVIKUMAR, E.H. RUBIN & E. GUPTA. 1999. In vitro activation of irinotecan to SN-38 by human liver and intestine. Anticancer Res. **19:** 2067–2071.

35. DRENGLER, R.L., J.G. KUHN, L.J. SCHAAF, G.I. RODRIGUEZ, M.A. VILLALONA CALERO, L.A. HAMMOND, J.A. STEPHENSON, JR., S. HODGES, M.A. KRAYNAK, et al. 1999. Phase I and pharmacokinetic trial of oral irinotecan administered daily for 5 days every 3 weeks in patients with solid tumors. J. Clin. Oncol. **17:** 685–696.
36. ZAMBONI, W.C., P.J. HOUGHTON, J. THOMPSON, P.J. CHESHIRE, S.K. HANNA, L.B. RICHMOND, X. LOU & C.F. STEWART. 1998. Altered irinotecan and SN-38 disposition after intravenous and oral administration of irinotecan in mice bearing human neuroblastoma xenografts. Clin. Cancer Res. **4:** 455–462.
37. ONISHI, Y., M. OGURO & H. KIZAKI. 1997. A lymphoma cell line resistant to 4-piperidinopiperidine was less sensitive to CPT-11. Cancer Chemother. Pharmacol. **39:** 473–478.
38. DODDS, H., S. CLARKE, M. FINDLAY, J. BISHOP, J. ROBERT & L. RIVORY. 2000. Clinical pharmacokinetics of the irinotecan metabolite 4-piperidinopiperidine and its possible clinical importance. Cancer Chemother. Pharmacol. **45:** 9–14.
39. RIVORY, L.P., J.F. RIOU, M.C. HAAZ, S. SABLE, M. VUILHORGNE, A. COMMERCON, S.M. POND & J. ROBERT. 1996. Identification and properties of a major plasma metabolite of irinotecan (CPT-11) isolated from the plasma of patients. Cancer Res. **56:** 3689–3694.
40. DODDS, H.M., M.C. HAAZ, J.F. RIOU, J. ROBERT & L.P. RIVORY. 1998. Identification of a new metabolite of CPT-11 (irinotecan): pharmacological properties and activation to SN-38. J. Pharmacol. Exp. Ther. **286:** 578–583.
41. HAAZ, M.C., L. RIVORY, C. RICHE, L. VERNILLET & J. ROBERT. 1998. Metabolism of irinotecan (CPT-11) by human hepatic microsomes: participation of cytochrome P-450 3A and drug interactions. Cancer Res. **58:** 468–472.
42. HAAZ, M.C., C. RICHE, L.P. RIVORY & J. ROBERT. 1998. Biosynthesis of an aminopiperidino metabolite of irinotecan [7-ethyl-10-[4-(1-piperidino)-1-piperidino]carbonyloxycamptothecine] by human hepatic microsomes. Drug Metab. Dispos. **26:** 769–774.
43. LOKIEC, F., B.M. DU SORBIER & G.J. SANDERINK. 1996. Irinotecan (CPT-11) metabolites in human bile and urine. Clin. Cancer Res. **2:** 1943–1949.
44. DODDS, H.M., J. ROBERT & L.P. RIVORY. 1998. The detection of photodegradation products of irinotecan (CPT-11, Campto, Camptosar), in clinical studies, using high-performance liquid chromatography/atmospheric pressure chemical ionisation/mass spectrometry. J.. Pharm. Biomed. Anal. **17:** 785–792.
45. PLATZER, P., T. THALHAMMER, G. HAMILTON, E. ULSPERGER, E. ROSENBERG, R. WISSIAK & W. JAGER. 2000. Metabolism of camptothecin, a potent topoisomerase I inhibitor, in the isolated perfused rat liver. Cancer Chemother. Pharmacol. **45:** 50–54.
46. DODDS, H., R. WUNSCH, E. GILLAM & L. RIVORY. 1999. Further elucidation of the pathways involved in the catabolism of the camptothecin analogue irinotecan. Proc. AACR **40:** 110.
47. ZANETTA, S., A. SANTOS, A. DEROUSSENT, T. CRESTEIL, E. RAYMOND, A. BOIJE, L. VERNILLET, M. RISSE, A. GOUYETTE & G. VASSAL. 1999. CYP3A4 and CYP3A5 metabolism of irinotecan (CPT-11) in humans. Proc. AACR **40:** 83–84.
48. DODDS, H.M., D.J. CRAIK & L.P. RIVORY. 1997. Photodegradation of irinotecan (CPT-11) in aqueous solutions: identification of fluorescent products and influence of solution composition. J. Pharm. Sci. **86:** 1410–1416.
49. REID, J., J. BUCKNER, L. SCHAAF, P. NOVOTNY, K. WRIGHT, D. KIMMEL & L. MILLER. 1999. Pharmacokientics of irinotecan (CPT-11) in recurrent glioma patients: results of an NCCTG phase II trial. Proc. ASCO **18:** 141a.
50. FRIEDMAN, H.S., W.P. PETROS, A.H. FRIEDMAN, L.J. SCHAAF, T. KERBY, J. LAWYER, M. PARRY, P.J. HOUGHTON, S. LOVELL, K. RASHEED, et al. 1999. Irinotecan therapy in adults with recurrent or progressive malignant glioma. J. Clin. Oncol. **17:** 1516–1525.
51. IYER, L., C.D. KING, P.F. WHITINGTON, M.D. GREEN, S.K. ROY, T.R. TEPHLY, B.L. COFFMAN & M.J. RATAIN. 1998. Genetic predisposition to the metabolism of irinotecan (CPT-11). Role of uridine diphosphate glucuronosyltransferase isoform 1A1 in the glucuronidation of its active metabolite (SN-38) in human liver microsomes. J. Clin. Invest. **101:** 847–854.

52. RIVORY, L.P. & J. ROBERT. 1995. Identification and kinetics of a beta-glucuronide metabolite of SN-38 in human plasma after administration of the camptothecin derivative irinotecan. Cancer Chemother. Pharmacol. **36:** 176–179.
53. GUPTA, E., T.M. LESTINGI, R. MICK, J. RAMIREZ, E.E. VOKES & M.J. RATAIN. 1994. Metabolic fate of irinotecan in humans: correlation of glucuronidation with diarrhea. Cancer Res. **54:** 3723–3725.
54. IYER, L., D. HALL, S. DAS, M.A. MORTELL, J. RAMIREZ, S. KIM, A. DI RIENZO & M.J. RATAIN. 1999. Phenotype-genotype correlation of in vitro SN-38 (active metabolite of irinotecan) and bilirubin glucuronidation in human liver tissue with UGT1A1 promoter polymorphism. Clin. Pharmacol. Ther. **65:** 576–582.
55. WASSERMAN, E., A. MYARA, F. LOKIEC, F. GOLDWASSER, F. TRIVIN, M. MAHJOUBI, J.L. MISSET & E. CVITKOVIC. 1997. Severe CPT-11 toxicity in patients with Gilbert's syndrome: two case reports. Ann. Oncol. **8:** 1049–1051.
56. ANDO, Y., H. SAKA, G. ASAI, S. SUGIURA, K. SHIMOKATA & T. KAMATAKI. 1998. UGT1A1 genotypes and glucuronidation of SN-38, the active metabolite of irinotecan. Ann. Oncol. **9:** 845–847.
57. WASSERMAN, E., A. MYARA, F. LOKIEC, M. RIOFRIO, P. BLEUZEN, J. SANTONI, F. TRIVIN, P. HERAIT, M. MAHJOUBI, J. MISSET & E. CVITKOVIC. 1998. Bilirubin (Bil) and SN-38 metabolism: pharmacodynamics of CPT-11. Proc. ASCO **17:** 185a.
58. RAYMOND, E., L. VERNILLET, V. BOIGE, A. HUA, M. DUCREUX, S. FAIVRE, C. JACQUES, M. GATINEAU, D. MIGNARD, J. VERGNIOL, et al. 1999. Phase I and pharmacokinetic (PK) study of irinotecan (CPT-11) in cancer patients (pts) with hepatic dysfunction. Proc. ASCO **18:** 165a.
59. GUPTA, E., X. WANG, J. RAMIREZ & M.J. RATAIN. 1997. Modulation of glucuronidation of SN-38, the active metabolite of irinotecan, by valproic acid and phenobarbital. Cancer Chemothe.r Pharmacol. **39:** 440–444.
60. TAKASUNA, K., Y. KASAI, Y. KITANO, K. MORI, R. KOBAYASHI, T. HAGIWARA, K. KAKIHATA, M. HIROHASHI, M. NOMURA, E. NAGAI, et al. 1995. Protective effects of kampo medicines and baicalin against intestinal toxicity of a new anticancer camptothecin derivative, irinotecan hydrochloride (CPT-11), in rats. Jpn. J. Cancer Res. **86:** 978–984.
61. NARITA, M., E. NAGAI, H. HAGIWARA, M. ABURADA, T. YOKOI & T. KAMATAKI. 1993. Inhibition of beta-glucuronidase by natural glucuronides of kampo medicines using glucuronide of SN-38 (7-ethyl-10-hydroxycamptothecin) as a substrate. Xenobiotica **23:** 5–10.
62. CIOTTI, M., N. BASU, M. BRANGI & I.S. OWENS. 1999. Glucuronidation of 7-ethyl-10-hydroxycamptothecin (SN-38) by the human UDP-glucuronosyltransferases encoded at the UGT1 locus. Biochem. Biophys. Res. Commun. **260:** 199–202.
63. TAKAHASHI, T., Y. FUJIWARA, M. MIYAZAKI, T. KURATA, T. OGURI, M. YOKOZAKI, T. ISOBE, S. ISHIOKA, M. YAMAKIDO, O. KATOH & P. MACKENZIE. 1998. The role of glucuronidation in 7-ethyl-10-hydroxycamptothecin (SN-38) resistance. Proc. ASCO **17:** 185a.

Pharmacology of Camptothecin Esters

JOACHIM G. LIEHR,[a,c] NICK J. HARRIS,[a] JOHN MENDOZA,[a]
AHMED E. AHMED,[b] AND BEPPINO C. GIOVANELLA[b]

[a]*The Stehlin Foundation for Cancer Research at Christus St. Joseph Hospital, Houston, Texas 77003, USA*

[b]*Department of Pathology, University of Texas Medical Branch at Galveston, Galveston, Texas 77555, USA*

ABSTRACT: An intact lactone ring of camptothecins is a structural requirement for their anticancer activity. Propionate esters of camptothecin (CPT) and 9-nitrocamptothecin (9NC), CZ48 and CZ112, respectively, have been synthesized as derivatives resistant to lactone hydrolysis and are chemotherapeutically active. In this study, we have examined the mechanism of action of CZ48 and CZ112 and their distribution, metabolism, and toxicity. CZ112 incubated in human plasma retained its lactone structure longer than 9NC ($t_{1/2}$: 10.5 and <1 hr for CZ112 and 9NC, respectively). This resistance to lactone hydrolysis was also observed in mouse plasma or albumin solutions. Neither CZ48 nor CZ112 inhibit topoisomerase I and thus are prodrugs dependent on hydrolysis to CPT or 9NC, respectively. Rates of hydrolysis of CZ48 to CPT are higher by homogenates of mouse liver, spleen, lung, and kidney than by plasma. Rates of hydrolysis by tumor cells in culture vary and were higher by breast cancer and melanoma cells than by colon cancer cells. On the basis of these and other data, it is proposed that CZ48 and CZ112 may act as anticancer agents by resisting hydrolysis to camptothecins while in circulation. Hydrolysis in tissues may release intact lactone in target tissues.

INTRODUCTION

Camptothecin (CPT) and its derivatives such as 9-nitrocamptothecin (9NC) are inhibitors of topoisomerase I.[1–4] Many of these derivatives, including 9NC, are currently being examined for their cancer chemotherapeutic activity.[5–8] The integrity of the lactone ring system of CPT derivatives has now been recognized as a key determinant for the chemotherapeutic efficacy of this class of drugs.[9] Wall and coworkers described the hydrolysis of the CPT lactone to the corresponding open salt with increasing pH consistent with the known alkaline hydrolysis of esters and lactones.[10–12] Moreover, the hydrolysis of CPT derivatives to the open salt forms is also favored in biological systems.[13,14] For instance, CPT or 9NC administered to patients is rapidly hydrolyzed while in circulation.[15] Only 2–5% of these drugs remain in the lactone form when incubated in plasma *in vitro*.[14,15] The reason for the rapid hydrolysis of CPT or 9NC to the open salt form *in vivo* or in plasma *in vitro* is the high-affinity binding of the salt form to serum albumin.[14,16] This affinity of albumin for the camp-

---

[c]Address for correspondence: Joachim G. Liehr, Ph.D., The Stehlin Foundation for Cancer Research at Christus St. Joseph Hospital, 1918 Chenevert, Houston, TX 77003. Voice: 713-756-5750; fax: 713-756-5783.

tothecin salts results in a rapid equilibration in the presence of albumin with the salt form prevailing. The rapid hydrolysis of CPT derivatives to the open salt forms, catalyzed by alkali or albumin binding, represents an inactivation process for this class of drugs, since the open salt forms of CPT derivatives carry only some toxicity and very little pharmacological activity.[8,10–12]

CAMPTOTHECIN ESTER CANCER DRUGS

CPT and 9NC esters have been synthesized in the hope of circumventing problems with rapid lactone hydrolysis as described above and have been examined for anticancer activity.[17] These ester derivatives have been prepared in the expectation that a bulky acyl substituent in the vicinity of the lactone moiety might interfere with albumin binding of the drug and thus might inhibit the conversion of the active lactone form of the drug into inactive salt. Moreover, lactone hydrolysis likely is facilitated by hydrogen bonding of the C-20 hydroxy group of CPT to the carbonyl oxygen. Therefore, acylation of this hydroxy group was expected to eliminate this hydrogen bonding and thus also to impede lactone hydrolysis. Series of CPT and 9NC esters were synthesized and examined for chemotherapeutic activity against tumor cells in culture and against human tumor xenografts in nude mice.[17] Consistent with expectations, the propionate esters of CPT and 9NC, CZ48 and CZ112, respectively, carried anticancer activity in these test systems (for a review of these results, see the text by Cao in this volume), whereas shorter or longer acyl ester chains were inactive (for structures, see FIG. 1).

In the following text, we will examine the mechanism of action of camptothecin esters and compare it with that of the parent CPT or 9NC, respectively. Moreover, we will describe their toxicity, metabolism, and distribution in relation to parent camptothecins to determine if esterification improves the anticancer activity of this class of antineoplastic drugs.

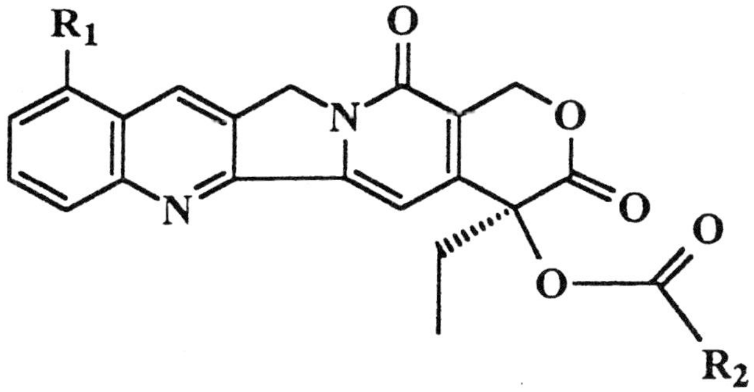

FIGURE 1. Structures of camptothecin esters. R_1 = H; R_2 = CH_2CH_3, camptothecin propionate ester (CZ48). R_1 = NO_2; R_2 = CH_2CH_3, 9-nitrocamptothecin propionate ester (CZ112).

STABILITY OF CAMPTOTHECIN ESTERS

The primary biochemical reason for the synthesis and pharmacological examination of camptothecin esters has been their postulated stability in biological fluids. Therefore, stability of esters has been the first parameter we have evaluated. CZ48 was incubated in a 4% solution of human serum albumin in phosphate-buffered saline at 37°C. After 4 hr, there was no detectable hydrolysis to the open salt form. In contrast, CPT lactone, incubated under the same conditions, rapidly hydrolyzed to salt as described previously.[14,16]

Incubations of CZ112 with mouse and human plasma have also been carried out to evaluate drug stability.[17] Free drug lactone concentrations in mouse and human plasma declined when incubated at 37°C ($t_{1/2}$ mouse: >50 hr, $t_{1/2}$ human: 10 hr). However, this decrease in lactone concentrations must have been mainly due to protein binding rather than to hydrolysis, because most of the initial drug was recovered upon acid digestion of the proteins. In contrast, the parent camptothecin drug 9NC rapidly hydrolyzed to the salt form in mouse or human plasma with half-lives established previously.[14,16] These data demonstrate that the propionate esters of CPT and 9NC, CZ48 and CZ112, respectively, are more stable than the parent camptothecin drugs in albumin solutions and in plasma *in vitro*. It is concluded that the ester chain in the vicinity of the lactone moiety inhibits albumin binding and thus makes these drugs resistant to hydrolysis.

TOPOISOMERASE I INHIBITION BY CAMPTOTHECIN ESTERS

CPT and many of its derivatives are capable of stabilizing the topoisomerase I–DNA complex and thus inhibit the action of this enzyme.[1–4] The inhibitory activity of the esters CZ48 and CZ112 has been examined using a topoisomerase I inhibition assay kit purchased from TopoGen, Inc. (Columbus, OH). Three different concentrations of these two ester test compounds did not show any detectable enzyme inhibition *in vitro*, whereas the parent compounds CPT and 9NC were fully active as described previously.[1–3,18] These data clearly demonstrate that the camptothecin esters CZ48 and CZ112 fail to inhibit topoisomerase I and thus are not pharmacologically active without metabolic activation to CPT and 9NC, respectively. Thus, these two camptothecin derivatives, which are chemotherapeutically active against human tumors in nude mice,[17] are prodrugs and require metabolic activation by esterase-mediated hydrolysis to the parent compounds.

IN VITRO METABOLISM OF CAMPTOTHECIN ESTERS

Camptothecin esters undergo hydrolysis to the parent drug substance when incubated with whole blood. For instance, 11 to 13% of 1 µg CZ112, incubated in 1 ml of whole dog or mouse blood at 37°C, has been converted to 9NC after 4 or 24 hr of incubation, respectively. Human blood hydrolyzes esters more efficiently. After 4 and 24 hr, 20% and 33% of CZ112 have been metabolized by whole human blood to 9NC, respectively.

TABLE 1. Metabolic conversion of CZ48 to CPT by rat or human liver homogenate

	CPT formed (percent of total drug recovered)	
Incubation time (hr)	Rat	Human
0	<0.1	<0.1
	<1.0	n.d.
4	7.1	n.d.
24	23.1	40.9
48	25.8	54.3

NOTE: CZ48 (40 ng) was incubated at 37°C in 1 ml homogenate prepared from 25 mg tissue. Metabolites were extracted and analyzed by high-pressure liquid chromatography. Amounts of total CPT formed are expressed as percent of total drug recovered.

Tissues also contain esterases and therefore hydrolyze camptothecin esters to camptothecin parent substance. In a series of incubations of CZ48 with homogenates of mouse liver, spleen, lung, and kidney, the highest metabolic conversion of propionate ester to CPT metabolite has been observed in hepatic tissue, consistent with the known high esterase activity in this tissue.[19] After 24 hr of incubation of CPT in liver homogenate, 28% of the dose was recovered as CPT salt and 34% in the lactone form. The remainder was unchanged CZ48. Other tissues contain less esterase activity, and, accordingly, their homogenates metabolized CZ48 to smaller amounts of CPT. Mouse spleen, lung, and kidney homogenate converted CZ48 to 6–8% CPT lactone and 9–17% CPT salt. The remaining 76–85% of the substrate remained unchanged.

Rat and human liver homogenates hydrolyzed CZ48 to CPT at differing rates. The rate of conversion of CZ48 by rat liver homogenates was less than that of mouse liver (TABLE 1). After 24 and 48 hr of incubation, 23–26% of radioactive drug substance had been hydrolyzed to CPT. In contrast, human liver homogenate metabolized CZ48 to CPT at double the rate observed in rat. These data demonstrate the esterase activity of tissues and plasma using camptothecin esters as substrates.

Tumor cells cultured in RPMI medium metabolized CZ112 to 9NC at different rates. The highest rates of metabolic conversion have been detected with human melanoma and human breast cancer cells (FIGS. 2 and 3). Moreover, the resulting 9NC metabolite was released into the medium mainly as lactone, the pharmacologically active form. In contrast, four colon cancer cell lines hydrolyzed the ester drug at a lower rate and converted a larger portion of the 9NC metabolite formed into the inactive salt form (FIG. 3). These differential metabolic rates are consistent with the better anticancer activity of camptothecins against breast cancer cells and xenografts in nude mice compared to colon cancers.[9,17,19]

IN VIVO METABOLISM OF CAMPTOTHECIN ESTERS

As part of an examination of the *in vivo* metabolism of camptothecin esters, nude mice were treated with 20 mg/kg CZ48. In a control experiment, other nude mice were treated with 2 mg/kg CPT. Plasma total CPT and CPT lactone concentrations

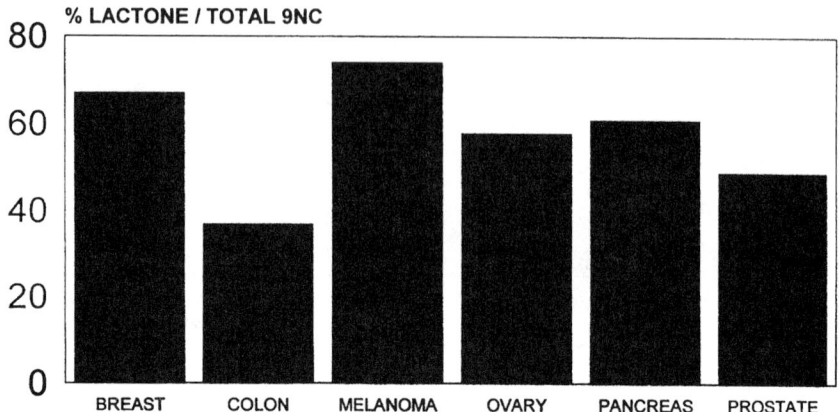

FIGURE 2. *In vitro* hydrolysis of CZ112 to 9NC lactone by human cancer cells in culture (4–6 different cell lines/organ site). The breast and colon cancer cell lines used are those shown in FIGURE 2. Data are expressed as percent 9NC lactone/total 9NC formed by hydrolysis of CZ112.

were determined by high-pressure liquid chromatography in each experiment, and values have been compared. CPT lactone levels from administered CPT initially exceeded those produced by ester hydrolysis of CZ48. However, these levels declined rapidly, whereas CPT lactone produced as metabolite of CZ48 persisted longer while in circulation in the mouse. *In vivo* tissue and tumor concentrations of CPT as a result of CPT or CZ48 administration are currently under investigation and will be reported in the future. These experiments demonstrate that a 10-fold higher dose of CZ48, which is well tolerated by the mice, produces comparable CPT lactone concentrations in plasma.

TOXICITY OF CAMPTOTHECIN ESTERS

The toxicity of CZ112 has been tested in nude mice and has been compared to that of 9NC. For instance, male mice survived single injections of up to 150 mg/kg CZ112. At doses above 100 mg/kg, some temporary body weight loss occurred, but the animals recovered. Upon repeated dosing (five daily injections/week, no injections on weekends) for 5 months, no male animals survived on 20 mg/kg CZ112. At 30 mg/kg for 30 days using the same regimen, 7/18 male mice survived.

The toxicity of CZ112 has also been examined in female nude mice, because esterase activity is known to be under hormonal control.[19] Female nude mice tolerated much higher doses of this ester drug. At single doses of 230 mg/kg CZ112, there was some initial body weight loss of the animals, but all animals survived. Upon repeated dosing (20 mg/kg per week CZ112, injected once daily on five days/week for five months), 4/5 female mice survived; at 30 mg/kg using the same regimen for 30 days 13/18 female animals survived.

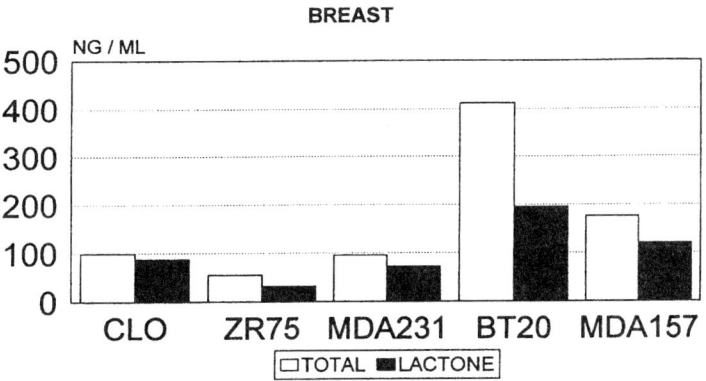

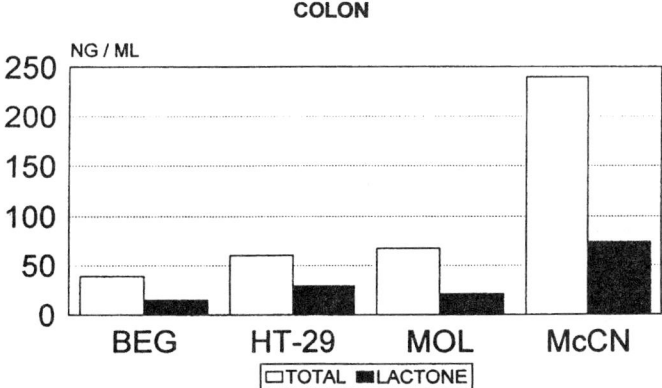

FIGURE 3. *In vitro* hydrolysis of CZ112 to 9NC by human breast (*upper panel*) and colon (*lower panel*) cancer cells in culture. Approximately 10^6 cells/ml of the cell lines indicated were incubated with 10 µM CZ112 for 24 hr in RPMI 1640 medium. Control incubations without cells produced <6 ng/ml total 9NC. Products formed were extracted from the medium, analyzed by HPLC (fluorescence detection) and expressed as ng/ml total 9NC (white) and 9NC lactone (black).

These data clearly indicate that toxicity of camptothecin esters is gender-dependent (androgen-dependent). The known regulation of esterase activity by androgen likely determines camptothecin ester toxicity.[19] It is concluded from these data that camptothecin esters are relatively nontoxic and are activated to toxic camptothecin metabolites by esterase.

CONCLUSION

Our data demonstrate that camptothecin esters, which have been shown to be chemotherapeutically active against human tumor xenografts in nude mice,[17] are prodrugs requiring metabolic activation by ester hydrolysis. A metabolic conversion to the active camptothecin metabolite occurs at comparatively low rates in blood. A higher hydrolysis rate than in blood has been observed in liver homogenate of various species consistent with the higher esterase activity in that organ.[19] Intermediate rates of parent camptothecin formation by hydrolysis of camptothecin ester drugs have been observed with homogenates of mouse kidney, spleen, and lung. In these incubations, camptothecin lactone and salt were formed in approximately equal amounts by most tissue homogenates, resulting in an improved lactone/salt equilibrium than has been observed when camptothecin itself has been administered.

Tumor cells convert camptothecin esters to active camptothecin metabolite at differing rates. High rates of metabolic conversion have been detected with several melanoma and breast cancer cell lines, much lower rates with four colon cancer lines. These results are consistent with the excellent response of melanoma and breast cancer xenografts in nude mice to this drug and the lower response of colon cancers in this system.[17]

Camptothecin esters are also much less toxic than camptothecins. The difference in toxicity between male and female mice likely is due to the gender difference in esterase activity, which is known to be androgen-regulated.[19] The low toxicity of the esters indicates that they act as a low-toxicity reservoir of prodrug, which may be converted by ester hydrolysis to the pharmacologically active and toxic camptothecin lactone.

In summary, camptothecin esters are prodrugs of low toxicity and are metabolically activated by esterases to parent camptothecins, which are both pharmacologically active and carry toxicity. Most of the ester drugs survive intact while in circulation and are then subject to tissue esterase action. Thus, these esters are a promising class of camptothecin.

ACKNOWLEDGMENTS

The authors wish to thank Betty Harris for the preparation of the manuscript and Dr. Z. Cao for assistance with FIGURE 1. Funding by SuperGen, Inc. and by the Friends of the Stehlin Foundation is gratefully acknowledged.

REFERENCES

1. HSIANG, Y.-H., R. HERTZBERG, S. HECHT & L.F. LIU. 1985. Camptothecin induces protein-linked DNA breaks via mammalian DNA topoisomerase I. J. Biol. Chem. **260:** 14873–14878.
2. HSIANG, Y.-H & L.F. LIU. 1988. Identification of mammalian DNA topoisomerase I as an intracellular target of the anticancer drug camptothecin. Cancer Res. **49:** 1722–1726.
3. JAXEL, C., K.W. KOHN, M.C. WANI, et al. 1989. Structure–activity study of the actions of camptothecin derivatives on mammalian topoisomerase. I. Evidence for a specific receptor site and a relation to antitumor activity. Cancer Res. **49:** 1465–1469.
4. HSIANG, Y.-H, L.F. LIU, M.E. WALL, et al. 1989. DNA topoisomerase I-mediated DNA cleavage and cytotoxicity of camptothecin analogues. Cancer Res. **49:** 4385–4389.
5. KINGSBURG, W.D., J.C. BOEHM, D.R. JAKAS, et al. 1991. Synthesis of water soluble (aminoalkyl) camptothecin analogues: inhibition of topoisomerase I and antitumor activity. J. Med. Chem. **34:** 98–107.

6. SAWADA, S., S. MATSUOKA, K. NOKATA, et al. 1991. Synthesis and antitumor activity of 20(S)-camptothecin derivatives: A-ring-modified and 7,10-disubstituted camptothecins. Chem. Pharmacol. Bull. **39:** 3183–3188.
7. STEHLIN, J.S., B.C. GIOVANELLA, E.A. NATELSON, et al. 1999. A study of 9-nitrocamptothecin (RFS-2000) in patients with advanced pancreatic cancer. Int. J. Oncol. **14:** 821–831.
8. SLICHENMEYER, W.J., E.K. ROWINSKY, R.C. DONEHOWER & S.H. KAUFMANN. 1993. The current status of camptothecin analogues as antitumor agents. J. Natl. Cancer Inst. **85:** 271–291.
9. GIOVANELLA, B.C., E. NATELSON, D. HARRIS, et al. 1996. Protocols for the treatment of human tumor xenografts with camptothecins. In The Camptothecins: From Discovery to the Patient. Ann. N.Y. Acad. Sci. **803:** 181–187.
10. WANI, M.C., A.W. NICHOLAS, G. MANIKUMAR & M.E. WALL. 1987. Plant antitumor agents. 25. Total synthesis and antileukemic activity of ring A substituted camptothecin analogues. Structure–activity correlations. J. Med. Chem. **30:** 1774–1779.
11. WANI, M.C., A.W. NICHOLAS & M.E. WALL. 1987. Plant antitumor agents. 28. Resolution of a key tricyclic synthon, 5'(RS)-1,5-dioxo-5'-hydroxy-2'H,5'H,6'H-6'-oxopyrano[3',4'f]$\Delta^{6,8}$-tetrahydroindolizine: total synthesis and antitumor activity of 20(S)- and 20-(R)camptothecin. J. Med. Chem. **30:** 2317–2319.
12. FASSBERG, J. & V.J. STELLA. 1992. A kinetic and mechanistic study of the hydrolysis of camptothecin and some analogues. J. Pharmacol. Sci. **81:** 676–684.
13. BURKE, T.G. 1996. Chemistry of the camptothecins in the blood stream. Drug stabilization and optimization of activity. In The Camptothecins: From Discovery to the Patient. Ann. N.Y. Acad. Sci. **803:** 29–31.
14. BURKE, T.G. & Z. MI. 1994. The structural basis of camptothecin interactions with human serum albumin: impact on drug stability. J. Med. Chem. **37:** 40–46.
15. LIEHR, J.G., A.A. AHMED & B. GIOVANELLA. 1996. Pharmacokinetics of camptothecins administered orally. In The Camptothecins: From Discovery to the Patient. Ann. N.Y. Acad. Sci. **803:** 157–163.
16. BURKE, T.G. & Z. MI. 1993. Preferential binding of the carboxylate form of camptothecin by human serum albumin. Anal. Biochem. **212:** 285–287.
17. CAO, Z., N. HARRIS, A. KOZIELSKI, et al. 1998. Alkyl esters of camptothecin and 9-nitroCamptothecin: synthesis, in vitro pharmacokinetics, toxicity, and antitumor activity. J. Med. Chem. **41:** 31–37.
18. GIOVANELLA, B.C., J.S. STEHLIN, M.E. WALL, et al. 1989. DNA topoisomerase I-targeted chemotherapy of human colon cancer in xenografts. Science **246:** 1046–1048.
19. SATOH, T. & M. HOSOKAWA. 1998. The mammalian carboxylesterases: from molecules to functions. In Annual Revue of Pharmacology and Toxicology. A.K. Cho, T.F. Blaschke, I.K. Ho & H.H. Loh, Eds.: 257–288. Annual Reviews. Palo Alto, CA.

The Clinical Development of 9-Aminocamptothecin

CHRIS H. TAKIMOTO[a] AND REBECCA THOMAS

Developmental Therapeutics Department, Medicine Branch, Division of Clinical Sciences, National Cancer Institute, Bethesda, Maryland 20889, USA

ABSTRACT: 9-Aminocamptothecin (9-AC) is a topoisomerase I–targeting agent first synthesized by Wani and Wall in 1986. Because of its potent *in vitro* effects and promising preclinical activity in colorectal cancer animal models, it was designated a high-priority compound for further drug development by the NCI. In 1993, 9-AC first entered clinical trials as a 72-hour intravenous (i.v.) infusion. Predictable myelosuppression was the major dose-limiting toxicity, and pharmacokinetic studies showed a relatively short plasma half-life and unstable lactone ring. Unfortunately, phase II studies using this schedule showed minimal or no activity in tumors such as colorectal and lung cancer. Modest activity was observed in ovarian cancer and in refractory lymphomas. Efforts to improve systemic drug exposure by utilizing alternative schedules of administration of 9-AC such as prolonged, continuous intravenous infusions have also been tested. However, phase II studies of 120-hour weekly infusions of 9-AC have not shown improved activity against solid tumors such as colorectal cancer. More recently, a daily times 5 days i.v. administration schedule has been tested. Currently, further development of intravenously administered 9-AC for the treatment of colorectal cancer is not promising. Thus, topotecan and irinotecan remain the only two successfully developed topoisomerase I–targeting drugs in the United States. This experience with 9-AC raises important questions regarding how to best select new topoisomerase I–targeting drugs for future clinical development.

INTRODUCTION

9-Aminocamptothecin (9-AC) is a water-insoluble camptothecin derivative that was first synthesized in 1986 by Wani and Wall (TABLE 1).[1] *In vitro* studies demonstrated that 9-AC was a highly active inhibitor of topoisomerase I enzyme activity with greater potency than topotecan or irinotecan.[2] In structure–activity studies, the ability of 9-AC to interfere with DNA topoisomerase I–mediated DNA cleavage was strongly correlated with its *in vivo* antitumor activity against murine L1210 lymphoblastic leukemia.[3,4] The antitumor activity of 9-AC was investigated further against a variety of human tumor xenografts in immunodeficient nude mice. When administered to mice as a subcutaneous suspension in Tween 80, 9-AC induced impressive durable complete responses, even in advanced bulky tumors.[5,6] In three human colon

---

[a]Address for correspondence: Chris H. Takimoto, M.D., Ph.D., Department of Medicine, Division of Medical Oncology, University of Texas Health Science Center at San Antonio, 7703 Floyd Curl Drive, MSC 7884, San Antonio, TX 78229. Voice: 210-567-4777; fax: 210-567-6687.
takimotoc@oncology.uthscsa.edu

TABLE 1. 9-Aminocamptothecin (9-AC) clinical development history

1986	Total synthesis of 9-AC by Drs. Wani and Wall.
1989	National Cancer Institute Decision Network selects 9-AC for high-priority clinical development.
1992	Suitable clinical formulation of 9-AC in dimethylacetamide developed.
1993	First Phase I trials of 9-AC infusion initiated.
1994	Cooperative research and development agreement (CRADA) signed between National Cancer Institute and Pharmacia & Upjohn.
1995	First Phase II trials of 9-AC initiated.
1997	United States marketing rights for 9-AC transferred to IDEC Pharmaceutical Corporation.
1999	IDEC terminates clinical development of 9-AC.

cancer xenografts, 9-AC was highly active with minimal systemic toxicity and produced the best antitumor responses compared to a panel of nine anticancer agents that included 5-fluorouracil, doxorubicin, melphalan, methotrexate, vincristine, vinblastine, and several nitrosourea compounds.[5] Additional activity against human tumor xenografts have been reported in malignant melanoma,[7] acute leukemia,[8] prostate,[9] breast,[10] ovarian,[11] and bladder cancers,[12] as well as in a central nervous system metastatic tumor model.[6]

In preclinical toxicology studies, the major dose-limiting toxicities were myelosuppression (predominantly neutropenia) and gastrointestinal toxicity. Animal pharmacokinetic studies performed in combination with these experiments were particularly revealing.[13] Intravenous injections of 9-AC that resulted in high peak plasma concentrations and rapid drug clearance were ineffective against human xenograft tumors, but still generated lethal toxicity. In contrast, subcutaneous injections of 9-AC suspensions that resulted in lower, more prolonged plasma concentrations of 9-AC lactone in the nanomolar range were associated with optimal antitumor efficacy and with minimal systemic toxicities.[13]

CLINICAL STUDIES

Because of this impressive preclinical activity, the National Cancer Institute selected 9-AC as a high-priority compound for further clinical development in 1989. Nevertheless, testing in humans was delayed by difficulties in formulating 9-AC in a vehicle suitable for intravenous administration. In 1993, a clinical formulation of 9-AC in dimethylacetamide (DMA) plus polyethylene glycol and phosphoric acid was developed for use in the initial phase I trials. More recently, Pharmacia & Upjohn has developed a newer colloidal formulation of 9-AC complexed with dimyristoylphosphatidylcholine and dimyristoylphosphatidylglycerol that is stable in standard intravenous solutions. This colloidal dispersion (CD) formulation has been used in more recent clinical trials.

TABLE 2. Phase I trials of 9-AC

Regimen and recommended Phase II doses	Dose-limiting toxicities	Drug formulation	Reference
0.84 mg/m²/d i.v. × 72 hr every 2 weeks, or	Neutropenia	DMA	14
1.13 mg/m²/d i.v. × 72 hr every 2 weeks with G-CSF	Neutropenia Some thrombocytopenia		
1.08 mg/m²/d i.v. × 72 hr every 3 weeks	Neutropenia Some thrombocytopenia	DMA	15
1.3 mg/m²/d i.v. × 72 hr every 3 weeks	Neutropenia	CD	16
0.48 mg/m²/d i.v. × 120 hr weekly for 3 of every 4 weeks	Neutropenia Diarrhea	DMA	17
0.60 mg/m²/d i.v. × 120 hr weekly for 2 of every 3 weeks	Neutropenia	DMA	
1.65 mg/m² i.v. over 24 hr weekly for 4 of every 5 weeks	Neutropenia	CD	18
1.1 mg/m²/d i.v. over 30 min daily × 5 days every 3 weeks	Neutropenia	CD	57
No recommended oral dose daily × 5 every 2 weeks	No dose-limiting toxicity determined	CD	22
1.1 mg/m²/d orally daily × 14 days every 3 weeks	Thrombocytopenia Neutropenia	PEG 1000	23
Special populations			
Pediatric solid tumors 1.25 mg/m²/d i.v. × 72 hr every 3 weeks	Neutropenia Thrombocytopenia	DMA	20
Acute leukemia 1.4 mg/m²/d c.i.v. over 7 days	Mucositis	CD	21

ABBREVIATIONS: i.v., intravenous; c.i.v., continuous intravenous infusion; DMA, dimethylacetamide formulation; CD, colloidal dispersion formulation; PEG 1000, polyethylene glycol 1000.

Phase I Studies

The initial phase I clinical trials of 9-AC used the DMA formulation administered as a 72-hr infusion every two[14] or three weeks (TABLE 2).[15,16] This schedule was selected because of the preclinical studies demonstrating that prolonged drug exposures were needed to see biologic effects.[5] In both of these studies, the major dose-limiting toxicity was neutropenia, with thrombocytopenia seen to a lesser extent. Other common toxicities included anemia, fatigue, nausea and vomiting, diarrhea, alopecia, and mucositis. 9-AC was not associated with pulmonary toxicity or hemorrhagic cystitis, and the diarrhea was much less severe than that seen with irinotecan. The recommended phase II dose on the every 2-week schedule was 0.84 mg/m^2 per day (35 µg/m^2 per hr) infused continuously over 72 hr without G-CSF; with G-CSF support, the dose could be increased to 1.13 mg/m^2 per day (47 µg/m^2 per hr).[14] On the every 3-week schedule, 1.08 mg/m^2 per day (45 µg/m^2 per hr) over 72 hr was well tolerated without the need for colony-stimulating factors.[15] No objective responses were seen in the 79 patients entered in both studies. More recently, other schedules of intravenous 9-AC administration have been developed, including a prolonged 120-hr infusion weekly,[17] a 24-hr infusion weekly for 4 of 5 weeks,[18] or a short intravenous infusion daily for 5 days every 3 weeks (TABLE 2).[19] On all of these schedules, the principal dose-limiting toxicity was myelosuppression, although gastrointestinal toxicities such as diarrhea were also observed in some of the prolonged infusion schedules.[17] For the daily times 5 schedule of 9-AC, the recommended phase II dose of 9-AC was 1.1 mg/m^2 per day infused over 15 min daily every 3 weeks.[19] Neutropenia and thrombocytopenia were dose limiting. Phase I trials in pediatric patients[20] and acute leukemia patients[21] have also been completed (TABLE 2). Oral formulations of 9-AC have also been developed and studied clinically. Mani *et al.* performed a phase I trial of orally administered 9-AC over a dose range of 0.2 to 0.68 mg/m^2 per day using the CD formulation.[22] This study was terminated because of wide interpatient variability in the plasma area-under-the-curve (AUC) without determining a recommended phase II dose. In another study, de Jonge and colleagues had better success using a polyethylene glycol (PEG) 1000 formulation of 9-AC in capsules administered over a dose range of 0.25 to 1.5 mg/m^2 per day for 7 or 14 days every 3 weeks.[23] The recommended phase II dose was 1.1 mg/m^2 per day daily for 14 days with neutropenia and thrombocytopenia being dose limiting. The oral bioavailability of these 9-AC PEG 1000 capsules was 48 ± 17.6%.[24]

Clinical Pharmacology

The pharmacokinetics of 9-AC have predominantly been studied in conjunction with phase I trials of this agent. Similar to most camptothecins, 9-AC contains a terminal lactone ring that is easily hydrolyzed by a rapid nonenzymatic chemical hydrolysis to form the more water soluble but less active hydroxy carboxylic acid species. At neutral and basic pH, the equilibrium for this hydrolysis very much favors the inactive carboxylate species. The pharmacokinetics of 9-AC have been examined using analytic assays that can measure both the lactone and carboxylate forms of the drug.[25-27] In pharmacokinetic studies, the amount of 9-AC that is present in plasma relative to the total drug (lactone + carboxylate) is quite low, with reported values ranging from 8% to 16% (TABLE 3).[18,20,24,28] This is consistent with earlier studies demonstrating greater instability of 9-AC lactone in human plasma compared with other camptothecin derivatives such as topotecan or irinotecan.[29] Other pharmacokinetic parameters for 9-AC lactone include a terminal elimination half-life commonly ranging from 4.5 to 10 hr,[18-21,28] a volume of distribution at steady state ranging from 58 to 325 l/m^2,[18-21,28] and a systemic clearance ranging from 11.3 to 55 l/(hr · m^2).[18-21,28] Urinary clearance accounts for 8.6 to 32.1% of the total dose administered.[19,28] As with other camptothecin derivatives, interpatient variability in plasma pharmacokinetics is quite high (TABLE 2). Preliminary reports suggest that patients receiving anticonvulsant medications may have increased clearance and lower plasma drug levels of 9-AC.[30] This may be due to increased meta-

TABLE 3. 9-AC pharmacokinetics[a]

Dose and schedule	Formulation	Compound	Terminal half-life (hr)	Volume of distribution at steady-state (l/m²)	CL (l/hr/m²)	Urinary excretion (%)	Percent lactone in plasma (%)	Reference
0.12–1.8 mg/m²/d i.v. over 72 hr	DMA	Lactone	4.47 ± 0.53	195 ± 114	24.5 ± 7.3	—	8.7 ± 4.7	28
		Total	8.38 ± 2.1	23.6 ± 10.6	—	32.1 ± 8.3 over 24 hr	—	
1.08 mg/m²/d i.v. over 72 hr	DMA	Lactone	42.2 ± 34.4	12.6 ± 3.6	55.2 ± 18.0	—	—	15
0.86–1.49 mg/m²/d i.v. over 72 hr[b]	DMA	Lactone	7.1 ± 3.5	135.3 ± 52.5	—	—	10.8 ± 3.6	20
		Total	8.1 ± 3.8	21.2 ± 13.3	—	—	—	
0.7–1.9 mg/m²/d i.v. over 24 hr	CD	Lactone	10.7 ± 6.71	111.0 ± 72.3	18.0 ± 9.0	—	7.99	18
0.9–1.55 mg/m²/d i.v. over 72 hr	CD	Lactone	22.5 ± 8.5	325 ± 145	30.3 ± 4.5	—	—	16
0.45–1.4 mg/m²/d c.i.v. over 7 days	CD	Lactone	4.3 ± 2.7	58.4 ± 23.3	11.3 ± 4.9	—	—	21
0.4–1.3 mg/m²/d i.v. over 15 min	CD	Lactone	7.0 ± 3.4	89 ± 69	15.7 ± 9.2	—	16 ± 6	19
		Total	7.7 ± 4.6	17.7 ± 6.0	2.36 ± 1.24	8.6 ± 4.0	—	

ABBREVIATIONS: i.v, intravenous; CIV, continuous intravenous infusion; DMA, dimethylacetamide formulation; CD, colloidal dispersion formulation.
[a]Values are means ± SD unless otherwise stated.
[b]Pediatric patients.

bolic clearance of 9-AC in patients receiving hepatic enzyme-inducing antiepileptic agents, such as phenytoin, carbamazepine, phenobarbital, primidone, felbamate, and valproic acid. However, hepatic metabolites of 9-AC have not been identified.[31] An alternative explanation may be the induction of transport proteins by these same agents that could lead to increased 9-AC clearance and biliary secretion in these patients.[32] In pharmacodynamic studies, 9-AC steady-state plasma concentrations[28,32] and AUC[18,19,33] correlated with the dose-limiting toxicity of neutropenia.

Phase II Studies

In phase II studies, 16 previously treated patients with metastatic colorectal cancer were treated with 72-hr infusions of 9-AC administered at 1.2–1.4 mg/m^2 per day for 72 hours every 2 weeks; however, no responses were observed, and the myelosuppressive toxicity was substantial (TABLE 4).[34] Grade 4 neutropenia occurred in 56% of patients and febrile neutropenia occurred in 31%. In another trial, 17 previously untreated patients with advanced colorectal cancer were treated with a lower dose of 9-AC 0.84 mg/m^2 per day for 72 hours every 2 weeks, but again, no responses were observed.[35] Clinical activity has been observed in recurrent and refractory ovarian cancer using the 72-hour infusion schedule. In two studies of 28 and 38 patients with platinum-treated ovarian cancer, the response rates were 21% and 19%, respectively.[36,37] Responses have also been observed in relapsed or refractory lymphoma following the administration of 9-AC at 0.96 mg/m^2 per day over 72 hours every 3 weeks with G-CSF support.[38] In 40 evaluable lymphoma patients, the partial response rate was 25% (95%CI 13–41%) with a median duration of response of 5 months (range 1–10) and a median survival time of 12.5 months. Objective responses rates of 3% to 13% have also been reported in central nervous system tumors, non-small cell lung cancer, and in breast cancer (TABLE 4).

Because preclinical studies suggest that low prolonged exposures to 9-AC are important for both antitumor efficacy and for minimizing toxicity, several prolonged infusion schedules of 9-AC have also been tested. The phase II results are just now becoming available (TABLE 4). When 9-AC was examined as a 120-hour infusion at 0.48 mg/m^2 per day (20 µg/m^2 per hr) for 120 hr every week for 3 of 4 weeks in 17 previously untreated patients with metastatic colorectal cancer, there were no responses.[39] Thus, although antitumor activity for 9-AC has been observed in ovarian cancer and refractory lymphoma, the activity of this agent in advanced colorectal cancer has been disappointing. Phase II results from the prolonged infusion in other tumors and for the daily times 5 schedule are still pending.

FURTHER CLINICAL DEVELOPMENT AND UNANSWERED QUESTIONS

In 1997, the Pharmacia & Upjohn Company transferred the development rights for 9-AC to IDEC Pharmaceuticals Corporation. Later in that same year, phase II testing of 9-AC using 1.1 mg/m^2 on an intravenous daily times 5 schedule was initiated. Results from these studies will be reported later this year. However, in a recent filing with the U.S. Securities and Exchange Commission, IDEC Pharmaceuticals notified the U.S. government that it was halting the development of 9-AC based on

TABLE 4. Phase II trials of 9-aminocamptothecin

Disease	Dose and schedule	No. entered/evaluable patients	Patients with prior chemotherapy	Overall response rate (%)	Response type	Median duration of response (months)	Median duration of survival (months)	Reference
Colorectal cancer	1.42 mg/m^2/d i.v. over 72 hr every 2 weeks with G-CSF	16/14	16	0 (95% CI 0–20)	0 PR	NA	9.5 (95% CI 7.3–12.9)	34
Colorectal cancer	0.84 mg/m^2/d i.v. over 72 hr every 2 weeks	17/17	0 for advanced disease 7 received adjuvant therapy	0	0 PR	NA	NA	35
Colorectal cancer	0.48 mg/m^2/d i.v. over 120 hr weekly for 3 of 4 weeks	18/17	0 for advanced disease 5 received adjuvant therapy	0	0 PR	NA	8 (range 0.75–14.5)	39
Ovarian cancer	0.84–1.13 mg/m^2/d i.v. over 72 hr every 2 weeks with G-CSF	28/28	28	21	6 PR	NA	NA	36
Ovarian cancer	0.84 mg/m^2/d i.v. over 72 hr every 2 weeks	46/38	46	19 (95% CI 6–38)	5 PR	NA	NA	37
Refractory Hodgkin's and non-Hodgkin's lymphoma	0.96 mg/m^2/d i.v. over 72 hr every 3 weeks with and without G-CSF	45/40	45	25 (95% CI 13–41)	10 PR	5 (range 1–10)	12.5	38
Breast cancer	1.1 mg/m^2/d i.v. over 72 hr every 2 weeks with G-CSF	18/15	18	13	2 PR	3.5–5	NA	58
Non-small cell lung cancer	1.42 mg/m^2/d i.v. over 72 hr every 2 weeks with G-CSF	58/54	0	8.6 (95% CI 2.9–19)	5 PR	2.25–7.0	5.4	59
Central nervous system tumors	0.85–1.78 mg/m^2/d i.v. over 72 hr every 2 weeks	99/39	NA	3	1 PR	NA	NA	60
Head and neck cancer	0.85–1.0 mg/m^2/d i.v. over 72 hr every 2 weeks	14/14	0	0	0 PR	NA	6 (1–9+)	61

ABBREVIATIONS: i.v., intravenous; CR, complete response; PR, partial response; CI, confidence interval; NA, data not available; G-CSF, granulocyte-colony-stimulating factor.

preliminary results from its phase II studies.[40] Thus, by any measure of effectiveness, the phase II data of antitumor activity of 9-AC has been disappointing, with only modest response rates reported in ovarian cancer and lymphoma. Of particular note is the lack of meaningful activity in advanced colorectal cancer, despite the impressive preclinical activity in human colon cancer xenograft models. One potential explanation for this discrepancy may be the inability to achieve the necessary plasma drug concentrations needed for antitumor efficacy. Because of the greater sensitivity of human bone marrow stem cells to 9-AC compared with murine bone marrow, dose-limiting myelosuppression makes it impossible to safely achieve the same plasma drug concentrations in humans that were associated with optimal antitumor efficacy in the mouse xenograft studies.[41]

For those interested in the clinical development of topoisomerase I targeting agents specifically, and cancer chemotherapy drug development in general, a key unanswered question is why has 9-AC been so much less clinically useful than its close camptothecin relatives, topotecan and irinotecan? This question is particularly vexing given the impressive preclinical activity of 9-AC.[5] At least three major reasons may explain some of the marked differences observed between the various camptothecin derivatives in clinical testing: (1) pharmacokinetic differences, (2) differences in molecular pharmacology, and (3) differences in clinically relevant resistance mechanisms.

Major pharmacokinetic differences exist between the various camptothecins (TABLE 5). For example, 9-AC is much less water soluble than topotecan or irinotecan, a property that initially delayed its clinical development. In addition, the amount of drug in plasma present in the active lactone form varies for the different analogues (TABLE 5), with the highest levels seen with SN-38 (51–64%)[42] and the lowest with 9-AC (9%).[28] This is largely due to the high plasma protein binding affinity of the open ring 9-AC carboxylate, which tends to shift the equilibrium away from the active lactone. In contrast, the protein binding of topotecan is much less; and for SN-38, the active metabolite of irinotecan, plasma protein binding effects tend to favor the stability of the active closed-ring lactone.[43] The clinical impact of this equilibrium has not been precisely characterized. The hydrolysis of 9-AC lactone to carboxylate is a reversible reaction; therefore, low lactone levels could theoretically be compensated for by higher total drug concentrations. However, higher total drug concentrations may potentially contribute to drug toxicity. Additional studies are needed to clarify these issues. Finally, the apparent half-life of irinotecan's active metabolite, SN-38, is longer than other analogues (TABLE 5), which may help to explain why irinotecan is active as a short infusion given every 3 weeks.

Differences also exist between the camptothecins at the molecular level. For example, SN-38 is a more potent inhibitor of topoisomerase I and can generate cleavable complexes in colon cancer cells that are more stable than those produced by topotecan or 9-AC.[44] The exact clinical significance of these differences must still be determined, but these factors may become increasingly important as we gain a better understanding of the determinants of tumor responsiveness to camptothecin therapy.

Finally, very little is known about clinically relevant resistance mechanisms and the camptothecins. For example, the role of the P-glycoprotein-associated multidrug resistance (MDR) phenotype in camptothecin resistance has not been clearly de-

TABLE 5. Comparative pharmacokinetics of 9-aminocamptothecin, topotecan, and irinotecan

Drug	Schedule	C_{max} (nM)	Half-life (hr)	Percent lactone in plasma (%)	Reference
9-AC	0.12–1.8 mg/m^2/d i.v. over 72 hr	3–10	4.5 ± 0.5	8.7 ± 4.7	28
Topotecan	0.5–2.5 mg/m^2 i.v. over 30 min	21–82	3.01 ± 0.54	16–20	62
CPT-11 (SN-38)	50–345 mg/m^2 i.v. over 90 min	21–89	11 ± 3.8	51 ± 3	63, 64

ABBREVIATIONS: 9-AC, 9-aminocamptothecin; CPT-11, irinotecan; i.v., intravenous; C_{max}, maximal plasma concentration.

fined, but differences between the various camptothecins have been observed. Irinotecan and SN-38 do not appear to be substrates for the MDR drug efflux pump,[45] and cross resistance to irinotecan is not seen in P388 leukemia cells expressing pleotropic drug resistance to vincristine and doxorubicin.[46] In recent comparison studies, MDR-expressing sublines were ninefold more resistant to topotecan and twofold more resistant to 9-AC compared with parental wild-type cells.[47] No increase in resistance to camptothecin or 10,11-methylenedioxycamptothecin was observed. While other investigators have confirmed these findings for topotecan, this degree of MDR-associated resistance is much less than the 200-fold change in sensitivity typically described for classic MDR substrates, such as doxorubicin or etoposide.[48–50] Topotecan may also be a substrate for other transport systems, such as the multidrug resistance-associated protein (MRP),[51] but the clinical relevance of all these studies are still uncertain. In human colon cancer xenografts that highly express MDR, irinotecan was still quite effective, even against a cell line resistant to topotecan.[52] These data suggest that different mechanisms of camptothecin resistance may be specific for certain camptothecin analogues. Further characterization of these specific mechanisms of resistance are required.

Novel mechanisms of transport resistance may also be important for the camptothecin derivatives. Transport-related cross resistance between mitoxantrone and a number of different camptothecins, including topotecan, SN-38, and 9-AC was observed in two different cell lines[53,54] The mitoxantrone resistant breast cancer cell line was 101-fold cross resistant to SN-38, and also showed decreased intracellular drug accumulation that was not related to the expression of P-glycoprotein or MRP. However, a novel new mitoxantrone transporter was recently characterized in these cells that may be responsible for camptothecin resistance.[55,56] The extent to which this newly identified protein alters camptothecin uptake and efflux must still be determined, but it represents another potentially important mechanism of camptothecin drug resistance in malignant cells.

In many respects, 9-AC more closely resembles topotecan than irinotecan. It is not a prodrug, it is directly active on topoisomerase I, and it is a weak MDR substrate with a relatively short half-life. Furthermore, it has some activity in ovarian cancer, and its clinical dose-limiting toxicity is myelosuppression. Given the growing number of new anticancer agents under development, however, it is unlikely that similar activity in the absence of a distinct advantage in efficacy or safety is enough justification for the further clinical development of a new camptothecin topoisomerase I-targeting agent.

CONCLUSIONS

Although the clinical development of 9-AC continues, the bright promise of this agent that was highlighted by the pioneering studies published by Giovanella and colleagues in *Science* in 1989[5] has not been sustained by recent clinical trial results. Final judgment regarding the fate of 9-AC must await the results of the phase II trials of prolonged infusions and daily times 5 administration schedules that are not yet fully available. However, this experience raises a key question for the development of new camptothecin analogues. Specifically, what are the major drug characteristics important for selecting new topoisomerase I targeting agents for further clinical development? The answer to this difficult but essential question lies in improving our knowledge of how these agents function at the molecular level, identifying the key determinants of clinical antitumor responsiveness, defining the important differences in their clinical pharmacology, and understanding the clinically relevant mechanisms of camptothecin drug resistance.

REFERENCES

1. WANI, M.C., A.W. NICHOLAS & M.E. WALL. Plant antitumor agents. 23. Synthesis and antileukemic activity of camptothecin analogues. J. Med. Chem. **29:** 2358–2363.
2. KINGSBURY, W.D., J.C. BOEHM, D.R. JAKAS, *et al.* 1991. Synthesis of water-soluble (aminoalkyl)camptothecin analogues: inhibition of topoisomerase I and antitumor activity. J. Med. Chem. **34:** 98–107.
3. JAXEL, C., K.W. KOHN, M.C. WANI, *et al.* 1989. Structure–activity study of the actions of camptothecin derivatives on mammalian topoisomerase I: evidence for a specific receptor site and a relation to antitumor activity. Cancer Res. **49:** 1465–1469.
4. HSIANG, Y.H., L.F. LIU, M.E. WALL, *et al.* 1989. DNA topoisomerase I-mediated DNA cleavage and cytotoxicity of camptothecin analogues. Cancer Res. **49:** 4385–4389.
5. GIOVANELLA, B.C., J.S. STEHLIN, M.E. WALL, *et al.* 1989. DNA topoisomerase I–targeted chemotherapy of human colon cancer in xenografts. Science **246:** 1046–1048.
6. POTMESIL, M., D. VARDEMAN, A.J. KOZIELSKI, *et al.* 1995. Growth inhibition of human cancer metastases by camptothecins in newly developed xenograft models. Cancer Res. **55:** 5637–5641.
7. PANTAZIS, P., H.R. HINZ, J.T. MENDOZA, *et al.* 1992. Complete inhibition of growth followed by death of human malignant melanoma cells in vitro and regression of human melanoma xenografts in immunodeficient mice induced by camptothecins. Cancer Res. **52:** 3980–3987.
8. JEHA, S., H. KANTARJIAN, S. O'BRIEN, *et al.* 1998. Activity of oral and intravenous 9-aminocamptothecin in SCID mice engrafted with human leukemia. Leuk. Lymphoma **32:** 159–164.
9. DE SOUSA, P.L., M.R. COOPER, A.R. IMONDI & C.E. MYERS. 1997. 9-Aminocamptothecin: a topoisomerase I inhibitor with preclinical activity in prostate cancer. Clin. Cancer Res. **3(2):** 287–294.
10. PANTAZIS, P., A.J. KOZIELSKI, D.M. VARDEMAN, *et al.* 1993. Efficacy of camptothecin congeners in the treatment of human breast carcinoma xenografts. Oncol. Res. **5:** 273–281.

11. PANTAZIS, P., A.J. KOZIELSKI, J.T. MENDOZA, et al. 1993. Camptothecin derivatives induce regression of human ovarian carcinomas grown in nude mice and distinguish between non-tumorigenic and tumorigenic cells in vitro. Int. J. Cancer **53:** 863–871.
12. KEANE, T.E., R.E. EL-GALLEY, C. SUN, et al. 1998. Camptothecin analogues/cisplatin: an effective treatment of advanced bladder cancer in a preclinical in vivo model system. J. Urol. **160:** 252–256.
13. POTMESIL, M., S.G. ARBUCK, C.H. TAKIMOTO, et al. 1996. 9-Aminocamptothecin and beyond. Preclinical and clinical studies. Ann. N.Y. Acad. Sci. **803:** 231–246.
14. DAHUT, W., N. HAROLD, C. TAKIMOTO, et al. 196. Phase I and pharmacologic study of 9-aminocamptothecin given by 72-hour infusion in adult cancer patients. J. Clin. Oncol. **14:** 1236–1244.
15. RUBIN, E., V. WOOD, A. BHARTI, et al. 1995. A phase I and pharmacokinetic study of a new camptothecin derivative, 9-aminocamptothecin. Clin. Cancer Res. **1:** 269–276.
16. EDER, J.P., JR., J.G. SUPKO, T. LYNCH, et al. 1998. Phase I trial of the colloidal dispersion formulation of 9-amino-20(S)-camptothecin administered as a 72-hour continuous intravenous infusion. Clin. Cancer Res. **4:** 317–324.
17. TAKIMOTO, C., W. DAHUT, H. HAROLD, et al. 1996. A phase I trial of a prolonged infusion of 9-aminocamptothecin (9-AC) in adult patients with solid tumors. Proc. Am. Soc. Clin. Oncol. **14:** 471.
18. SIU, L.L., A.M. OZA, E.A. EISENHAUER, et al. 1998. Phase I and pharmacologic study of 9-aminocamptothecin colloidal dispersion formulation given as a 24-hour continuous infusion weekly times four every 5 weeks. J. Clin. Oncol. **16:** 1122–1130.
19. HERBEN, V.M.M., R. VAN GIJN, J.H.M. SCHELLENS, et al. 1999. Phase I and pharmacokientic study of a daily times 5 short intravenous infusion schedule of 9-aminocamptothecin in a colloidal dispersion formulation in patients with advanced solid tumors. J. Clin. Oncol. **17:** 1906–1914.
20. LANGEVIN, A.M., D.T. CASTO, P.J. THOMAS, et al. 1998. Phase I trial of 9-aminocamptothecin in children with refractory solid tumors: a Pediatric Oncology Group study. J. Clin. Oncol. **16:** 2494–2499.
21. VEY, N., H. KANTARJIAN, H. TRAN, et al. 1999. Phase I and pharmacologic study of 9-aminocamptothecin colloidal dispersion formulation in patients with refractory or relapsed acute leukemia. Ann. Oncol. **10:** 577–583.
22. MANI, S., L. IYER, L. JANISCH, et al. 1998. Phase I clinical and pharmacokinetic study of oral 9-aminocamptothecin (NSC-603071). Cancer Chemother. Pharmacol. **42:** 84–87.
23. DE JONGE, M.J., C.J. PUNT, A.H. GELDERBLOM, et al. 1999. Phase I and pharmacologic study of oral (PEG-1000) 9-aminocamptothecin in adult patients with solid tumors. J Clin. Oncol. **17:** 2219.
24. SPARREBOOM, A., M.J. DE JONGE, C.J. PUNT, et al. 1998. Pharmacokinetics and bioavailability of oral 9-aminocamptothecin capsules in adult patients with solid tumors. Clin. Cancer Res. **4:** 1915–1919.
25. TAKIMOTO, C.H., R.W. KLECKER, W.L. DAHUT, et al. 1994. Analysis of the active lactone form of 9-aminocamptothecin in plasma using solid-phase extraction and high-performance liquid chromatography. J. Chromatogr. B Biomed. Appl. **655:** 97–104.
26. VAN GIJN, R., V.M. HERBEN, M.J. HILLEBRAND, et al. 1998. High-performance liquid chromatographic analysis of the investigational anticancer drug 9-aminocamptothecin, as the lactone form and as the total of the lactone and the hydroxycarboxylate forms, in micro-volumes of human plasma. J. Pharmacol. Biomed. Anal. **17:** 1257–1265.
27. LOOS, W.J., A. SPARREBOOM, J. VERWEIJ, et al. 1997. Determination of the lactone and lactone plus carboxylate forms of 9-aminocamptothecin in human plasma by sensitive high-performance liquid chromatography with fluorescence detection. J. Chromatogr. B Biomed. Sci. Appl. **694:** 435–441.
28. TAKIMOTO, C.H., W. DAHUT, M.T. MARINO, et al. 1997. Pharmacodynamics and pharmacokinetics of a 72-hour infusion of 9-aminocamptothecin in adult cancer patients. J. Clin. Oncol. **15:** 1492–501.
29. MI, Z., H. MALAK & T.G. BURKE. 1995. Reduced albumin binding promotes the stability and activity of topotecan in human blood. Biochemistry **34:** 13722–13728.

30. GROSSMAN, S.A., F. HOCHBERG, J. FISHER, et al. 1998. Increased 9-aminocamptothecin dose requirements in patients on anticonvulsants. NABTT CNS Consortium. The New Approaches to Brain Tumor Therapy. Cancer Chemother. Pharmacol. **42:** 118–26.
31. TAKIMOTO, C.H., W. DAHUT, N. HAROLD, et al. 1996. Clinical pharmacology of 9-aminocamptothecin. Ann. N.Y. Acad. Sci. **803:** 324–326.
32. MINAMI, H., T.E. LAD, M.K. NICHOLAS, et al. 1999. Pharmacokinetics and pharmacodynamics of 9-aminocamptothecin infused over 72 hours in phase II studies. Clin. Cancer Res. **5:** 1325–1330.
33. DE JONGE, M.J., J. VERWEIJ, W.J. LOOS, et al. 1999. Clinical pharmacokinetics of encapsulated oral 9-aminocamptothecin in plasma and saliva. Clin. Pharmacol. Ther. **65:** 491–499.
34. SALTZ, L.B., N.E. KEMENY, W. TONG, et al. 1997. 9-Aminocamptothecin by 72-hour continuous intravenous infusion is inactive in the treatment of patients with 5-fluorouracil-refractory colorectal carcinoma. Cancer **80:** 1727–1732.
35. PAZDUR, R., E. DIAZ-CANTON, W.P. BALLARD, et al. 1997. Phase II trial of 9-aminocamptothecin administered as a 72-hour continuous infusion in metastatic colorectal carcinoma. J. Clin. Oncol. **15:** 2905–2909.
36. MCCARTHY, N., G. SAROSY, L. MINASIAN, et al. 1999. Phase II and pharmacokinetic (PK) study of 9-aminocamptothecin (9AC) in recurrent epithelial ovarian cancer. Proc. Am. Soc. Clin. Oncol. **18:** 363a.
37. SPEYER, J., H. HOCHSTER, J. MANDELI, et al. 1999. Phase II study of 72 hr 9-aminocamptothecin (9AC) infusion in second-line therapy of ovarian cancer (a NYGOG and ECOG study). Proc. Am. Soc. Clin. Oncol. **18:** 363a.
38. WILSON, W.H., R. LITTLE, D. PEARSON, et al. 1998. Phase II and dose-escalation with or without granulocyte colony-stimulating factor study of 9-aminocamptothecin in relapsed and refractory lymphomas [published erratum appears in J. Clin. Oncol. 1998 Aug; 16(8): 2895]. J. Clin. Oncol. **16:** 2345–2351.
39. PAZDUR, R., D.C. MEDGYESY, R.J. WINN, et al. 1998. Phase II trial of 9-aminocamptothecin (NSC 603071) administered as a 120-hr continuous infusion weekly for three weeks in metastatic colorectal carcinoma. Invest. New Drugs **16:** 341–346.
40. IDEC PHARMACEUTICALS CORPORATION. 1999. Letter to Stockholders, July 22. San Diego, CA.
41. ERICKSON-MILLER, C.L., R.D. MAY, J. TOMASZEWSKI, et al. 1997. Differential toxicity of camptothecin, topotecan and 9-aminocamptothecin to human, canine, and murine myeloid progenitors (CFU-GM) in vitro. Cancer Chemother. Pharmacol. **39:** 467–472.
42. RIVORY, L.P., E. CHATELUT, P. CANAL, et al. 1994. Kinetics of the in vivo interconversion of the carboxylate and lactone forms of irinotecan (CPT-11) and of its metabolite SN-38 in patients. Cancer Res. **54:** 6330–5333.
43. BURKE, T.G. & Z. MI. 1994. The structural basis of camptothecin interactions with human serum albumin: impact on drug stability. J. Med. Chem. **37:** 40–46.
44. TANIZAWA, A., A. FUJIMORI, Y. FUJIMORI & Y. POMMIER. 1994. Comparison of topoisomerase I inhibition, DNA damage, and cytotoxicity of camptothecin derivatives presently in clinical trials. J. Natl. Cancer Inst. **86:** 836–842.
45. JANSEN, W.J., T.M. HULSCHER, J. VAN ARK-OTTE, et al. 1998. CPT-11 sensitivity in relation to the expression of P170-glycoprotein and multidrug resistance-associated protein. Br. J. Cancer **77:** 359–365.
46. TSURUO, T., T. MATSUZAKI, M. MATSUSHITA, et al. 1988. Antitumor effect of CPT-11, a new derivative of camptothecin, against pleiotropic drug-resistant tumors in vitro and in vivo. Cancer Chemother. Pharmacol. **21:** 71–74.
47. CHEN, A.Y., C. YU, M. POTMESIL, et al. 1991. Camptothecin overcomes MDR1-mediated resistance in human KB carcinoma cells. Cancer Res. **51:** 6039–5044.
48. HENDRICKS, C.B., E.K. ROWINSKY, L.B. GROCHOW, et al. 1992. Effect of P-glycoprotein expression on the accumulation and cytotoxicity of topotecan (SK&F 104864), a new camptothecin analogue. Cancer Res. **52:** 2268–2278.
49. MATTERN, M.R., G.A. HOFMANN, R.M. POLSKY, et al. 1993. In vitro and in vivo effects of clinically important camptothecin analogues on multidrug-resistant cells. Oncol. Res. **5:** 467–474.

50. HOKI, Y., A. FUJIMORI & Y. POMMIER. 1997. Differential cytotoxicity of clinically important camptothecin derivatives in P-glycoprotein-overexpressing cell lines. Cancer Chemother. Pharmacol. **40:** 433–438.
51. JONSSON, E., H. FRIDBORG, K. CSOKA, et al. 1997. Cytotoxic activity of topotecan in human tumour cell lines and primary cultures of human tumour cells from patients. Br. J. Cancer **76:** 211–219.
52. HOUGHTON, P.J., P.J. CHESHIRE, J.C. HALLMAN, et al. 1993. Therapeutic efficacy of the topoisomerase I inhibitor 7-ethyl-10-(4-[1-piperidino]-1-piperidino)-carbonyloxy-camptothecin against human tumor xenografts: lack of cross-resistance in vivo in tumors with acquired resistance to the topoisomerase I inhibitor 9-dimethylaminomethyl-10-hydroxycamptothecin. Cancer Res. **53:** 2823–2829.
53. YANG, C.J., J.K. HORTON, K.H. COWAN & E. SCHNEIDER. 1995. Cross-resistance to camptothecin analogues in a mitoxantrone-resistant human breast carcinoma cell line is not due to DNA topoisomerase I alterations. Cancer Res. **55:** 4004–4009.
54. KELLNER, U., L. HUTCHINSON, A. SEIDEL, et al. 1997. Decreased drug accumulation in a mitoxantrone-resistant gastric carcinoma cell line in the absence of P-glycoprotein. Int. J. Cancer **71:** 817–824.
55. DOYLE, L.A., W. YANG, L.V. ABRUZZO, et al. 1998. A multidrug resistance transporter from human MCF-7 breast cancer cells. Proc. Natl. Acad. Sci. USA **95:** 15665–15670.
56. MIYAKE, K., L. MICKLEY, T. LITMAN, et al. 1999. Molecular cloning of cDNAs which are highly overexpressed in mitoxantrone-resistant cells: demonstration of homology to ABC transport genes. Cancer Res. **59:** 8–13.
57. HERBEN, V.M., R. VAN GIJN, J.H. SCHELLENS, et al. 1999. Phase I and pharmacokinetic study of a daily times 5 short intravenous infusion schedule of 9-aminocamptothecin in a colloidal dispersion formulation in patients with advanced solid tumors. J. Clin. Oncol. **17:** 1906–1914.
58. KRAUT, E.H., S.P. BALCERZAK, D. YOUNG, et al. 2000. A phase II study of 9-aminocamptothecin in patients with refractory breast cancer. Cancer Invest. **18:** 28–31.
59. VOKES, E.E., R.H. ANSARI, G.A. MASTERS, et al. 1998. A phase II study of 9-aminocamptothecin in advanced non-small-cell lung cancer [see comments]. Ann. Oncol. **9:** 1085–1090.
60. HOCHBERG, F., S.A. GROSSMAN, T. MIKKELSEN, et al. 1998. Efficacy of 9-aminocamptothecin (9-AC) in adults with newly diagnosed glioblastoma multiforme (GBM) and recurrent high grade astrocytomas. Proc. Am. Soc. Clin. Oncol. **17:** 388a.
61. LAD, T., F. ROSEN, R. ARIETTA, et al. 1998. Phase II trial of 9-aminocamptothecin (9AC/DMA) in patients with advanced squamous cell head and neck cancer. Proc. Am. Soc. Clin. Oncol. **17:** 392a.
62. ROWINSKY, E.K., L.B. GROCHOW, C.B. HENDRICKS, et al. 1992. Phase I and pharmacologic study of topotecan: a novel topoisomerase I inhibitor. J. Clin. Oncol. **10:** 647–656.
63. ROWINSKY, E.K., L.B. GROCHOW, D.S. ETTINGER, et al. 1994. Phase I and pharmacological study of the novel topoisomerase I inhibitor 7-ethyl-10-[4-(1-piperidino)-1-piperidino]carbonyloxycamptothecin (CPT-11) administered as a ninety-minute infusion every 3 weeks. Cancer Res. **54:** 427–436.
64. ROTHENBERG, M.L., J.G. KUHN, H.A. BURRIS III, et al. 1993. Phase I and pharmacokinetic trial of weekly CPT-11. J. Clin. Oncol. **11:** 2194–2204.

Alternative Administration of Camptothecin Analogues

C.F. VERSCHRAEGEN,[a] K. JAECKLE, B. GIOVANELLA, V. KNIGHT, AND B.E. GILBERT

Section of Gynecologic and Medical Therapeutics and Department of Neurooncology, The University of Texas M.D. Anderson Cancer Center; Department of Molecular Physiology and Biophysics and Department of Molecular Virology and Microbiology, Baylor College of Medicine; and Stehlin Foundation for Cancer Research, Houston, Texas 77030, USA

ABSTRACT: The binding of camptothecin (CPT) to the DNA-topoisomerase complex is reversible, but it needs to be maintained for maximal inhibitory activity. It is also dependent on the chemical structure of CPT. The lactone form is thought to be necessary for the activity. In human serum, the equilibrium between lactone and carboxylate is in favor of the latter. For these reasons, alternative administration of CPT analogues is being evaluated. The ideal compound would remain in lactone form and would expose the host for long periods of time to its effects. Oral administration of irinotecan (CPT-11) and topotecan (TPT) is discussed by other investigators. We studied oral rubitecan and reported a low lactone to total drug area under the plasma concentration-time curve (AUC_P) ratio (14.7%), with low plasma concentration over time despite repeated administrations and the presence of an enterohepatic cycle. Aerosolization of a liposomal formulation of rubitecan is currently under study. Six patients have been treated once a day for 5 days every 3 weeks. The dose was 6.7 µg/kg/day. Plasma levels are dose for dose higher than those after oral administration, but the ratio of lactone versus total drug is low. No toxicity was observed. The study will continue with increasing doses and lengths of administration. Intrathecal administration of topotecan has been studied in a phase I trial in children. Doses of 0.4 mg are tolerated without toxicity, and clinical responses have been seen in patients with refractory meningial carcinomatosis. Phase II studies are planned. Intraperitoneal (ip) administration of topotecan has been studied in a phase I trial as a 24-hour infusion in 5% dextrose at pH 3.5 every 21 days. Dose-limiting toxicity is 4 mg/m^2. Toxic effects are neutropenia, anemia, emesis, fever, and pain. Five of 10 patients with ascites had symptomatic relief. Pharmacokinetic analysis demonstrates a second-order kinetics with elimination half-lives of 0.49 and 2.7 hours. The peritoneal to plasma AUC ratio was 31.2. Intramuscular, transdermal, and subcutaneous administrations have been extensively studied in the mouse.

INTRODUCTION

Camptothecin (CPT) and its analogues target the topoisomerase-I enzyme (topo-I). Topo-I relaxes DNA by cleaving a single strand of a duplex DNA and allowing passage of the other strand through the nick before religation. Unwinding of the

[a]M.D. Anderson Cancer Center, 1515 Holcombe Boulevard, Box 401, Houston, TX 77030. Voice: 713-792-7959; fax: 713-745-1541.
cverschr@mdanderson.org

DNA is a prerequisite for processing the genetic information. Camptothecin stabilizes the normally transient covalent linkage (also called "cleavable complex") between the topo-I and the DNA strand. Because malignant cells often contain greater amounts of topo-I than do normal cells, they are usually more sensitive to the toxic effects of CPT.[1,2] The alkaloid CPT is the parent compound of topotecan (TPT), irinotecan (CPT-11), exatecan (DX8951f), rubitecan (9-nitrocamptothecin [9NC], RFS2000), 9-aminocamptothecin (9AC), silatecan, and other analogues.[3] The three initial compounds are watersoluble derivatives of CPT, and the other ones are water insoluble.[4,5] CPT and analogues are in a pH-dependent equilibrium between a closed lactone E-ring and an open carboxylate form. The lactone ring is the active compound required for binding with the topo-I–DNA complex.[6–10] However, at physiologic pH in human serum, most of the CPT is in carboxylate form.[11] In human serum, the AUC of the lactone form is between 0 and 16% of the AUC of both forms combined. This observation may be the reason for the low therapeutic index observed with these compounds in humans.[12]

The preponderance of preclinical and clinical data indicates that cytotoxic activity of TPT resides in the E-ring lactone.[13] However, correlations between the degree of neutropenia and plasma concentrations of lactone and open-ring forms have suggested that the open-ring carboxylate may contribute to myelosuppression.[14] At pH 6, more than 80% of the total TPT is in the lactone form, but at physiologic pH in the presence of human albumin, TPT is rapidly hydrolyzed to the carboxylate form.[15] A progressive loss of the lactone form in plasma is observed from the start of TPT infusion.

The active metabolite of CPT-11 is SN-38.[16] A carboxylesterase catalyzes the conversion of CPT-11 to SN-38 (7-ethyl-10-hydroxycamptothecin).[17,18] Carboxylesterase activity is usually higher in tumor cells, with lymphoma, small cell lung cancer, endometrial cancer, and mesothelioma containing the highest carboxylesterase activity. The carboxylesterase activity correlates with the antitumor activity.[17] In vitro studies have indicated that SN-38 has 100- to 1,000-fold greater antitumor activity than does CPT-11 itself. SN-38 is inactivated by glucuronidation.[19] A total of 16 metabolites have been identified in human bile, and 8 appear in the urine. TPT and CPT-11 are commercially available. DX8951f and 9NC are currently in phase II studies. The other analogues are either in the preclinical stage or in phase I studies.[20–26] DX8951f has a fluorine on the C-11 carbon of the A-ring, which stabilizes the molecule. Preliminary analyses show an increased percentage of lactone in the plasma. However, it has only been used intravenously.[27] 9NC is administered orally. Results of phase I and II have already been published.[12,28]

The puzzling question with CPT analogues is the following. When tested against human tumors in nude mice models, these drugs have the capacity to cure the affected animals. By comparison with other cytotoxic drugs,[2] CPT analogues are at least 100 times more potent. Once tumors have been eradicated, they usually do not recur. In mice, 50% of the drug present in serum is in the lactone form versus only 10% in human serum. In humans, the therapeutic index falls dramatically, and anticancer responses are observed in less than 20% of patients. There also is a fair percentage of stable disease that lasts usually 6 months. In fact, with the amount of lactone that reaches the tumor in humans, it is fairly surprising that any responses are observed. The clinical activity of TPT is most likely related to the higher concentration of lactone observed at physiologic pH (around 30%), but it is compounded by the rapid elimination from the plasma.[29,30]

This paper reviews other novel routes of administration that have been tested clinically and preclinically.

AEROSOLIZED ADMINISTRATION OF LIPOSOMAL 9-NITROCAMPTOTHECIN

Previous work has shown that certain drugs delivered to the respiratory tract in a liposome formulation may have advantages of noninvasive administration, including high pulmonary concentrations, often rapid entry into the systemic circulation, reduced toxicity, and reduced dosage requirements compared to oral and parenteral administration.[17,18] Dilauroylphosphatidylcholine (DLPC) aerosol formulations of beclomethasone and cyclosporin have already been administered in clinical settings.[31–33]

Pharmacokinetic studies of liposome aerosols in mice with CPT showed high concentrations of CPT in the lungs, which were rapidly disseminated to the liver, tumor, brain, and other organs.[34] 9-NC–DLPC liposome (LGNC) aerosols have demonstrated a favorable therapeutic index (significantly reduced tumor growth rate and shrinkage without serious side effects) in treating three different human cancer xenografts, breast, colon, and lung, in a nude mouse model.[35] The liposome formulation may help keep the E-ring closed for penetration in tumor cells. In animal models, equivalent activity of L9NC compared to the nonliposomated 9-NC is seen at one fifth or less of the dose. Toxicity profiles in the mouse indicate a maximum tolerated dose of approximately 4 mg/kg when given orally; however, the highest aerosol dose tested to date of 307 μg/kg/day was nontoxic. Such activity was noted in the absence of weight loss or other evident toxicity.[36]

Patients were eligible if they had primary or metastatic cancer in the lungs, had failed standard chemotherapy regimens for their disease, had normal bone marrow function and normal hepatic and renal function, had no known respiratory disease other than cancer, and had an acceptable pulmonary function defined as >50% FEV1, >50% FEV1/FVC, >50% TLC, and >50% DLCO of predicted values. Standard exclusion criteria applied. Treatment in the feasibility cohort consisted of 0.2 mg/ml of 9NC in aerosol reservoir for 60 minutes (= daily dose of 6.7 μg/kg/day) per day for 5 days, then observation for 2 weeks. Drug was administered using an AeroTech II nebulizer (CIS-US, Bedford, MA) flowing at 10 L of compressed air/min with a reservoir containing 10 ml of L9NC and administered through a mouth-only face mask.[37] To date, only the feasibility study has been completed, with six patients having been treated. Pulmonary function tests were repeated 1 hour after completion of aerosol on day 1 of treatment and again on days 5 and 21. No dose-limiting toxicity was observed during the first course of treatment in patients completing the feasibility cohort. Pharmacology samples were obtained from all patients during treatment. Five patients gave blood samples and four patients had bronchoalveolar lavage.

Stabilization of disease was observed in two patients who received 4 and 10⁺ courses, and a mixed response in one patient. Three patients had progressive disease after two courses.

Maximum concentration of drug (C_{max}) (lactone + carboxylate forms) was observed 1 hour (range, 30 min to 2 hours) after completion of aerosol and was 37.7 ng/ml (range 59.1–15.5 ng/ml). At 24 hours, the concentration was still 6 ng/ml. Lactone was measured in two patients. The percentage of lactone was highest during the aerosol and reached 11.6 and 22.8%. After aerosol completion, lactone percentage decreased to below 10%. Ratio of lactone AUC versus total drug AUC was 3.2% and 3.5%.

Patients receiving 2 mg/m^2 of 9NC orally, which is roughly the equivalent of 50 μg/kg, had a total drug C_{max} of 158 ng/ml at 4 hours and a lactone C_{max} of 18 ng/ml at 1 hour (11%). The AUC ratio of lactone versus total drug was 14%.

If these data are extrapolated, systemic absorption of 9NC after aerosolization is 60% higher than that after oral administration. However, lactone versus total drug ratio does not seem to improve. The level of lactone detection, however, was around 1 ng/ml, and the error in the measurement may be significant. It will be important to analyze lactone levels at higher doses of L9NC. Concentration of 9NC in bronchoalveolar lavage is at least 10 times higher than plasma levels. Final results are pending.

INTRATHECAL ADMINISTRATION OF CAMPTOTHECINS

Neoplastic meningitis remains a significant diagnostic and treatment challenge for clinical oncologists, and the long-term outcome for most patients with leptomeningeal metastases from an underlying solid tumor or recurrent leptomeningeal leukemia or lymphoma is poor. Systemic chemotherapy may be helpful in specific conditions, such as gestational trophoblastic disease, to eradicate brain disease, but is usually of little help because the penetration of most drugs into the cerebrospinal fluid (CSF) is limited by the blood brain barrier. This may not be true for topotecan. Following systemic intravenous administration of 10 mg/m^2 over 10 minutes in a nonhuman primate model, topotecan penetrated the CSF, and lactone concentration reached 30%.[38] Direct intrathecal instillation of anticancer drugs is another approach that has been used to circumvent the pharmacologic sanctuary imposed by the blood brain barrier. Because few anticancer agents can safely be administered by the intrathecal route, the effectiveness of this form of regional therapy is limited. In recent years the development of several promising new intrathecal agents (e.g., diaziquone, mafosfamide, and DTC-101)[39–41] has been possible through use of a unique nonhuman primate model.[42] Intrathecal topotecan has successfully been tested in this model. Pharmacokinetic studies performed following a direct intraventricular dose of 0.1 mg demonstrated that 450-fold greater CSF exposure could be achieved with 1/100th the systemic dose.[43] No systemic or neural toxicity, with the exception of transient pleocytosis in 30% of animals, was observed following intraventricular topotecan administration. Further studies to evaluate the long-term toxicity of weekly intralumbar injections of topotecan were performed in three animals that received 0.1 mg of topotecan via lumbar puncture weekly for 4 weeks. This dose was well tolerated, without evidence of myelosuppression, neurotoxicity, or pleocytosis. These preclinical studies served as the basis for a phase I study of intrathecal topotecan in patients with neoplastic meningitis, who were over 3 years of age.[44]

sensitive malignancies confined to the peritoneal cavity. Persistence of the active lactone form in the peritoneal cavity would be a definite advantage.

Two phase I studies have been looking at one administration of topotecan (either over 24 hours or over 1 hour) every 3 weeks. The maximum tolerated doses were 3 and 20 mg/m^2, respectively. In the first phase I trial 15% of the total dose was given as an intraperitoneal bolus in 2 L of 5% dextrose in water, and the remainder was given as a continuous intraperitoneal infusion over 24 hours. Dose-limiting toxicity was neutropenia. Other toxicities included leukopenia, anemia, emesis, fever, and abdominal pain. No objective responses were achieved; 5 of 10 patients with ascites had a decrease in fluid accumulation with administration of intraperitoneal TPT. Elimination of TPT from the peritoneal cavity followed second-order kinetics with first- and second-phase half-lives of 0.49 and 2.7 hours, respectively. Plasma pharmacokinetics fitted first-order kinetics with a half-life of 3.9 hours. The $AUC_{peritoneal} : AUC_P$ ratio was 31.2.[47]

In the second study, TPT was administered i.p. with 1 L of normal saline over 1 hour. Dose-limiting toxicity was skin rash and fever with hypotension in 30% of patients at 30 mg/m^2, whereas hematologic toxicity was grade 2 or less. Other toxicities included nausea, vomiting, and abdominal pain. The ratio between lactone and carboxylate was 1:5 in the peritoneal fluid and in the plasma. Topotecan reached peak plasma levels 6 hours after i.p. instillation. The ratio of i.p. versus i.v. peak levels ranged from 125–250.[48]

Intraperitoneal administration of topotecan results in substantial exposure of the peritoneal cavity to increased drug concentration without compromising systemic exposure; this may be beneficial for the treatment of patients with peritoneal carcinomatosis.

A third study looked at intraperitoneal administration of TPT 1.5 mg/day for 5 consecutive days. The $AUC_{peritoneal} : AUC_P$ ratio was 23. The elimination of TPT from the peritoneal cavity was rapid (1–2 hours), and peak plasma levels occurred between 0.4 and 2 hours. The local peritoneal tolerance appears to be excellent, and no systemic effects have been noted.[49]

The same study looked at intraperitoneal administration of 9AC (0.42 mg/m^2/day given every other day for 6 days). The $AUC_{peritoneal} : AUC_P$ ratio was 7. Elimination of 9AC and time to peak plasma levels paralleled the ones for TPT. Again, at these doses, tolerance was excellent.[49]

Intraperitoneal irinotecan has been studied in mouse models and compared to intravenous and oral administration. Oral administration resulted in greater tumor inhibition than did the i.p. route.[50] Intravenous administration was worse than i.p. administration both in terms of survival of the animals and pharmacokinetically. Peritoneal clearance of CPT-11 was 10-fold lower after i.p. versus i.v. administration, resulting in longer exposure to CPT-11 for the i.p. administration.[51]

TRANSDERMAL ADMINISTRATION OF CAMPTOTHECINS

Transdermal administration has been tested in nude mice bearing different human tumors. Drugs tested were CPT and 9NC. Drugs were formulated in patches or used with a liposoluble vehicle. Vehicles used were vaseline, cottonseed oil, and 20% DMSO. A human topoisomerase-I inhibitor-sensitive breast cancer was extensively

Intrathecal topotecan was administered twice weekly during a 4- to 6-week induction, followed by a consolidation phase of 4 weekly doses, then a monthly maintenance phase. The starting dose was 0.025 mg. In the first cohort of patients, weekly intrapatient dose escalations to 0.05, 0.1, and 0.2 mg were done. Subsequent cohorts were treated without escalation at 0.2 mg and 0.4 mg. A total of 12 patients were treated. Patient characteristics were as follows: median age 13 years (range 3–19), meningeal spread of medulloblastoma/primitive neuroectodermal tumor (5 patients), rhabdomyosarcoma (2 patients), glioma (2 patients), acute lymphoblastic leukemia (ALL, 1 patient), retinoblastoma (1 patient), and germinoma (1 patient). Non-dose-limiting toxicities included nausea, vomiting, headache, and transient leukopenia. Another adverse event consisted of staring with myoclonic jerking after the third dose ($n = 1$). Peak topotecan levels in two patients with indwelling Ommaya reservoirs treated at the 0.2 mg dose level were 6.1 and 6.8 µM. Topotecan lactone concentrations >0.1 µM were present in the CSF longer than 8 hours. The terminal elimination half-life was 2.8 hours. In a study of CSF penetration of topotecan after systemic administration, the elimination half-life was 4.8 hours.[45]

Two patients had some benefit following intrathecal topotecan. One patient with ALL and one with leptomeningeal gliomatosis had stable disease for more than six maintenance cycles with intrathecal topotecan. In summary, intrathecal administration of topotecan is well tolerated at doses up to 0.4 mg and is associated with some antitumor activity. A phase II study of topotecan in children with neoplastic meningitis is planned.

A plasma and CSF pharmacokinetics study of intrathecal 9AC and CPT-11 in a nonhuman primate model was also performed. 9AC, 0.2 mg/kg (4 mg/m^2) or 0.5 mg/kg (10 mg/m^2), was infused intravenously over 15 minutes, and irinotecan, 4.8 mg/kg (96 mg/m^2) or 11.6 mg/kg (225 mg/m^2), was infused over 30 minutes. Plasma and CSF samples were obtained at frequent intervals over 24 hours. Lactone and total drug forms of 9AC, irinotecan, and the active metabolite of irinotecan, SN-38, were quantified by reverse-phase HPLC. The lactone form of 9AC accounted for 26% of the total drug in plasma. The CSF penetration of 9AC was reflected by a peak concentration of 11–21 nM (0.5 mg/kg dose) at 30–45 minutes after administration, but the ratio of the $AUC_{CSF} : AUC_P$ was only 3.5%. AUC_P of the lactone form of SN-38 was around 2.0% of the AUC_P of irinotecan lactone. The lactone form of irinotecan accounted for 26% of the total drug in plasma, and the lactone form of SN-38 accounted for 55% of the total SN-38 in plasma. The $AUC_{CSF} : AUC_P$ ratio for irinotecan lactone was 14%. SN-38 lactone and carboxylate could not be measured in CSF. CSF penetration of 9AC and SN-38 is substantially less than that of topotecan, which has an $AUC_{CSF} : AUC_P$ ratio of 32%.[46]

Further study of intrathecal CPT is warranted in an attempt to identify effective new agents that will expand the limited armamentarium of anticancer agents that are available for intrathecal administration.

INTRAPERITONEAL ADMINISTRATION OF CAMPTOTHECINS

Intraperitoneal (i.p.) administration of topoisomerase inhibitors may have pharmacologic benefits over i.v. administration especially for topoisomerase-I inhibitor-

TABLE 1. Transdermal administration of camptothecin (CPT) and 9-nitrocamptothecin (9NC) in a nude mouse model

Treatment twice a week	Dose (mg/kg of CPT)	Dose (mg/kg of 9NC)	Animals surviving (n)	Days to maximum tumor inhibition
Controls	0	0	3/27 (9NC) 4/20 (CPT)	None
Intragastric	2	2	3/4 (CPT) 2/4 (9NC)	30
Transdermal	5–10	5–10	24/24 (9NC) 27/33 (CPT)	30 for 9NC 40 for CPT
Transdermal vaseline carrier		6 and 7.5	11/14	28
Transdermal cotton-seed oil carrier		5, 6, and 7.5	14/16	28
Transdermal 20% DMSO carrier		7.5	3/4	28

tested (TABLE 1). Results show that transdermal administration is as good as oral administration. Patches were selected for further study. Other human tumors tested with 9NC patches included colon, melanoma, and lung tumors. Patches of 9NC were applied twice a week on the skin until the tumors disappeared. The dose of 9NC for the patches was 7.5 mg/kg twice a week. Antitumor activity was comparable to oral doses (through direct intragastric injections) of 9NC 1.5 mg/kg for 3 days every 4 days.

Weekly intramuscular injections were tested at low doses of 9NC (0.75–1 mg/kg) either as a liposome or mixed with cottonseed oil. Tumor inhibition was best with 9NC in cottonseed oil.

CONCLUSIONS

Camptothecins are drugs that are well suited for various modes of administration. In animal models, longer exposure seems to produce more antitumor activity. The CPTs are absorbed systemically through the gastrointestinal tract, lungs, and skin. When administered through the peritoneal cavity or the intrathecal space, systemic absorption is present but reduced, leaving high concentrations of drugs in these body cavities.

The main problem that remains to be solved is the equilibrium of lactone versus carboxylate forms, which in humans favors the inactive (carboxylate) form. To date, alternative administrations have not helped to shift equilibrium to the lactone form. In the future, new delivery systems such as liposomes, polyethylene glycol esters, or polymers as well as new derivatives need to be studied in an attempt to stabilize the lactone form.

REFERENCES

1. LIEBES, L., M. POTMESIL, T. KIM, et al. 1998. Pharmacodynamics of topoisomerase I inhibition. Western blot determination of topoisomerase I and cleavable complex in patients with upper gastrointestinal malignancies treated with topotecan. Clin. Cancer Res. **4:** 545.
2. GIOVANELLA, B.C., J.S. STEHLIN, M.E. WALL, et al. 1989. DNA topoisomerase I-targarted chemotherapy of human color cancer in xenografts. Science **246:** 1046.
3. ROTHENBERG, M.L. 1997. Topoisomerase I inhibitors: review and update. Ann. Oncol. **8:** 837.
4. VERSCHRAEGEN, C.F., A.P. KUDELKA & J.J. KAVANAGH. 1998. Topoisomerase-I inhibitors in gynaecologic tumours. [Review]. Ann. Acad. Med. Singapore **27:** 683.
5. BALAT, O., & C. VERSCHRAEGEN. 1995. Topoisomerase I inhibitors in gynecologic cancer. Expert Opin. Invest. Dr. **4:** 1217.
6. JAXEL, C., K.W. KOHN, M.C. WANI, et al. 1989. Structure-activity study of the actions of camptothecin derivatives on mammalian topoisomerase I: evidence for a specific receptor site and a relation to antitum or activity. Cancer Res. **49:** 1465.
7. NABIEV, I., F. FLEURY, I. KUDELINA, et al. 1998. Spectroscopic and biochemical characterisation of self-aggregates formed by antitumor drugs of the camptothecin family: their possible role in the unique mode of drug action. Biochem. Pharmacol. **55:** 1163.
8. CHOURPA, I., J.F. RIOU, J. M. MILLOT, et al. 1998. Modulation in kinetics of lactone ring hydrolysis of camptothecins upon interaction with topoisomerase I cleavage sites on DNA. Biochemistry **37:** 7284.
9. CARRIGAN, S.W., P.C. FOX, M.E. WALL, et al. 1997. Comparative molecular field anaylsis and molecular modeling studies of 20-(S)-camptothecin analogs as inhibitors of DNA topoisomerase I and anticancer/antitumor agents. J. Comp. Aided Mol. Designs **11:** 71.
10. RIVORY, L.P. & J. ROBERT. 1995. Molecular, cellular, and clinical aspects of the pharmacology of 20(S) camptothecin and its derivatives. Pharmacol. Ther. **68:** 269.
11. GABR, A., A. KUIN, M. AALDERS, et al. 1997. Cellular pharmacokinetics and cytotoxicity of camptothecan and topotecan at normal and acidic pH. Cancer Res. **57:** 4811.
12. VERSCHRAEGEN, C.F., E.A. NATELSON, B.C. GIOVANELLA, et al. 1998. A phase I clinical and pharmacological study of oral 9-nitrocamptothecin, a novel water-insoluble topoisomerase I inhibitor. Anti-Ca. Dr. **9:** 36.
13. HERTZBERG, R.P., M.J. CARANFA, K.G. HOLDEN, et al. 1989. Modification of the hydroxy lactone ring of camptothecin: inhibition of mammalian topoisomerase I and biological activity. J. Med. Chem. **32:** 715.
14. MOERTEL, C., A. SCHUTT, R. REITEMEIER, et al. 1972. Phase II study of camptothecin in the treatment of advanced gastrointestinal cancer. Cancer Chemother. Rep. **56:** 95.
15. DENNIS, M.J., J.H. BEIJNEN, L.B. GROCHOW, et al. 1997. An overview of the clinical pharmacology of topotecan. [Review]. Semin. Oncol. **24:** S5.
16. KAWATO, Y., M. AONUMA, Y. HIORTA, et al. 1991. Intracellular roles of SN-38, a metabolite of the camptothecin derivative CPT-11, in the antitumor effect of CPT-11. Cancer Res. **51:** 4187.
17. DANKS, M., C. MORTON, C. PAWLIK, et al. 1998. Overexpression of a rabbit liver carboxylesterase sensitizes human tumor cells to CPT-11. Cancer Res. **58**.
18. HAAZ, M., L RIVORY, C. RICHE, et al. 1997. The transformation of irinotecan (CPT-11) to its active metabolite SN-38 by human liver microsomes. Differential hydrolysis for the lactone and carboxylate forms. Naunyn Schmiedebergs Arch. Pharmacol. **356:** 257.
19. GUPTA, E., T.M. LESTINGI, R. MICK, J. RAMIREZ, et al. 1994. Metabolic fate of irinotecan in humans: correlation of glucuronidation with diarrhea. Cancer Res. **54:** 3723.
20. PRATESI, G., M. TORTORETO, C. CORTI, C., et al. 1995. Successful local regional therapy with topotecan of intraperitoneally growing human ovarian carcinoma xenografts. Br. J. Cancer **71:** 525.
21. ECKHARDT, S.G., S.D. BAKER, J.R. ECKARDT, et al. 1998. Phase I and pharmacokinetic study of GI147211, a water-soluble camptothecin analogue, administered for five consecutive days every three weeks. Clin. Cancer Res. **4:** 595.

22. HALUSKA, P., E. RUBIN & C. VERSCHRAEGEN. 1999. Topoisomerase-I inhibitors in gynecologic tumors. Hem/Oncol. Clin. No. Am. **13:** 43.
23. MATSUI, S., W. ENDO, C. WRZOSEK, et al. 1997. New DNA topoisomerase I inhibitor (TI), BNPI 1100, induces cytotoxicity through a dual mechanism in HCT-8 human ileocecal carcinoma cells (Meeting abstract). Proc. Ann. Meet. Am. Assoc. Cancer Res. **38:** A110.
24. SUGARMAN, S.M., Y. ZOU, K. WASAN, et al. 1996. Lipid-complexed camptothecin: formulation and initial biodistribution and antitumor activity studies. Cancer Chemother. Pharmacol. **37:** 531.
25. MITSUI, I., E. KUMAZAWA, Y. HIROTA, et al. 1995, A new water-soluble camptothecin derivative, DX-8951f, exhibits potent antitumor activity against human tumors in vitro and in vivo. Japanese J. Cancer Res. **86:** 776.
26. STEVENSON, J.P., D. DEMARIA, J. SLUDDEN, et al. 1999. Phase I pharmacokinetic study of the topoisomerase I inhibitor GG211 administered as a 21-day continuous infusion. Ann. Oncol. **10:** 339.
27. KUMAZAWA, E., T. JIMBO, Y. OCHI, et al. 1998. Potent and broad antitumor effects of DX-8951f, a water-soluble camptothecin derivative, against various human tumors xenografted in nude mice. Cancer Chemother. Pharmacol. **42:** 210.
28. VERSCHRAEGEN, C.F., F. GUPTA, E. LOYER, et al. 1999. A phase II clinical and pharmacological study of oral 9-nitrocamptothecin in patients with refractory epithelial ovarian, tubal or peritoneal cancer. AntiCa. Dr. **10:** 375.
29. HERBEN, V.M., W.W. TEN BOKKEL HUININK, et al. 1996. Clinical pharmaco-kinetics of topotecan. Clin. Pharm. **31:** 85.
30. VAN WARMERDAM, L.J., G.J. CREEMERS, S. RODENHUIS, et al. 1996. Pharmacokinetics and pharmacodynamics of topotecan given on a daily-times-five schedule in phase II clinical trials using a limited-sampling procedure. Cancer Chemother. Pharmacol. **38:** 254.
31. WALDREP, J.C., B.E. GILBERT, V. KNIGHT, et al. 1997. Pulmonary delivery of beclomethasone liposome aerosol in volunteers. Tolerance & safety. Chest **111:** 316.
32. ENGLUND, J.A., P.A. PIEDRA, Y.M. AHN, et al. 1994. High-dose, short-duration ribavirin aerosol therapy compared with standard ribavirin therapy in children with suspected respiratory syncytial virus infection [see comments]. J. Pediatr. **125:** 635.
33. GILBERT, B.E., P.R. WYDE, G. LOPEZ-BERESTEIN, et al. 1994. Aerosolized amphotericin B-liposomes for treatment of systemic Candida infections in mice. Anti Ag. 7& Chemother. **38:** 356.
34. KOSHKINA, N.V., B.E. GILBERT, J.C. WALDREP, et al. 1999. Distribution of camptothecin after delivery as a liposome aerosol or following intramuscular injection in mice. Cancer Chemother. Pharmacol. **44:** 187.
35. KNIGHT, V., N.V. KOSHKINA, J.C. WALDREP, et al. 1999. Anticancer effect of 9-nitrocamptothecin liposome aerosol on human cancer xenografts in nude mice. Cancer Chemother. Pharmacol. **44:** 177.
36. KNIGHT, V., E.S. KLEINERMAN, J.C. WALDREP, et al. 2000. 9 Nitrocamptothecin liposome aerosol treatment of human cancer subcutaneous xenograft and pulmonary cancr metastases in mice. Ann. N.Y. Acad. Sci .
37. VERSCHRAEGEN, C., B. GILBERT, A. HUARINGA, et al. 2000. Feasibility, phase I and pharmacological study of aerosolized liposomal 9 nitro-(20S)-camptothecin (L9NC) in patients with advanced malignancies in the lungs. Proc. Am. Soc. Clin. Oncol. **19:** A904.
38. BLANEY, S.M., D.E. COLE, F.M. BALIS, et al. 1993. Plasma and cerebrospinal fluid pharmacokinetic study of topotecan in nonhuman primates. Cancer Res. **53:** 725.
39. BERG, S.L., F.M. BALIS, S. ZIMM, et al. 1992. Phase I/II trial and pharmacokinetics of intrathecal diaziquone in refractory meningeal malignancies. J. Clin. Oncol. **10:** 143.
40. BLANEY, S.M., F.M. BALIS & D.G. POPLACK. 1991. Pharmacologic approaches to the treatment of meningeal malignancy. Oncology (Huntington) **5:** 107.
41. CHAMBERLAIN, M.C., S. KHATIBI, J.C. KIM, et al. 1993. Treatment of leptomeningeal metastasis with intraventricular administration of depot cytarabine (DTC 101). A phase I study. Arch. Neurol. **50:** 261.
42. MCCULLY, C.L., F.M. BALIS, J. BACHER, et al. 1990. A rhesus monkey model for continuous infusion of drugs into cerebrospinal fluid. Lab. Anim. Sci. **40:** 520.

43. BLANEY, S.M., D.E. COLE, L. GODWIN, *et al.* 1995. Intrathecal administration of topotecan in nonhuman primates. Cancer Chemother. Pharmacol. **36:** 121.
44. BLANEY, S., R. HEIDEMAN, D. COLE, *et al.* 1998. A phase I study of intrathecal topotecan. Proc. Am. Assoc. Cancer Res. **39:** A2198.
45. BAKER, S.D., R.L. HEIDEMAN, W.R. CROM, *et al.* 1996. Cerebrospinal fluid pharmacokinetics and penetration of continuous infusion topotecan in children with central nervous system tumors. Cancer Chemother. Pharmacol. **37:** 195.
46. BLANEY, S.M., C. TAKIMOTO, D.J. MURRY, *et al.* 1998. Plasma and cerebrospinal fluid pharmacokinetics of 9-aminocamptothecin (9-AC), irinotecan (CPT-11), and SN-38 in nonhuman primates. Cancer Chemother. Pharmacol. **41:** 464.
47. PLAXE, S.C., R.D. CHRISTEN, J. O'QUIGLEY, *et al.* 1998. Phase I and pharmacokinetic study of intraperitoneal topotecan. Invest. New Dr. **16:** 147.
48. BOS, A., E. VRIES, *et al.* 1999. Phase I and pharmacokinetic study of intraperitoneal topotecan. Proc. Am. Soc. Clin. Oncol. **18:** A1404.
49. HORNREICH, G., L. LIEBES, E. NEWMAN, *et al.* 1999. Pharmacokinetics of intraperitoneal 9-amincamptothecin or topotecan in phase I trials. Proc. Am. Soc. Clin. Oncol. **18:** A671.
50. CHOI, S.H., Y. TSUCHIDA & H.W. YANG. 1998. Oral versus intraperitoneal administration of irinotecan in the treatment of human neuroblastoma in nude mice. Ca Let **24:** 15.
51. GUICHARD, S., E. CHATELUT, I. LOCHON, *et al.* 1998. Comparison of the pharmacokinetics and efficacy of irinotecan after administration by the intravenous versus intraperitoneal route in mice. Cancer Chemother. Pharmacol. **42:** 165.

Topotecan (Hycamptin) and Topotecan-Containing Regimens in the Treatment of Hematologic Malignancies

MILOSLAV BERAN[a] AND HAGOP M. KANTARJIAN

The Department of Leukemia, Division of Medicine, The University of Texas, M.D. Anderson Cancer Center, 1515 Holcombe Boulevard/Box 61, Houston, Texas 77030-4095, USA

ABSTRACT: Single-agent topotecan is an active drug in chemotherapy-naive MDS and CMML and, to a lesser degree, in refractory/relapsed acute leukemias, low-/intermediate-grade lymphoma, and myeloma. Its combination with cytosine arabinoside induces complete remissions in high-risk MDS/CMML. A triple-combination regimen of cyclophosphamide, cytosine arabinoside, and topotecan (CAT) was extensively tested in refractory/relapsed as well as in untreated AML. By proving effective in inducing complete remission in newly diagnosed AML at rates comparable to those achieved by anthracycline-cytosine arabinoside regimens, for example, CAT offers a useful treatment alternative. Topotecan combined with paclitaxel is promising in low-/intermediate-grade lymphomas. The activity of topotecan justifies further evaluation of topotecan-containing combination regimens, particularly in MDS/CMML and acute leukemias.

INTRODUCTION

As a new group of antineoplastic agents, topoisomerase I inhibitors have been in clinical trials for more than 10 years. Most currently used agents are semisynthetic derivatives of a plant alkaloid (camptothecin, CPT) extracted from *Camptotheca acuminata*. The low activity, poor watersolubility, and high toxicity of CPT have been successfully improved in semisynthetic derivatives, several of which are now extensively studied in clinical trials in a wide variety of tumors including hematologic malignancies. Although first phase I trials in leukemia and lymphoma were conducted with CPT-11,[1] the bulk of the data has been accumulated in trials with topotecan (TPT). The experience with topotecan in hematologic malignancies is the subject of this review.

SINGLE AGENT TOPOTECAN

TABLE 1 summarizes hematologic diseases in which experience with TPT was gathered either in a setting of salvage therapy or in previously untreated patients for whom there was no generally accepted standard of care.

---

[a]Voice: 713-792-7305; fax: 713-794-4297.
mberan@mdanderson.org

ACUTE LEUKEMIA AND BLASTIC PHASE CHRONIC MYELOGENOUS LEUKEMIA

The first two trials in acute myelogenous leukemia (AML) included some patients with acute lymphoblastic leukemia (ALL) and blastic phase of chronic myelogenous leukemia (CML).[2,3] Selecting a continuous, 5-day infusion regimen as potentially advantageous with regard to the drug pharmacokinetics and tentative mechanisms of action, both groups reported similar dose-limiting toxicities, median tolerated doses (MTD), and antileukemic activity. In both studies, the dose- limiting toxicities were severe mucositis, diarrhea, and mild nausea and vomiting. Myelosuppression-related fevers and infections were observed in three quarters of the patients. The MTD of 10 mg/m^2 continuous i.v. infusion (CIV) over 5 days (2 mg/day) found in the M.D. Anderson study[2] was identical to the MTD determined in the study of Rowinsky et al. (10.5 mg/m^2 CIV over 5 days).[3] In the M.D. Anderson study, which included 27 patients, responses were seen in 5 of 17 patients with AML or AUL (29%) with two complete (CR) and two partial (PR) remissions. The leukemic burden was reduced in all patients. The study of Rowinsky et al. included 17 patients, 8 with AML and documented one PR.[3] These reports provide evidence of the antileukemic activity of TPT using continuous infusion for 5 days. To further evaluate the importance of the TPT schedule, a phase I/II trial of short daily infusion was carried out in a similar population of patients with refractory acute leukemia. Dose-limiting toxicities consisted of high fever, rigors, precipitous anemia, and hyperbilirubinemia, but no mucositis or diarrhea. With MTD of 4.5 mg/m^2 daily for 5 days, the equitoxic dose of TPT was two times higher with short infusion. Antileukemic effects but no complete or partial responses were noted.[4]

Although no final conclusion could be drawn, one was left with the impression that CIV may be the preferable mode of administration. Single-agent TPT undoubtedly proved its activity in AML, and continuous infusion was selected for most subsequent studies. The studies just referred to also provided insight into the activity of the drug in two other leukemias, ALL and blastic and accelerated (AP) phases of CML. Evidence of activity of TPT in ALL was initially indicated from reports of Uckum et al.[5] who observed prolongation of survival by TPT treatment of SCID mice grafted with lethal numbers of human ALL cells. In a total of 12 heavily pretreated patients with ALL, included in the aforementioned trials, antileukemic activity, measured by decrease in circulating and bone marrow blasts was noted in all patients with suggestion of dose-related response. These effects were not maintained, however with return of progressive disease within 4 weeks.[3,4] Interesting and potentially important data were obtained in chemotherapy-naive patients with high-risk ALL. In 13 patients, TPT was given initially as a single dose using therapeutic window approach.[6] TPT was administered at 2.1 mg/m^2 CI over 24 hours for 5 days to 15 previously untreated adult patients with high risk ALL. After evaluation of response to TPT, all patients subsequently received standard treatment for ALL. Hematologic improvement in six patients with normal platelet or neutrophil counts but no CR's suggest that single agent TPT has modest effect in untreated adult high risk ALL, probably insufficient to be included in therapeutic regimens of this disease at the schedule used.

TABLE 1. Experience with topotecan in hematological malignancies: therapeutic situation

Regimen	Salvage	Frontline
Single agent topotecan	AML, ALL, CML-BP, lymphoma (NHL), myeloma, MDS, CMML	MDS, CMML
Combination regimens	AML, ALL, CML-BP/AP, MDS, CMML, NHL	MDS, CMML, AML, CML-BP/AP

TABLE 2. Topotecan in NHL: response by grade and previous therapy[a]

Histologic grade	No prior therapy	Response no. (%)
Low (LGL)	1	1/3 (33)
	>1	4/21 (19)
	ALL	5/24 (21)
Intermediate (IGL)	1	10/24 (42)
	>1	2/16 (12)
	ALL	12/40 ( )

[a]Modified from Preti et al.[7]

Experience with TPT in the blastic phase of CML is limited to few patients treated in phase I studies.[2,3] One of three patients[2] and one of four[3] of these patients, respectively, achieved CR/chronic phase lasting 5 and 6 months, respectively. The results were promising enough to include TPT in novel combination chemotherapy regimens for AML and the blastic phase of CML.

NON-HODGKIN'S LYMPHOMA (NHL)

In a phase II study,[7] 74 patients with refractory/relapsed lymphoma (35 indolent and 43 more aggressive non-Hodgkin's lymphoma) were treated with TPT by 30 minutes i.v. injection on 5 consecutive days at a dose of 1.5 mg/m^2/day without growth factor support ($n = 35$) or 2.0 mg/m^2/day with growth factor support ($n = 39$). Of 71 evaluable patients, 3 achieved CR and 14 PR for an overall response rate of 24%. Major toxicities were hematologic with grade 4 neutropenia in 40%, grade 4 thrombocytopenia in 33%, and grade 3 anemia in 31% of cycles. Responses were mostly partial, and response rates correlated with prior therapy. The results summarized in TABLE 2 suggest a potential role of TPT in the treatment of lymphomas and present a rationale for the development of combination regimens.

TABLE 3. Response to topotecan in multiple myeloma[a]

SWOG response criteria	Patients (n)	%
Remission	1	2.8
Partial remission	6	13.9
Stable	2	4.6
No response	20	46.5
Progressive disease	10	23.2
Not evaluable	4	9.3

[a]Kraut et al.[14]

CHRONIC LYMPHOCYTIC LEUKEMIA (CLL)

In a single phase II study reported by O'Brien et al.,[8] 12 patients with refractory B-CLL (median age 63 years; Rai 3-4, 42%; prior fludarabine therapy, 100%; fludarabine refractory, 33%) received an i.v. bolus of 2 mg/m^2 of TPT daily for 5 days. There were no significant responses and only modest and transient decreases in lymphocyte counts. Myelosuppression was common and the only significant toxicity. While failing to document antileukemic activity, the study gave some insight into the tentative mechanism of action of TPT. Although measurable levels of the target enzyme topoisomerase I are found in B-CLL cells (ref. 9 and Beran, unpublished data), and DNA-protein cross-binding was demonstrated *in vitro*, this per se was not sufficient for toxicity in a slow cycling population of B-CLL cells.[10] The finding is in line with evidence that progression through the cell cycle is required for the lethal action of TPT.[11-13]

MULTIPLE MYELOMA

Encouraged with the activity of topoisomerase I inhibitor CPT-11 in B-cell lymphoproliferative disorders,[1] the Southwest Oncology Group conducted a phase II study in resistant or relapsing myelomas. Kraut et al.[14] reported results in 46 patients treated with short (30-minute) i.v. infusion of 1.25 mg TPT daily on a 5 days every 3 weeks schedule. The results in 43 evaluable patients are summarized in TABLE 3. Most toxicities were hematologic with grade 3 and 4 thrombocytopenia in 21 of 43 patients and granulocytopenia in 40 of 43 patients. There were no complete remissions, 1 remission and six partial remissions by Southwest Oncology Group criteria. Although the response rate was low, any activity in therapy-resistant disease such as myeloma is encouraging. Significant myelosuppression on limited dose escalation was seen in most patients, and further exploration of TPT in this patient population would require modification of the regimen and possibly inclusion of growth factor support. Whether higher doses will be more effective is unknown, but it may be worthwhile to explore TPT in combination regimens using less myelosuppressive drugs.

TABLE 4. Response to topotecan in high risk MDS (n = 30) and CMML (n = 30) by prior therapy[a]

Prior therapy	Number CR/total (%)		
	CMML	MDS	Total
No	2/12 (17)	1/7 (14)	3/9 (16)
Yes	6/18 (33)	10/33 (43)	16/41 (39)
Total	8/30 (27)	11/30 (37)	19/60 (32)

[a]Beran et al.[16,17]

MYELODYSPLASTIC SYNDROMES AND CHRONIC MYCLOMOCYTIC LEUKEMIA

The myelodysplastic syndromes (MDS) are a heterogeneous group of stem cell disorders characterized by bone marrow failure and highly variable prognoses. In patients considered high risk (HR) according to the FAB classification (HR MDS), the median survival of untreated patients is between 6 and 12 months. Importantly, there is no generally accepted standard of care beyond supportive care, except in a minority of patients eligible for allogeneic bone marrow transplantation.[15] The use of the investigational drug TPT was encouraged by its activity in acute leukemias as well as the knowledge that the target of the drug, topoisomerase I (topo I), is present in all cells regardless of the stage of cell cycle, a factor to be considered in slowly proliferating cells of MDS patients. The first trial included a total of 60 patients, 30 with high risk MDS (RAEB and RAEB-t) and 30 with CMML.[16,17] Approximately half the patients were previously treated and the rest received supportive care only. The treatment schedule was derived from AML phase I studies, and TPT was given as a continuous i.v. infusion of 10 mg/m^2 for 5 days. Up to two courses were given for induction, and in responding patients additional courses at reduced doses were allowed. The results, which were encouraging particularly in previously untreated patients, are summarized in TABLE 4. The overall CR rate was 30%. Complete remission was more frequent in untreated patients (43% for MDS and 33% for CMML). Significant side effects such as severe mucositis (23%), diarrhea (17%), fever of unknown origin (85%), and documented infections (47%) were major complications, undoubtedly related to the high dose of the drug. Disappearance of chromosomal abnormalities including +8 and −5/−7 in patients achieving CR were particularly encouraging.

Because of severe myelosuppression, oral prophylaxis with antibacterial, antifungal, and antiviral antibiotics was necessary. Most MDS patients (80%) achieved their best response with the first course. Progression into AML shortly after therapy was uncommon, and in most patients failing to respond, the disease remained stable. Up to 10 cycles were given without cumulative toxicity; some patients, however, received none or only one or two continuation courses. In CMML, the response rate was slightly lower, particularly in the salvage setting, but some patients continued to benefit from several courses of therapy. The overall response in these disorders was highly favorable and led to the inclusion of TPT in combination therapies. With a median follow-up of 31 months, the median duration of CR was 7.5 months and the

TABLE 5. Responses to topotecan + Ara-C in 86 patients with high risk MDS and Cytogenic, and history of previous malignancy[a]

Category	Patients (n)	CR (%)	p value
RAEB	25	80	
RAEBt	34	47	
CMML	27	44	0.01
Diploid	40	50	
inv16, t(8;21)	3	100	
−5/−7	21	71	
±8	9	67	
Other	13	31	NS

[a]Beran et al.[18]

median survival was 10.5 months. The impact on survival could not be documented in this single arm, phase II study design. Reduction of the TPT dose to 1.5 mg/m^2 per day for 5 days in a maintenance treatment setting abolished most of the nonhematologic side effects and is a dose to explore in further trials.

TOPOTECAN COMBINATIONS

Combination of TPT and Cytosine Arabinoside (Ara-C) for MDS and CMML (TA)

Based on the promising activity of TPT in MDS, the combination of ara-C, the most active agent in AML, and TPT was explored in patients with previously untreated diseases.[18] Topotecan was given as a continuous infusion (1.25 mg/m^2 per 24 hours) and ara-C as a short infusion (1g/m^2 i.v. daily) for 5 days. Up to two induction courses were given, and patients achieving CR could receive up to 6 monthly maintenance courses at a 50% daily dose reduction. In a report on 86 patients, the overall CR rate was 56% with a very low induction treatment-associated mortality of 7%. The CR rate was slightly higher in MDS (61%) than in CMML (44%) and not significantly different in subcategories of patients with primary and secondary disease and in patients with different karyotypes (TABLE 5). The median CR duration was 50 weeks for MDS and 33 weeks for CMML. The median survival was 60 weeks for MDS and 44 weeks for CMML.[18] These results were comparable to the responses obtained by other intensive anti-leukemia combination chemotherapy regimens, such as idarubicin/ high dose ara-C or FLAG.[19] The potential advantage of the TPT–ara-C combination may be better tolerance as evidenced by a <10% induction mortality.[18,19] hematologic remissions were associated with conversion of abnormal to diploid karyotype in all but a few patients. As with other anti-leukemic regimens, the significance of the remission status and the impact of this treatment on the natural history of the disease remain to be determined. Landmark analysis of the survival of patients who were alive 6 weeks after the first course of induction with the TA regimen showed a significant survival advantage in patients achieving complete remission (Beran et al., unpublished data). With a word of caution that better survival may be due to a more favorable natural history of such patients, the results suggest the benefit of achieving a CR state. Particularly encouraging was the high remission rate in patients with a karyotype associated with a poor prognosis.[18] As with other anti-leukemic types of chemotherapy, maintaining remission remains a major challenge. It is unlikely that improvement will be achieved with more intensive induction and/or maintenance chemotherapy.[19] The low mortality of induction regimens such as TA favors the use of this regimen to induce CR prior to, for example, allogeneic bone marrow transplantation, because a long-term disease-free survival of 20–25%[15] in HR MDS/CMML patients, transplanted on presentation, is still unsatisfactory.

TOPOTECAN COMBINATIONS IN ACUTE MYELOGENOUS LEUKEMIA

Several two-drug combinations have been investigated in the treatment of acute leukemias. In primary refractory or relapsed patients, responses were observed using combinations of TPT and intermediate dose ara-C.[20] In this study, TPT was given as a short infusion, and in escalating doses, daily for 5 days along with ara-C 1 g/m^2 per day for 5 days. The highest dose of TPT was 7.5 mg/m^2/day x 5 days. The MTD of TPT was 4.75 mg/m^2 per day and 7.0 mg/m^2 per day i.v. over 30 minutes for 5 days in low and high risk patients, respectively, when given along with a 30-minute infusion of 1 g/m^2 per day of ara-C daily for 5 days. Clinical responses were seen in 4 of 39 patients with AML, 3 of 6 patients with ALL, and 1 of 8 patients with CML-blastic phase. The dose-limiting toxicity was mucositis.[20]

Several interesting observations from preclinical studies were the basis for the design of TPT combinations with other drugs. The importance of drug scheduling was inferred from observations in animal models that treatment with topo I– followed by topo II–targeting drugs results in synergistic or additive antitumor activity.[21–23] In malignant ascitic cells and peripheral white blood cells of patients treated with topo I–targeting drugs, downregulation of topo I was accompanied by upregulation of topo II.[24–26] This could potentially increase the sensitivity of cells to topo II–targeting agents. Topotecan toxicity was enhanced by combination with DNA-damaging agents, such as cyclophosphamide or cisplatinum, to a greater extent than with antimetabolites.[27] Furthermore, besides causing DNA damage, treatment of cells with cyclophosphamide was reported to induce an increased level of topo I[28] in addition to damage to DNA, both thought to favor the subsequent use of TPT after pretreatment with cyclophosphamide. In addition, this approach was supported by the observation that topo I inhibitors also interfere with repair of DNA damage.[13,29]

A pilot phase I–II study of VP-16 followed by TPT and TPT followed by VP-16 was carried out in refractory/resistant acute leukemias and included 12 and 15 patients in each arm, respectively. Whereas anti-leukemic activity of both arms was comparable, the TPT followed by VP-16 was clearly more toxic,[30] confirming the data obtained in the SCID mouse model of human AML (S. Jeha and M. Beran, in preparation). Only one CR was obtained (TPT → VP-16 schedule). The combination of these two drugs was also explored by Crump et al.,[31] who treated 10 refractory/relapsed AML/BC CML with 1.5 mg/m^2 CIV infusion of TPT over 24 hours for 5 days followed on days 6–8 by 100 mg/m² per day of i.v. etoposide. At this dose level, considered too close to MTD to be escalated, one CR was observed in a patient with CML-BC. This concept of timed sequential chemotherapy was further investigated by Mainwaring et al.[32] in 16 patients with relapsed/refractory acute leukemia (14 AML/AUL, 2 ALL). Treatment with TPT (1.5 mg/m² i.v. over 30 minutes daily for 3 days) was followed by etoposide (100 mg/m² per day) and mitoxantrone (10 mg/m² per day) on days 4-5 and 9-10. A "CR" was defined as clearance of circulating blasts and a decrease of bone marrow blasts below 5%, but it did not require complete normalization of peripheral blood counts. Such "CR" was observed in 7 of 14 patients (50%) with AML/AUL and both patients with ALL. While demonstrating significant anti-leukemic activity and no undue toxicity resulting in early death, this treatment did not induce "true" complete remissions in this heavily pretreated patient population. Similar to findings in solid tumors,[33,34] these studies provided no definite evidence that in this patient population, the expected responses are improved by sequential administration of these drugs. Finally, in a pilot study designed to assess toxicity and potential activity of a combination of cyclophosphamide (300 mg/m² per day over 2 hours) on days 1–4 with TPT (1.25 mg/m² CIV) starting 2 hours after the first dose of cyclophosphamide, 14 patients with refractory/relapsed AML were treated. The regimen was well tolerated, with no grade III/IV toxicities; the anti-leukemic activity, however, was not satisfactory with only transient suppression of leukemic cells. Neither CR nor PR was observed (Beran et al., unpublished data).

TRIPLE DRUG TOPOTECAN COMBINATIONS

Cyclophosphamide, Topotecan, and ara-C (CAT) in Leukemia, CML-BC, and MDS

Documented activity of the TPT–ara-C combination in MDS/CMML patients[18] and activity of cyclophosphamide in leukemia[35,36] along with preclinical data suggesting potential benefits of the combination of DNA-damaging agents with TPT[27,37] led to the design of the CAT regimen. When explored first in refractory/resistant acute leukemias, it consisted of cyclophosphamide (C) 500 mg i.v. every 12 hours over 3 hours on days 1–3, topotecan (T) 1.25 mg/m² CIV over 24 hours, days 2–6, and ara-C (A) 2 g/m² i.v. daily over 4 hours, days 2–6.[35] It was first studied in salvage setting in AML, ALL, and blast crisis of CML. Initial results are summarized in TABLE 6. The regimen was well tolerated, and CR remissions were observed in heavily pretreated patients with AML and CML-A/BC. The results were analyzed according to the stratification system for evaluating and selecting therapies in patients with relapsed/refractory AML, which determines the expected responses in patients with varying treatment histories.[39] The response rates in AML and CML BC/AP were according to expectations. In ALL, it seemed less active, and 1 CR in 11 patients with ALL was disappointing.[38]

In its modified version (cyclophosphamide 300 mg/m² every 12 hours, days 1-3) (ara-C 1 g/m² i.v. daily, days 2-6, and TPT 1.5 g/m² CIV over 24 hours daily, days 2-6), the CAT regimen was investigated first in previously untreated patients with an unfavorable prognosis karyotype AML aged <71 years. Treatment was well tolerated with only one induction death (6%). The CR rate was a surprising 83%, and

TABLE 6. Topotecan, cyclophosphamide, and ARA-C in refractory/relapsed AML, ALL and CML BP/AP[a]

Disease	Patients (n)	Number CR (%)
AML	52	10 (19)
ALL	11	1 (7)
CML-AP	11	2 (18)
CML-BP	17	7 (41)

[a]Cortes et al.[38] AP, accelerated phase; BP, blastic phase of CML. Cortes et al., unpublished data.

TABLE 7. Treatment of newly diagnosed AML with CAT. Patient characteristics and response to induction chemotherapy in "favorable" and "unfavorable" cytogenetic category[a]

Characteristics		Favorable (n = 96)			Unfavorable (n = 60)		
		Total no.	CR (%)	ED (%)	Total no.	CR (%)	ED (%)
Age (yr)	≤64	60	44 (73)	2 (3)	42	22 (52)	5 (12)
	>64	16	11 (68)	3 (19)	18	5 (28)	8 (44)
PS	≤2	72	53 (74)	3 (4)	50	24 (40)	7 (14)
	>2	4	2 (50)	2 (50)	7	0	6 (86)
AHD	0	51	36 (70)	5 (10)	33	18 (54)	6 (30)
	>0	24	18 (75)	0	29	9 (30)	7 (26)
Karyotype							
inv16, t(8;21)		11	10 (91)	1 (9)	—	—	
Diploid		65	45 (69)	4 (6)	—	—	
±8		—	—		5	3 (60)	0
−5/−7, 11Q		—	—		37	15 (40)	8 (22)
Others		—	—		18	9 (50)	5 (28)
Total				5 (6.5)	60	27 (45)	13 (22)

the regimen was subsequently investigated in the setting of frontline treatment of all newly diagnosed HR MDS and AML (excluding acute promyelocytic leukemias). Preliminary analyses of the results were reported separately for a "good prognosis" karyotype, that is, diploid, t(8;21), inv16 (40), and a "poor prognosis" karyotype including all other patients.[41] TABLE 7 summarizes the updated results of CAT induction therapy (Kantarjian et al., in preparation). The rate of CR was higher and treatment-associated mortality lower in patients with a "favorable" karyotype. Although final assessment and comparison of response rates to other high dose chemotherapeutic regimens such as idarubicin + high dose ara-C (IA), FLAG, or FLAG with idarubicin (FLAG-Ida) await appropriate covariate-adjusted analyses, it appears that CAT is equivalent to anthracycline–high dose ara-C regimens. With a lower overall mortality and lack of cardiotoxicity it may be a useful alternative antileukemic induction regimen.

In patients with HR MDS, the preliminary comparison with TA indicates that the addition of cyclophosphamide did not increase response rates, while it may have increased toxicity.[19] Again, final judgment must come from an appropriate covariate adjusted analysis after a longer follow-up.

TOPOTECAN COMBINATIONS IN NON-HODGKIN'S LYMPHOMA

Responses of low and intermediate grade non-Hodgkin's lymphomas, refractory to or relapsing after an anthracycline-containing regimen, to either TPT[7] or paclitaxel[42] were reported. Combination of TPT and paclitaxel in refractory/relapsed/diffuse large B-cell, peripheral T-cell, follicular center-cell grade 3, and anaplastic large cell lymphomas is currently under study.[39] Preliminary results with this regimen (paclitaxel 200 mg/m^2 i.v. over 3 hours on day 1, TPT 1 mg/m^2 short i.v. infusion, daily, days 1–5) were recently reported.[43] Responses were assessed after three courses and evaluated separately in primary refractory and resistant diseases. Of a total of 33 patients, 14 achieved PR and 3 achieved CR. Responses (CR + PR) were observed in 72% of patients with relapsed and 27% in primary refractory disease.[43] The regimen was well tolerated, appears more active than either single agent, and is comparable to cyclophosphamide/paclitaxel. The study continues to accrue patients.

The combination of TPT (1.5 mg/m^2 per day, days 1–5) followed by oral etoposide 50 mg twice daily, days 6–12 every 28 days for six courses, was investigated in 22 patients with relapsed/refractory intermediate grade non-Hodgkin's lymphoma. Most patients received only one prior regimen (CHOP), and 17 achieved CR or PR. Upon relapse, 12 patients were classified as being at low/low intermediate and seven at high intermediate risk according to the International Prognostic Index. Treatment was associated with significant hematologic toxicity (grade III/IV neutropenia in 19 of 22 patients and thrombocytopenia in 6 of 12 patients), preventing delivery of the scheduled etoposide dose in 16 of 22 patients. Only 4 of 20 patients received the scheduled 6 cycles. Nonhematologic toxicity was mild. Because of the marked myelosuppression associated with only modest activity (4 PR, no CR), this regimen will unlikely find use in the salvage treatment of non-Hodgkin's lymphoma.

SUMMARY AND CONCLUSIONS

The activity of single agent topotecan was documented in relapsed/refractory acute leukemias, accelerated and blastic phases of CML, MDS, myeloma, and low/intermediate grade lymphoma. Topotecan was particularly active in previously untreated, high-risk MDS and CMML. The combination of TPT with ara-C was highly effective in high risk MDS/CMML, and a regimen of cyclophosphamide, ara-C, and topotecan (CAT) was effective in refractory/relapsed AML and CML-AP/blastic phase. In newly diagnosed AML, the activity of the CAT regimen is comparable to that of other high intensity induction regimens, such as combinations of high dose ara-C with anthracyclines (idarubicin–ara-C) or with fludarabine (FA, FLAG) and FLAG + idarubicin (FLAG-Ida). In HR MDS and AML, TPT will likely continue to be explored as an alternative drug to, for example, anthracycline antibiotics or fludarabine in combination regimens. Its value as a single agent, particularly in MDS/CMML, will continue to be assessed when oral preparation becomes available. Of particular interest is the use of oral TPT and its combinations in postremission management of MDS, CMML, and elderly patients with AML. The optimal delivery of TPT, such as the length of administration (short versus continuous infusions), dose intensity, and sequencing in combination with other drugs, needs to be further explored. Better assessment of the value of TPT in the treatment of lymphomas awaits the results of ongoing clinical trials.

REFERENCES

1. OHNO, R., K. OKADA, T. MASAOKA, et al. 1990. An early phase Ii study of CPT-11. A new derivative of camptothecin for the treatment of leukemia and lymphoma. J. Clin. Oncol. **8**: 1907–1912.
2. KANTARJIAN, H.M., M. BERAN, A. ELLIS, et al. 1993. Phase I study of topotecan, a new topoisomerase I inhibitor in patients with refractory or relapsed acute leukemia. Blood **81**: 1146–1151.
3. ROWINSKY, E.K., A.A. ADJEI, R.C. DONEHOWER, et al. 1994. Phase I and pharmacodynamic study of the topoisomerase I-inhibitor topotecan in patients with refractory acute leukemia. J. Clin. Oncol. **12**: 2193–2203.
4. ROWINSKY, E.K., S.H. KAUFMANN, S.D. BAKER, et al. 1996. A phase I and pharmacological study of topotecan infused over 30 minutes for five days in patients with refractory acute leukemia. Clin. Cancer Res. **2**: 1921–1930.
5. UCKUM, F.M., C.F. STEWARD, G. REAMAN, et al. 1995. In vitro and in vivo activity of topotecan against human 8-lineage acute lymphoblastic leukemia cells. Blood **85**: 2817–2828.
6. GORE, S.D., E.K. ROWINSKY, C.B. MILLER, et al. 1998. A phase II "window" study of topotecan in untreated patients with high risk adult acute lymphoblastic leukemia. Clin. Cancer Res. **4**: 2677–2689.
7. PRETI, H.H. et al. 2000. J. Clin. Oncol. In press.
8. O'BRIEN, S., H. KANTARJIAN, A. ELLIS, et al. 1995. Topotecan in chronic myelogenous leukemia. Cancer **75**: 1104–1108.
9. POTMESIL, M., Y.H. HSIANG, L.F. LIU, et al. Resistance of human leukemic and normal lymphocytes to drug-induced DNA cleavage and low levels of DNA topoisomerase II. Cancer Res. 48.
10. ANDREEFF, M., Z. DARPYNKIEWICZ, T.L. SHARPLESS, et al. 1980. Discrimination of human leukemia subtypes by flow cytometric analysis of cellular DNA and RNA. Blood **55**: 282.
11. DEL PINO, G., J.S. SKIERSKI & A. DARPYNKIEWICZ. 1991. The concentration dependent diversity of effects of DNA topoisomerase I and II inhibitors on the cell cycle of HL-60 cells. Exp. Cell Res. **195**: 485–491.
12. VALKOV, N.I. & D.A. SULLIVAN. 1997. Drug resistance to DNA topoisomerase I and II inhibitors in human leukemia, lymphoma and multiple myeloma. Sem. Hematol. **34**: 48–62.
13. POMMIER, Y., P. PAURGUIER, Y. URASAKI, et al. 1999. Topoisomerase I inhibitors: selectivity and cellular resistance. Drug Resistance Updates **2**: 307–318.
14. KRAUT, E.H., J.J. CROWLEY, J.L. WADE, et al. 1998. Evaluation of topotecan in resistant and relapsing multiple myeloma: a Southwest Oncology Group Study. J. Clin. Oncol. **16**: 589–592.

15. APPELBAUM, F.R. & J. ANDERSON. 1998. Allogeneic bone marrow transplantation for myelodysplastic syndromes: outcomes analysis according to IPSS score. Leukemia **12:** 25–29.
16. BERAN, M., H.M. KANTARJIAN, S. O'BRIEN, *et al.* 1996. Topotecan, a topoisomerase I inhibitor, is active in the treatment of myelodysplastic syndrome and chronic myelomonocytic leukemia. Blood **88:** 2473–2479.
17. BERAN, M., E. ESTEY, S.M. O'BRIEN, *et al.* 1998. Results of topotecan single-agent therapy in patients with myelodysplastic syndromes and chronic myelomonocytic leukemia. Leukemia Lymphoma **31:** 521–531.
18. BERAN, M., E. ESTEY, S. O'BRIEN, *et al.* 1999. Topotecan and cytarabine is an active combination regimen in myelodysplastic syndromes and chronic myelomonocytic leukemia. J. Clin. Oncol. **17:** 2819–2830.
19. BERAN, M. 2000. Intensive chemotherapy of patients with high-risk myelodysplastic syndrome. Int. J. Hematol. **72:** 139–150.
20. SEITER, K., E.J. FELDMAN, H.D. HALICKA, *et al.* 1997. Phase I clinical and laboratory evaluation of topotecan and cytarabine in patients with acute leukemia. J. Clin. Oncol. **15:** 44–51.
21. MATSUMOTO, N., S. NAKANO, T. ESAKI, *et al.* 1995. Sequence-dependent modulation of anticancer drug activities by 7-ethyl-10-hydroxycamptothecin in an HST-1 human squamous carcinoma cell line. Anticancer Res. **15:** 405–410.
22. EDER, J.P., M. IKEBE, N. WONG, *et al.* 1996. CPT-11/topoisomerase II (topo II) inhibitor combination therapy: molecular pharmacology and therapeutic response. Proc. Am. Assoc. Cancer Res. **37:** abstr. 430.
23. WHITACRE, C.M., E. ZBOROWSKA, N.H. GORDON, *et al.* 1997. Topotecan increases topoisomerase IIa levels and sensitivity to treatment with etoposide in a schedule-dependent process. Cancer Res. **57:** 1425–1428.
24. ECKARDT, J.R., H.A. BURRIS, D.D. VON HOFF, *et al.* 1994. Measurement of tumor topoisomerase I and II levels during the sequential administration of topotecan and etoposide. Proc. Am. Soc. Clin. Oncol. **13:** abstr. 358.
25. RUBIN, E., V. WOOD, A. BHARTI, *et al.* 1995. A phase I and pharmacokinetic study of a new camptothecin derivative, 9-aminocamptothecin. Clin. Cancer Res. **1:** 269–276.
26. MURREN, J.R., S. ANDERSON, J. FEDELE, *et al.* 1997. Dose-escalation and pharmacodynamic study of topotecan inn combination with cyclophosphamide in patients with refractory cancer. J. Clin. Oncol. **15:** 148–157.
27. KAUFMANN, S.C., D. PEEREBOOM, C.H.-A. BUCKWALTER, *et al.* 1996. Cytotoxic effects of topotecan combined with various anticancer agents in human cancer cell lines. J. Natl. Cancer Inst. **88:** 734–741.
28. MURREN, J.R., S. ANDERSON, J. FEDELE, *et al.* 1997. Dose-escalation and pharmacodynamic study of topotecan in combination with cyclophosphamide in patients with refractory cancer. J. Clin. Oncol. **15:** 148–157.
29. THIELMAN, H.W., O. POPANDA, R. GERSBACH, *et al.* 1993. Various inhibitors of DNA topoisomerases diminish repair-specific DNA incision in UV-irradiated human fibroblasts. Carcinogenesis **14:** 2341–2351.
30. VEY, N., H. KANTARJIAN, M. BERAN, *et al.* 1999. Combination of topotecan with cytarabine or etoposide in patients with refractory or relapsed acute myeloid leukemia: results of a randomized phase I/II study. Invest. New Drugs **17:** 89–95.
31. CRUMP, M., J. LIPTON, D. HEDLEY, *et al.* 1999. Phase I trial of sequential topotecan followed by etoposide in adults with myeloid leukemia: a National Cancer Institute of Canada Clinical Trials Group Study. Leukemia **13:** 343–347.
32. MAINWARING, M.G., J.J. LYNCH, V. REDDY, *et al.* 1999. Phase II study of timed sequential chemotherapy with topotecan followed by mitoxantrone + etoposide in the treatment of refractory leukemia and lymphoma. Blood **10:** 509a (abstr. 2280).
33. HAMMOND, L.A., J.R. ECKARDT, R. GANAPATHI, *et al.* 1998. A phase I and translational study of sequential administration of the topoisomerase I and II inhibitors topotecan and Etoposide. Clin. Cancer Res. **4:** 1459–1467.
34. GUPTA, E., D. TOPPMEYER, R. ZALNEK, *et al.* 1998. Clinical evaluation of sequential topoisomerase targeting treatment in advanced malignancies. Cancer Therapeutics **1:** 292–301.

35. Hoogstraaten, B. 1960. Cyclophosphamide (Cytoxan) in acute leukemia: preliminary report. Cancer Chemother. Rep. **8:** 116–119.
36. Pierce, M., N. Shore, A. Sitarf, *et al.* 1966. Cyclophosphamide therapy in acute leukemia of childhood. Cooperative study conducted by members of Children's Cancer Cooperative Group A. Cancer **19:** 1551–1560.
37. Johnson, R.K., F.L. McCabe & Y. Yu. 1992. Combination regimens with topotecan in animal tumor models. Ann. Oncol. **3:** 85.
38. Cortes, J., E. Estey, M. Beran, *et al.* 2000. Cyclophosphamide, ara-C and topotecan (CAT) for patients with refractory or relapsed acute leukemia. Leukemia Lymphoma **36:** 479–484.
39. Estey, E., S. Kornblau, S. Pierce, *et al.* 1996. A stratification system for evaluating and selecting therapies in patients with relapsed or primary refractory acute myelogenous leukemia. Blood **88:** 756.
40. Estey, E., H. Kantarjian, F.J. Giles & M. Beran. 1998. Treatment of newly-diagnosed AML and MDS with cyclophosphamide, ara-C, topotecan. Blood **92:** 951.
41. Beran, M., F.J. Giles, J.E. Cortes, *et al.* 1999. Comparison of the cyclophosphamide ©, Ara-C (A), topotecan (T)(CAT) regimen to ara-C plus topotecan or idarubicin (I) as initial therapy for patients with adverse abnormal karyotype acute myeloid leukemia (AML). Blood **94:** 4213.
42. Younes, A., J.P. Ayoub, A. Sarris, *et al.* 1997. Paclitaxel activity for the treatment of non-Hodgkin's lymphoma: final report of a phase II trial. Br. J. Haematol. **96:** 328–332.
43. Younes, A., N. Okpara, J.E. Romaguera, *et al.* 1999. Phase II study of paclitaxel plus topotecan with G-CSF support for the treatment of relapsed and refractory aggressive non-Hodgkin's lymphoma. Blood **94:** 270b, abstr. 4421.
44. Crump, M., R. Meyer, S. Conban, *et al.* 1994. Phase II study of topotecan + etoposide in patients with aggressive histology non-Hodgkin's lymphoma (NHL). Blood **94:** abstr. 2353.

DX-8951f: Summary of Phase I Clinical Trials

R. DE JAGER, P. CHEVERTON, K. TAMANOI, J. COYLE, M. DUCHARME,
N. SAKAMOTO, M. SATOMI, M. SUZUKI, AND
THE DX-8951f INVESTIGATORS

Daiichi Pharmaceutical Corporation (USA); Daiichi Pharmaceutical Limited (UK); Daiichi Pharmaceutical Co., Ltd. (Japan); Phoenix International Life Sciences Inc. (Canada)

ABSTRACT: Exatecan mesylate (DX-8951f) is a new hexacyclic camptothecin analogue with favorable attributes compared to topotecan and CPT-11, including watersolubility, greater potency against topoisomerase I, lack of esterase-dependent activation, broad antitumor activity, and low cross-resistance against MDR-1 overexpressing tumors. In preclinical studies, the compound demonstrated a favorable toxicology profile with hematologic dose-limiting toxicity and moderate gastrointestinal toxicity, linear pharmacokinetics, P450 hepatic metabolism (CYP3A4 and CYP1A2), and predominately fecal excretion. The results of six U.S. and European phase I clinical trials as well as two Japanese studies are presented including total DX-8951 and lactone DX-8951 pharmacokinetics. The toxicity profile was similar for all schedules of administration. Hematologic toxicity was dose-dependent and reversible. Neutropenia was dose-limiting in minimally pretreated patients, whereas neutropenia and thrombocytopenia were dose-limiting in heavily pretreated patients. Non-hematologic toxicity included moderate gastrointestinal toxicity (nausea, vomiting>diarrhea), transient elevation of hepatic transaminases, asthenia, and alopecia. Two cases of acute pancreatitis not predicted by preclinical toxicology were also observed. Antineoplastic activity was detected in several solid tumor types: non-small cell lung cancer, extrapulmonary small cell cancer, colorectal cancer, hepatocellular cancer, and sarcoma. Antitumor activity was seen in CPT-11 and topotecan-resistant tumors. Pharmacokinetics were linear within the dose range tested. A pharmacokinetic/pharmacodynamic model predictive of DX-8951f–induced neutropenia in individual patients was developed. The daily ×5, every 3-week schedule with the drug administered as a 30-minute intravenous infusion was selected for future phase II clinical trials based on its superior antitumor activity.

INTRODUCTION

Exatecan mesylate (DX-8951f, Daiichi Pharmaceutical Co., Ltd., Japan) was synthesized to impart greater antitumor efficacy and less toxicity than those of existing camptothecin analogues such as CPT-11 and topotecan. DX-8951f: (1,5,9,5)-1-amino-9-ethyl-5-fluoro-1,2,3,9,12,15-hexahydro-9-hydroxy-4-methyl-10H-benzo(de) pyrano (3,4: 6,7) indolizino (1,2-b) quinoline-10,13-dione monomethanesulfonate (salt), dihydrate is a water-soluble, fluorinated, hexacyclic camptothecin derivative that, unlike CPT-11, does not require metabolic activation. The anhydrous

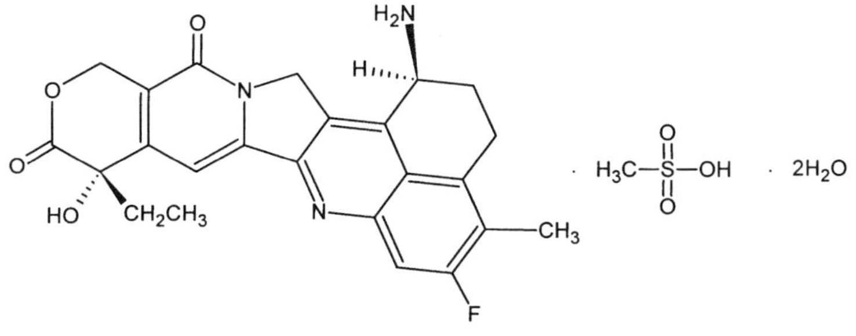

DX-8951f: Monomethanesulfonate dihydrate
DX-8951:   Anhydrous free base

Molecular Weight: 567.59 (DX-8951f, monomethanesulfonate dihydrate)
                    435.45 (DX-8951, anhydrous free base)

FIGURE 1. Chemical structure of DX-8951f.

free-base form of the drug is referred to as DX-8951. The chemical structure is shown in FIGURE 1. Similar to other camptothecin derivatives, the lactone form of DX-8951 is hydrolyzed into an open-ring hydroxy-acid form. The two species coexist in solution according to a reversible pH-dependent equilibrium. DX-8951f was approximately 3 times more potent than SN-38, the active metabolite of CPT-11, 10 times more potent than topotecan, and 20 times more potent than camptothecin as an inhibitor of topoisomerase I activity *in vitro*, and 5 times more potent than SN-38 as an inhibitor of DNA synthesis. The inhibition of human topoisomerase I by the lactone form was about 300-fold more potent than that by the hydroxy-acid form.

In cell-based cytotoxicity assays, DX-8951f was 7–30 times more active than SN-38 or topotecan against a wide range of breast, lung, gastrointestinal, prostate, brain, and pediatric tumor cell lines. DX-8951f was also effective in inhibiting the growth of clonogenic cells from human head and neck, liver, non-small cell lung, breast, colon, and ovarian and prostate tumors *in vitro*. DX-8951f has shown activity *in vivo* against a wide range of human tumor xenografts in nude mice, including gastric, pancreatic, colon, breast, ovary, and lung tumors.[1–5] In addition, DX-8951f exhibited potent antitumor activity in an intracranial xenograft of human RH 30 rhabdomyosarcoma, murine lung and liver metastasis models, and early and late disease models of human acute myelogenous leukemia.[6,7] Several *in vitro* and *in vivo* experiments using human tumor cell lines and drug-resistant variants have demonstrated that DX8951f, unlike SN-38 or topotecan, is not affected by mechanisms of drug resistance based on the overexpression of P glycoprotein or the decrease in levels of topoisomerase I mRNA or protein.[8] DX-8951f is not a substrate for the P glycoprotein multidrug carrier associated with the MDR phenotype, whereas topotecan and SN-38 are weak substrates. Studies in the *in vivo* homologous Meth A mouse fibrosarcoma model demonstrated that a cyclical dosing pattern gave superior antitumor activity, at lower doses of DX-8951f, than was seen with single dose administration.

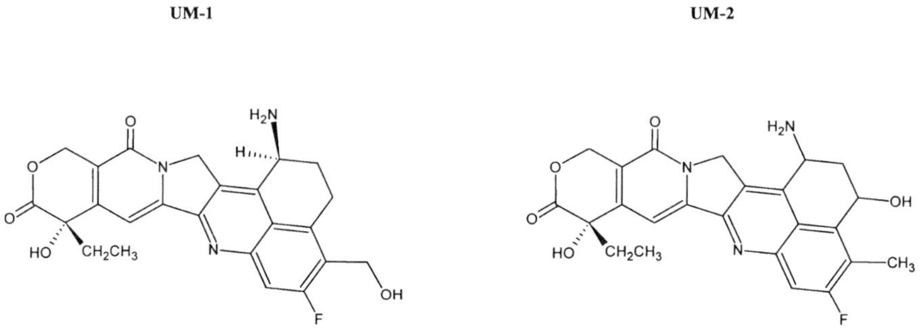

FIGURE 2. DX-8951f metabolites.

Preclinical pharmacologic and toxicologic studies were performed in rodents and dogs. ^{14}C-DX-8951f and high-performance liquid chromotography were used for differential quantification of total drug and lactone. Pharmacokinetic studies in mice and dogs showed that the t½ for lactone and total DX-8951 was similar, that the area under the concentration time curve (AUC) for the lactone was approximately 50% of the total drug AUC, and that the AUC was linearly related to the dose. The distribution of DX-8951 into tissues was reported in all species tested. Very low levels were detected in brain tissue. Therefore, DX-8951 does not appear to cross the intact blood brain barrier. DX-8951 is highly bound to plasma proteins.

In vitro, the observed plasma protein binding values were approximately 93% in the rat, 86% in the dog, 96% in the monkey, and 97% in man. Metabolic in vitro studies using human liver microsomes indicate that CYP3A4 and CYP1A2 of the P450 superfamily of enzymes play key roles in the metabolism of DX-8951, resulting in the formation of two hydroxylated metabolites, UM-1 and UM-2 (FIG. 2).[9,10]

Antitumor activity of both metabolites is much less potent than that of DX-8951f. The principal route of excretion was the feces (70–90%), whereas 10–25% of the drug was recovered in the urine. The toxicity profile was consistent across animal species: hematologic toxicity (anemia, neutropenia, lymphopenia, and thrombocytopenia), gastrointestinal toxicity (vomiting, diarrhea), and alopecia. Hematologic toxicity was schedule- and dose-dependent. Neutropenia was the dose-limiting toxicity. The dog was the most sensitive species. The human equivalent of the 1/3 dog toxic dose low was used to determine the starting dose for each corresponding schedule of administration in human clinical trials.

GLOBAL PHASE I CLINICAL DEVELOPMENT

DX-8951f was tested according to a parallel and integrated phase I clinical development plan in the United States, Europe, and Japan with the goal of selecting a single best dosing regimen for future phase II studies. To achieve this goal, a core protocol was established to standardize clinical data evaluation including: toxicity and efficacy criteria; definitions of dose-limiting toxicity (DLT) and maximal tolerated dose (MTD); inclusion and exclusion criteria; and supportive therapy. Data were ex-

TABLE 1. Parallel development in 3 regions

PRT 001, 30 min, every 3 weeks
Institute Gustave Roussy (France)
National Cancer Center East (Japan)
PRT 002, 30 min, daily 5 days, every 3 weeks
Institute for Drug Development (USA)
National Cancer Center Hospital (Japan)
PRT 003, 24 hr, every 3 weeks
MD Anderson Cancer Center (USA)
PRT 004, 24 hr, weekly
Memorial Sloan-Kettering Cancer Center (USA)
PRT 005, Cont., 5 days – 21 days
Institute for Drug Development (USA)
PRT 006, 30 min, weekly
The Churchill, Oxford Radcliffe Hospital (UK)
Vrije Universiteit Amsterdam (The Netherlands)

changed in a timely manner among the three regions so that all investigators had access to the data necessary for decision-making as dose escalation was in progress. Data collection and processing were done in compliance with the ICH guidelines.[11]

Six phase I studies were conducted outside of Japan according to three schedules of administration and two durations of intravenous infusion (TABLE 1). Two studies were duplicated in Japan. However, these Japanese studies included the pharmacokinetics of DX-8951 lactone as well as total DX-8951, whereas the other studies were limited to the measurement of total DX-8951 due to logistical considerations.

STUDY OBJECTIVES

For each dosage regimen and duration of infusion of DX-8951f, the objectives of the studies were to determine the MTD, DLT, toxicity profile, pharmacokinetics, and pharmacodynamics; to detect evidence of antitumor activity; and to define a dose for phase II studies. The selection of a single dosage regimen for phase II studies was to be based on a comparison of the results of the six individual phase I clinical trials.

STARTING DOSE AND DOSE ESCALATION

For each study, the starting dose was chosen as 1/3 of the toxic dose low for the corresponding schedule of administration in the dog, which was the most sensitive species. There was no standardization of the method of dose escalation. A modified Fibonacci method was used in studies PRT 001, 006, and the two Japanese studies, whereas a modified continual reassessment method was used in studies PRT 002, 003, 004, and 005.[12,13] No significant differences were noted between the two methods in terms of number of dose escalation steps. MTDs were determined separately for minimally (MP) and heavily pretreated patients (HP). HP patients were defined as those who had received more than six courses of alkylating-agent–containing chemotherapy (or more than four courses of carboplatin), radiation therapy to more than 25% of hematopoietic reserves, and two or more courses of mitomycin C or nitrosurea. All toxic effects were graded according to the National Cancer Institute Common Toxicity Criteria. DLT was defined as: febrile ($\geq 38.5°C$) or 5-day grade 4 neutropenia; other grade 4 hematologic toxicity; grade 4 vomiting with maximum supportive care; any grade 3 nonhematologic toxicity (excluding nausea and vomiting); any grade 3 or higher adverse event requiring intensive care treatment; or the inability to start a second course after a 2-week delay due to toxicity. The MTD was defined as the dose at which 20% of patients experienced DLT during the first course.

PHARMACOKINETIC AND PHARMACODYNAMIC ANALYSIS

The pharmacokinetics of DX-8951 were determined in all phase I studies (PRT001 to PRT006) using standard noncompartmental and compartmental pharmacokinetic methodologies.[14–17] The latter methodology was used in addition to noncompartmental analysis in order to obtain additional protein kinase (PK) parameters, a better understanding of the pharmacokinetics of the drug, as well as more information on the relationship between the pharmacokinetics of the drug and its pharmacological effects as it relates to toxicity.

Compartmental PK/PD analyses were performed with a population methodology (IT2S) in order to obtain more robust estimations of the individual PK and PK/PD parameters.[18] No evidence of nonlinear pharmacokinetics (e.g., "hockey-stick" profiles, change in elimination of the drug between different study days) could be seen when looking at each individual patient plots of plasma concentrations versus time following administration of the drug by different regimens. Discrimination between different pharmacokinetic models was performed for each study by minimizing the Akaike information criterion test and optimizing both the fitted versus the observed concentrations versus time and the weighted residuals versus the observed values relationship. The most appropriate pharmacokinetic model to describe DX8951 plasma concentrations and excreted urinary amounts for each study is presented in FIGURE 3.

When the drug was given by a 24-hour infusion and concentrations available for 24 hours after a dose (PRT003), the quality of the fitting was as good using a two- or three-compartment model. Therefore, the first model was chosen because it is simpler. When DX-8951f was given as a 24-hour infusion and concentrations available for only 6 hours after a dose, a single compartment model fitted the data as well as the two- or three-compartment one. These observations are not surprising, as a 24-hour–hour constant infusion may mask a distribution phase (hence, a two-compartment appears as good as a three-compartment), and the lack of plasma observations after 6 hours prevents one from capturing the terminal elimination phase of the drug (hence, a one-compartment appears as good as a three-compartment). The relationship between the pharmacokinetics of DX8951 and its pharmacological effects on platelets and neutrophils was investigated using regression analysis. These clearly indicated that DX8951 exposure (i.e., the area under the plasma concentration time

TABLE 2. Distribution of Patients ($n = 165$)

Schedule		30-min infusion	24-h infusion
d 1 q3wk	(E)	12	22
	(J)	15	
d 1-5 q3wk	(US)	36	25[a]
	(J)	28	
wk ×3 q4wk	(E)	35	27

[a] 5–21 day CIVI.

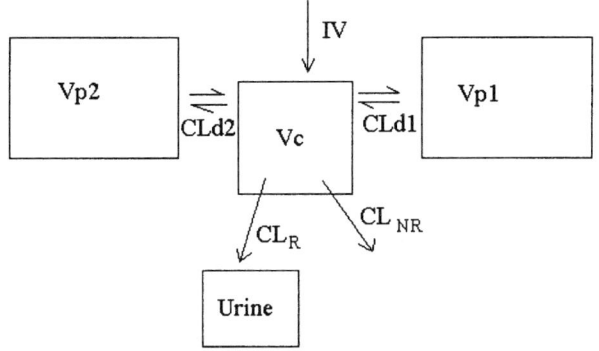

IV: Intravenous administration rate (mg/h); Vc: Central volume of distribution (L);
CLd1: distributional clearance between Vp1 and Vc (L/h);
Vp1: First peripheral volume of distribution (L);
CLd2: distributional clearance between Vp2 and Vc (L/h);
Vp2: Second peripheral volume of distribution (L);
CL_R: Renal clearance (L/h); CL_{NR}: non-renal clearance (L/h);

FIGURE 3. Structural pharmocokinetic model for DX-8951.

curve [AUC]) was related to the decrease in the neutrophil and platelet counts in every subject. All neutrophil and platelet counts were therefore modeled in each subject using the indirect response PK/PD model.[14]

PATIENT DISTRIBUTION

A total of 201 patients were enrolled in phase I studies: 127 patients received DX-8951f as a 30-minute infusion and 74 patients were treated by intermittent 24-hour or continuous 5–21-day infusions. The distribution by study is shown in TABLE 2. The 5–21 day continuous infusion study was still ongoing at the time of this writing.

TOXICITY

The toxicity profile was similar for all schedules of administration. Hematologic toxicity was dose-dependent and predictable. Neutropenia was dose-limiting in MP

TABLE 3. Comparison of PK models for 30-minute and 24-hour continuous infusions

Study	Administration regimen of DX8951	Sampling strategy	Most appropriate PK model to describe plasma concentrations of DX8951
PRT002	30-minute constant infusion daily for 5 consecutive days	Multiple plasma samples on day 1 and day 5 (until 24 hours after each dose), Cmin on days 2, 3, and 4	3-compartment linear PK model
PRT003	24-hour continuous infusion every 3 weeks	Multiple plasma samples during infusion and for 24 hours following first infusion	2-compartment linear PK model
PRT004	24-hour continuous infusions every week for 3 weeks	Multiple plasma samples during infusion and 6 hours after the infusion on weeks 1 and 3.	1-compartment linear PK model

TABLE 4. DX-8951f: phase I studies MTDs

Schedule	MTD (mg/m^2/day)	>MTD (mg/m^2/day)	Prior treatment
d1, q 3wk (30-min)	5.33	7.1	MP/HP
d1-5, q 3wk (30-min)	0.5	0.6	MP
	0.3	0.4	HP
wk ×1, q 3wk (24-hr)	2.4	3.0	HP
	<2.4	3.6	HP
wk ×3, q 4wk (24-hr)	1.0	1.2	MP
	<0.8	0.8	HP
5-21d CIVI q 4wk (24-hr)	0.23	0.30	MP
	0.23	ND	HP
wk ×3, q 4wk (30-min)	2.75	3.13	MP
	2.06	2.35	HP

patients, whereas neutropenia and thrombocytopenia were dose-limiting in HP patients. Neutrophil and platelet count nadirs occurred between days 10 and 15, with recovery by day 22 in most patients receiving DX-8951f in 3-week courses. In studies in which DX-8951f was given according to a 4-week course, nonhematologic toxicity consisted mostly of mild to moderate (Grade 1 or 2) gastrointestinal toxicity (nausea/vomiting, diarrhea, stomatitis, asthenia, fever, and alopecia). Nausea and vomiting were controlled by standard antiemetic drugs (compazine, ondansetron). Transient and reversible elevation of serum transaminases were also observed. In addition, there were two cases (1%) of acute pancreatitis. Nonhematologic toxicities for the daily ×5, every 3 weeks (30-minute infusion) schedule are shown in TABLE 3.

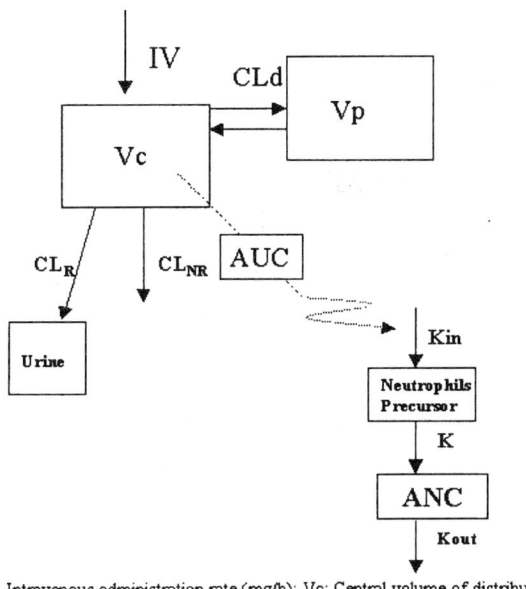

IV: Intravenous administration rate (mg/h); Vc: Central volume of distribution (L);
CLd: distributional clearance between Vp and Vc (L/h);
Vp: peripheral volume of distribution (L);
CL_R: Renal clearance (L/h); CL_{NR}: non-renal clearance (L/h);
AUC: Predicted total exposure of the drug following an administered dose (mcg.h/L)
Kin: Zero-order formation rate constant; K: first-order formation rate constant
ANC: Absolute neutrophil counts; Kout: First-order elimination rate constant of neutrophils

FIGURE 4. Structural pharmocokinetics pharmacodynamics model for DX-8951.

Values for the MTDs and stopping doses (>MTD) are listed in TABLE 4. The MTDs for MP patients were greater than the MTDs for HP patients except for the single-dose, every 3 weeks (30-minute) regimen for which a single MTD was determined for MP and HP patients. This study involved only 12 patients, and the MTD was close to the SD. The number of dose escalation steps in each study reflected the MTD/SD ratios and did not correlate with the dose escalation method. It was not possible to evaluate the impact of the modified continual reassessment method in these studies because of the small number of patients and because the opinion of investigators prevailed over the modified continual reassessment method-assigned doses at toxic dose levels.

ANTINEOPLASTIC ACTIVITY

Antitumor activity was detected in several solid tumor types including partial responses in non-small cell lung cancer, extrapulmonary small cell cancer, colorectal cancer, hepatocellular cancer, and sarcoma. Disease stabilization, including minor responses, was seen in colorectal cancer, hepatocellular cancer, prostate cancer, and peritoneal cancer. In particular, antitumor activity was seen in CPT-11–resistant and topotecan-resistant cancers.[19–31] The daily ×5 (30-minute), weekly ×3 and the 5–21

TABLE 5. Phase I studies: average PK parameters

Parameter	Pharmacokinetic methodology	
	Noncompartmental	Population compartmental
CL (L/h per m^2)	1.87 (67%)	1.63 (64%)
Fe (%)	N/C	9.9 (60%)
Vc (L per m^2)	N/C	6.4 (28.7%)
Vss (L per m^2)	17 (39%)	17.65 (28.9%)
T$_{1/2}$ (h)	9.1 (54%)	12.3 (60%)

TABLE 6. PK parameters: single dose, q3 weeks (n = 15)

Dose (mg/m^2)	Plasma		Urinary excretion	
	$\dfrac{AUC_{lactone}}{AUC_{total}}$	$\dfrac{AUC_{UM-1}}{AUC_{DX-8951}}$	DX-8951 (%)	UM-1 (%)
3	0.29 ± 0.12	0.04 ± 0.01	6.3 ± 1.6	10.5 ± 1.2
5	0.33 ± 0.05	0.05 ± 0.01	7.6 ± 3.0	15.6 ± 2.1
6.65	0.28 ± 0.09	0.04 ± 0.01	11.0 ± 5.3	19.2 ± 4.6
Total	0.30 ± 0.08	0.04 ± 0.01	8.7 ± 4.2	16.0 ± 4.5

H. Minami (ASCO, 1999.)

day (continuous infusion) regimens appeared to be more active than the single-dose regimens or the 24-hour intermittent regimens. There was no correlation between the number of patients showing antitumor effects and the dose intensity of the regimen used in individual studies. The daily ×5 (30-minute) regimen, which appeared to be the best in terms of antineoplastic activity, was selected for phase II trials, whereas the corresponding MTDs for MP and HP patients were selected as phase II doses.[32]

PHARMACOKINETICS AND PHARMACODYNAMICS

A summary of the average PK parameters along with their interindividual variability for all phase I studies can be found in TABLE 5. The pharmacokinetics of DX-8951 were linear within the range of doses tested. Plasma C$_{max}$ and AUC were linearly related to dose. There was no accumulation of the drug in the plasma over 5 days with the daily ×5 regimen in most patients. Clearance and Vss were dose-independent. Both total DX-8951 and its lactone form were measured only in the single-dose, every 3 weeks (30-minute) study conducted in Japan (TABLE 6). The lactone AUC was 30% of the AUC of the total DX-8951. The plasma AUC of the UM-1 metabolite was 4% of the total DX-8951 AUC. In the urine, 25% of the drug was recovered as DX-8951 with a 2:1 ratio between the UM-1 metabolite and DX-8951. Pharmacokinetic parameters were not different whether calculated by a noncompartmental or a compartmental method. The interindividual variability was within expected range. The PK model

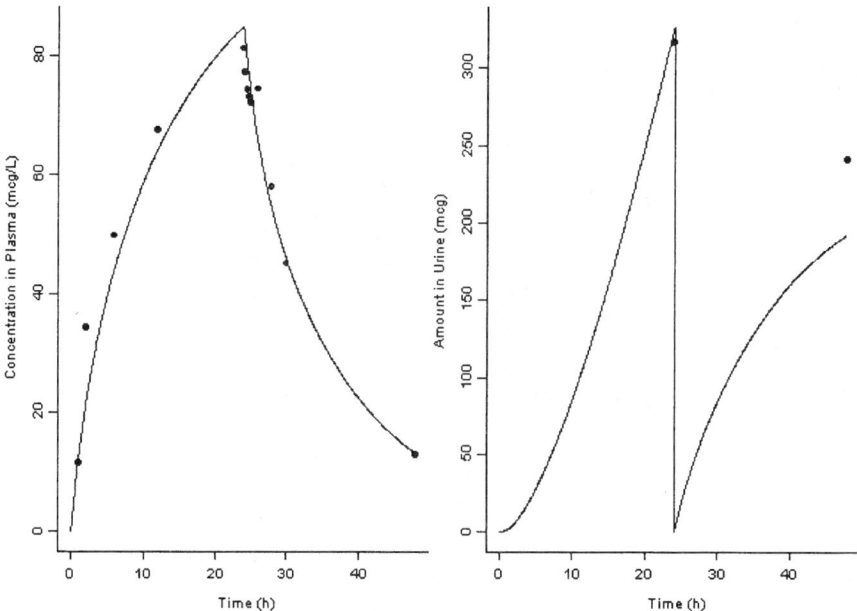

FIGURE 5. Comparison of predicted and observed plasma and urine concentations in a representative patient (PRT 003).

used in every study was explaining the observed plasma concentrations and excreted urinary amounts very well, as demonstrated by a representative patient from PRT003 (24-hour infusion) and PRT002 (5 days of daily administration): The pharmacokinetic/pharmacodynamic (PK/PD) correlation has been analyzed so far for the daily ×5 (30-minute) and single-dose (24-hour continuous infusion) studies. Using a population PK/PD method (IT2S), results were best described by a sigmoid E-max method or an E-max method. For PRT003, the relationship between the pharmacokinetics of the drug and the evolution in absolute neutrophil counts could be described by the PD parameters in TABLE 6. The neutrophil counts were associated with a normal elimination half-life of 15.2 hours (calculated as 0.693/Kout). The observed decrease in neutrophil counts started to occur (Tlag) on average 34 and 54 hours after the beginning of the first and second administration of DX8951, respectively. The duration of the inhibition in neutrophil production (Trel) by DX8951 appeared to be on average 352 and 342 hours for the first and second administration of the drug, respectively. The evolution in the absolute neutrophil counts in each subject was well explained by the PK/PD model, as demonstrated by the graph (FIG. 6) of the observed and fitted neutrophil counts versus time, coming from a representative patient. This PK/PD model may be very useful clinically and for future studies, as it may be able to predict in a given patient what dosing regimen of DX8951 would minimize the decrease in the absolute neutrophil counts.

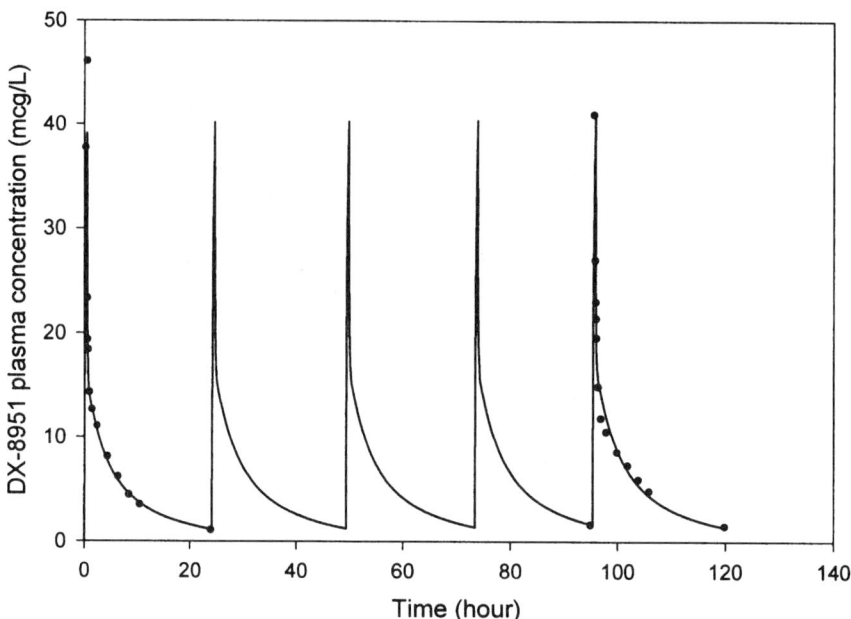

FIGURE 6. Comparison of predicted and observed plasma concentrations in a representative patient (PRT 002).

CONCLUSION

DX-8951f is a new camptothecin derivative that was selected for phase I clinical trials based on favorable characteristics identified during preclinical development, including broad spectrum *in vitro* and *in vivo* antitumor activity, the relative absence of cross-resistance with CPT-11 and topotecan, and a better safety profile than that of CPT-11. These preclinical observations were predictive of the results of the human phase I clinical studies. The safety profile, which is the same for all schedules tested, has been established. Neutropenia is the principal DLT. Thrombocytopenia may be associated with neutropenia in HP patients at the MTD. Gastrointestinal toxicity was moderate, consisting of nausea and vomiting controlled by standard anti-emetics In contrast to CPT11, severe diarrhea was not observed with DX-8951f. Other non–dose-limiting toxicities include asthenia, transient elevation of transaminases, moderate alopecia, fever, and mucositis. In addition to the favorable safety profile of DX-8951, the drug exhibited linear pharmacokinetics within the dose range listed, and antitumor activity was detected including that against CPT-11 and topotecan-resistant tumors. Based on the favorable results obtained in phase I clinical development, disease-oriented phase II studies of DX-8951f were initiated. The daily ×5, every 3 weeks schedule, with the drug administered as an (30-minute) intravenous infusion showed the most antitumor activity and was selected for phase II clinical trials.

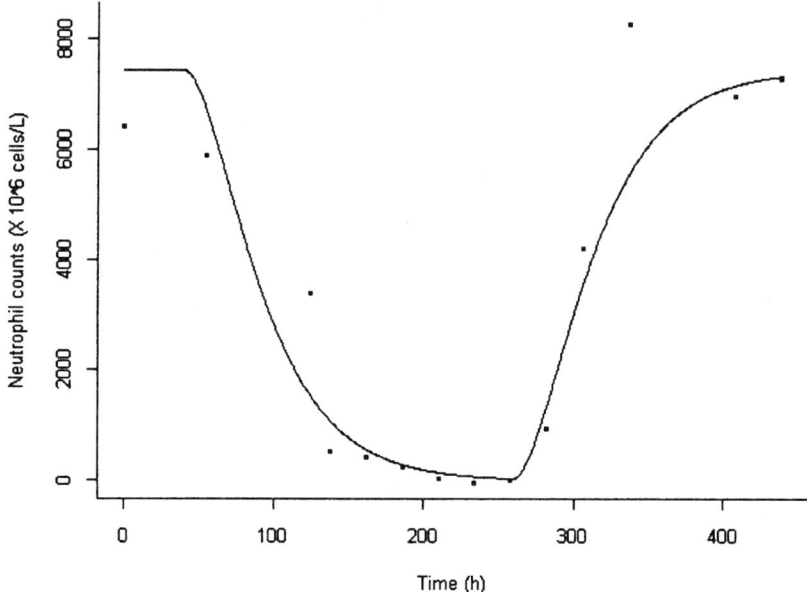

FIGURE 7. Comparison of predicted and observed values of ANC versus time.

TABLE 7. Correlation between the pharmacokinetic parameters and neutrophil counts

PD parameter	Patient average	Interindividual variability
Tlag 1	34.2 h	66%
Tlag 2	54.2 h	77%
Trel 1	352 h	20%
Trel 2	342 h	19%
Kout	0.046 h^{-1}	15
Emax	80%	N/C
AUC50	550 mcg.h/L	64%
K	38.6 h^{-1}	412%

APPENDIX: INVESTIGATORS

JEAN-PIERRE ARMAND, MD, ANDRE RAYMOND, MD, ERIC ROWINSKY, MD, and THOMAS JOHNSON, MD, *Institut Gustave Roussy, Villejuif, France*

CHARLES GEYER, MD and DANIEL VON HOFF, MD, *Cancer Treatment & Research Center, San Antonio, Texas*

MELANIE ROYCE, MD, PAULO HOFF, MD, and RICHARD PAZDUR, MD, *MD Anderson Cancer Center, Houston Texas*

LEONARD SALTZ, MD and SUNIL SHARMA, MD, *Memorial Sloan Kettering Cancer Center, New York*

DENNIS TALBOT, MD, *Oxford Radcliffe Hospital, Oxford, England*
EPIE BOVEN, MD, *Vrije Universiteit Amsterdam, Amsterdam, Netherlands*
YASUTSUNA SASAKI, MD and HIRONOBU MINAMI, MD, *National Cancer Center Hospital East, Tokyo, Japan*
TOMOHIDE TAMURA, MD and YASUHIRO SHIMADA, MD, *National Cancer Center Hospital, Tokyo, Japan*

REFERENCES

1. KUMAZAWA, E. & A. TOHGO. 1998. Antitumor activity of DX-8951f: a new camptothecin derivative. Exp. Opin. Invest. Drugs **7:** 625–632.
2. MITSUI, I., E. KUMAZAWA, Y. HIROTA, *et al.* 1995. A new water-soluble camptothecin-derivative, DX-8951f, exhibits potent antitumor activity against human tumors *in vitro and in vivo*. Jpn J. Cancer Res. **86:** 776–786.
3. TAKIGUCHI, S., A. TOHGO, *et al.* 1997. Antitumor effect of DX-8951, a novel campotothecin analog, on human pancreatic tumor cells and their CPT-11-resistant variants cultured *in vitro* and xenografted into nude mice. Jpn J. Cancer Res. **88:** 760–769.
4. LAWRENCE, R.A., E. IZBICKA, R.L. DE JAGER, *et al.* 1999. Comparison of DX-8951f and topotecan effects on tumor colony formation from freshly explanted adult and pediatric human tumor cells. Anti-Cancer Drugs **10:** 655–661.
5. KUMAZAWA, E., T. JIMBO, Y. OCHI & A. TOHGO. 1998. Potent and broad antitumor effects of DX-8951f, a water-soluble campothecin derivative, against various human tumors xenografted in nude mice. Cancer Chemother. Pharmacol. **42:** 210–220.
6. GONZALES, P., J. MARTY, S.D. STRINGER, *et al.* 2000. In vivo antitumor activity of DX-8951F against an intracranial sarcoma tumor model. Proc. Am. Assoc. Cancer Res. **41:** 1349.
7. VEY, N., F.J. GILES, H. KANTARJIAN, *et al.* 2000. The topoisomerase I inhibitor DX-8951f is active in a severe combined immunodeficient mouse model of human acute myelogenous leukemia. Clin. Cancer Res. **6:** 731–736.
8. JOTO, N., M. ISHII, M. MINAMI, *et al.* 1997. DX-8951f, a water-soluble campothecin analog, exhibits potent antitumor activity against a human lung cancer cell line and its SN-38 resistant variant. Int. J. Cancer **72:** 680–686.
9. OGUMA, T., Y. OSHIMA & M. NAKAOKA. 2000. Sensitive high-performance liquid chromatographic method for the determination of the lactone and lactone plus hydroxyacid forms of a new camptothecin derivative, DX-8951, in human plasma using fluorescence detection. J. Chromatogr. **740:** 237–245.
10. OGUMA, T., T. KONNO, A. INABA & M. NAKAOKA. 2000. Determination of DX-8951 and its main metabolite in human plasma and urine by high-performance liquid chroatography/atmospheric pressure chemical ionization tandem mass spectrometry. Biomed. Chromatogr. Submitted.
11. NATIONAL CANCER INSTITUTE. 1988. Guidelines for reporting of adverse drug reaction. Bethesda, MD, Division of Cancer Treatment, National Cancer Institute.
12. O'QUIGLEY, J., M. PEPE & L. FISHER. 1990. Continual reassessment method: a practical design for phase I clinical trials in cancer. Biometrics **46:** 33–48.
13. GOODMAN, S.N., M.L. ZAHURAK & S. PIANTADOSI. 1995. Some practical improvements in the continual reassessment method for phase I studies. Stat. Med. **14:** 1149–1161.
14. DAYANEKA, N.L., V. GARG & W.J. JUSKO. 1993. Comparison of four basic models of indirect pharmacodynamic responses. J. Pharmacokinet. Biopharm. **21:** 457–478.
15. GIBALDI, M. & D. PERRIER. 1982. Pharmacokinetics. 2nd Ed. Marcel Dekker Inc. New York.
16. WILLIAMS, M.L., I.W. WAINER, C.P. GRANVIL, *et al.* 1999. Pharmacokinetics of R- and (S)-cyclophosphamide and their dechloroethylated metabolites in cancer patients. Chirality **11:** 301–308.
17. YAMAOKA, K., T. NAKAGAWA & T. UNO. 1978. Application of Akaike's information criterion (AIC) in the evaluation of linear pharmacokinetic equations. J. Pharmacokinet. Biopharm. **6:** 165–175.

18. COLLINS, D. & A. FORREST. 1995. IT2S user's guide. State University of New York at Buffalo. Buffalo, New York.
19. JOHNSON, T., C. GEYER, R. DE JAGER, et al. 1998. Phase I and pharmacokinetic (PK) study of DX-8951f, a novel hexacyclic camptothecin (CPT) analog, on a daily for 5 days every 3 week schedule. Proc. Am. Soc. Clin. Oncol. **17:** 196a.
20. ROYCE, M., P.M. HOFF, R. BRITO, et al. 1998. Phase I trial of DX-895IF, a novel camptothecin analogue, administered by a 24-hour continuous infusion. Proc. Am. Soc. Clin. Oncol. **1:** 197a.
21. DAVIDSON, K., E. IZBICKA, R. LAWRENCE, et al. 1998. Anticancer activity of DX-8951f, a water soluble camptothecin analog against human tumor specimens taken directly from adult and pediatric patients. Proc. Am. Soc. Clin. Oncol. **17:** 197a.
22. JOHNSON, T., C. GEYER, R. DE JAGER, et al. 1998. A phase I and pharmacokinetic (PK) study of DX8951f, a novel hexacyclic camptothecin (CPT) analog, on a 30 minute infusion for 5 days every 3 week schedule. 10th NCI-EORTC Symposium on New Drugs in Cancer Therapy, Abstract 245.
23. HOFF, P.M., Y. LASSERE, M. ROYCE, et al. 1998. Phase I study of the new camptothecin analogue DX-8951f administrated by 24-hour continuous infusion. 10th NCI-EORTC Symposium on New Drugs in Cancer Therapy, Abstract 246.
24. ROWINSKY, E., T. JOHNSON, C. GEYER, et al. 1999. A phase I and pharmacokinetic (PK) study of DX-8951f, a hexacyclic camptothecin (CPT) analog on a daily ×5 day schedule. Proc. Am. Soc. Clin. Oncol. **18:** 632a.
25. ROYCE, M., Y. LASSERE, P. HOFF, et al. 1999. A phase I and pharmacokinetic (PK) study of DX-8951f, a hexacyclic camptothecin (CPT) analog administered by 24-hour continuous infusion to patients with advanced solid tumors. Proc. Am. Soc. Clin. Oncol. **18:** 682a.
26. SHARMA, S., N. KEMENY, G.K. SCHWARTZ, et al. 1999. A phase I study of topoisomerase I inhibitor DX-8951f given as a continuous infusion over 24 hours every three weeks. Proc. Am. Soc. Clin. Oncol. 18: 683a.
27. DE JAGER, R., T. OGUMA, T. KAJIMURA, et al. 1999. Comparison of DX-8951f of clinical and pre-clinical toxicokinetics (TK). Proc. Am. Soc. Clin. Oncol. **18:** 686a.
28. GEYER, C., L. HAMMOND, T. JOHNSON, et al. 1999. A phase I and pharmacokinetic study with escalation of both treatment duration and dose: dose schedule optimization of the hexacyclic camptothecin (cpt) analog DX-8951f. Proc. Am. Soc. Clin. Oncol. **18:** 813a.
29. BOVEN, E., M. SATOMI, M. SUZUKI, et al. 1999. Phase I and pharmacokinetic studies of DX08951f in patients with advanced tumours. 10th Conference on DNA Topoisomerse in Therapy, Abstract S30.
30. GONZALES, P., J. MARTY, S.D. STRINGER, et al. 2000. In vivo antitumor activity of DX-8951F against an intracranial sarcoma tumor model. Proc. Am. Assoc. Cancer Res. **41:** 1349.
31. GARRISON, M., L.A. HAMMOND, C. GEYER, et al. 2000. A Phase I and pharmacokinetic study of the camptothecin (CPT) analog DX-8951f (exetecan mesylate): escalating infusion and dose. Proc. Am. Soc. Clin. Oncol. **19:** 765.
32. ROWINSKY, E.K., T.R. JOHNSON & C.E. GEYER CE. 2000. DX-8951f (exatecan mesylate), a hexacyclic camptothecin anolog on a daily 5 schedule: a phase I and pharmacokinetic study in patients with advanced solid malignancies. J. Clin. Oncol. **18:** 3151–3163.

Cellular and Molecular Responses to Topoisomerase I Poisons

Exploiting Synergy for Improved Radiotherapy

SHIGEKI MIYAMOTO,[a] TONY T. HUANG,[a] SHELLY WUERZBERGER-DAVIS,[a] WILLIAM G. BORNMANN,[b] JOHN J. PINK,[c] COLLEEN TAGLIARINO,[c] TIMOTHY J. KINSELLA,[c] AND DAVID A. BOOTHMAN[c,d]

[a]*Department of Pharmacology, University of Wisconsin-Madison, Madison, Wisconsin 53792, USA*

[b]*Preparative Synthesis Core Facility, Memorial Sloan-Kettering Cancer Center, New York, New York 10021, USA*

[c]*Departments of Radiation Oncology & Pharmacology, Case Western Reserve University, Cleveland, Ohio 44106-4942, USA*

ABSTRACT: The efficacy of topoisomerase (Topo) I–active drugs may be improved by better understanding the molecular and cellular responses of tumor compared to normal cells after genotoxic insults. Ionizing radiation (IR) + Topo I–active drugs (e.g., Topotecan) caused synergistic cell killing in various human cancer cells, even in cells from highly radioresistant tumors. Topo I poisons had to be added either during or immediately after IR. Synergy was caused by DNA lesion modification mechanisms as well as by concomitant stimulation of two pathways of cell death: necrosis (IR) + apoptosis (Topo I poisons). Cumulative data favor a mechanism of synergistic cell killing caused by altered DNA lesion modification and enhanced apoptosis. However, alterations in cell cycle regulation may also play a role in the synergy between these two agents in certain human cancers. We recently showed that NF-κB, a known anti-apoptotic factor, was activated in various cancer cells after poisoning Topo I using clinically active drugs. NF-κB activation was dependent on initial nuclear DNA damage followed by cytoplasmic signaling events. Cytoplasmic signaling leading to NF-κB activation after Topo I poisons was diminished in cytoplasts (lacking nuclei) and in CEM/C2 cells that expressed a mutant Topo I protein that did not interact with Topo I–active drugs. NF-κB activation was intensified in S-phase and blocked by aphidicolin, suggesting that activation was a result of double-strand break formation due to Topo I poisoning and DNA replication. Dominant-negative IκB expression augmented Topo I poison-mediated apoptosis. Elucidation of molecular signal transduction pathways after Topo I drug–IR combinations may lead to improved radiotherapy by blocking anti-apoptotic NF-κB responses. Recent data also indicate that synergy caused by IR + Topo I poisons is different from radiosensitization by β-lapachone (β-lap), a "reported" Topo I and II-α poison *in vitro*. In fact, β-lap does not kill cells by poisoning either Topo I or II-α *in vivo*. Instead, the compound is "activated" by an IR (damage)–inducible enzyme,

---

[d]Address for correspondence: David A. Boothman, 10900 Euclid Avenue (BRB-326 East), Laboratory of Molecular Stress Responses, Case Western Reserve University, Cleveland, OH 44106-4942. Voice: 216-368-0840; fax: 216-368-1142.
dab30@po.cwru.edu

NAD(P)H:quinone oxidoreductase (NQO1), a gene cloned as x-ray-inducible transcript #3, xip3. Unlike the lesion modification pathway induced by IR + Topo I drugs, β-lap kills cells via NQO1 futile cycle metabolism. Downstream apoptosis caused by β-lap appears to be noncaspase-mediated, involving calpain or a calpain-like protease. Thus, although Topo I poisons or β-lap in combination with IR both synergistically kill cancer cells, the mechanisms are very different.

INTRODUCTION

Topoisomerase I Poisons

Topoisomerase I (Topo I) is a nuclear enzyme that unwinds genomic supercoiled DNA by nicking a single DNA strand, passing the intact strand through the nick, and then ligating the break. Topo I activity, thereby, decreases the linking number of DNA by one. Thus, Topo I unwinds supercoiled DNA, functioning mainly during RNA transcription and DNA replication, as well as in viral encapsulation, HIV replication, genetic recombination, and chromosomal condensation/decondensation.[1]

Drugs active against Topo I can cause lethality through an enzyme-mediated nicking reaction. Camptothecin (CPT) and its analogues reversibly stabilize DNA-Topo I "cleavable" complexes.[2] Precisely how stabilization of cleavable complexes leads to cell responses and subsequent death is under intense investigation. Because CPT-mediated cell death is largely S-phase specific in many, but not all, cells,[3] it was hypothesized that DNA replication forks collide with DNA–Topo I complexes. This collision then results in several potentially toxic problems for the cell, including replication fork arrest, topologically (or strain)-induced DNA double-strand breaks, inhibition of transcription, stabilization of the p53 tumor suppressor, and subsequent p53-mediated apoptosis. Concentration-dependent G_1 and/or G_2 cell cycle checkpoint arrests, as well as nonapoptotic cell death responses, are also observed after Topo I poisons.[4–6] Most CPT-mediated cell death models predict that Topo I poisons would be clinically efficacious if continuously administered over long periods of time, similar to 5-fluorouracil (which inhibits thymidylate synthase), another S-phase-specific drug.[6] Interestingly, however, most animal studies and clinical trials to date have not reported major differences in anti-tumor activity based on treatment schedules,[7] and many current clinical trials are retesting the theory that CPT is S-phase specific *in vivo* and should be given under prolonged, continuous routes of administration. Recently, we discovered dramatic S-phase-specific activation of NF-κB, a transcription factor, in various human cancer cells following brief (1–2 hr) exposures to CPT analogues (e.g., topotecan, TPT). Because NF-κB is an antiapoptotic factor that can induce downstream genes that protect against cell death, this cellular response to Topo poisons (also found with Topo II-α poisons) may be a leading factor in mitigating the efficacy of these drugs. These recent findings will be discussed below.

β-Lapachone

β-Lapachone (β-lap) is a naturally occurring 1,2-naphthoquinone initially isolated from the bark of the Lapacho tree, native to South America. We showed that this drug was a radiosensitizing agent against radioresistant human cancer cells, including human laryngeal carcinoma (HEp-2) and malignant melanoma (U1-Mel) cell lines.[8,9] Using cell-free assays, β-lap inhibited Topo I by catalytic inhibition, a mechanism quite different from that of CPT, TPT, 9-aminocamptothecin (9-AC), or irinotecan (CPT-11).[10–12] β-Lap administration did not (a) stabilize Topo I–DNA cleavable complexes *in vivo*[12] or *in vitro*[10]; (b) result in formation of DNA single-strand nicks *in vivo*[13]; or (c) lead to the damage-mediated stabilization (induction) of wild-type p53.[14] The fact that β-lap did not produce DNA single-strand nicks in human or hamster cancer cells[13] was indirectly confirmed by the absence of wild-type p53 induction in breast or prostate cancer cells.[11,14] Whereas assays *in vitro* indirectly suggested that Topo I and/or Topo II-α may be intracellular targets of β-lap, it seemed likely that it was not the mechanism through which this compound killed cells.[14–16] We reported that the cytotoxicity caused by β-lap in MCF-7 breast cancer cells could be solely accounted for by apoptotic responses.[14] Further investigation revealed that β-lap probably does not act on Topo I or Topo II-α *in vivo*, but is instead activated to induce a novel noncaspase-mediated apoptotic response directed by the NQO1 damage-inducible enzyme, also referred to as xip3.[17,18]

NF-κB Activation Responses

The NF-κB/Rel family of transcription factors regulates expression of genes critical for apoptosis, as well as many other genes.[19–21] NF-κB exists as dimeric complexes composed of p50, p65 (RelA), c-Rel, RelB, or p52. NF-κB associates with members of the IκB family of proteins, such as IκBα, which localizes NF-κB in the cytoplasm.[22,23] Dissociation from IκBα is essential for NF-κB to enter the nucleus and activate gene expression. Several signaling cascades that control NF-κB activation converge at an IκB kinase (IKK) complex, responsible for site-specific phosphorylation of IκBα.[24–27] Phosphorylation of IκBα causes multi-ubiquitination of IκBα and its subsequent degradation by the 26S proteasome.[28,29] This sequence of events can be induced without *de novo* protein synthesis by multiple extracellular stimuli.

NF-κB activation pathways typically originate from ligand–receptor interactions at the cell membrane. However, NF-κB can also be activated by certain DNA-damaging agents. We hypothesized that a signal may be transferred from the nucleus to the cytoplasm to activate NF-κB after DNA damage in the nucleus.[30] Devary *et al*.[31] showed that enucleated cells (i.e., cytoplasts) retained full capacity to activate NF-κB after UV irradiation, showing that nuclear DNA damage is not required for NF-κB activation after this cytotoxic stress. In contrast, NF-κB activation by certain DNA-damaging agents, including CPT, correlated with their capacity to induce DNA breaks.[32] The requirement of damaged DNA in the nucleus for activation was not examined. One of our objectives was to determine whether or not nuclear events associated with the DNA-damaging action of CPT or TPT were required for activation of cytoplasmically located NF-κB complexes. We also examined the influence of NF-κB activation in CPT-mediated apoptosis. We discovered a series of nuclear events induced by CPT/TPT that converged with cytoplasmic signaling events responsible for the activation of NF-κB. These signal transduction responses provided an anti-apoptotic function.

MATERIALS AND METHODS

Chemicals and Cell Treatments

9-Amino-20(RS)camptothecin (9-AC) was obtained from Monroe E. Wall (Research Triangle Park, NC) as previously described. Topotecan (TPT, MW: 421.4) was a gift from SmithKline Beecham (King of Prussia, PA) and was made fresh in DMSO. CPT, VP16, calpain inhibitor I (ALLN), DMSO, bacterial LPS, PMA, cycloheximide, aphidicolin, and cytochalasin B were purchased from Sigma Chemical Co. Human recombinant TNFα was from CalBiochem. IgGs against IκBα (C21), c-Rel (C), p65 (A and C20), Rel-B (C-19), p52 (I-18), and p50 (NLS) were purchased from Santa Cruz Biotechnology. A monoclonal anti-Flag antibody was purchased from Kodak, horseradish peroxidase-conjugated anti-rabbit and anti-mouse antibodies and protein A were obtained from Amersham. β-Lap (M_r: 242.3, see top insert, FIG. 1) and camptothecin (M_r: 348.3) were obtained and prepared as described.[9,11] Both drugs were dissolved in DMSO, concentrations determined, and stock aliquots stored at –20°C.[3,8,14,17] Exact concentrations of drugs were determined using spectrophotometric analysis.[14,17] Stored vials were used only once.

Tissue Culture Techniques

Human malignant melanoma (U1-Mel) cells were generously provided by Dr. J. B. Little (Dept. Radiation Therapy, Harvard Medical School, Boston, MA). Their initial plating and growth to confluence-arrest were described.[8,14,33,34] Cells were free of mycoplasma contamination, and contaminated cells were found to be a major cause of artifacts in nearly all of the endpoint investigated in this study, as we recently described for cellular responses to IR.[35] Culture conditions for 70Z/3 and 70Z/3-CD14 murine pre-B cells were described.[36] CEMp and CEM/C2 human T-cell lines were kindly provided by Dr. Y. Pommier (NIH) and maintained in RPMI-1640 medium (Cellgro, Mediatech) supplemented with 10% fetal bovine serum (FBS, HyClone Laboratory, Inc.), 1000 units of penicillin G (Sigma Chemical Co., St. Louis, MO), and 0.5 mg/ml streptomycin sulfate (Sigma) in an humidified 5% CO_2–95% air incubator. HeLa human cervical carcinoma cells and PC-3 human prostate carcinoma cells were maintained in DMEM (Cellgro) supplemented with 10% FBS and antibiotics as above in a 10% CO_2–90% air incubator. The human kidney embryonic fibroblast 293 (HEK293) was maintained in the latter medium on 0.1% (wt/vol) gelatin-coated plastic culture dishes.

Survival Determinations

Typically, 5.0×10^5 cells from subconfluent cultures were plated onto 25 cm^2 tissue culture flasks. All flasks were letter-coded, and experiments performed double-blind. Cells were fed every 2–3 days until growth arrest by confluency was achieved, usually in 5–7 days. Cells were then fed every other day for an additional 7–10 days. One day before each experiment, cells were shifted to DME containing 0.2% FCS to further arrest U1-Mel cells. Confluence-arrested U1-Mel cells demonstrated ≤6% [^{3}H]thymidine-labeled nuclei and ~85% G_0/G_1, 4% S-phase, and 11% G_2/M cells.[8,9,34] Following IR exposure and β-lap or Topo I poison post-treatments (e.g., with 9-AC, CPT, or TPT), colony-forming assays were performed using 10-fold lim-

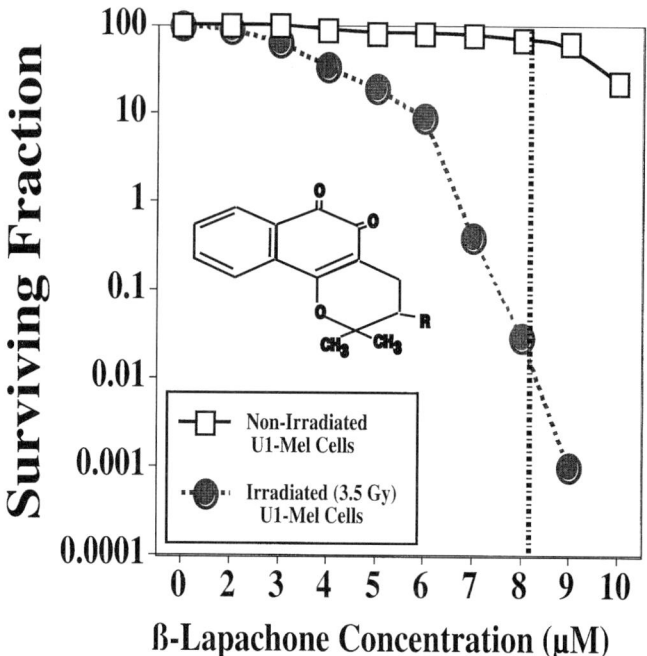

FIGURE 1. β-Lap synergistically enhances the cytotoxicity of low serum-treated, confluent U1-Mel cells. Radioresistant human malignant melanoma (U1-Mel) cells were grown to confluency and shifted to medium containing a low (0.2%) percentage of fetal bovine serum, where >85% G_0/G_1 and fewer than 5% S-phase (incorporating [^{3}H]thymidine into their DNA) were noted.[8,9,33,34] Arrested cells were then treated with 3.5 Gy IR or mock irradiated. Immediately after IR exposure, cells were treated with or without various concentrations of β-lap as described in MATERIALS AND METHODS. Control cells were treated with an equivalent percentage of DMSO for each dose of drug, and no dose of DMSO used in the experiment caused growth inhibition or lethality. *Top insert*: structure of β-lap. A number of R-substituted derivatives have been made, and these do not affect the activity of this compound; however, many alter the solubility or other pharmacokinetic properties.[41,60] *Bottom insert, open square*: nonirradiated U1-Mel cells treated with various concentrations of β-lap alone for 4 hr; *solid circle*: U1-Mel cells treated with IR followed immediately with various concentrations of β-lap for 4 hr. Colony-forming ability assays were then performed and analyzed as described in MATERIALS AND METHODS. The vertical dashed line indicates the approximate cut-off between physiologically relevant doses of β-lap found for mice.[41] Results are similar to those previously published.[9] Any concentration of β-lap above ~8 µM would be nonphysiological, achieved in tissue culture but not in mice at the maximum tolerated dose (MTD) of the drug.

iting dilution analyses. All colony-forming assays were performed at least seven times in duplicate. Survival curves were normalized for toxicity due to IR or drug exposures alone, as well as variations in initial viable cells plated. A colony consisted of 100 or more normal-appearing cancer cells. Data were obtained, analyzed, and graphed.[8,9,34]

Topo I Enzyme Assays

Purified calf thymus Topo I or Topo I crude extracts from isolated nuclei of U1-Mel cells were used in enzymatic assays.[9] Loss of Form I relative to total DNA loaded onto each lane of the agarose gels was quantitated.[9]

SDS-K⁺ Topo I Complex Assays

A modification of the SDS-KCl assay was used to quantify DNA–Topo I complexes via glass fiber filter binding as previously described.[12,13]

Flow Cytometry

Changes in cell cycle distribution were recorded and cell death measured.[14] Data were analyzed by ModFit LT (Verity Software House). Statistical evaluations (p values) were calculated using the Student's t test. For FACS sorting of G_1, S, and total cell fractions for EMSA analyses, 70Z/3 cells were first treated with agents, stained with Hoechst 33342 at the final concentration of 10 µg/ml for 15 min at 37°C in RPMI growth medium, and sorted using FACStar^{PLUS} (Becton Dickinson) at 4°C. Cells (10^6) were purified, and total cell extracts prepared for EMSA analysis.[14]

Northern Blot Analyses

Northern blot analyses on control or IR-treated cells were performed as previously described.[34] Equal loading of Northern blots was accomplished by ethidium-stained gels and by 36B4 transcript levels.[34]

Electrophoretic Mobility Shift and Supershift Assays

The Igκ-κB oligonucleotide probe and conditions for electrophoretic mobility shift (EMSA) were described previously.[36] For supershift assays, 1 µg of IgG antibodies specific to NF-κB proteins (Santa Cruz Biotechnology) were added to nuclear extracts for 20 min on ice before addition of radiolabeled probe. The AP-1 site used for control EMSA reactions was obtained from Promega.

Enucleation

Cytochalsin B–mediated enucleation was performed as previously described.[37] Cytoplasts were incubated with prewarmed growth media for 30 min, 37°C for recovery. Enucleation efficiency varied from ~75%–95% for PC-3 and HeLa cells.[14]

Transient Transfections

Cells (HEK293, HeLa, or PC-3) were transiently transfected using a standard calcium phosphate precipitation method.[38] CEMp and CEM/C2 cells were transfected with DEAD-Dextran method.[39] An NF-κB-dependent luciferase reporter construct (3xκB-Luc) and the negative control construct (3xMκB-Luc) have been recently described.[40] Twenty-four hours after transfection, cells were treated with TPT (30 µM) or CPT (10 µM) for 2 hr, rinsed twice with growth medium, and further incubated without drugs for 6 hr before termination of the cultures. Positive control samples were treated with TNFα (10 ng/ml) for a total of 8 hr. Control samples were transfected with the LacZ cDNA under the control of the cytomegalovirus promoter in the pCMX vector (CMV-LacZ). For CEMp and CEM/C2 cells, total proteins were used for normalization. Full-length human IKKα cDNA was provided by Dr. I. M. Verma (Salk Institute). Full-length human IKKβ cDNA was cloned as previously described.[40] IKKα and IKKβ with a Lys-to-Ala substitution at the conserved ATP-binding site were generated by PCR mutagenesis and confirmed by DNA sequencing. The mutant genes were placed under the control of the CMV promoter in the pcDNA3.1(+) expression vector (Clontech). HEK293 cells were transfected with these constructs by calcium phosphate precipitation.

Retrovirus Construction and Infection

Production and infection of HA-tagged wild-type and HA-tagged S32/36A mutant IκBα expression constructs were described previously.[36] Other IκBα deletion mutants were generated by PCR-mediated mutagenesis and confirmed by sequencing. Stable pools were selected with hygromycin (1 mg/ml, Boehringer Mannheim), and the expression levels of the corresponding proteins were examined by either anti-IκBα (C21, a COOH-terminal epitope) or anti-HA antibodies.

Generation of a Green Fluorescent Protein–IκBα Fusion Construct

NH_2-terminally fused green fluorescent protein (GFP)-IκBα was generated by subcloning PCR-amplified human IκBα (MAD3) into *Hin*dIII-*Bam*HI sites of the pEGFP vector (Clontech), such that the entire MAD3 coding sequence was in frame with the GFP-coding sequence. Stable HEK293 cell clones were generated by G418 selection and subsequent FACS sorting.

RESULTS

Investigation of β-Lap Radiosensitization Led to Studies Using Topo I–Active Poisons

Our initial studies began with the observation that β-lap could work effectively as a radiosensitizer, even against the most radioresistant (in the literature) human cancer cell lines (e.g., Hep-2 or U1-Mel cells).[8,12] FIGURE 1 illustrates the ability of this drug to dramatically sensitize IR-exposed confluent U1-Mel cells. The data were similar to those previously published for various human cancer cells.[8,9,13] Confluent and low serum (0.2% fetal calf serum)–treated radioresistant U1-Mel cells were irradiated (3.5 Gy) or mock-irradiated (0 Gy), and then immediately exposed to DMSO (0.1%) or to various concentrations of β-lap in 0.1% DMSO (FIG. 1). Cells treated with DMSO alone showed no growth inhibition or lethality. As previously observed,[8,9] IR-exposed U1-Mel cells treated with various concentrations of β-lap for 4 hr showed significant lethality, far more than mock-irradiated, β-lap-treated cells. Confluent, low serum–exposed U1-Mel cells were fairly resistant to β-lap up to 9 μM. At concentrations of β-lap above 9 μM, however, significant lethality (90% lethality) was observed from exposure to the drug alone. Pharmacokinetic data showed, however, that levels of β-lap above 8 μM were nonphysiological, wherein only 5–8 μM β-lap was achieved in the bloodstream, normal tissue, or tumor tissue of mice at the MTD[41] (also, unpublished data). Cells treated with 3.5 Gy and immediately assayed for survival (immediately re-seeded and, not allowing for potentially lethal damage recovery, PLDR[8,33] resulted in 30% survival, which dramatically increased to over 60% survival in the 4-hr post-treatment period before redilution and sparse reseeding of irradiated cells onto plates to promote log-phase growth in medium containing 10% fetal calf serum.

A few very important characteristics about the use of β-lap as a radiosensitizer led us to the recent elucidation of this drug's mechanism of action *in vivo*. First and foremost, the drug had to be administered either during IR treatment with exposure for at least 4 hr, or the drug had to be applied immediately after IR exposure for at least 4 hr.[9] Pretreatment of cells for 4 hr with various concentrations of β-lap below 8 μM had little or no effect on the survival of IR-treated U1-Mel cells. Furthermore, the duration of drug exposure had to be at least 4–5 hr, with logarithmic decreases in radiosensitization with decreasing time; for example, a 2-hr exposure of drugs had little radiosensitizing effect.[9]

We also investigated the intracellular mechanism of action of β-lap using control or IR-treated cells in an attempt to better understand the reasons for radiosensitization. One important observation was made: when cells were treated with IR or UV, β-lap exposure of confluent and low serum (arrested) U1-Mel or other cancer cells resulted in enhanced tritiated thymidine uptake, indicative of increased unscheduled DNA synthesis (UDS).[12,42,43] We reasoned that since only DNA ligase inhibitors were known to cause enhanced UDS,[42] this drug must prevent the final steps of DNA repair. We then tested the ability of β-lap to inhibit DNA ligases using bacterial, yeast, and eukaryotic sources of the enzyme. Interestingly and unexpectedly, the compound did not inhibit DNA ligases using any of these enzyme sources. We noted, however, that β-lap prevented alkaline phosphatase activity when mixed with cell extracts from irradiated, but not control, U1-Mel cells (unpublished data). We suspect that this inhibition of kinases by β-lap exposure was the result of loss of energy (ATP) within the cell or extracts, caused by NQO1 activity (see below).

Because the final steps of topoisomerases are to re-ligate the broken ends of DNA after their unwinding activities, and since β-lap did not inhibit DNA ligases, we then tested the effects of β-lap on purified Topo I or Topo II-α enzymes, as well as nuclear extracts from irradiated or nonirradiated cells. Addition of β-lap did not affect Topo II-α activity; however, the compound inhibited Topo I from human extracts.[9,11] We also noted an apparent activation of Topo I using chick erythrocyte Topo I, which was the result of an aberrant Topo I–mediated nicking reaction.[9,11] Recently, inhibition of Topo II-α by preincubation of enzyme with β-lap has been reported[15]; however, inhibitory effects were observed only *in vivo*, and other labs (including our own) have not reproduced these effects.[9] Collectively, our data prompted us to hypothesize that modulation of Topo I by any mechanism might result in enhanced cell killing follow IR.[9,44] We, therefore, tested CPT (a prototype Topo I poison) for its ability to radiosensitize various human cancer cells under conditions identical to those described above using β-lap.

Topo I Poisons Also Caused Radiosensitization Similar to That of β-Lap

On the basis of our results with β-lap and our discovery that this drug affected Topo I, we tested CPT and TPT for their abilities to sensitize Hep-2 or U1-Mel cells to IR under conditions identical to those described above for β-lap. We were the first to discover that camptothecin could synergistically kill cancer cells when combined with IR.[9] Later, we showed similar effects using 9-AC or TPT.[44–46] All Topo I poisons tested thus far have similar radiosensitizing effects on radioresistant human cancer cells as described below for TPT or CPT.

We reasoned that if β-lap worked as a radiosensitizer by influencing Topo I, then clinically relevant Topo I poisons should work in a similar manner with similar kinetics and characteristics. Much to our surprise, we discovered that exposure of low serum–exposed, IR-treated, confluent U1-Mel or Hep-2 cells with CPT or TPT caused a significant enhancement of cell death beyond lethality caused by either IR or Topo I poison alone.[8] Furthermore, cell death responses were kinetically similar to those observed with β-lap: (a) the drugs had to be administered immediately after IR exposure; (b) a 4-hr post-treatment was optimal; (c) longer exposure of cells to Topo I poisons alone caused considerable toxicity, thereby masking the abilities of these compounds to radiosensitize cells; and (d) pretreatment with Topo I poisons had little or no affect on cell killing following IR—the two drugs were additive and not synergistic under pretreatment conditions.

Mechanistically, both β-lap and CPT-related Topo I poisons (CPT, 9-AC, or TPT) caused enhanced sensitization of IR-treated cells in very similar fashions.[44–46] Post-IR exposures of U1-Mel cells with either CPT or β-lap led to increases in total DNA strand breaks (measured by alkaline elution) and in the formation of DSBs (measured by neutral elution).[13] Interestingly, post-IR exposures with either TPT or β-lap caused the formation of new DSBs and SSBs that could not be explained by IR exposure alone.[12,13] These lesions appeared to arise from lesion modification mechanisms and not from simple inhibition of DNA repair. Exposure of cells to β-lap alone at any doses tested did not result in DNA breaks. Increased DNA break formation following TPT + IR was accompanied by a rather dramatic enhancement (>30-fold) of Topo I–DNA complex formation, as measured using standard DNA filtration methods.[13] In contrast, β-lap + IR caused much lower levels of DNA–protein complex formation (only threefold increases), and the complexes could not be confirmed to include the Topo I protein.[13] As we will discuss later, the mechanism of action of β-lap-mediated radiosensitization was entirely different from that caused by Topo I poisons + IR. However, these data suggested at the time that β-lap and Topo I poisons were both good radiosensitizers and that they may still work by the same mechanisms of action.[44–46] Although some differences were noted between the radiosensitizing abilities of β-lap compared to Topo I poisons, these data were not inconsistent with the notion that β-lap may act as a radiosensitizer via modification of Topo I. Furthermore, we proposed that Topo I poisons caused radiosensitization via a lesion modification mechanism, wherein Topo I binds to SSBs created by IR and cleaves the DNA-forming DSBs that have Topo I enzyme linked to the DNA damage ends.[9,12,45–47] To date, all available data appear consistent with this mechanism of radiosensitization for classical Topo I poisons (TPT, CPT, and 9-AC). However, further research elucidating this mechanism is needed.

Interestingly, other studies by Chen et al.[47,48] showed that pretreatments with Topo I poisons before IR exposures resulted in synergistic cell killing, effects not observed in many other laboratories.[9,44–46,49–52] These data,[47,48] using Chinese hamster DC3F or MCF-7 cells, are in contrast with the studies discussed above and may be caused by increased apoptosis resulting from the combination treatment or from altered cell cycle regulation. These data indicate that there are possibly multiple mechanisms in tumor cells for enhanced lethality due to Topo I poisons + IR, including altered cell cycle regulation effects. Furthermore, other studies[51,53] have shown only additive effects of IR + Topo I poisons, underscoring the need for studies of the molecular factors that influence radiosensitization of human cancer cells.

Radiosensitization by β-Lap Is Not Similar to Other Typical Topo I Poisons

Another major difference between β-lap and more typical Topo I poisons (i.e., CPT and its analogues) was that β-lap did not cause DNA–Topo I complex formation when cells were treated with the drug alone, as did CPT or its derivatives.[10,12] The compound also catalytically inhibited DNA Topo I instead of forming DNA–Topo I–drug ternary complexes,[10,11] as was the case with typical Topo I poisons.[2] Although we did find that SSBs and DSBs were enhanced by β-lap in IR-treated cancer cells, DNA–Topo I complex formation increased only slightly above background; in cell extracts, this filtration method actually measures protein–DNA complexes and is not specific for DNA–Topo I protein complexes. Thus, although the kinetics of enhanced IR lethality appeared to be similar, the two drugs (β-lap compared to TPT or CPT) appeared to worked quite differently.

Other differences between CPT-related Topo I poisons and β-lap were also apparent. Although both drugs caused apoptosis in various human cancer cells, (a) β-lap was far more efficient at inducing cell killing by apoptosis, and, unlike CPT or other Topo I-active poisons, lethality caused by this drug was due entirely to apoptosis in various human cancer cells[14]; and (b) β-lap caused an extremely steep dose–response cytotoxicity curve in confluent or log-phase cells, compared to CPT or TPT, which exhibited some cell cycle dependency on overall cell killing; interestingly, the ability of CPT or TPT alone to induce apoptosis did not appear to be cell cycle-mediated[14,54]; (c) β-lap caused little or no cell cycle checkpoint alterations and no induction (i.e., stabilization) of wild-type p53, whereas dramatic p53 stabilization responses were noted following CPT, 9-AC, or TPT[14]; (d) β-lap treatment caused entirely different intracellular proteolysis during apoptosis (i.e., β-lap induced atypical PARP cleavage producing an ~60 kDa polypeptide) in an apparent noncaspase-, calpain-, or calpain-like-mediated pathway[3,14]; CPT analogues caused classic caspase-mediated apoptosis[3]; and (e) β-lap killed cells independent of p53 status and was blocked by dicoumarol cotreatments, which had little or no effect on classical Topo I poisons such as TPT, CPT, or 9-AC[3,17]; interestingly, CPT analogues also killed cells by p53-independent pathways.[3,11,18]

β-Lap Works through xip3, Also Known as NQO1

Recent data from our laboratory have elucidated the mechanism of action of β-lap in human cancer cells when the drug was used without IR. Various assays *in vitro* implicated several DNA repair and metabolism enzymes as potential key targets (e.g., Topo I, Topo II-α, or DNA polymerase β) for this drug (reviewed in Ref. 17). Until recently, however, key intracellular enzymes required for the compound's cytotoxic activity had not been elucidated. The fact that dicoumarol (out of several inhibitors tested) could prevent β-lap-mediated toxicity strongly suggested that

NAD(P)H:quinone oxidoreductase (NQO1, also known as DT diaphorase or xip3) was a key intracellular determinant in lethality caused by this drug.[17] Dicoumarol is a fairly specific inhibitor of NQO1 as discussed.[17] Furthermore, we discovered two cell lines, LNCaP human prostate cancer and MDA-MD-468 human breast cancer cells, that were inherently resistant to β-lap-mediated apoptosis and cytotoxicity. In contrast, DU-145 human prostate and MCF-7 human breast cancer cells were sensitive to this drug.[3,17,18] Interestingly, these cell lines were not appreciably different in their sensitivities to CPT or Topo II-α poisons.[3,18] Further studies demonstrated that LNCaP and MDA-MB-468 cells were deficient in NQO1 expression, whereas MCF-7 and DU-145 cells expressed high levels of the protein and enzyme. Thus, NQO1 levels correlated with sensitivity to β-lap, and toxicity in DU-145 and MCF-7 cells after drug exposure was prevented by dicoumarol. However, unlike menadione, which is detoxified by NQO1, β-lap was "activated" by this two-electron reductase.

As final proof that β-lap exposure alone (without IR) killed cells through NQO1, LNCaP and MDA-MB-468 (NQO1-deficient) cells were transfected with CMV-controlled NQO1, and various expressing and nonexpressing transfectants were analyzed for lethality to β-lap compared to menadione, as well as to CPT-mediated lethality.[17,18] These studies clearly demonstrate that NQO1 is a major determinant of cell sensitivity to β-lap, since NQO1-transfected LNCaP or MDA-MB-468 cells became very sensitive to the drug, and this sensitivity was blocked by dicoumarol. Once again, sensitivity to the drug correlated well with specific and atypical intracellular apoptotic proteolysis, namely atypical PARP cleavage and degradation of p53 and pRb, consistent with a noncaspase-mediated, calpain or calpain-like cysteine protease activation pathway.[3,14]

NQO1 Is a Damage-Inducible Protein, Possibly Explaining β-Lap's Ability to Radiosensitize Cells

Treatment of U1-Mel cells with IR (3.5 Gy) resulted in a dramatic increase in NQO1 transcript levels (FIG. 2). Peak levels of NQO1 were noted 4–8 hr post-IR. In dose–response experiments, NQO1 levels were significantly induced by as little as 1.0 Gy,[34] a clinically relevant dose of IR. Interestingly, LNCaP cells, which lack NQO1 expression, were one of few cancer cells that were not radiosensitized by β-lap.[8,9] Work is ongoing in our laboratory to demonstrate that β-lap sensitizes cells via the IR induction of its intracellular activating enzyme, NQO1. Thus, although the kinetics of radiosensitization of β-lap + IR compared to IR + CPT (or TPT or 9-AC) appear to be similar, the actual mechanism of cell killing is very different.

We recently demonstrated that when NQO1-expressing cells were exposed to β-lap, an NQO1-mediated futile cycling of the compound was apparent[17] (also unpublished data). The rate-limiting intracellular substrate of this NQO1-dependent reaction was apparently intracellular loss of NAD(P)H levels, and we theorize ultimate loss of energy balance in the cell. Thus, addition of β-lap to cell extracts may lead to a complete loss of energy via NQO1-dependent futile cycling of the drug, thereby explaining the inhibition of alkaline phosphatase previously observed in ligase reaction assays (unpublished data). An NQO1-dependent mechanism of β-lap-mediated radiosensitization also explains the temporal sequence of addition of β-lap required during or immediately after IR exposures, since IR-induced NQO1 expression reached peak levels in 4 hr. A two-hour exposure of β-lap, which was shown to have

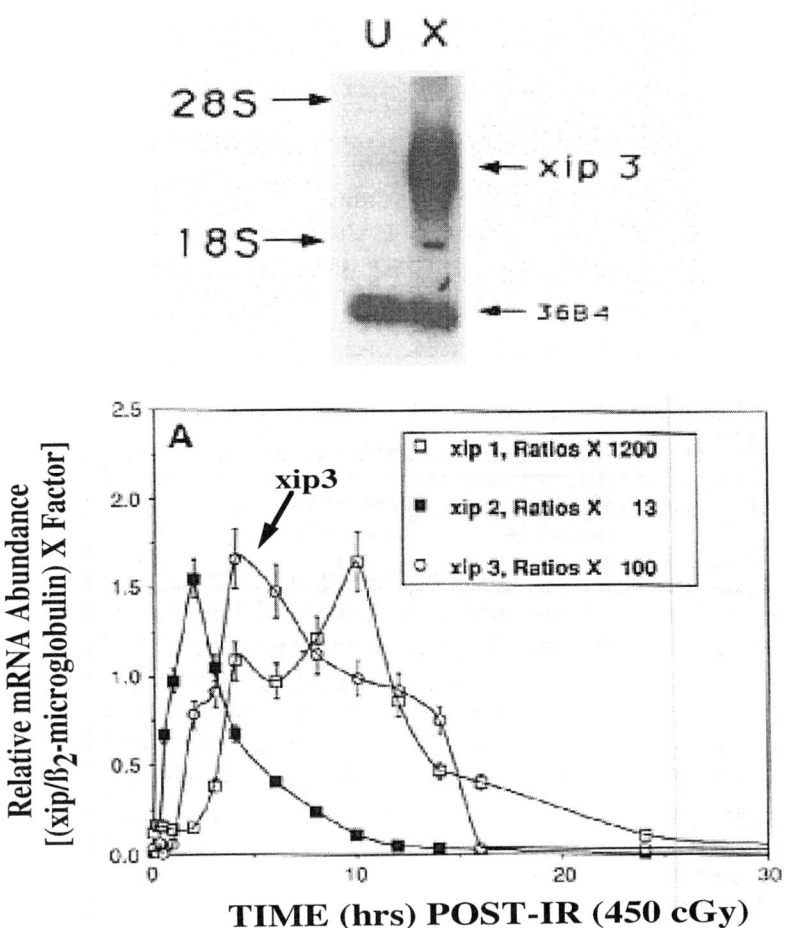

FIGURE 2. NQO1 is an IR-inducible transcript in low serum-exposed, confluent U1-Mel cells. *Left panel*: Confluent U1-Mel cells were treated with 3.5 Gy IR, total RNA was extracted 5 hr later, and specific transcript levels were analyzed by Northern blot analyses using random-primed NQO1 or 36B4 cDNAs as probes. 36B4 transcript levels remain unaltered after IR exposure and were used as a loading standard. *Right panel*: the kinetics of NQO1 induction in U1-Mel cells after 4.5 Gy with respect to β_2-microglobulin (or 36B4); the relative levels were multiplied by an arbitrary factor of 100 to graph the data. Similar responses were observed after 3.5 Gy. Peak NQO1 levels were observed between 4–5 hr post-IR exposure. The induction kinetics of NQO1 in U1-Mel cells were consistent with cellular responses to β-lap, which is activated by this IR (damage)-inducible enzyme (see FIG. 1, text). (From Boothman *et al.*[34]; reprinted with permission from the *Proceedings of the National Academy of Science, USA.*)

little effect on radiosensitization,[9] may not have been sufficient time for NQO1 expression and/or for complete futile cycling of the drug. Short exposures thereby allow cell recovery. In contrast, a 4-hr period of futile cycling of β-lap would result in a critical (threshold) loss of energy leading to activation of calpain or calpain-like apoptosis.[13,14] Research in our laboratory is currently directed towards elucidating the exact mechanism of β-lap-mediated radiosensitization, a mechanism we theorize will involve NQO1 (or xip3) as a major factor in the response.

NF-κB Signaling after Topo I Poisons

Because NF-κB is implicated in the control of apoptosis, we analyzed the mechanisms of NF-κB activation by DNA-damaging agents. We were also interested in elucidating the potential nuclear-to-cytoplasmic signaling pathways activated by Topo I poisons, since inactive NF-κB is present in the cytoplasm, and the majority of DNA damage is induced in the nucleus. Our rationale was that study of the NF-κB activation mechanism by DNA-damaging agents may provide novel targets for anticancer drug development, which may be used in combination with radiation or chemotherapy treatment to increase their efficacy. Since NF-κB can also be activated by oxidative stress in the cells (reviewed in Ref. 40), we began our studies using CPT, a well-characterized Topo I poison that causes DNA strand breaks without simultaneous generation of oxidative stress in the cell.

Exposure of various murine or human cancer cell lines with CPT resulted in NF-κB activation, as measured by EMSA and κB-reporter gene assays.[40] We treated 70Z/3 murine pre-B cells, CEM T leukemic, PC-3 prostate cancer, HEK293 embryonic kidney fibroblast, and HeLa cervical cancer cell lines. We found that in all cell lines tested, NF-κB activation by CPT was dose-dependent, detectable at 10 ng/ml, saturating at 10 μg/ml. The NF-κB activation profile was transient (peaking at 1–2 hr, undetectable by 6–8 hr) in treated cells despite continuous CPT exposure. Pretreatment with cycloheximide did not interfere with this pathway, indicating that this activity stimulated by CPT does not require *de novo* protein synthesis. A similar pattern of the NF-κB activation response was observed when these cells were treated with TPT. Induction of NF-κB DNA-binding activity by CPT or TPT treatment resulted in increased NF-κB-dependent transcription of a luciferase reporter gene. Thus, CPT or TPT activation of NF-κB occurs without *de novo* protein synthesis and may utilize pre-existing regulatory component(s).

The primary molecular target of CPT or TPT is Topo I enzyme, but CPT-sensitive Topo I is present both in the nucleus and mitochondria.[55] To determine the requirement of an intact nucleus for NF-κB activation by CPT, we enucleated PC-3 and HeLa cells by the cytochalasin B-mediated enucleation procedure.[37] Although enucleation did not affect the activation of NF-κB by PMA or TNF, the NF-κB response after CPT or TPT was dramatically diminished in the cytoplasts. These observations indicated that the presence of intact nucleus was essential for efficient NF-κB activation by CPT. To our knowledge, this is the first direct demonstration of the requirement of intact nucleus for any NF-κB activation pathways.

Next, we addressed whether direct interaction of CPT and a Topo I–DNA complex is necessary for activation of NF-κB by examining the human CEM/C2 cells, which express a CPT-resistant mutant Topo I enzyme.[56] This mutant Topo I enzyme contains two amino acid substitutions, Met370 to Thr and Asp722 to Ser. The latter mutation makes Topo I enzyme ~1000-fold resistant to CPT (or TPT)-mediated inhibition of the re-ligation of DNA nicks, making it incapable of efficiently inducing DNA damage after CPT treatment *in vivo*.[57] We compared CPT-induced NF-κB activity in CEM/C2 and the parental CEMp cells by EMSA. Time-course and dose–response studies, as well as κB-dependent luciferase reporter assays, clearly demonstrated that CEM/C2 cells could not mount an NF-κB response after CPT treatment. Activation of NF-κB in CEM/C2 cells by TNF-α or other DNA-damaging agents, such as VP16 and IR, indicated that the lack of NF-κB activation was specific to CPT.

CPT inhibition of the re-ligation step during the Topo I reaction induces stabilization of the cleavable complexes, resulting in the generation of Topo I-associated SSBs. These SSBs were reversible, but could be converted into DSBs during S-phase, when the replication fork collides with the cleavable complex.[5] Therefore, we next evaluated whether SSBs or DSBs were critical for NF-κB activation by CPT. Cells were treated with aphidicolin for 30 min, then exposed to CPT for 2 hr and cell extracts examined for NF-κB activation. EMSA analyses showed that aphidicolin selectively blocked activation of NF-κB by CPT, but not by other inducing agents, such as bacterial lipopolysaccharide (LPS) or TNF-α. These results suggested that DSBs, not SSBs, were critical for NF-κB activation after CPT. These data also implied that this activation pathway was coupled to S-phase. We, therefore, enriched 70Z/3-CD14 cells in S-phase by FACS sorting after cells were stimulated with CPT or LPS for 2 hr. Compared to similarly obtained G_1 cell populations, NF-κB activation was 2.8-fold higher in the S-phase population, when equivalent amounts of cell extracts were analyzed by EMSA. LPS stimulation did not show any significant differences in NF-κB activation between S and G_1 cells. These findings demonstrated that CPT activation of NF-κB was cell cycle coupled, and predominantly took place during S-phase of the cell cycle in a DSB-dependent fashion.

Our data, thus far, are consistent with the onset of an NF-κB activation pathway initiated by DSBs in the nucleus (FIG. 3). Even though inactive NF-κB/IκBα complexes are largely present in the cytoplasm in a preinduction state, our recent studies demonstrated that these complexes continually shuttle between the nucleus and the cytoplasm.[58] These observations raised the possibility that the release of NF-κB from IκBα may take place within the nucleus after DNA damage, rather than in the cytoplasm. To evaluate this possibility, we first accumulated the inactive NF-κB complexes in the nucleus by treating cells with the nuclear export inhibitor leptomycin B (LMB). Cells were then treated with CPT. Under these conditions, NF-κB activation was not induced.[58] Moreover, we found that NF-κB activation by CPT requires (i) degradation of IκBα by the ubiquitin–proteasome pathway; (ii) inhibition of CPT-induced IκBα degradation by proteasome inhibitors caused accumulation of IκBα in the cytoplasm; (iii) mutation of the IκB kinase phosphorylation sites on IκBα blocked NF-κB activation by CPT; (iv) dominant-negative mutants of IκB kinases, IKKα and IKKβ, blocked CPT activation of NF-κB; (v) CPT activation of NF-κB was deficient in IKKα$^{-/-}$, IKKβ$^{-/-}$, or IKKγ$^{-/-}$ cells; and (vi) IKKα and IKKβ are not shuttling between the nucleus and the cytoplasm.[40] Although we cannot completely discount the possibility that some posttranslational modification may be imposed on inactive NF-κB/IκBα complexes in the nucleus after DNA damage, our observations are consistent with the hypothesis that DSBs initiate a nuclear-to-cytoplasmic signaling pathway to activate the IKK complex in the cytoplasm to ul-

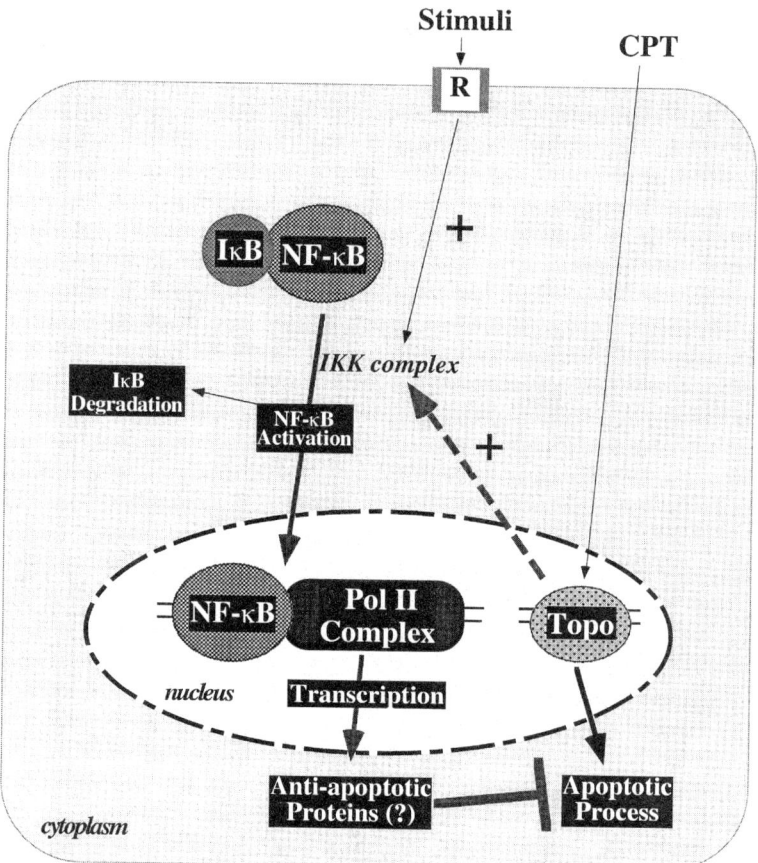

FIGURE 3. A model depicting a putative "nuclear-to-cytoplasmic" signal transduction pathway activated by Topo I poisons. See discussion section and the paper by Huang et al.[40] for further details.

timately induce degradation of IκBα to release NF-κB in the cytoplasm. Once in the nucleus, NF-κB appears to regulate expression of anti-apoptotic genes (FIG. 3), since inhibition of NF-κB activation by expression of a dominant-negative IκBα mutant protein enhanced apoptotic responses in certain cancer cells after CPT treatment.[58]

DISCUSSION AND CONCLUSIONS

The studies summarized here highlight the need to better understand the cellular and molecular responses of normal compared to tumor tissues to cytotoxic agents (such as IR, Topo I poisons, β-lap, and combinations of these agents). The Topo I poison-mediated activation of NF-κB could be a very important anti-apoptotic response that affects efficacy of therapy using Topo I poisons, with or without other cytotoxic agents (e.g., IR). Our laboratories are currently working to better understand the unique S-phase-specific signal transduction pathways induced by CPT analogues that simultaneously activate apparently functionally opposing p53 and NF-κB transcriptional responses (FIG. 3). These coordinate cellular responses presumably evolved in eukaryotic cells to halt the cell cycle in G_1 and/or G_2 (dependent on dose and timing) to allow time for repair and recovery (p53-dependent), but also possibly to stimulate transcriptional responses that lead to enhanced cell survival (NF-κB mediated). Manipulating these pathways will presumably allow for enhanced cytotoxic effects and possibly methods for greatly improving therapy. We speculate that manipulating these pathways could be accomplished through the use of tissue- and tumor-specific expression of dominant-negative IκB or through the use of proteasome inhibitors. Both of these methods should prevent NF-κB activation by sequestering NF-κB in the cytosol of tumor cells, thereby preventing nuclear translocation of this transcription factor. Alternatively, by dissecting the components and biochemical reactions involved in the putative nuclear-to-cytoplasmic signaling pathway, inhibitors specific to NF-κB activation induced by DSBs may be developed. Overall, these findings highlight the need for further investigation and elucidation of the molecular responses occurring in normal compared to tumor cells following the combination of IR and Topo I poison exposures.

Interestingly, β-lap exposure of human cancer cells does not lead to induction of NF-κB.[59] In fact, administration of this drug actually suppresses NF-κB activation responses,[59] which we theorize occurs via the futile cycling of this drug and loss of energy balance within exposed cells expressing NQO1.[17] Thus, β-lap holds special interest as a radiosensitizer in that the overall enhanced IR-mediated cytotoxicity is equivalent to that of the Topo I poisons, but is not susceptible to the same downstream protective responses. In fact, not only are NF-κB responses suppressed, but p53 and pRb are specifically degraded.[3,14] p53 and pRb are apparently substrates for the downstream activated calpain or calpain-like protease that is activated following β-lap exposure[3] (also, Tagliarino et al., unpublished data). Thus, apoptotic responses are stimulated following β-lap exposure, simultaneously with suppression of anti-apoptotic responses (mediated by NF-κB downregulation). Furthermore, identification of NQO1 as a principal target or activating enzyme within the cell is a major step towards improving specificity of radiosensitization with this drug.

ACKNOWLEDGMENTS

Support for this work was provided by Grant #DAMD17-98-1-8260 from the U.S. Department of Defense (DOD) Breast Cancer Initiative, and Grant #R01-CA83196 to D.A.B.; a postdoctoral research fellowship (DAMD17-001-0194) to J.J.P. from the DOD Breast Cancer Initiative; and a predoctoral fellowship (DAMD18-00-2354) to C.T. from the DOD Breast Cancer Initiative. This work was also funded by a Howard Hughes Medical Institute grant awarded from the University of Wisconsin-Madison Medical School, grants from the NIEHS Center, University of Wisconsin-Madison and the UW Comprehensive Cancer Center, and NIH Grant R01-CA85542 to S.M.

REFERENCES

1. WANG, J.C. 1996. DNA topoisomerases. Ann. Rev. Biochem. **65:** 635–692.
2. HERTZBERG, Y.-H., M.G. LIHOU & L.F. LIU. 1989. Arrest of replication forks by drug-stabilized topoisomerase I–DNA cleavable complexes as a mechanism of cell killing by camptothecin. Cancer Res. **49:** 5077–5082.
3. PINK, J.J., S. WUERZBERGER-DAVIS, C. TAGLIARINO, et al. 2000. Activation of a cysteine protease in MCF-7 and T47D breast cancer cells during β-lapachone-mediated apoptosis. Exp. Cell Res. **255:** 144–155.
4. AVEMANN, K., R. KNIPPERS, T. KOLLER & J.M. SOGO. 1988. Camptothecin, a specific inhibitor of type I DNA topoisomerase, induces DNA breakage at replication forks Mol. Cell. Biol. **8:** 3026–3034.
5. HSIANG, Y.H., M.G. LIHOU & L.F. LIU. 1989. Arrest of replication forks by drug-stabilized topoisomerase I–DNA cleavable complexes as a mechanism of cell killing by camptothecin. Cancer Res. **49:** 5077–5082.
6. ZHANG, H., P. D'ARPA & L.F. LIU. 1990. A model for tumor cell killing by topoisomerase poisons. Cancer Cells **2:** 23–27.
7. GROCHOW, L.B., E.K. ROWINSKY, R. JOHNSON, et al. 1992. Pharmacokinetics and pharmacodynamics of topotecan in patients with advanced cancer. Drug Metab. Dispos. **20:** 706–713.
8. BOOTHMAN, D.A., S. GREER & A.B. PARDEE. 1987. Potentiation of halogenated pyrimidine radiosensitizers in human carcinoma cells by β-lapachone (3,4-dihydro-2,2-dimethyl-2H-naphtho[1,2-b]pyran-5,6-dione), a novel DNA repair inhibitor. Cancer Res. **47:** 5361–5366.
9. BOOTHMAN, D.A., D.K. TRASK & A.B. PARDEE. 1989. Inhibition of potentially lethal DNA damage repair in human tumor cells by β-lapachone, an activator of topoisomerase I. Cancer Res. **49:** 605–612.
10. LI, C.J., L. AVERBOUKH & A.B. PARDEE. 1993. β-Lapachone, a novel DNA topoisomerase I inhibitor with a mode of action different from camptothecin. J. Biol. Chem. **268:** 22463–22468.
11. PLANCHON, S.M., S. WUERZBERGER, B. FRYDMAN, et al. 1995. β-Lapachone-mediated apoptosis in human promyelocytic leukemia (HL-60) and human prostate cancer cells: a p53-independent response. Cancer Res. **55:** 3706–3711.
12. BOOTHMAN, D.A., M. WANG, R.A. SCHEA, et al. 1992. Posttreatment exposure to camptothecin enhances the lethal effects of X-rays on radioresistant human malignant melanoma cells. Int. J. Radiat. Oncol. Biol. Phys. **24:** 939–948.
13. BOOTHMAN, D.A. & A.B. PARDEE. 1989. Inhibition of radiation-induced neoplastic transformation by beta-lapachone. Proc. Natl. Acad. Sci. USA **86:** 4963–4967.
14. WUERZBERGER, S.M., J.J. PINK, S.M. PLANCHON, et al. 1998. Induction of apoptosis in MCF-7:WS8 breast cancer cells by β-lapachone. Cancer Res. **58:** 1876–1885.
15. FRYDMAN, B., L.J. MARTON, J.S. SUN, et al. 1997. Induction of DNA topoisomerase II-mediated DNA cleavage by β-lapachone and related naphthoquinones. Cancer Res. **57:** 620–627.
16. DOLAN, M.E., B. FRYDMAN, C.B. THOMPSON, et al. 1998. Effects of 1,2-naphthoquinones on human tumor cell growth and lack of cross-resistance with other anticancer agents. Anticancer Drugs **9:** 437–448.
17. PINK, J.J., S.M. PLANCHON, C. TAGLIARINO, et al. 2000. NAD(P)H:quinone oxidoreductase (NQO1) activity is the principal determinant of β-lapachone cytotoxicity. J. Biol. Chem. **275:** 5416–5424.
18. PLANCHON, S.M., J.J. PINK, C. TAGLIARINO, et al. 2000. β-Lapachone-induced apoptosis in human prostate cancer cells: involvement of NQO1/xip3. Exp. Cell Res. Submitted.
19. BAEUERLE, P.A. & D. BALTIMORE. 1996. NF-κB—Ten years after. Cell **87:** 13–20.
20. VERMA, I.M., J.K. STEVENSON, E.M. SCHWARZ, et al. 1995. Rel/NF-κB/IκB family: intimate tales of association and dissociation. Genes Dev. **9:** 2723–2735.
21. SONENSHEIN, G.E. 1997. Rel/NF-κB transcription factors and the control of apoptosis. Sem. Cancer Biol. **8:** 113–119.

22. BEG, A.A., S.M. RUBEN, R.I. SCHEINMAN, et al. 1992. IκB interacts with the nuclear localization sequences of the subunits of NF-κB: a mechanism for cytoplasmic retention. Genes Dev. **6:** 1899–1913.
23. GANCHI, P.A., S.C. SUN, W.C. GREENE & D.W. BALLARD. 1992. IκB/MAD-3 masks the nuclear localization signal of NF-κB p65 and requires the transactivation domain to inhibit NF-κB p65 DNA binding. Mol. Biol. Cell **3:** 1339–1352.
24. DIDONATO, J.A., M. HAYAKAWA, D.M. ROTHWARF, et al. 1997. A cytokine-responsive IκB kinase that activates the transcription factor NF-κB. Nature **388:** 548–554.
25. MERCURIO, F., H. ZHU, B.W. MURRAY, et al. 1997. IKK-1 and IKK-2: cytokine-activated IκB kinases essential for NF-κB activation. Science **278:** 860–866.
26. WORONICZ, J.D., X. GAO, Z. CAO, et al. 1997. IκB kinase-β: NF-κB activation and complex formation with IκB kinase-a and NIK. Science **278:** 866–869.
27. ZANDI, E., D.M. ROTHWARF, M. DELHASE, et al. 1997. The IκB kinase complex (IKK) contains two kinase subunits, IKKα and IKKβ, necessary for IκB phosphorylation and NF-κB activation. Cell **91:** 243–252.
28. ALKALAY, I., A. YARON, A. HATZUBAI, et al. 1995. Stimulation-dependent IκBα phosphorylation marks the NF-κB inhibitor for degradation via the ubiquitin-proteasome pathway. Proc. Natl. Acad. Sci. USA **92:** 10599–10603.
29. CHEN, Z., J. HAGLER, V.J. PALOMBELLA, et al. 1995. Signal-induced site-specific phosphorylation targets IκBα to the ubiquitin-proteasome pathway. Genes Dev. **9:** 1586–1597.
30. STEIN, B., M. KRAMER, H.J. RAHMSDORF, et al. 1989. UV-induced transcription from the human immunodeficiency virus type 1 (HIV-1) long terminal repeat and UV-induced secretion of an extracellular factor that induces HIV-1 transcription in nonirradiated cells. J. Virol. **63:** 4540–4544.
31. DEVARY, Y., C. ROSETTE, J.A. DIDONATO & M. KARIN. 1993. NF-κB activation by ultraviolet light not dependent on a nuclear signal. Science **261:** 1442–1445.
32. PIRET, B. & J. PIETTE. 1996. Topoisomerase poisons activate the transcription factor NF-κB in ACH-2 and CEM cells. Nucl. Acids Res. **24:** 4242–4248.
33. BOOTHMAN, D.A., I. BOUVARD & E.N. HUGHES. 1989. Identification and characterization of X-ray-induced proteins in human cells. Cancer Res. **49:** 2871–2878.
34. BOOTHMAN, D.A., M. MEYERS, N. FUKUNAGA & S.W. LEE. 1993. Isolation of x-ray-inducible transcripts from radioresistant human melanoma cells. Proc. Natl. Acad. Sci. USA **90:** 7200–7204.
35. YANG, C.R., C. WILSON-VAN PATTEN, S.M. PLANCHON, et al. 2000. Coordinate modulation of Sp1, NF-κB, and p53 in confluent human malignant melanoma cells after ionizing radiation FASEB J. **14:** 379–390.
36. MIYAMOTO, S., B. SEUFZER & S. SHUMWAY. 1998. Novel IκBα degradation process in WEHI231 murine immature B cells. Mol. Cell. Biol. **18:** 19–29.
37. POSTE, G. 1972. Enucleation of mammalian cells by cytochalasin B. I. Characterization of anucleate cells. Exp. Cell Res. **73:** 273–286.
38. CAO, Z.D., J. XIONG, M. TAKEUCHI, et al. 1996. TARF6 is a signal transducer for interleukin-1. Nature **383:** 443–446.
39. CHIAO, P.J., S. MIYAMOTO & I.M. VERMA. 1994. Autoregulation of IκBα activity. Proc. Natl. Acad. Sci. USA **91:** 28–32.
40. HUANG, T.T., S.M. WUERZBERGER-DAVIS, B.J. SEUFZER, et al. 2000. NF-κB activation by camptothecin: a linkage between nuclear DNA damage and cytoplasmic signaling events. J. Biol. Chem. **275:** 9501–9509.
41. GLEN, V.L., P.R. HUTSON, N.J. KEHRLI, et al. 1997. Quantitation of β-lapachone and 3-hydroxy-β-lapachone in human plasma samples by reversed-phase high-performance liquid chromatography. J. Chromatogr. B Biomed. Sci. Appl. **692:** 181–186.
42. BOORSTEIN, R.J. & A.B. PARDEE. 1984. β-Lapachone greatly enhances MMS lethality to human fibroblasts. Biochem. Biophys. Res. Commun. **118:** 828–834.
43. BOORSTEIN, R.J. & A.B. PARDEE. 1983. Coordinate inhibition of DNA synthesis and thymidylate synthase activity following DNA damage and repair. Biochem. Biophys. Res. Commun. **117:** 30–36.
44. LAMOND, J.P., M. WANG, T.J. KINSELLA & D.A. BOOTHMAN. 1996. Radiation lethality enhancement with 9-aminocamptothecin: comparison to other topoisomerase I inhibitors. Int. J. Radiat. Oncol. Biol. Phys. **36:** 369–376.

45. LAMOND, J.P., M.P. MEHTA & D.A. BOOTHMAN. 1996. The potential of topoisomerase I inhibitors in the treatment of CNS malignancies: report of a synergistic effect between topotecan and radiation. J. Neurooncol. **30:** 1–6.
46. LAMOND, J.P., M. WANG, T.J. KINSELLA & D.A. BOOTHMAN. 1996. Concentration and timing dependence of lethality enhancement between topotecan, a topoisomerase I inhibitor, and ionizing radiation. Int. J. Radiat. Oncol. Biol. Phys. **36:** 361–368.
47. CHEN, A.Y., P. OKUNIEFF, Y. POMMIER & J.B. MITCHELL. 1997. Mammalian DNA topoisomerase I mediates the enhancement of radiation cytotoxicity by camptothecin derivatives. Cancer Res. **57:** 1529–1536.
48. CHEN, A.Y., H. CHOY & M.L. ROTHENBERG. 1999. DNA topoisomerase I-targeting drugs as radiation sensitizers. Oncology (Huntington) **13:** 39–46.
49. SAUER, R. & A. HEUSER. 1997. [Topoisomerase I inhibitor with potential radiosensitizing effect]. Strahlenther Onkol. **173:** 125–130.
50. MATTERN, M.R., G.A. HOFMANN, F.L. MCCABE & R.K. JOHNSON. 1991. Synergistic cell killing by ionizing radiation and topoisomerase I inhibitor topotecan (SKF 104864). Cancer Res. **51:** 5813–5816.
51. MARCHESINI, R., A. COLOMBO, C. CASERINI, et al. 1996. Interaction of ionizing radiation with topotecan in two human tumor cell lines. Int. J. Cancer **66:** 342–346.
52. LANZA, A., S. TORNALETTI, M. STEFANINI, et al. 1993. The sensitivity to DNA topoisomerase inhibitors in L5178Y lymphoma strains is not related to a primary defect of DNA topoisomerases. Carcinogenesis **14:** 1759–1763.
53. BALOSSO, J., N. GIOCANTI & V. FAVAUDON. 1991. Additive and supraadditive interaction between ionizing radiation and pazelliptine, a DNA topoisomerase inhibitor, in Chinese hamster V-79 fibroblasts. Cancer Res. **51:** 3204–3211.
54. PINK, J.J., S.M. PLANCHON, C. TAGLIARINO, et al. 2000. NAD(P)H:quinone oxidoreductase activity is the principal determinant of β-lapachone cytotoxicity [In Process Citation]. J. Biol. Chem. **275:** 5416–5424.
55. LIN, J.H. & F.J. CASTORA. 1995. Response of purified mitochondrial DNA topoisomerase I from bovine liver to camptothecin and m-AMSA. Arch. Biochem. Biophys. **324:** 293–299.
56. FUJIMORI, A., Y. HOKI, N.C. POPESCU & Y. POMMIER. 1996. Silencing and selective methylation of the normal topoisomerase I gene in camptothecin-resistant CEM/C2 human leukemia cells. Oncol. Res. **8:** 295–301.
57. FUJIMORI, A., W.G. HARKER, G. KOHLHAGEN, et al. 1995. Mutation at the catalytic site of topoisomerase I in CEM/C2, a human leukemia cell line resistant to camptothecin. Cancer Res. **55:** 1339–1346.
58. HUANG, T.T., N. KUDO, M. YOSHIDA & S. MIYAMOTO. 2000. A nuclear export signal in the N-terminal regulatory domain of IκBα controls cytoplasmic localization of inactive NF-κB/IκBα complexes. Proc. Natl. Acad. Sci. USA **97:** 1014–1019.
59. MANNA, S.K., Y.P. GAD, A. MUKHOPADHYAY & B.B. AGGARWAL. 1999. Suppression of tumor necrosis factor-activated nuclear transcription factor-κB, activator protein-1, c-Jun N-terminal kinase, and apoptosis by β-lapachone. Biochem. Pharmacol. **57:** 763–774.
60. PLANCHON, S.M., S.M. WUERZBERGER-DAVIS, J.J. PINK, et al. 1999. Bcl-2 protects against β-lapachone-mediated caspase-3 activation and apoptosis in human myeloid leukemia (HL-60) cells [In Process Citation]. Oncol. Rep. **6:** 485–492.

In Vitro Antitumor Activity of 9-Nitro-Camptothecin as a Single Agent and in Combination with other Antitumor Drugs

RALPH J. BERNACKI, PAULA PERA, PETER GAMBACORTA, YSEULT BRUN, AND WILLIAM R. GRECO

Department of Pharmacology and Therapeutics, Roswell Park Cancer Institute, Buffalo, New York 14263, USA

ABSTRACT: Preclinical studies at Roswell Park Cancer Institute by Minderman, Cao, and Rustum (unpublished results) showed that a combination of SN-38 and 5-FU against HCT-8 human colon carcinoma cells *in vitro* was synergistic, with the best interaction occurring when the drugs were added sequentially, SN-38 first. Their *in vivo* studies using HCT-8 tumor xenografts implanted s.c. in nude athymic mice demonstrated superior efficacy for a sequential i.v. administration of CPT-11, 24 hr before 5-FU. On the basis of these studies, our group has begun to evaluate effects of RFS2000 (9-nitro-20(S)-camptothecin) (9-NC) in combination with a series of other antitumor agents. Using a panel of human tumor cell lines including A121 ovarian cancer, HCT-8 colon cancer, H-460 NSCLC, HT-1080 fibrosarcoma, and MCF7 mammary cancer, we found that a 2-hr exposure to 9-NC resulted in ID_{50} values of <1.0 µM, whereas continuous exposure to drug resulted in ID_{50} values of <1.0 nM. Tumor growth inhibitory activities of 5-FU, gemcitabine, and paclitaxel were determined for comparison. Combinations of these agents were evaluated with 9-NC using the human HCT-8 colon tumor cell line. Concurrent and sequential combinations of 9-NC with 5-FU had some regions of the concentration–effect surface with local synergy and some with local antagonism. However, sequential combination of 9NC or SN-38 followed by 5-FU, 24 hr later appeared to be highly synergistic at high dose–effect levels (i.e., ID_{90}), suggesting that sequential drug administration may be more efficacious at high effect level and that the order of drug addition is very important. Overall, our results were similar to that found earlier by Rustum's group with CPT11 (or SN-38) and 5-FU, suggesting that sequential combination of 9-NC (or other camptothecin analogues) followed by 5-FU has potential for the treatment of cancer in man.

INTRODUCTION

In 1966, Wall *et al.* identified the plant alkaloid camptothecin (CPT) as the active antitumor ingredient extracted from the *Camptotheca* tree.[1] Subsequently, a number of water-soluble semisynthetic derivatives of CPT (e.g., irinotecan or CPT-11) and insoluble derivatives [e.g., 9-amino- (9-AC) and 9-nitro-CPT (9-NC)] have been reported to show clinical activity.[2] On the basis of the findings of Rustum's group,[3] we evaluated combinations of 9-NC with other active chemotherapeutic drugs (i.e., paclitaxel, gemcitabine, and 5-fluorouracil), in an effort to identify drug combinations and conditions with potential for the treatment of cancer in man.

MATERIALS AND METHODS

Human Tumor Cell Lines

HT-1080/DR4 fibrosarcoma (HT-1080), MCF7-R mammary cancer (MCF7-R), HCT-8 colon cancer, A121 ovarian cancer, and H-460 NSCLC were propagated as monolayers in RPMI-1640 containing 5% FCS, 5% NuSerum IV, 20 mM HEPES, 2 mM L-glutamine at 37°C in a 5% CO_2 humidified atmosphere.

Drugs

9-Nitro-camptothecin (9-NC), RFS 2000, was provided by Supergen Inc., San Ramon, CA. All other agents were purchased from Sigma Chemical Co., Saint Louis, MO.

Growth Inhibition Assay in 96-Well Microtiter Plates

Assessment of cell growth inhibition was determined according to the methods of Skehan et al.[4] Briefly, cells were plated from 400–1200 cells/well in 96-well plates and incubated at 37°C 15–18 hr before drug addition to allow for cell attachment. Cells were exposed to drug for 2 hr (short term), followed by two washings in complete medium. Tumor cells were further incubated in complete medium for a total of four to six cell doublings (72 hr). For continuous exposure, cells were incubated in the presence of compound for a total of four to five cell doublings. At the end of the growth period, cells were fixed (100 µl of ice-cold 50% TCA) and stained (50 µl of 0.4% sulforhodamine B (SRB)), and optical density was measured at 570 nm.

Combination Studies

Combination studies of 9-NC and various agents were performed in one of two ways. Concurrent, continuous exposure or a 2-hr exposure to 9-NC followed by a second 2-hr exposure to the second compound 24 hr later. HCT-8 cells were plated in five 96-well plates. 9-NC and the second compound (drug B) were added to the cell plates after an overnight incubation in the following manner: 9-NC with drug B, in five fixed-ratio binary mixtures (1:4, 1:2, 1:1, 2:1, 4:1) at the predicted IC_{50} values, were prepared. These drug solutions were then serially diluted over a 6-log range and added to the cell plates. For continuous exposure, plates were then incubated for 72 hr. For sequential exposure compound preparation, drug B was substituted by growth medium. Cells were exposed to 9-NC for 2 hr, followed by two washings in complete medium. Twenty-four hours later, 9-NC was substituted by growth medium, and cells were exposed to drug B for 2 hr. Cell growth inhibition was assessed as outlined above.

Data Analysis

Data were fitted with the Sigmoid-E_{max} concentration–effect model with nonlinear regression, weighted by the reciprocal of the square of the predicted response. The concentration of drug, which resulted in 50% growth inhibition (ID_{50}), was calculated. A universal response surface approach was used to more fully analyze drug

TABLE 1. Effect of short-term and continuous exposure of 9-nitrocamptothecin (9-NC), 5-fluoruracil (5-FU), and gemcitabine on human tumor cell growth

Cell line[a]	9-NC ID$_{50}$ (μM ± SE)		5-FU ID$_{50}$ (μM ± SE)		Gemcitabine ID$_{50}$ (μM ± SE)	
	Short term[b]	Continuous exposure[b]	Short term[b]	Continuous exposure[b]	Short term[b]	Continuous exposure[b]
A121	0.02 ± 0.001	0.004 ± 0.00007	421 ± 12	5.8 ± 0.30	0.1 ± 0.004	0.002 ± 0.00007
H-460	0.05 ± 0.007	0.002 ± 0.0002	65 ± 5.6	1.8 ± 0.14	0.2 ± 0.03	0.003 ± 0.0001
HT-1080	3.3 ± 0.19	0.006 ± 0.0008	74 ± 1.9	1.5 ± 0.20	0.7 ± 0.02	0.003 ± 0.0003
HT-1080/DR4	0.1–1.0[c]	0.003 ± 0.00008	135 ± 5.3	2.3 ± 0.20	0.3 ± 0.01	0.002 ± 0.00007
MCF7-S	0.03 ± 0.0009	0.002 ± 0.00003	20 ± 1.5	0.9 ± 0.05	0.5 ± 0.05	0.003 ± 0.00007
MCF7-R	0.60 ± 0.08	0.003 ± 0.004	471 ± 55	6.2 ± 0.90	0.1 ± 0.005	0.002 ± 0.0002
LCC6-WT	nd[d]	0.009 ± 0.0008	nd	1.1 ± 0.15	nd	0.002 ± 0.0002
LCC6-MDR	nd	0.005 ± 0.00005	nd	1.8 ± 0.30	nd	0.001 ± 0.0001

[a] A121, ovarian; HCT-8, colon carcinoma H460-NSCLC; HT-1080, human fibrosarcoma cell line; /DR4 doxorubicin-selected MDR (MRP/LRP-phenotype); MCF7-S, breast; MCF7-R, doxorubicin resistant; LCC6, mammary; LCC6-MDR, Pgp transfected.
[b] Following an overnight incubation, cells were exposed to compounds for 2 hr (short term), followed by two washings in complete medium. Cells were further incubated in complete medium for a total of 4–5 cell doublings. For continuous exposure, cells were incubated in the presence of compound for a total of 4–5 cell doublings (120 hr for HT1080/DR4, 96 hr for all other lines).
[c] Percent growth inhibition was 50% ±3 over the indicated concentration range.
[d] Not done.

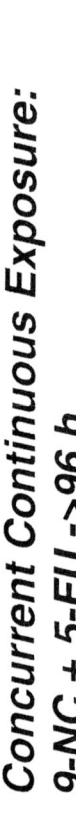
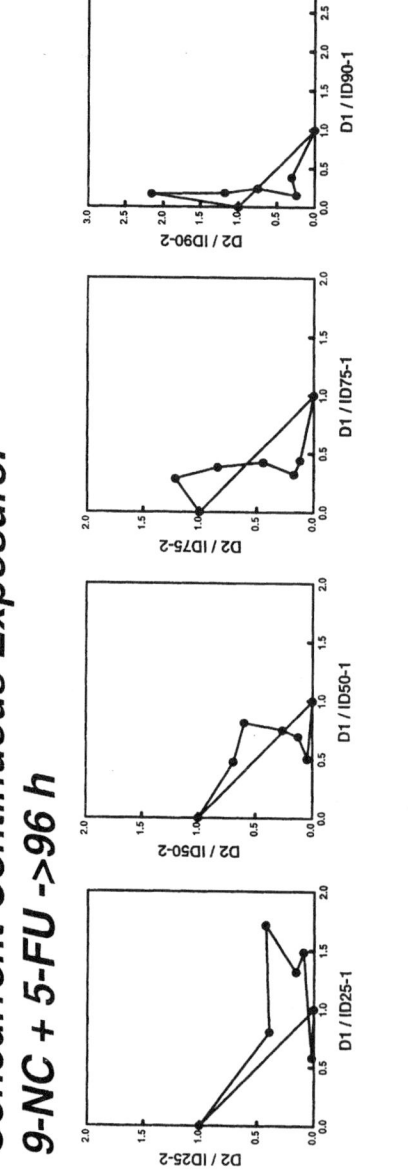
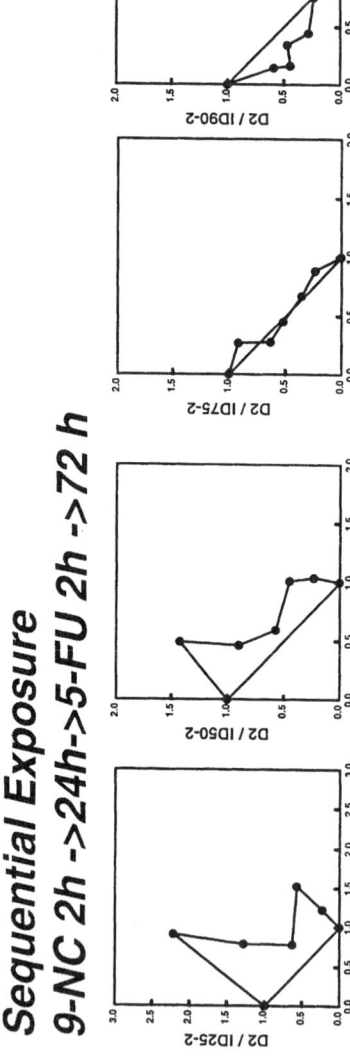

FIGURE 1. Effect of sequential exposure of 9-NC followed by 5-FU in human colon cell line HCT-8.

combination effects. This adaptation consists of deriving composite models for joint drug effect for the cases of interaction (synergism, antagonism), which include interaction parameters. This approach is mathematically consistent with the traditional isobologram but is more objective and more easily automated.[5]

RESULTS AND CONCLUSIONS

Tumor cell exposure to 9-NC resulted in growth arrest, which was time and dosage dependent. There was greater variation and more apparent Pgp (but not MRP)-mediated drug resistance to 9-NC following short-term (2 hr) compared to continuous drug exposure (TABLE 1). Concurrent combination of 9-NC with 5-FU, gemcitabine, or paclitaxel suggested that the most synergistic drug combination against human HCT-8 colon cancer cells was 9-NC with 5-FU. Sequential combination of 9-NC or SN-38 followed by 5-FU, 24 hr later, appeared to be most synergistic at high (e.g., 90%) growth inhibitory levels (FIG. 1). Each set of figures is composed of four isobols at ID_{25}, $_{-50}$, $_{-75}$, and $_{-90}$. ID_{90} represents the concentration of drug (D) needed for 90% growth inhibition, ID_{50}, for 50%, and so forth. The axes represent 9-NC (D1) and 5-FU (D2), respectively. The data demonstrate the degree of tumor cell growth inhibition resulting from treatment with a range of ratios of drug concentrations added to the cells. Starting from the left the ratios of D1:D2 are 1:0, 4:1, 2:1, 1:1, 1:2, 4:1, and 0:1. Data points lying above the diagonal line suggest an antagonistic interaction. Those found on the line suggest an additive response, and those below are synergistic. All the 9NC/5FU combinations at high effect level (i.e., 90% growth inhibition) appear to be consistently synergistic. Recent studies have demonstrated that the sequential administration of 9-NC followed 24 hr later by 5FU to nude athymic mice implanted with human HCT-8 colon tumor xenograft resulted in outstanding therapeutic benefit. Overall, our results demonstrate that combinations of 9-NC and 5-FU were synergistic at high dose effect levels and suggest that sequential combination of 9-NC followed by 5-FU has potential for the treatment of cancer in man.

REFERENCES

1. WALL, M.E., M.C. WANI, C.E. COOK, et al. 1966. Plant antitumor agents. The isolation and structure of camptothecin, a novel alkaloidal leukemia and tumor inhibitor from *Camptotheca acuminata*. J. Am. Chem. Soc. **88:** 3888.
2. TAKIMOTO, C.H. & S.G. ARBUCK. 1996. The camptothecins. *In* Cancer Chemotherapy and Biotherapy. 2nd edit. Chabner & Longo, Eds.
3. MATSUI, S., W. ENDO, C. WRZOSEK, et al. 1999. Characterization of a synergistic interaction between a thymidylate synthase inhibitor, ZD 1694, and a novel lipophilic topoisomerase I inhibitor karenitecin, BNP 1100: mechanisms and clinical implications. Eur. J. Cancer **35:** 984–993.
4. SKEHAN, P., R. STORENG, D. SCUDIERO, et al. 1990. New colorimetric cytotoxicity assay for anticancer-drug screening. J. Natl. Cancer Inst. **82:** 1107–1112.
5. FAESSEL, H.M., H.K. SLOCUM, R.C. JACKSON, et al. 1998. Super in vitro synergy between inhibitors of dihydrofolate reductase and inhibitors of other folate-requiring enzymes: the critical role of polyglutamylation. Cancer Res. **58:** 3036–3050.

p53 and p21 Are Major Cellular Determinants for DNA Topoisomerase I-Mediated Radiation Sensitization in Mammalian Cells

ALLAN Y. CHEN,[a,c] PAUL B. SCRUGGS,[a] LING GENG,[a]
MACE L. ROTHENBERG,[b] AND DENNIS E. HALLAHAN[a]

[a]*Department of Radiation Oncology,* [b]*Division of Hematology/Medical Oncology, Vanderbilt University Medical Center, The Vanderbilt Clinic, Nashville, Tennessee 37232-5671, USA*

INTRODUCTION

The role of combined modality therapy with chemotherapy and radiation has become increasingly important in the treatment of various human malignancies.[1,2] Recent progress in the development of novel chemotherapeutic agents has presented a great opportunity for identifying new chemoradiation regimens with better treatment efficacy towards cancers. Mammalian DNA topoisomerase I (topo-I) is a major cytotoxic target of many newly developed chemotherapeutic drugs including camptothecin (CPT) derivatives.[3,4] Instead of direct inhibition of the catalytic activity of enzyme, topo-I drugs exert their cytotoxic effect by inducing enzyme-mediated DNA damages.[3,4] The presence of elevated levels of topo-I in cancer cells renders it a favored anticancer target.[3,4] Recent studies have indicated that topo-I is also a target for radiation sensitization (RS).[5–7] The topo-I-mediated radiosensitization is unique in its being schedule-dependent, cell cycle phase-specific, cell line-dependent, but not strictly dependent on cytotoxicity of drugs.[7,8] In an attempt to identify cellular factors that are involved in topo-I-mediated RS, we investigated whether inhibition of active DNA metabolism, p53- or p21-regulatory pathway alters the induction of RS by topo-I drugs.

METHODS AND MATERIALS

Cell Lines. The Chinese hamster CHO cells, human HeLa and MCF-7 cells were obtained from Dr. T. Dermody (Vanderbilt University Medical School) and Dr. J.B. Mitchell (National Cancer Institute, NCI). The MCF-7/E6 subline, generated by transfection with the HPV16-E6 gene,[9] was a gift from Dr. A.J. Fornace (NCI). The human colon cancer HCT-116 (parental) and its isogenic HCT-116 (p21–/–) and HCT-116 (p53–/–) cell lines, generated by homogeneous recombination,[10] were provided by Dr. B. Vogelstein (Johns Hopkins Oncology Center).

---

[c]Address for correspondence: Allan Y. Chen, MD, PhD, Department of Radiation Oncology, Vanderbilt University Medical Center, 1301 22nd Ave. S., The Vanderbilt Clinic, Nashville, TN 37232-5671. Voice: 615-322-2555; fax: 615-343-0161.
Allan.chen@mcmail.vanderbilt.edu

TABLE 1. Modulation of camptothecin (CPT)-induced radiation sensitization by inhibitors of various DNA metabolism in CHO cells[a]

Treatment	SER[a]
No drug	1.0
1.0 µM CPT	1.4
1.0 µM CPT + aphidicolin	1.1
1.0 µM CPT + cordycepin	1.4
1.0 µM CPT + cyclohexamide	1.7
1.0 µM CPT + 2,4-dinitrophenol	1.5

[a]Radiation survival clonogenic assays were conducted with CHO cells co-treated with 1 µM of CPT and various inhibitors for 30 minutes prior to irradiation.
[b]SER, sensitization enhancement ratio = radiation dose at 10% Sv of control curve divided by radiation dose at 10% Sv of drug-treated curve.

TABLE 2. Modulation of camptothecin (CPT)-induced radiation sensitization by p53 and p21 in various human cells[a]

	Cells line	SER[b]
Breast cancer	MCF-7	1.3
	MCF-7/E6	0.9
Cervical cancer	HeLa	1.0
Colon cancer	HCT-116 (parental)	2.0
	HCT-116 (p53-/-)	1.6
	HCT-116 (p21-/-)	1.0

[a]Radiation survival clonogenic assays were conducted with cells of various cell lines treated with or without 1 µM of CPT prior to irradiation.
[b]SER, sensitization enhancement ratio = radiation dose at 10% Sv of control curve divided by radiation dose at 10% Sv of drug-treated curve.

Clonogenic Survival Assay. Overnight cultures of $0.5 - 1 \times 10^6$ per 100-mm dish exponentially growing cells were treated with drug and radiation of various protocols. Cells were then trypsinized, rinsed, counted, and plated for colony formation. Following 1–2 weeks of incubation, colonies were fixed and stained with crystal violet. All survival points were done in triplicate.

SUMMARY

We found that CPT induced RS in a time-dependent manner. In CHO cells, the maximal level of RS was induced immediately after drug incubation and gradually diminished in the next 4–8 hours. Cotreatment with replication inhibitor-aphidicolin, but not inhibitors for transcription and protein synthesis, partially reversed the CPT-induced RS (TABLE 1). These results suggest that the interactions between drug-trapped topo-I cleavable complexes and replication fork precede the initiation of RS. Three independent lines of experiments indicate that p53 and p21 regulatory pathways are involved in topo-I-mediated RS in human cells (TABLE 2). First, human HeLa cells, which contain a disrupted p53 function due to the endogenously existing HPV16-E6 protein, are resistant to CPT-induced RS. Second, in contrast to parental MCF-7 cells, HPV16-E6-transfected MCF-7/E6 cells are resistant to CPT-induced RS. Third, the level of RS induced by CPT in parental HCT-116 colon cancer cells decreases in its isogenic p53 knockout cells and diminishes in its isogenic p21 knockout cells. Our finding is consistent with a model that the RS process is initiated by sublethal cellular damages induced by topo-I poisons. Downstream, the topo-I-mediated sublethal damage may activate DNA damage responses including p53- and p21-regulatory pathways and eventually leads to RS.

REFERENCES

1. HELLMAN, S. 1997. Principles of cancer management: Radiation therapy. *In* Cancer: Principles and Practice of Oncology, V.T. DeVita, S. Hellman & S.A. Rosenberg, Eds. : 307–332. J.B. Lippincott Co. Philadelphia, PA.
2. ROTMAN, M., H. AZIZ & T.H. WASSERMAN. 1998. Chemotherapy and radiation. *In* Cancer: Principles and Practice of Radiation Oncology, C.A. Perez & L.W. Brady, Eds. : 705–722. J.B. Lippincott Co. Philadelphia, PA.
3. CHEN, A.Y. & L.F. LIU. 1994. DNA topoisomerases: essential enzymes and lethal targets. Annu. Rev. Pharmacol. Toxicol. **34:** 191–218.
4. POMMIER, Y., P. POURQUIER; Y. FAN, *et al.* 1998. Mechanism of action of eukaryotic DNA topoisomerase I and drugs targeted to the enzyme. Biochim. Biophys. Acta **1400:** 83–105.
5. MATTERN, M.R., G.A. HOFMANN, F. MCCABE, *et al.* 1991. Synergistic cell killing by ionizing radiation and topoisomerase I inhibitor topotecan (SK&F 104864). Cancer Res. **51:** 5813–5816.
6. BOOTHMAN, D.A., N. FUKUNAGA & M. WANG. 1994. Down-regulation of topoisomerase I in mammalian cells following ionizing radiation. Cancer Res. **54:** 4618–4626.
7. CHEN, A.Y., P. OKUNIEFF, Y. POMMIER, *et al.* 1997. Mammalian DNA topoisomerase I mediates the enhancement of radiation cytotoxicity by camptothecin derivatives. Cancer Res. **57:** 1529–1536.
8. CHEN, A.Y., H. CHOY & M.L. ROTHENBERG. 1999. DNA topoisomerase I-targeting drugs as radiation sensitizers. Oncology **13:** 39–46.
9. Fan, S., M.L. Smith, D.J. Rivet, II, *et al.* 1995. Disruption of p53 function sensitizes breast cancer MCF-7 cells to cisplatin and pentoxifylline. Cancer Res. **55:** 1649–1654.
10. Bunz, F., A. Dutriaux; C. Lengauer, *et al.* 1998. Requirement for p53 and p21 to sustain G2 arrest after DNA damage. Science **282:** 1497–1501.

The Homocamptothecin, BN 80927, Is a Potent Topoisomerase I Poison and Topoisomerase II Catalytic Inhibitor

DANIÈLE DEMARQUAY,[a] HÉLÈNE COULOMB, MARION HUCHET, LAURENCE LESUEUR-GINOT, JOSÉ CAMARA, OLIVIER LAVERGNE, AND DENNIS BIGG

Institut Henri Beaufour, Les Ulis, France

Homocamptothecins (hCPTs, FIG. 1) represent a new family of camptothecin (CPT) analogues in which insertion of a methylene (-CH2-) spacer between the alcohol moiety and carbonyl group of the classical six-membered α-hydroxylactone ring results in a seven-membered β-hydroxylactone ring[1] which undergoes slow and irreversible hydrolytic ring-opening, providing higher plasma concentrations of the active lactone form. Homocamptothecins have been shown to be highly potent antitumor drugs *in vitro* and *in vivo*,[2] acting via a classical topoisomerase (topo) I poisoning mechanism.[3] Structure activity studies[4] led to the selection of a difluorinated hCPT, BN 80915, which is now in clinical trials. Interestingly, we found another promising homocamptothecin, BN 80927,[5] which shows inhibitory effects on topo II activity in addition to its topo I poisoning activity.

RESULTS

BN 80927 (FIG. 1) was compared to SN38 (the active metabolite of CPT-11) or VP-16 (etoposide) in the *in vitro* studies summarized here. BN 80927 is a very stable homocamptothecin, because about 90% of its lactone form remains after 3 hours' incubation in human plasma. In cell-free systems, BN 80927, like other hCPTs, inhibits topo I-mediated supercoiled-DNA relaxation.[5] It was confirmed to be a topo I poison, because it stabilizes topo I-cleavable complexes in HT29 cells as revealed on an immunoblot using topo I-directed antibody (*in vivo* complexes of topo [ICT] assay). Quantitative experiments were performed using DNA-protein-complexes (DPC) assay in living HT29 cells. In this assay, topo I and topo II can be trapped in a covalent complex with DNA by adding denaturants while the enzyme is actively engaged in breaking and resealing steps on DNA. Radiolabeled ^{3}H-DNA-^{14}C-protein-complexes can be quantified after KCL/SDS coprecipitation. The amount of labeled DNA in the precipitate is a measure of DNA molecules covalently bound to proteins. We demonstrated that after 1 hour of incubation of HT29 cells with drugs, the amount of BN 80927-induced DPCs is about threefold higher than that induced by SN38. The DPC levels then reach a plateau that is somewhat higher for BN 80927 than for SN38. Furthermore, the DPCs induced by BN 80927 are more stable than those induced by SN38, as shown by reversion experiments.

---

[a]Institut Henri Beaufour, 5 avenue du Canada, 91966 Les Ulis, France. Fax: 33 1 69 07 38 02.
daniele.demarquay@beaufour-ipsen.com

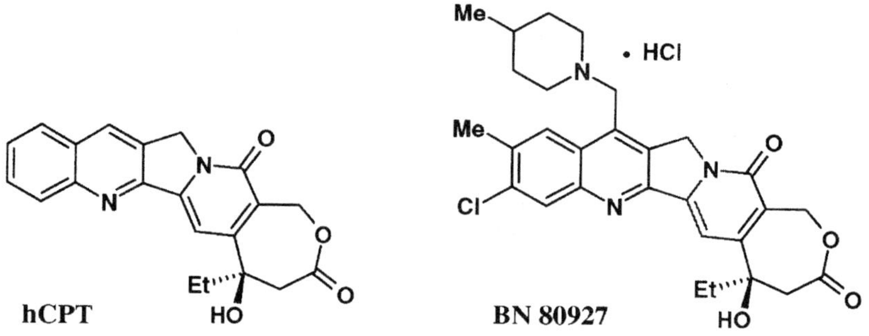

FIGURE 1. Chemical structure of homocamptothecin (hCPT) and its derivative, BN 80927.

In addition to its topo I poisoning activity, BN 80927 shows topo II inhibitory activity; it inhibits topo II-mediated supercoiled-DNA relaxation as well as DNA decatenation. In these two assays it appears more potent than etoposide. However, in contrast to etoposide, it does not stabilize topo II-cleavable complexes, as shown by ICT experiments. Therefore, BN 80927 should be considered a topo II catalytic inhibitor.

CONCLUSION

BN 80927 is a novel, highly stable, homocamptothecin that is both a potent topo I poison and a catalytic inhibitor of topo II. As such, it was of obvious interest to investigate whether this unusual combination leads to a different profile of activity compared to that of pure topo I poisons. Further studies, entailing cytotoxicity experiments on a panel of human tumor cells and xenograft experiments of human prostate adenocarcinoma cells, were undertaken to address this point and are shown in the companion poster (Huchet *et al.*, this volume).

REFERENCES

1. LAVERGNE, O., L. LESUEUR-GINOT, F. PLA RODAS, *et al.* 1997. BN 80245: an E-ring modified camptothecin with potent antiproliferative and topoisomerase I inhibitory activities. Bioorg. Med. Chem. Lett. **7:** 2235–2238.
2. LESUEUR-GINOT, L., D. DEMARQUAY, R. KISS, *et al.* 1999. Homocamptothecin, an E-ring modified camptothecin with enhanced lactone stability, retains topoisomerase I-targeted activity and antitumor properties. Cancer Res. **59:** 2939–2943.
3. BAILLY, C., A. LANSIAUX, L. DASSONNEVILLE, *et al.* 1999. Homocamptothecin, an E-ring modified camptothecin analogue, generates new topoisomerase I-mediated DNA breaks. Biochemistry **38:** 15556–15556.
4. LAVERGNE, O., L. LESUEUR-GINOT, F. PLA RODAS, *et al.* 1998. Homocamptothecins: synthesis and antitumor activity of novel E-ring-modified camptothecin analogues. J. Med. Chem. **41:** 5410–5419.
5. LAVERGNE, O., J. HARNETT, A. ROLLAND, *et al.* 1999. BN 80927: a novel homocamptothecin with inhibitory activities on both topoisomerase I and topoisomerase II. Bioorg. Med. Chem Lett. **9:** 2599–2602.

The Dual Topoisomerase Inhibitor, BN 80927, Is Highly Potent against Cell Proliferation and Tumor Growth

MARION HUCHET,[a] DANIÈLE DEMARQUAY,[a,c] HÉLÈNE COULOMB,[a]
PHILIP KASPRZYK,[b] MARK CARLSON,[b] JEFFREY LAUER,[b]
OLIVIER LAVERGNE,[a] AND DENNIS BIGG[a]

[a]*Institut Henri Beaufour, Les Ulis, France*

[b]*Biomeasure Inc., Milford, Massachusetts, USA*

BN 80927 belongs to a novel family of camptothecin (CPT) analogues, the homocamptothecins (hCPTs),[1] developed on the concept of topoisomerase (topo) I inhibition and characterized by the unique feature of a seven-membered β-hydroxylactone ring. The lower reactivity of the lactone ring results in enhanced plasma stability compared to that of conventional camptothecin analogues such as topotecan and irinotecan. BN 80927, in addition to its topo I poisoning activity, has been shown to be a topoisomerase II catalytic inhibitor.[2] We report here the results of studies evaluating the antiproliferative activity of BN 80927 in a panel of human tumor cell lines, including cells overexpressing P-glycoprotein (PgP). We also evaluated the cytotoxicity of BN 80927 on resting cells, because human tumors are a heterogeneous population of cells including cells that are not actively proliferating. Finally, we report the antitumor activity in xenograft models after oral administration of BN 80927.

BN 80927 IS A POTENT INHIBITOR OF TUMOR CELL PROLIFERATION

The cytotoxic activity of BN 80927 was evaluated on a panel of human tumor cell lines corresponding to different target tissues. Cultured cells were exposed to drugs for 72 hours and subjected to a WST colorimetric assay (Boehringer Mannheim) to evaluate 50% inhibitory concentrations (IC50 values, given with 95% confidence limits). We chose to report here the BN 80927 IC50 values compared to SN38 and topotecan (TPT) of three representative tumor cell lines (HT29, DU145, and HL60), as indicated in TABLE 1. BN 80927 shows high antiproliferative activity with a profile similar to that of benchmarks but with greater potency. A possible effect of PgP and multidrug resistant-associated protein (MRP) overexpression on the activity of BN 80927 was also investigated. TABLE 2 lists the resistance factor (Rf) corresponding to the ratio of IC50 values of the resistant strain HL60dnr (daunorubicin) and HL60adr (adriamycin) with respect to the sensitive parental leukemia cell line (HL60). A lower Rf is obtained for BN 80927 compared to benchmarks in both pairs

[c]*Institut Henri Beaufour, 5 avenue du Canada, 91966 Les Ulis, France. Fax: 33 1 69 07 38 02.*
daniele.demarquay@beaufour-ipsen.com

TABLE 1. *In vitro* cytotoxicity against human tumor cell lines

Cell line		IC$_{50}$ (nM) [95% confidence limits]					
Name	Tissue	BN 80927		SN-38		TPT	
HT29	Colon	21	[11.5–38]	110	[80–140]	210	[140–310]
DU145	Prostate	3.13	[1.56–6]	18	[12–25]	53	[29–97]
HL60	Leukemia	7.4	[1.8–30]	8.37	[1–6.4]	nd	

TABLE 2. Cytotoxicity against resistant cell lines (Resistance factor [Rf] = IC50$_R$/IC50$_S$)

Cell lines couple	Rf BN 80927	Rf SN38
HL60adr/HL60	0.18	1.21
HL60dnr/HL60	4.3	9.93

of cell lines. HL60dnr and HL60adr, respectively, overexpress PgP and MRP; such a low Rf suggests that BN 80927 is not a suitable substrate for these glycoproteins. Moreover, BN 80927 performs better than SN38 in terms of its cytotoxicity on the resistant strains. These results may be of clinical relevance in the context of second-line chemotherapy.

BN 80927 SHOWS CYTOTOXIC ACTIVITY TOWARDS RESTING HT29 CELLS

This study evaluates the effect of BN 80927, compared to SN38 and CPT, on resting cells that are common in human tumors. We examined drug cytotoxicity as a function of cell transition from quiescence to the proliferative state. To accurately determine whether quiescent cells are sensitive to those agents, we briefly exposed synchronous G0/G1 HT29 cell populations to the three drugs with concentrations ranging from 0.64 to 400 nM. Cytotoxicity was assessed 3 days after drug removal.

Neither CPT nor SN38 shows cytotoxic activity on resting cells. In contrast, BN 80927 has potent cytotoxicity activity on resting HT29 cells. VP16, also tested in this model with concentrations varying from 80 to 10,000 nM, showed no activity.

BN 80927 INDUCES TUMOR REGRESSION IN XENOGRAFT MODELS

In vivo, BN 80927 was evaluated in preliminary xenograft studies against PC3 and DU145 transplantable prostate tumors in mice after oral administration. Impressive antitumor activity was found in both models. BN 80927, administered orally, was more efficacious than topotecan or irinotecan administered intraperitoneally in a classical schedule.

CONCLUSION

The results presented here clearly show the high potency of BN 80927 on inhibition of cell growth. BN 80927 was more potent than benchmarks on a wide panel of human tumor cell lines. Furthermore, BN 80927 has higher cytotoxic effects on cells exhibiting multidrug-resistant phenotypes. Because overexpression of the multidrug-resistant proteins PgP and MRP is a limitation to the successful chemotherapy of human tumors, these results suggest that treatment with BN 80927 may be effective not only for primary but also for recurrent tumors resistant to first-line chemotherapy. Another interesting finding that may contribute to clinical efficacy is the potent antiproliferative activity of BN 80927 against resting HT29 cells. The combination of topo I and topo II inhibitory activities along with the effect of BN 80927 on resting and chemoresistant cells may explain its excellent *in vivo* activity in xenograft models compared to established benchmarks. Thus, BN 80927 appears to be a promising antitumor compound with unique features in terms of biological profile and plasma stability.

REFERENCES

1. LAVERGNE, O., L. LESUEUR-GINOT, F. PLA RODAS, *et al.* 1998. Homocamptothecins: synthesis and antitumor activity of novel E-ring-modified camptothecin analogues. J. Med. Chem. **41:** 5410–5419.
2. LAVERGNE, O., J. HARNETT, A. ROLLAND, *et al.* 1999. BN 80927: a novel homocamptothecin with inhibitory activities on both topoisomerase I and topoisomerase II. Bioorg. Med. Chem Lett. **9:** 2599–2602.

Ubiquitin, SUMO-1, and UCRP in Camptothecin Sensitivity and Resistance

SHYAMAL D. DESAI,[a] YONG MAO,[a] MEI SUN,[a] TSAI-KUN LI,[a] JIAXI WU,[b] AND LEROY F. LIU[a,c]

[a]*Department of Pharmacology, UMDNJ-Robert Wood Johnson Medical School, Piscataway, New Jersey 08854, USA*

[b]*Department of Pharmacology and Therapeutics, Roswell Park Cancer Institute, Buffalo, New York 14263, USA*

In our earlier studies we observed that cells treated with the anticancer drug camptothecin (CPT), topoisomerase I (topo I), is rapidly multi-ubiquitinated and destroyed by 26S proteasome.[1] Many tumor cells are found to be defective in this process. Recently, we have also reported that topoisomerase I is conjugated to another ubiquitin-like protein, SUMO-1 (small ubiquitin modifiers), in response to CPT treatment.[2] Here we report upregulation of yet another ubiquitin-like protein in many tumor cells. This protein is identified as the interferon-inducible protein called ISG15 (interferon-stimulatory gene product 15) or UCRP (ubiquitin cross-reactive protein) using antiserum specific to UCRP in Western blot analysis. Interestingly, UCRP was greatly elevated in the cell line transformed with SV40 T-antigen (2RA), but not in its untransformed parental cell line, WI38, suggesting that accumulation of UCRP might be related to oncogenic transformation. We also observed a correlation between CPT hypersensitivity and UCRP upregulation in a panel of colorectal and breast cancer cell lines. By contrast, SUMOylation of topo I is not significantly different in these cancer cell lines.

UCRP is a 15-kD protein and is composed of two domains, each of which bears striking homology to ubiquitin.[3] These two domains are linked to each other with insertion of an extra proline residue at the junction.[3] It was found to be induced upon interferon treatment.[3] Induction of this protein is correlated with the appearance of resistance to viral infections.[3] Interestingly, UCRP is constitutively elevated in humans with the inherited disease ataxia telangiectasia as a result of constitutive activation of NFκB.[4]

SUMO-1 is also a 15-kD protein and has an 18% sequence similarity to ubiquitin.[5] Both SUMO-1 and UCRP are conjugated to target substrates in a way similar but not identical to that of ubiquitin.[3,5] It is well demonstrated that ubiquitin-conjugated substrates are targeted for destruction by 26S proteasome,[5] but the function of SUMO-1 and UCRP conjugation to the target protein has not yet been understood. It has been proposed that SUMO-1 conjugation is required for cellular trafficking or for antagonizing ubiquitination in order to prevent its target destruction.[6] Whether SUMO-1 conjugation to topo I upon CPT treatment is to facilitate or to prevent its

---

[c]*Department of Pharmacology, UMDNJ-Robert Wood Johnson Medical School, 675 Hoes Lane, Piscataway, New Jersey 08854. Voice: 732-235-5484; fax: 732-235-4073.*
   lliu@umdnj.edu

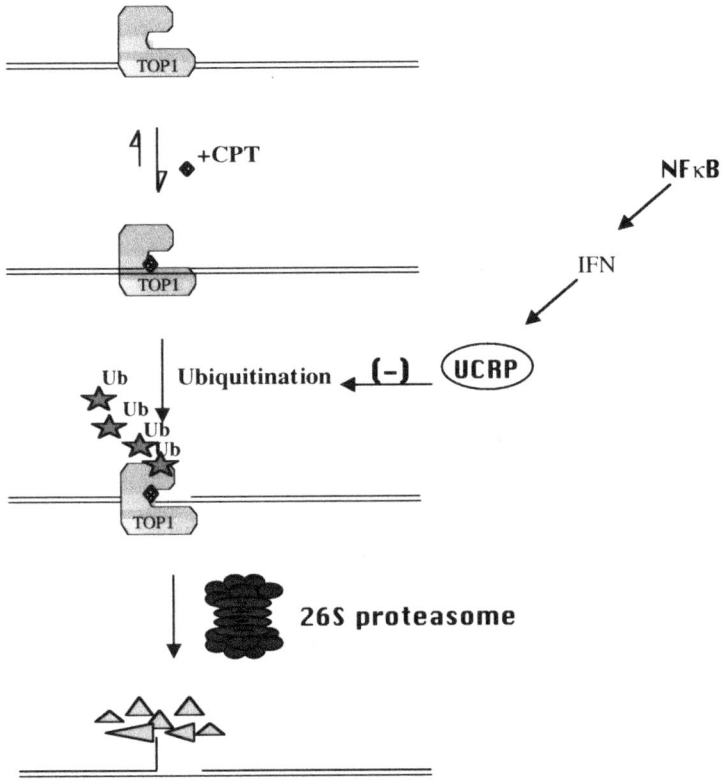

FIGURE 1. A speculative model for the role of UCRP in topo I downregulation.

destruction is unclear. Whether UCRP is conjugated to topo I upon CPT treatment is not yet known. Indeed, most of the substrates conjugated to SUMO-1 (including topoisomerase I) are shown to be conjugated to ubiquitin for their destruction via 26S proteasome.[5] Also, most of the SUMO-1 substrates are known to reside in subnuclear domains, called ND10.[6] These structures are disorganized in promyelocytic leukemia patients.[5] Components of ND10 and also UCRP/ISG15 are induced by interferons.[3,6] Interestingly, NFκB is activated upon CPT treatment, which in turn regulates expression of the IFN-β gene.[4] It has been reported that interferons increase S-phase population and therefore enhance CPT-11 sensitivity.[7] Based on these observations and our data, we hypothesize that in some tumor cells due to constitutive activation of NFκB, interferons are overproduced, leading to UCRP upregulation. Because UCRP is structurally similar to ubiquitin, it might possibly interfere with the normal ubiquitin-mediated destructive process of topo I upon CPT treatment (FIG. 1). This defective topo I downregulation in turn could lead to hypersensitivity of CPT in some tumor cells.

REFERENCES

1. DESAI, S.D., L.F. LIU., D. VAZQUEZ-ABAD & P. D'ARPA. 1997. Ubiquitin-dependent destruction of topoisomerase I is stimulated by the antitumor drug camptothecin. J. Biol. Chem. **272:** 24159–24164.
2. MAO, Y., M. SUN., S.D. DESAI & L.F. LIU. 2000. SUMO-1 conjugation to DNA topoisomerase I: possible repair response to topoisomerase-mediated DNA damage. Proc. Natl. Acad. Sci. USA. In press.
3. LOEB, K.R. & A.L. HAAS. 1992. The interferon-inducible 15-kDa ubiquitin homolog conjugates to intracellular proteins. J. Biol. Chem. **267:** 7806–7813.
4. SIDDOO-ATWAL, C., A.L. HAAS & M.P. ROSIN. 1996. Elevation of interferon beta-inducible proteins in ataxia telangiectasia cells. Cancer Res. **56:** 443–447.
5. KRETZ-REMY, C. & R.M. TANGUAY. 1999. SUMO/sentrin: protein modifiers regulating important cellular functions. Biochem. Cell Biol. **77:** 299–309.
6. CHELBI-ALIX, M.K. & H. DE THE. 1999. Herpes virus induced proteasome-dependent degradation of the nuclear bodies-associated PML and Sp100 proteins. Oncogene **18:** 935–941.
7. OHWADA, S., I. KOBAYASHI, M. MAEMURA, *et al.* 1996. Interferon potentiates antiproliferative activity of CPT-11 against human colon cancer xenografts. Cancer Lett. **110:** 149–154.

A Spectrophotometric Study of the pH-Dependent and DNA Binding Properties of Topotecan

STEVEN E. MILLER AND DANIEL S. PILCH[a]

Department of Pharmacology, UMDNJ-Robert Wood Johnson Medical School, Piscataway, New Jersey 08854, USA

INTRODUCTION

Camptothecin (CPT) and its derivatives are among the most promising new anticancer agents.[1] The cytotoxic activities of these compounds are derived from their abilities to stimulate topoisomerase I (TOP1)-mediated DNA cleavage.[1] Topotecan (TPT) and irinotecan (CPT-11) are two CPT derivatives that currently are in clinical use. In contrast to the water-insoluble noncharged CPT derivatives (e.g., 9-nitrocamptothecin [9NCPT]), TPT and CPT-11 are positively charged at physiological pH and are thus soluble in water. Currently, little is known about the specific molecular interactions that govern the biological activities of the camptothecins. Here, we report spectrophotometric investigations of the pH-dependent and DNA binding properties of TPT.

THE 9-[(DIMETHYLAMINO)METHYL] FUNCTIONALITY OF TPT DESTABILIZES THE PHENOLIC FORM OF THE DRUG

Absorption spectra of TPT at 37°C and pH values ranging from 3.2 to 11.9 are shown in FIGURE 1A. Increasing the pH from 4.0 to 8.2 results in the induction of a new peak at 415 nm. This pH-dependent transition corresponds to the conversion from the phenolic to the phenoxide form of TPT.[2,3] The absorption spectrum of 10-hydroxycamptothecin (10HCPT), a chemically identical compound to TPT except for a proton at the 9-position rather than a (dimethylamino)methyl functionality, exhibits a similar pH-dependent behavior. Note that the peak at 415 nm undergoes a pronounced red shift as the pH increases from 8.2 to 11.9 (FIG. 1A). This spectral shift corresponds to the deprotonation of the 9-[(dimethylamino)methyl] moiety.

FIGURE 1B shows the titration curve at 430 nm extracted from the family of absorption spectra shown in FIGURE 1A. Inspection of this curve reveals the two OH⁻-induced transitions noted above, namely, conversion of the phenolic to the phenoxide form of the drug followed by deprotonation of the 9-[(dimethylamino)methyl] moiety. Each of these pH-dependent transitions can be fit independently with the equation shown below to yield the associated pK_a value.

---

[a]Department of Pharmacology, UMDNJ-Robert Wood Johnson Medical School, 675 Hoes Lane, Piscataway, New Jersey 08854. Voice: 732-235-3352; fax: 732-235-4073.
  pilchds@umdnj.edu

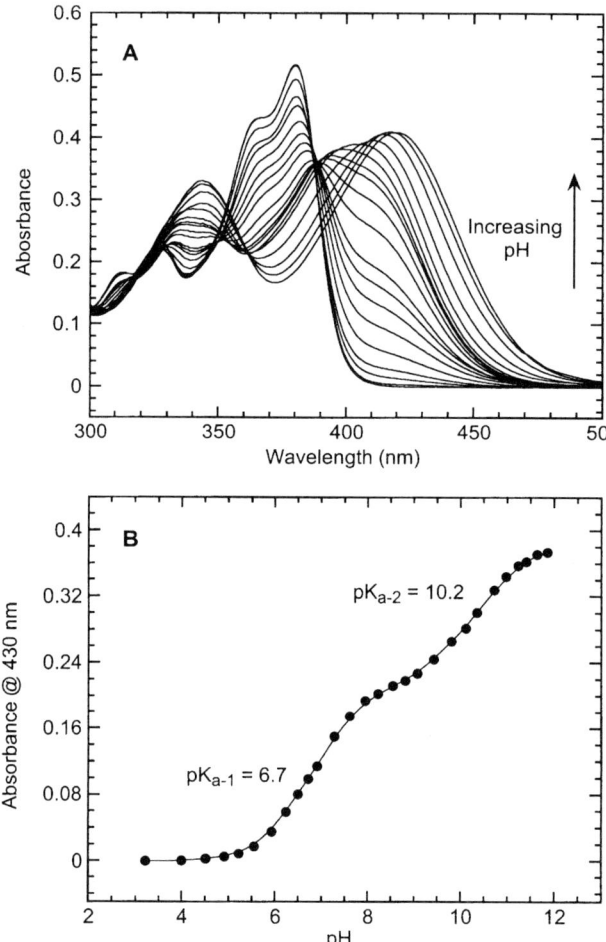

FIGURE 1. (**A**) Absorption spectra of 20 μM TPT at differing values of pH and a temperature of 37°C. From bottom to top at 430 nm, the spectra correspond to pH values of 3.2, 4.5, 5.2, 5.6, 5.9, 6.2, 6.5, 6.7, 6.9, 7.3, 7.6, 8.0, 8.2, 8.8, 9.4, 10.1, 10.7, 11.2, and 11.9. (**B**) Absorbance of TPT at 430 nm plotted as a function of pH. In these experiments, solutions were allowed to equilibrate overnight at 37°C prior to the recording of their absorption spectra. The buffer contained 10 mM sodium phosphate, 10 mM sodium acetate, 10 mM Borate, and 0.1 mM EDTA.

$$A = \frac{(A_{max} - A_{min})(10^{pH-pK})}{1 + (10^{pH-pK})} + A_{max}$$

This analysis yields pK_a values of 6.7 ± 0.1 and 10.2 ± 0.1 for conversion of the phenolic to the phenoxide form and deprotonation of the 9-[(dimethylamino)methyl] moiety, respectively. A similar analysis of the pH-dependent absorbance profile of 10HCPT reveals a pK_a of 8.5 ± 0.1 for conversion of the phenolic to the phenoxide form. Thus, the 9-[(dimethylamino)methyl] moiety destabilizes the phenolic form of the TPT, reducing the pK_a for its conversion to the phenoxide form by 1.8 units relative to 10HCPT.

COMPLEXATION WITH DOUBLE-HELICAL DNA STABILIZES THE PHENOLIC FORM OF TOPOTECAN

FIGURE 2A shows the absorption spectra of TPT obtained by incremental titration of the poly[d(A-T)]$_2$ duplex into a solution of TPT at pH 6.0 and 25°C. Upon the addition of the DNA, the peaks at 315, 330, 360, and 380 nm undergo a reduction in intensity as well as a red shift. These DNA-induced spectral changes are indicative of an interaction between TPT and the host DNA duplex. Another spectral change induced by the addition of the DNA is the disappearance of the peak 415 nm. Recall that this peak corresponds to the phenoxide form of TPT, which, at pH 6.0, comprises ≈20% of the total TPT in solution. Thus, the DNA-induced disappearance of the peak at 415 nm suggests that DNA binding induces the conversion of the phenoxide to the phenolic form of TPT. In other words, DNA preferentially binds and stabilizes the phenolic form of TPT.

Further inspection of FIGURE 2A reveals that the absorption spectra share isosbestic points at 388 and 406 nm, an observation indicative of a single absorbance-detectable mode of TPT binding. In the section that follows we describe how DNA-induced changes in the absorption properties of TPT can be analyzed to provide quantitative estimates for TPT-DNA association constants (K_a) as well as binding site sizes (n).

TOPOTECAN BINDS TO THE POLY[d(A-T)]$_2$ AND POLY[D(G-C)]$_2$ DUPLEXES WITH A SIMILAR AFFINITY AND AN ASSOCIATED SITE SIZE THAT IS CONSISTENT WITH AN INTERCALATIVE MODE OF INTERACTION

FIGURE 2B shows the Scatchard plots derived from the absorbance titrations of TPT with the poly[d(A-T)]$_2$ (FIG. 2A) and poly[d(G-C)]$_2$ (spectra not shown) duplexes. These plots were fitted (*solid lines*) with the McGhee-von Hippel equation[4] shown below, in which ν is the ratio of bound drug to DNA base pairs and L is the concentration of free drug.

$$\frac{\nu}{L} = K_a(1 - n\nu)\left(\frac{1 - n\nu}{1 - (n-1)\nu}\right)^{n-1}$$

These analyses yielded K_a values of 14,900 ± 400 and 14,500 ± 300 M^{-1} for TPT binding to poly[d(A-T)]$_2$ and poly[d(G-C)]$_2$, respectively. Thus, TPT exhibits similar affinities for the two host DNA duplexes. The McGhee-von Hippel analyses also yielded binding site sizes of 1.3 ± 0.3 and 1.4 ± 0.3 base pairs for TPT complexation with poly[d(A-T)]$_2$ and poly[d(G-C)]$_2$, respectively. These binding site sizes are consistent with the nearest-neighbor exclusion binding properties that are characteristic of DNA intercalation.

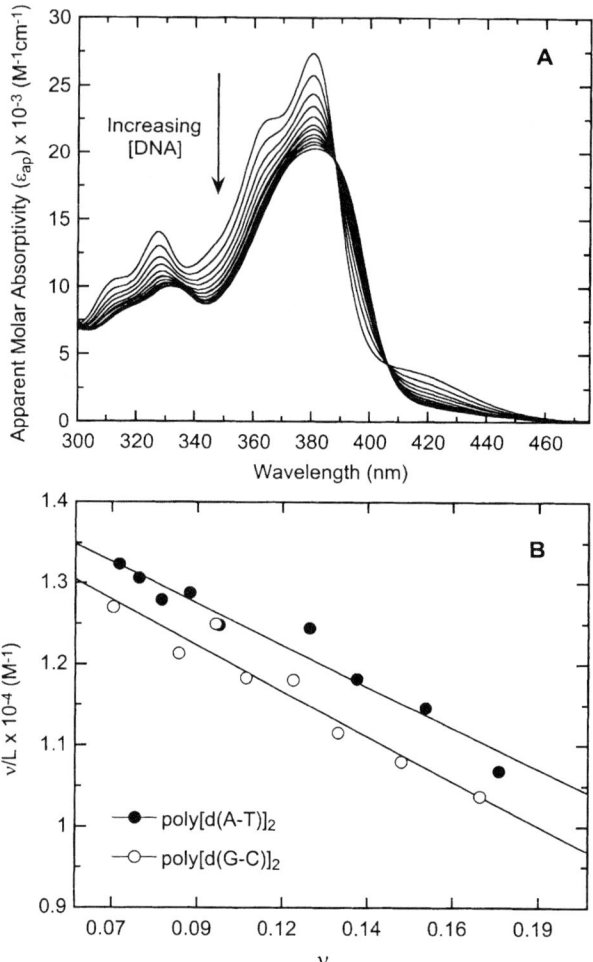

FIGURE 2. (**A**) Absorbance titration at 25°C of TPT (20 µM) with the poly[d(A-T)]$_2$ duplex. From top to bottom at 380 nm, the absorption spectra correspond to base pair/drug ratios of 0, 1, 2, 3, 4, 5, 6, 7, 8, 9, 10, and 12. Titration was conducted in pH 6.0 buffer containing 5 mM sodium cacodylate and 0.1 mM EDTA. (**B**) Scatchard plots derived from absorbance titrations at 25°C of TPT with either poly[d(A-T)]$_2$ (*solid circles*) or poly[d(G-C)]$_2$ (*open circles*). *Solid lines* represent nonlinear least square fits of the data with the McGhee-von Hippel equation shown in the text.

In summary, we have used spectrophotometric techniques to demonstrate that the tertiary amine moiety at the 9-position of TPT destabilizes the phenolic form of the drug. We also show that duplex DNA preferentially binds and stabilizes the phenolic form of TPT. In addition, TPT binds to d(A-T)$_n$·d(T-A)$_n$ and d(G-C)$_n$·d(C-G)$_n$ sequences with a similar affinity and an associated site size that is consistent with an intercalative mode of interaction. Such drug-DNA interactions may be of general importance in the formation and stabilization of ternary drug-DNA-TOP1 cleavable complexes involving camptothecin derivatives.

ACKNOWLEDGMENTS

This work was supported by grants from the National Cancer Institute (CA39962), the American Chemical Society (RPG CDD-98334), and the New Jersey Commission on Cancer Research (00-64-CCR-S).

REFERENCES

1. CHEN, A.Y. & L.F. LIU. 1994. DNA topoisomerases: essential enzymes and lethal targets. Annu. Rev. Pharmacol. Toxicol. **34:** 191–218.
2. FASSBERG, J. & V.J. STELLA. 1992. A kinetic and mechanistic study of the hydrolysis of camptothecin and some analogues. J. Pharm. Sci. **81:** 676–684.
3. CHOURPA, I., J.-M. MILLOT, G.D. SOCKALINGUM, et al. 1998. Kinetics of lactone hydrolysis in antitumor drugs of camptothecin series as studied by fluorescence spectroscopy. Biochim. Biophys. Acta **1379:** 353–366.
4. McGHEE, J.D. & P.H. VON HIPPEL. 1974. Theoretical aspects of DNA-protein interactions: co-operative and non-co-operative binding of large ligands to a one-dimensional lattice. J. Mol. Biol. **86:** 469–489.

Kinetics of *in Vitro* Hydrolysis of Homocamptothecins As Measured by Fluorescence

D. CHAUVIER,[a] I. CHOURPA,[b] D.C.H. BIGG,[c] AND M. MANFAIT[a,d]

[a]*Unité MéDIAN, IFR53, CNRS FRE 2141, UFR de Pharmacie, 51096 Reims, Cedex, France*

[b]*Laboratoire de Chimie Analytique, UFR de Pharmacie, 31 av. Monge, 37200 Tours, France*

[c]*Institut Henri Beaufour, 5 av. du Canada, 91966 Les Ulis, France*

The antitumor activity of camptothecin (CPT) was limited by the rapid pH-dependent conversion into the E-ring open (carboxylate) form, inactive and clinically toxic. At the same time, the reactivity of this ring appeared crucial in view of the activity loss with nonhydrolyzable analogues.

The action of CPTs correlated with stabilization of so-called cleavable complexes between DNA and nuclear topoisomerase I. The role of the lactone/carboxylate interconversion in drug–target contacts upon formation of the cleavable complexes remains unclear.

A novel CPT analogue with a seven-membered β-hydroxylactone ring, homocamptothecin (hCPT, Institut Beaufour, France) was the first to provide slow hydrolysis with inhibition of topoisomerase I and cytotoxic activity comparable to that of CPT.[1]

The study reported here aimed to investigate the β-hydroxylactone reactivity in cleavable complexes. One of the probable partners, DNA was modeled using both the nucleic acids (2' deoxynucleotides 5' monophosphate: dTMP, dCMP, dGMP) and double-stranded specific 30-mer oligonucleotides (Eurogentec, Belgium) corresponding to either strong camptothecin-induced or camptothecin-independent topoisomerase I cleavage sites in SV40.[2] Intrinsic fluorescence of hCPT was used to study the hydrolysis reactions of free drug with a large excess of targets.

The steady-state fluorescence measurements allowed both real-time and noninvasive quantification of hydrolysis kinetics for a submicromolar solution of hCPT in a DNA cleavage buffer. First of all, the fluorescence emission spectra of both intact and E-ring open forms of hCPT were recorded at the same pH and excitation conditions (FIG. 1). Then, the intensity ratio of the emission at two wavelengths was followed as a function of time. The lactone-form fraction was calculated from the spectral parameters, as previously described for CPTs.[3] The experimental precision obtained was satisfactory (about 5%).

---

[d]Address for correspondence: M. Manfait, Unité MéDIAN, IFR53, CNRS FRE 2141, UFR de Pharmacie, 51 rue Cognacq Jay, 51096 Reims, Cedex, France. Voice: (33)326913574; fax: (33)326913550.

michel.manfait@univ-reims.fr

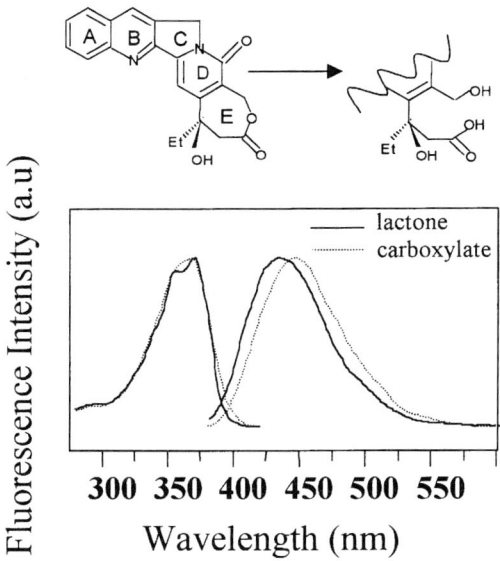

FIGURE 1. Fluorescence excitation (*left*) and emission (*right*) spectra for two forms of hCPT.

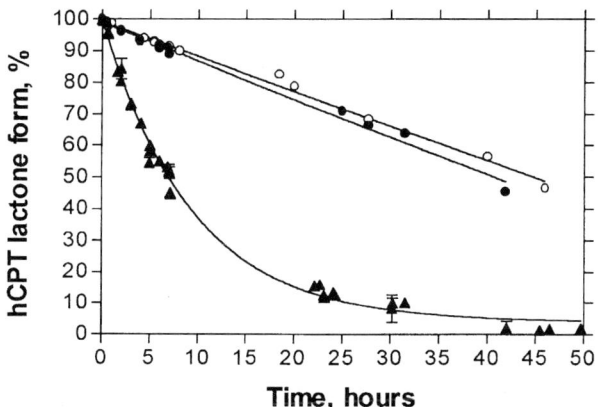

FIGURE 2. Kinetics of lactone hydrolysis for hCPT in the DNA cleavage buffer at pH 7.55 (●) or 8.25 (▲), free and with oligonucleotide (pH 7.55, O).

The results on free drug hydrolysis at different pHs confirmed the enhanced stability of the β-hydroxylactone compared to α-hydroxylactone (FIG. 2), both exhibiting pH-dependent half-lives. In contrast to hydrolysis of CPT, known to reach equilibrium at ca. 20% of lactone, the hCPT hydrolysis appeared total.

No modification in the drug's fluorescence emission was observed immediately after adding nucleotides or DNA. The long-time observation of the hCPT–DNA complexes indicated that the presence of DNA did not induce any changes in the hydrolysis kinetic of the β-hydroxylactone ring. This was unlike the case with CPTs, for which the lactone-form stabilization in the presence of specific nucleotide[4] or GC-containing DNA sequences[5,6] has been reported. Nevertheless, for CPT, the DNA-induced stabilization of lactone was indeterminant for cleavable complexe formation *in vitro*.[5]

While providing a pool of the active form of CPT, such "lactone protection" should not be necessary for hCPT, which is intrinsically more stable. The β-hydroxylactone/carboxylate equilibrium in ternary cleavable complexes is under investigation in our group.

REFERENCES

1. LESUEUR-GINOT, L. *et al.* 1999. Homocamptothecin, an E-ring modified camptothecin with enhanced lactone stability, retains topoisomerase I-targeted activity and antitumour properties. Cancer Res. **59:** 2939–2943.
2. JAXEL, C. *et al.* 1991. Effect of local DNA sequence on topoisomerase I cleavage in the presence or absence of camptothecin. J. Biol. Chem. **266:** 20418–20423.
3. CHOURPA, I. *et al.* 1998. Kinetics of lactone hydolysis in antitumour drugs of camptothecin series as studied by fluorescence spectroscopy. Biochim. Biophys. Acta **1379:** 353–366.
4. YAO, S. *et al.* 1998. Topotecan lactone selectivity binds to double and single-stranded DNA in the absence of topoisomerase I. Cancer Res. **58:** 3782–3786.
5. CHOURPA, I. *et al.* 1998. Modulation of kinetics of lactone ring hydrolysis of camptothecins upon interaction with topoisomerase I cleavage sites on DNA. Biochemistry **37:** 7584–7291.
6. YANG, D. *et al.* 1998. DNA interactions of two clinical camptothecin drugs stabilize their active lactone forms. J. Am. Chem. Soc. **120:** 2979–2980.

The Combinatorial Synthesis of Racemic Homosilatecan Libraries via a Cascade Radical Annulation

WU DU,[a] ANA E. GABARDA, DAVID BOM, AND DENNIS P. CURRAN

Department of Chemistry, University of Pittsburgh, Pittsburgh, Pennsylvania 15260, USA

Isolated from the Chinese tree, *Camptotheca accuminata,* in 1966 by Wani and Wall, camptothecin (CPT) has been a prominent lead for anticancer drug development for more than three decades. Despite its excellent *in vitro* activity, CPT failed in clinical trial because of its *in vivo* hydrolysis, which gives an inactive carboxylate.[1–3] Susceptibility of the lactone functionality of CPT results from the intramolecular hydrogen bonding between the lactone carbonyl and the α-hydroxy group. However, this structural feature is needed for binding of CPT to the receptor. Thus, to have a stable lactone while maintaining activity remains a challenge in this field.

Lipophilic CPT analogues were found to achieve lactone stabilization through lipid bilayer partitioning.[4–6] Developed in our group, 7-silylcamptothecins (silatecans)[7] were found to have highly improved blood stabilities, and one of them, DB-67, was selected for preclinical development. Homocamptothecins, another class of E-ring analogues having a methylene spacer between the hydroxy and the carbonyl groups, were also found to have considerably improved blood stabilities.[8] The combination of these two features resulted in homosilatecans that showed high lipophilicity and markedly improved human blood stabilities.[9] We report here our synthesis of homosilatecan libraries for further structure-activity relationship studies.

Synthesis of the racemic DE fragment is illustrated in Scheme 1. From commercially available starting material (**1**), intermediate (**2**) was prepared after five steps, and it was used in our synthesis of silatecan. Dihydroxylation followed by oxidative cleavage of the resulted diol gave ketone (**3**). Then, a Reformatsky reaction on ketone (**3**) followed by acid-catalyzed lactonization gave lactone (**4**). The TMS-iodide exchange was achieved using ICl as the iodination reagent. The reaction gave a high yield based on 50% recovery of the starting lactone (**4**). Finally, the methoxy group was deprotected by TMSI generated *in situ* to give the desired iodopyridone (**6**) (DE fragment) in 65% yield (Scheme 1).

N-Alkylation of iodopyridone (**6**) with different propargyl bromides (**7**) gave compounds (**8**) that were subjected to a cascade radical annulation with different aryl isonitriles (**9**) to give racemic homosilatecans (**10**) with two elements of diversity (Scheme 2).

More than 100 racemic homosilatecans (**10**) were prepared by this radical annulation reaction by either the traditional way or a Hewlett-Packard solution phase syn-

[a]Voice: 412-624-4946; fax: 412-624-9861.
wudu+@pitt.edu

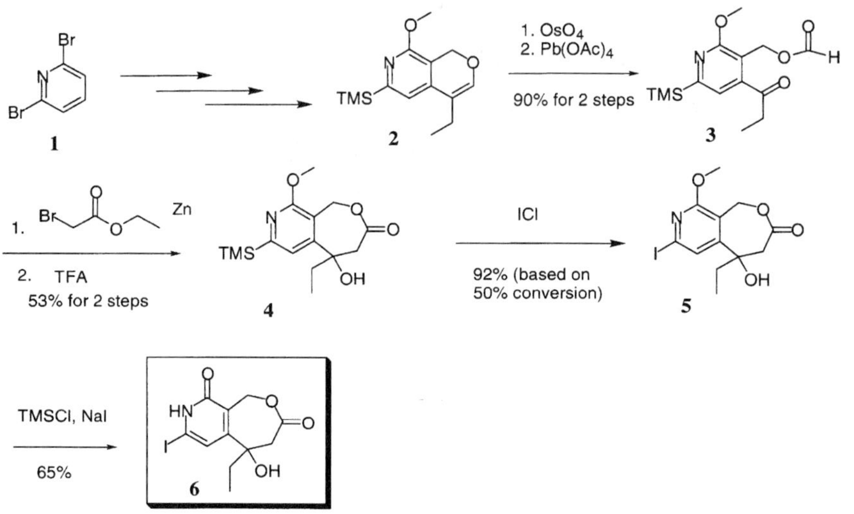
1. OsO4
2. Pb(OAc)4
90% for 2 steps
1. Zn
2. TFA
53% for 2 steps
ICl
92% (based on
50% conversion)
TMSCl, NaI
65%
1
2
3
4
5
6

SCHEME 1. Synthesis of intermediate 6.

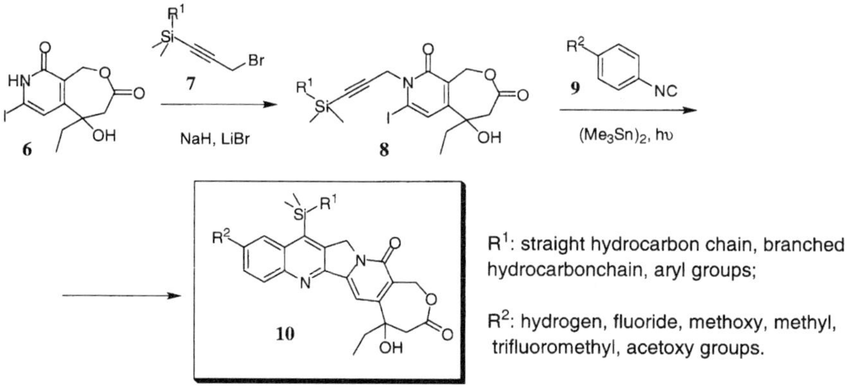
7
NaH, LiBr
8
9
(Me3Sn)2, hυ
6
10
R1: straight hydrocarbon chain, branched
hydrocarbonchain, aryl groups;
R2: hydrogen, fluoride, methoxy, methyl,
trifluoromethyl, acetoxy groups.

SCHEME 2. Synthesis of homosilatecans by a cascade radical cyclization.

thesizer. The automated purification protocol includes, first, a solid phase extraction on silica gel plug to remove the tin, excess aryl isonitriles, and other impurities. Then the crude products (**10**) were further purified by Gilson reversed-phase serial HPLC to give **10** with >95% purity by LC-MS. Some products were also characterized by ^{1}H-NMR and high resolution MS.

In conclusion, we have developed a practical method for the preparation of diverse homosilatecan analogues. The automated purification has allowed fast sample isolation with high purity and in satisfactory yield. More than 100 racemic homosilatecan analogues were prepared. Bioassay of these analogues will provide important information concerning the structure-activity relationship of this family of anticancer agents. Our goal is to identify analogues with high blood stability and anticancer activity for clinical development.

ACKNOWLEDGMENT

We thank the National Institutes of Health for funding this work.

REFERENCES

1. HERTZBERG, R.P., M.J. CARANFA & S.M. HECHT. 1989. Biochemistry **28**: 4629.
2. HSIANG, Y-H. & L.F. LIU. 1988. Cancer Res. **48**: 1722.
3. JAXEL, C., K.W. KOHN, M.C. WANI, et al. 1989. Cancer Res. **49**: 5077.
4. MI, Z. & T.G. BURKE. 1994. Biochemistry **33**: 10325.
5. BURKE, T.G., A.E. STAUBUS, A.K. MISHRA & H. MALAK. 1992. J. Am. Chem. Soc. **114**: 8318.
6. BURKE, A., T.G. MISHRA, A.K. WANI & M. WALL. 1993. Biochemistry **32**: 5352.
7. JOSIEN, H., S.-B.KO, D. BOM, D. & D.P. CURRAN. 1998. Chem. Eur. J. **4**: 67.
8. LAVERGNE, O., L. LESUEUR-GINOT, F.P. RODAS, et al. 1998. J. Med. Chem. **41**: 5410.
9. BOM, D., D.P. CURRAN, A.J. CHAVAN, et al. 1999. J. Med. Chem. **42**: 3018.

Combined Radiation and 9-Nitrocamptothecin (Rubitecan) in the Treatment of Locally Advanced Pancreatic Cancer

K. R. KEMP, J. G. LIEHR, AND B. GIOVANELLA

Stehlin Foundation for Cancer Research, 1918 Chenevert, Houston, Texas 77003, USA

The mechanism of camptothecin (CPT) and its analogues as topoisomerase I inhibitors has been well elucidated. As with most chemotherapeutic agents, once their mechanism of action is defined, it becomes common practice to combine them with a second treatment modality. The goal of combined modalities that act through different cellular pathways is to obtain either an additive or a synergistic effect, ultimately achieving improved tumor toxicity. In no area is this philosophy better illustrated then in the approach to locally advanced pancreatic cancer.

There are two primary reasons that we continue to pursue new treatments for this disease. First, clinical studies have shown that the current standardized chemotherapy for pancreatic cancer, Gemcitabine, has only a 23.8% clinical response rate.[1] Secondly, in 1998 the incidence of pancreatic cancer equalled the number of deaths, thus emphasizing our current inadequacies of treatment.[2]

Radiation is a logical modality to combine with chemotherapy because of its DNA injury through ionization. In the last few years, multiple studies have been published on the antitumor effect of CPT in addition to radiation. For example, 9-nitrocamptothecin has enhanced radiation lethality.[3] However, we do not know how to optimally dose the radiation with CPT and its analogues. This study was designed to address this question.

METHODS

Three-month-old nude homozygous Swiss mice belonging to the NIH high fertility strain were used. These mice were bred and raised at the Stehlin Foundation and maintained under strict pathogen-free conditions. They were kept one to three per cage with ad lib feeding and daily supplementation of vitamins, ampicillin, and gentamicin. The pancreatic cancer cells were obtained from the American Type Culture Collection. For inoculation, each mouse was anesthetized with intraperitoneal Avertin. Ten million cells were then injected subcutaneously in the right hind leg of each animal. Dr. Z. Cao formulated the Rubitecan (9-nitrocamptothecin, 9NC) at the Stehlin Foundation for Cancer Research. The stock suspension was prepared by combining 50 mg of drug with 25 cc of cottonseed oil. The 0.25 mg/kg dosage was made by combining 0.63 cc stock plus 19.4 cc cottonseed oil. All groups received 5-day per week intragastric injections of the Rubitecan for 6 weeks. Radiation treatments were performed in the Radiation Oncology Department of St. Joseph Hospital, Houston, Texas. Electron beam radiation was given once weekly, with the first treatment given the same week in which the Rubitecan dosing started. Radiation doses and number of fractionations were randomly selected for each experimental group. After anesthetizing the mice, the right hind limb was positioned for treatments. Tumors were irradiated with 12 MeV electrons produced by a Siemens Linear Accelerator at a dose rate of 2.76 Gy/min at 100 SSD. The depth was prescribed at the midplane depth of the tumor. A 0.5-cm bolus was used to increase the surface dose. Dose variation was ± 2%. In each experimental group, the mice were randomized into one of four groups. These groups included treatments of Rubitecan only, radiation only, Rubitecan plus radiation, or control. Randomization was performed by a computer program designed by Doug Coil at the Stehlin Foundation for Cancer Research. The tumors were measured weekly using calipers to assess antitumor activity. On average, they measured 140 mm^3 at the start of therapy. The mice were weighed weekly. Each experimental group was followed between 15 and 18 weeks after tumor injection.

RESULTS

In the first experimental group (FIG. 1), Rubitecan (0.25 mg/kg) was injected via intragastric route five times per week for 6 weeks. Radiation was given as 500 rads once a week only during the first 2 weeks of treatment. The combined effect of the two treatments was less than the additive effect of the two treatments alone. In the second experimental group, the same Rubitecan dosing was used; however, the radi-

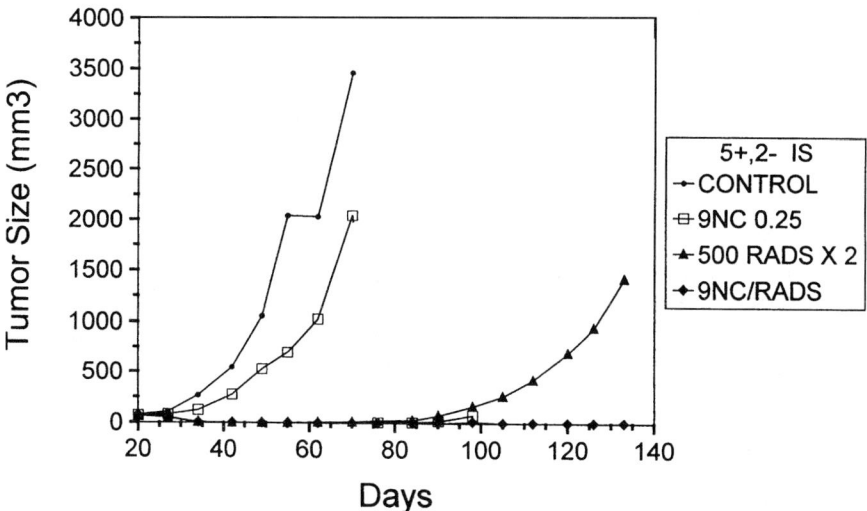

FIGURE 1. Response of a pancreatic cell line (MiaPaca$_2$) to Rubitecan and radiation treatment. Days are measured from the time of tumor injection. Radiation was administered as 500 rads on days 22 and 29.

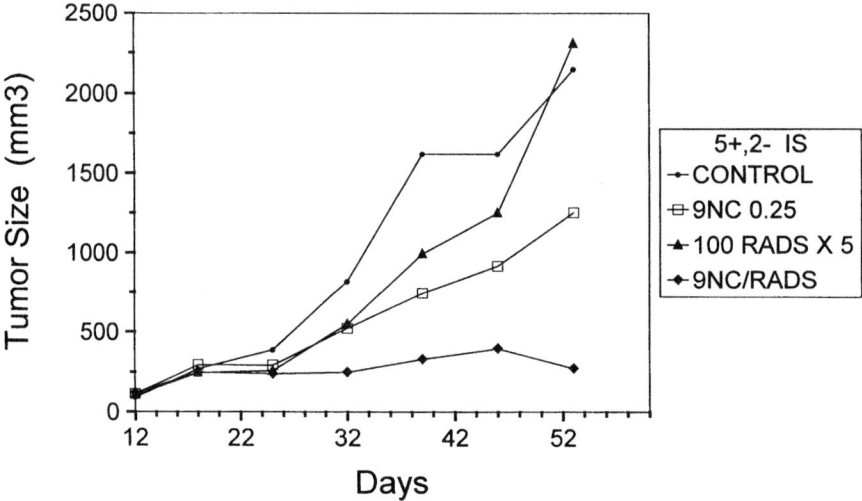

FIGURE 2. Response of a pancreatic cell line (MiaPaca$_2$) to Rubitecan and radiation treatment. Days are measured from the time of tumor injection. Radiation was administered as 100 rads on days 20, 27, 34, 41, and 48.

ation was administered as 200 rads weekly for 3 weeks. Again the combined effect was less than the additive effect. In the third experiment (FIG. 2), radiation was administered as 100 rads weekly for 5 weeks, while the Rubitecan was again dosed the same as before. This combination was equivalent to the additive effect of the two treatments alone.

DISCUSSION

As cancer researchers strive to find better therapies, we realize that there are multiple hurdles to overcome. One such hurdle is to find optimum dosing patterns of newly discovered modalities. This study proves that a variety of administration schedules can be chosen; however, not all are equally effective. In the first experiment, the high dose radiation given in two fractions proved antagonistic in the combination therapy. This likely occurs because of the instantaneous cell death caused by the radiation, which masks the effect of prolonged Rubitecan dosing. Conversely, in the last experiment, when the period of radiation treatments was spread over 5 weeks and at lower doses, we do see an additive effect of Rubitecan and radiation. This likely occurs because the repeated sublethal ionizing injury to the DNA leads to an increased number of DNA + topoisomerase I complexes, thus causing maximum susceptibility to the effect of Rubitecan. In the future, the design of clinical protocols for combined radiation and Rubitecan treatments should include low daily radiation dosing spanning several weeks instead of single fraction high dose therapies.

REFERENCES

1. ROTHENBERG, M. 1996. New developments in chemotherapy for patients with advanced pancreatic cancer. Oncology **10:** 18–22.
2. AMERICAN CANCER SOCIETY. 1998. Cancer Facts and Figures, 1998. :14.
3. LAMOND, J. *et al.* 1996. Radiation lethality enhancement with 9-aminocamptothecin: comparison to other topoisomerase I inhibitors. Int. J. Radiation Oncol. Biol. Phys. **36:** 369–376.

Preclinical and Phase I Clinical Studies with Ckd-602, a Novel Camptothecin Derivative

J.H. LEE,[a] J.M. LEE,[a] K.H. LIM,[a] J.K. KIM,[a] S.K. AHN,[a] Y.J. BANG,[b] AND C.I. HONG[a]

[a]*CKD Research Institute, CKD Pharmaceutical Corporation, Seoul 152-600, Korea*
[b]*Department of Hematooncology, Seoul National Univ. Hospital, Seoul, Korea*

INTRODUCTION

CKD-602, 7-[2-(*N*-isopropylamino)ethyl]-(20S)-camptothecin, is a novel camptothecin derivative antitumor agent under development by Chong Kun Dang Pharm., Seoul, Korea (FIG. 1).[1] Like other camptothecin derivatives, CKD-602 is a potent inhibitor of topoisomerase I, and successfully overcomes the poor watersolubility and toxicity of the parent drug.

PRECLINICAL STUDIES

Preclinical studies of CKD-602 demonstrated broad antitumor activity against various human tumor cell lines, and the results were equal or superior to those of camptothecin (CPT) and topotecan (TPT), a clinically active antitumor drug.[2,3] CKD-602 was less active than CPT against L1210 *in vitro*; the IC_{50} value was 0.55 μg/ml and 0.2 μg/ml, respectively. However, it showed superior *in vivo* antitumor activity to CPT against L1210 (ILS% was 168 and 110, respectively), and superior to TPT against L1210 leukemia (ILS% was 168 and 127, respectively), P388 leukemia, Lewis lung carcinoma, and B16 melanoma. CKD-602 treatment resulted in tumor regression, extensive tumor growth delays even in highly resistant CX-1 colon tumor (the IR% of CKD-602 was 88, whereas that of TPT was 70), and a broader therapeutic dosage range than TPT ([R/E]max value was 1.33 and 3.44, respectively). Preliminary studies showed that the intermittent dosing schedule showed superior antitumor activity to a single dose schedule.[4] In studies of CKD-602 against a panel of human tumor xenografts comprised of colon and breast carcinoma, greater activity and higher [R/E]max values were obtained than with TPT.

PHASE I CLINICAL STUDIES

A phase I and pharmacologic study was undertaken to determine the maximum-tolerated dose, the principal toxicities, and the pharmacologic behavior of CKD-602, a semisynthetic analogue of camptothecin with broad preclinical antitumor activity. Thirty-minute infusions of CKD-602 were performed daily for 5 consecutive days every 3 weeks in patients with advanced solid malignancies at doses ranging from 0.5–0.9 mg/m^2/day. Throughout the different doses, grade 3 and 4 neutropenia occurred in most courses; however, neutropenia was brief with rarely associated fever.

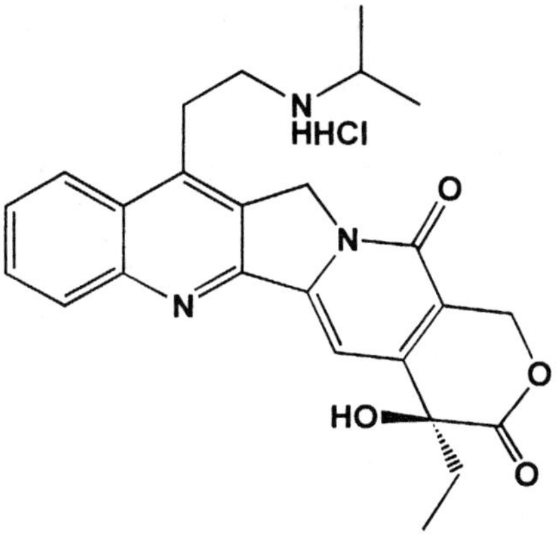

FIGURE 1. Chemical structure of CKD-602.

At doses of 0.7 and 0.9 mg/m^2/day, CKD-602 also induced mild depression in the hematocrit level, which was suitable grade 2 or 3; however, precipitous drops requiring transfusional therapy did not occur in all courses. Anemia, vomiting, and diarrhea were infrequent and modest in severity. Responses were observed in ovarian and stomach carcinoma. Drug disposition in plasma was described by a three-compartment or noncompartment model, with renal elimination accounting for 33.1–50.3% of drug disposition, and the accumulation index, which was compared with the AUC on day 1, varied from 1.13–1.27.

CONCLUSION

The maximum tolerated dose was 0.7 mg/m^2/day when CKD-602 was administered daily for 5 consecutive days every 3 weeks. Dose-limiting toxicity was shown to be neutropenia, and no other severe toxicity was observed. Partial responses were observed in patients with stomach and ovarian cancer. The results warrant further clinical development of CKD-602. Phase II clinical trials with gastric, ovarian, colon, and small cell lung cancer patients are ready to begin.

REFERENCES

1. JEW, S.S. et al. 1996. Inventors; Chong Kun Dang Corp., assignee. 1996. WO96/2166. Date of publication: July 18.
2. LEE, J.-H. et al. 1998. Antitumor activity of 7-[2-(N-isopropylamino)ethyl]-(20S)-camptothecin, CKD602, as a potent topoisomerase I inhibitor. Arch. Pharm. Res. **22**: 581–590.
3. LEE, J.-H. et al. 1998. Antitumor activities of CKD602, a novel camptothecin derivative [abstr]. Proc. Am. Assoc. Cancer Res. **39**: Abstr. No. 2071.
4. LEE, J.-H. et al. 1999. Toxicity, pharmacokinetics and cell-killing kinetics of CKD-602, a novel camptothecin agent. Proc. Am. Assoc. Cancer Res. **40**: Abstr. No. 716.

Action of Topoisomerase Targeting Drugs on Non-Hodgkin's Lymphoma and Leukemia
Correlation of Clinical and Cell Culture Studies

J.S. NAIR,[a] R. KANCHERLA,[b] K. SEITER,[b] F. TRAGANOS,[c] AND Y.-C. TSE-DINH[a]

[a]*Department of Biochemistry and Molecular Biology,* [b]*Zalmen A. Arlin Cancer Institute,*
[c]*Brander Cancer Institute, New York Medical College, Valhalla, New York 10595, USA*

In two phase I clinical studies, patients with non-Hodgkin's lymphoma (NHL) were treated with a combination of topotecan and etoposide (VP16), whereas patients with acute leukemia were treated with a combination of topotecan and ara-C (TA study) or topotecan, ara-C, and mitoxantrone (TAM study). The NHL patients were given 1–2.5 mg/m^2/day of topotecan for 30 minutes intravenously followed by 150 mg/m^2/day of VP16 for 3 hours over 5 days. Peripheral blood samples were collected from patients before treatment, immediately after topotecan and VP16 on day 1 and 3, and post-treatment on day 5, in sarkosyl to trap the topoisomerase (topo)–DNA covalent complexes for the In Vivo Link assay[1] and in EDTA for preparation of leukocyte RNA. In the TA study, patients were treated with 1 g/m^2/day of ara-C for 2 hours followed by 4.75–7.0 mg/m^2/day of topotecan for 30 minutes over 5 days with blood sampled at pre-treatment and post-topotecan on all 5 days. In the TAM study, patients were treated with 1 g/m^2/day of ara-C for 2 hours over 5 days, 3–4 mg/m^2/day of topotecan for 30 minutes from day 2–5 after ara-C, and 20–50 mg/m^2/day of mitoxantrone on day 6. Blood samples were collected pre-treatment, post-topotecan on days 3 and 5, post-treatment on day 7, and off-treatment on day 15.

Formation of covalent topo–DNA complexes was found to vary between patients. A significant correlation was noted between the clinical response and the formation of drug-induced covalent complex in NHL patients. All patients with complete and partial remission formed a drug-induced covalent complex, whereas some patients with stable or progressive disease also formed the complex. The formation of protein–DNA covalent complex appeared to be necessary but not sufficient for clinical response. The responders were more likely to form topo–DNA covalent complex than the nonresponders ($p = 0.0237$). In the TA study, correlation was not possible, as none of the patients clinically responded to the treatment. In the TAM study, covalent complex formation was examined only in two patients. One of these patients responded to treatment and was found to form the covalent complex at all expected time points.

Semiquantitative cDNA-polymerase chain reaction (PCR) was performed to examine the levels of topo I, topo IIα, and IIβ mRNA. The signal intensity of the PCR product obtained for actin was used to normalize the signal intensities of topogenes. The mRNA levels of topo I and IIβ did not show a large change during the course of treatment compared to the respective pre-treatment levels. However, topo I and IIβ mRNA levels of the responding NHL patients stayed at a higher level throughout treatment as compared to the nonresponders (FIG. 1A). A consistent decline in the level of topo IIα mRNA in the peripheral blood leukocytes of both NHL and leuke-

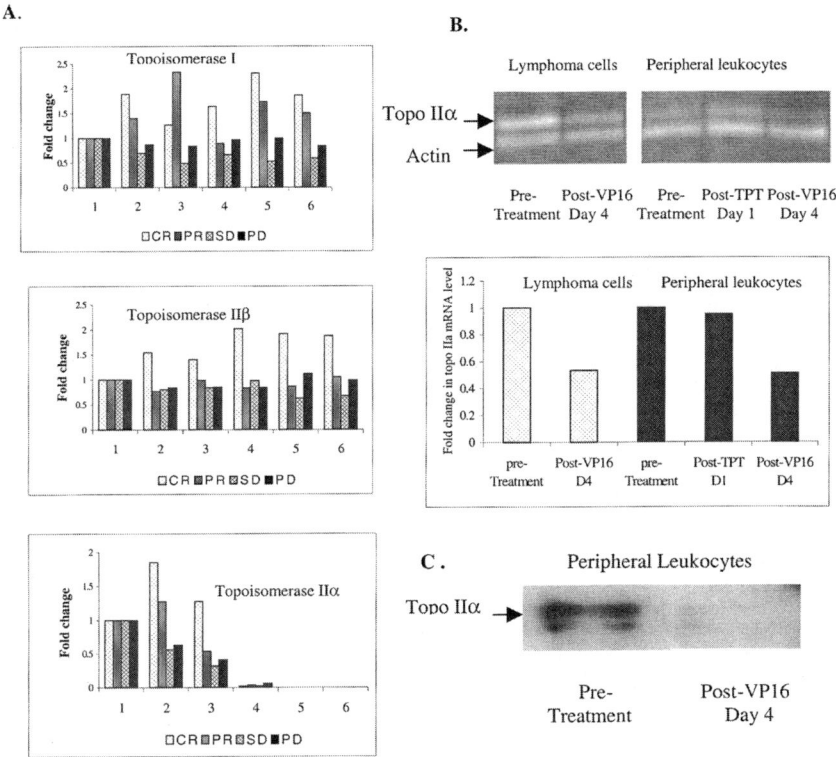

FIGURE 1. Expression of topoisomerases in patients with non-Hodgkin's lymphoma (NHL) during treatment. (**A**) Summary of change in mRNA levels for topoisomerase I, IIα, and IIβ in peripheral lymphocytes of 20 NHL patients as determined by semiquantitative cDNA-polymerase chain reaction (PCR). PCR products were analyzed by gel electrophoresis. Signal intensities from ethidium bromide-stained bands were normalized to the corresponding actin signal intensity and then divided by the pre-treatment level. The samples correspond to: (1) pre-treatment, (2) day 1 post topotecan, (3) day 1 post VP16, (4) day 3 post topotecan, (5) day 3 post VP16, and (6) day 5 post VP16. Patients were grouped according to clinical response. CR, complete response; PR, partial response; SD, stable disease; PD, progressive disease. (**B**) Comparison of topo IIα mRNA levels in lymphoma cells and peripheral leukocytes of an NHL patient during treatment. (**C**) Western blot analysis of the topo IIα protein level in peripheral leukocytes of the NHL patient studied in **B**. Equal concentration of nuclear extracts as determined by the BioRad assay were loaded, and the transfer was confirmed by Ponceau S staining of the blot.

mia patients was observed over the course of treatment. To determine the effect in the cancer cells in NHL, lymphoma cells were collected from one patient at three time points along with the peripheral blood during treatment. The pattern of topo IIα mRNA levels was similar in the lymphoma and peripheral leukocytes (FIG. 1B). Consistent with the decrease in the topo IIα mRNA level, a decrease in the topo IIα protein level was also observed in the peripheral leukocytes as determined by West-

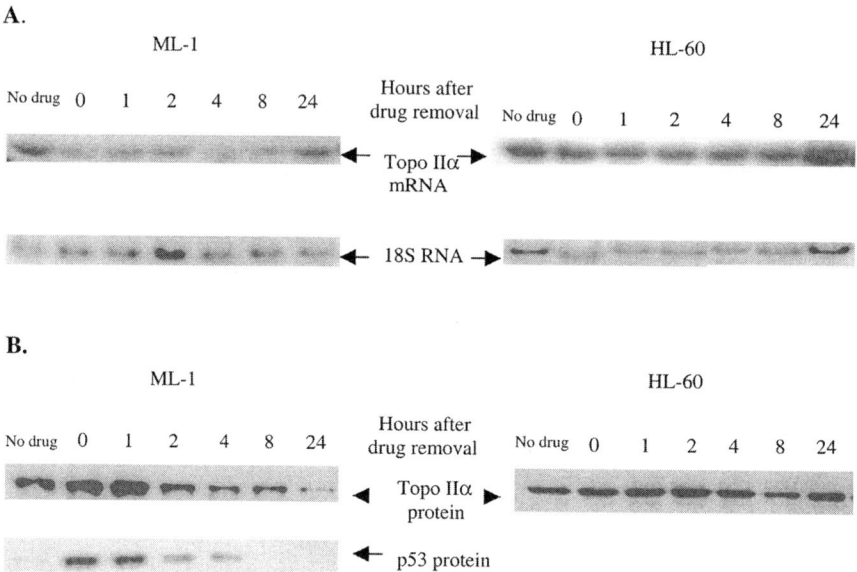

FIGURE 2. Effect of camptothecin treatment on the expression level of topo IIα in ML-1 and HL-60 leukemia cell lines. (**A**) Northern blot analysis of the topo IIα mRNA level. Signal from the 18S RNA was used as a standard for loading. (**B**) Western blot analysis of the topo IIα protein level in the two cell lines and the induction of p53 in ML-1 cells.

ern blot analysis (FIG. 1C). Similar decreases in topo IIα mRNA and protein levels were also observed in the leukemia patients (data not shown).

The decrease in the topo IIα level could be due to either the death of all the proliferating cells or the downregulation of topo IIα gene transcription by the increase in the p53 level in response to drug-induced DNA damage. It has been reported that p53 can downregulate the transcription of the topo IIα gene by binding to its basal promoter region.[2,3] To determine the effect of wild-type p53 on the expression level of topo IIα, two leukemic cell lines, ML-1 (wild-type p53) and HL-60 (p53 null), were selected. The cells were treated with 100–200 nM camptothecin for 1 hour to induce similar degrees of apoptosis as measured by flow cytometry, PARP cleavage, and DNA fragmentation. The drug was then removed and the cells were allowed to recover. The expression levels of topo IIα mRNA and protein were determined by Northern and Western blots (FIG. 2). In ML-1, p53 protein was induced followed by a decrease of topo IIα mRNA and protein levels from the pre-treatment level. In HL-60, topo IIα mRNA and protein levels remained relatively the same as pre-treatment levels (FIG. 2). It is therefore possible that the decrease in topo IIα mRNA in both NHL and leukemia patients after treatment with topotecan could result from the increase in the p53 level, although other mechanisms of downregulation of topo IIα could not be ruled out entirely. The transient nature of the increase in topo IIα expression after camptothecin treatment and its subsequent decrease should be considered in designing schedules for combination therapy using inhibitors of both topo I and topo II.

REFERENCES

1. SUBRAMANIAN, D. et al. 1995. Analysis of topoisomerase I/DNA complexes in patients administered topotecan. Cancer Res. **55:** 2097–2103.
2. SANDRI, M.I. et al. 1996. p53 regulates the minimal promoter of the human topoisomerase II alpha gene. Nucl. Acids Res. **24:** 4464–4470.
3. WANG, Q., G.P. ZAMBETTI & D.P. SUTTLE. 1997. Inhibition of DNA topoisomerase II alpha gene expression by the p53 tumor suppressor. Mol. Cell Biol. **17:** 389–397.

Improvement of Therapeutic Index of Low-Dose Topotecan Delivered per os

GRAZIELLA PRATESI, MICHELANDREA DE CESARE, AND FRANCO ZUNINO

Istituto Nazionale Tumori, Via Venezian 1, 20133 Milan, Italy

INTRODUCTION

The relevance of prolonged exposure in drug treatment with camptothecins was recently summarized.[1] Prolonged drug exposure may be more easily achieved by oral administration than by parenteral routes. Bioavailability and pharmacokinetics for oral topotecan have been investigated according to various treatment regimens.[1,2] A multicenter randomized phase III study of i.v. versus oral topotecan in patients with advanced ovarian carcinoma reported similar efficacy and lower myelotoxicity with oral than with i.v. administration.[3] However, the preclinical profile of i.v. versus oral topotecan was never investigated in comparative studies.

The aim of this study was to compare the antitumor potential of topotecan, administered orally, on a panel of human tumors xenografted subcutaneously (s.c.) in athymic nude mice. The tumors were representative of several histotypes and responded differently to i.v. topotecan (FIG. 1). The comparison was carried out under various treatment conditions.

MATERIALS AND METHODS

Athymic Swiss nude mice 9–12 weeks old (Charles River, Calco, Italy) were used throughout the study. Tumor lines were established and maintained in our laboratory according to previously described technical procedures.[4]

Topotecan, kindly supplied by Smith-Kline Beecham Pharmaceuticals, was dissolved in sterile, distilled water and delivered in a volume of 10 µl/kg of body weight. The drug was administered by gavage or intravenously using the same schedule, that is, every fourth day for four times (q4dx4). Many dose levels were investigated, and the maximum tolerated dose (MTD) was considered the one that induced one death in the group of treated mice, or a body weight loss ≥15%. A daily schedule using very low doses of topotecan was also investigated for the oral route. Percentage tumor volume inhibition (TVI%) in treated over control mice was assessed.

RESULTS AND CONCLUSIONS

The antitumor efficacy of topotecan delivered i.v. or per os q4dx4 against a panel of human tumor xenografts is reported in FIGURE 1. The MTD of topotecan by either route was used (TABLE 1). Oral topotecan was significantly more effective than i.v. drug against four tumor lines, NCI-H460, JCA-1, POVD, and U87, all of which were

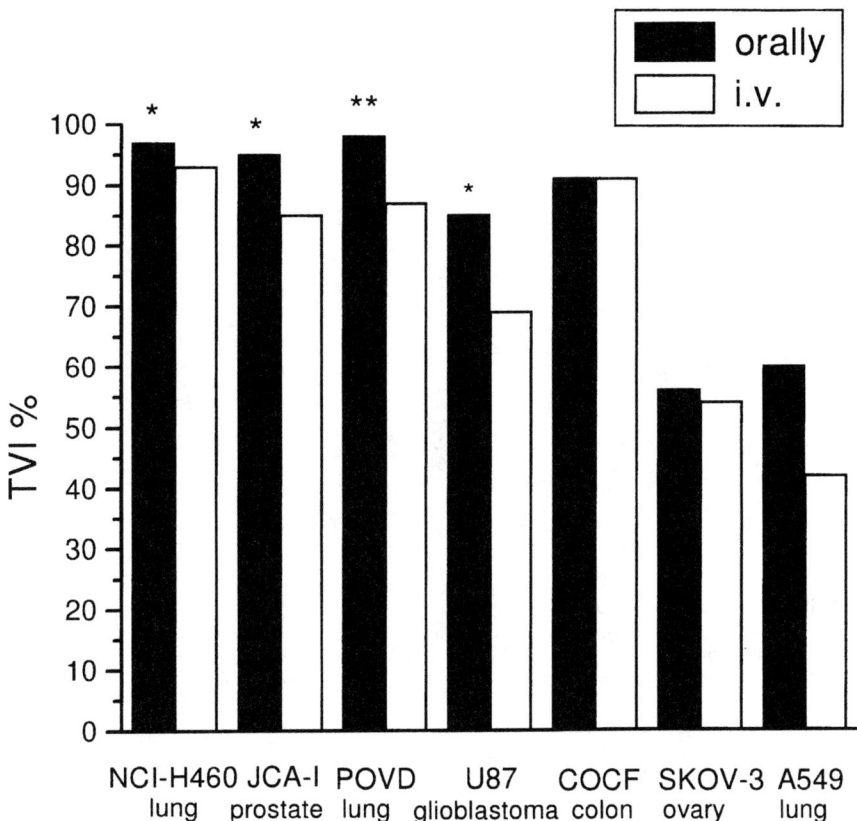

FIGURE 1. Antitumor activity of topotecan (15 mg/kg, q4dx4) against human tumor xenografts (in abscissa). The percentage of tumor volume inhibition (TVI%) in treated versus control mice is reported in ordinata. *$p <0.05$, **$p <0.01$ between the two treated groups, by Student's t test.

responsive (TVI>70%) to the drug, whereas a comparable antitumor effect was achieved in the CoCF tumor and in the two resistant tumors (TVI<70%), SKOV-3 and A549.

A more detailed study was performed against the very sensitive NCI-H460 lung tumor (TABLE 1). Using the schedule q4dx4, a large range of doses was used and the MTD was similar for topotecan delivered according to the two routes, that is, 15 mg/kg/injection for a total of 60 mg/kg. At this dose level, the oral drug was more effective than the i.v. drug. Moreover, daily treatment with low doses of oral topotecan allowed a higher cumulative dose to be delivered without toxicity (100 vs 60 mg/kg) and a much greater efficacy to be achieved, that is, 2 of 10 versus 0 of 8 complete responses and a $\log_{10}$ cell kill value of 6 versus 2.1. The same therapeutic regimen (daily, up to 100 mg/kg) was highly effective even against the A549 tumor (87% TVI), which was resistant to the drug given by the intermittent schedule (FIG. 1).

TABLE 1. Antitumor activity of topotecan against two non–small cell lung carcinoma xenografts

Tumor (D.T.)[a]	Route[b]	Schedule[c]	Total dose (mg/kg)	TVI%[d]	LCK[e]	CR[f] (80 d)	Body weight[g] loss %	Lethal[h] toxicity
NCI-H460 (4.2 ± 1.1)	Oral	q4d×4	20	80	1.3	0/8	0	0/4
			36	91	1.7	0/8	0	0/4
			60	98	2.1	0/8	8	0/4
			72	ND	ND	ND	ND	2/4
	i.v.	q4d×4	40	65	0.5	0/8	6	0/4
			60	93	2	0/8	10	1/4
	Oral	qd×5/w for 10 wk	60	87	2.4	0/8	0	0/4
			100	99	6.0	2/8	0	0/4
A549 (8.6 ± 1.9)	Oral	q4d×4	60	60	0.5	0/2	10	1/10
	i.v.	q4d×4	60	42	0.5	0/12	8	1/6
	Oral	qd×5 for 5 wk	50	63	1.6	0/8	4	0/4
			100	87	2.4	0/8	14	0/4

[a]Doubling time in nude mice. Mean day ± SD.
[b]Treatment started when tumors were visible and not measurable (<100 mm^3).
[c]Every 4 days for 4 times, q4d×4; daily for 5 days/week, qd×5/w.
[d]Tumor volume inhibition percentage in treated versus control mice. The best value is reported.
[e]Log$_{10}$ cell kill to reach 1,000 mm^3 in the NCI-H460 and 500 mm^3 in the A549.
[f]CR, complete response, i.e., no evidence of tumor at day 80.
[g]Mean body weight loss percentage: the highest value induced by treatments is reported.
[h]Number of toxic deaths/total number of treated mice.

In conclusion, the study in a panel of human tumor xenograft indicated that using an intermittent schedule (q4dx4) oral topotecan was at least as active as i.v. topotecan. Moreover, a therapeutic advantage could be achieved in the highly responsive tumors. The comparable activity achieved by i.v. and oral topotecan in a clinical study may reflect the low sensitivity of advanced pretreated tumors[3]; the MTD of topotecan was the same with the oral or i.v. route despite low drug availability (25%, data not shown). Finally, the results indicated that daily oral treatment with low doses of topotecan allowed a higher cumulative drug dose without toxicity and achieved greater antitumor efficacy, thus resulting in an improved therapeutic index.

REFERENCES

1. GERRITS, C.J.H., M.J.A. DE JONGE, J.H.M. SCHELLENS et al. 1997. Topoisomerase I inhibitors: the relevance of prolonged exposure for present clinical development. Br. J. Cancer **76:** 952–962.
2. SCHELLENS, J.H.M., G.J. CREEMERS, J.H. BEIJNEN et al. 1996. Bioavailability and pharmacokinetics of oral topotecan: a new topoisomerase I inhibitor. Br. J. Cancer **73:** 1268–1271.

3. GORE, M., G. RUSTIN, H. CALVERT *et al.* 1998. A multicentre, randomised, phase III study of topotecan (T) administered intravenously or orally for advanced epithelial ovarian carcinoma. Proc. Am. Soc. Clin. Oncol. **17:** 349a.
4. PRATESI, G., C. MANZOTTI, M. TORTORETO *et al.* 1989. Effects of 5-FU and cis-DDP combination on human colorectal tumor xenografts. Tumori **75:** 60–65.

Camptothecin Dose, Schedule, and Timing of Administration for Clinical Radiation Sensitization

TYVIN A. RICH[a] AND ALEXANDER V. KIRICHENKO

Department of Radiation Oncology, University of Virginia Health Sciences Center, Charlottesville, Virginia 22908, USA

INTRODUCTION

Radiation sensitization by camptothecin (CPT) *in vivo* is related to the dose and frequency of CPT administration.[1] Reasons for the superiority of fractionated treatments over single treatment may be related to the repeated formation of stabilized DNA–topoisomerase I (Topo I)-cleavable complexes with relatively frequent CPT administration.[2] These findings are consistent with the observation that DNA–Topo I–CPT cleavable complexes are in constant equilibrium between CPT trapping and dissociation and depend on the constant presence of the drug.[3] Our results are also consistent with those of Houghton *et al.*,[4] who showed that fractionated compared to single-dose CPT increases cytotoxicity in human xenografts. These data provide a rationale for using fractionated treatment of both CPT and external irradiation in the clinic. Clinical treatment schedules that have been tried include CPT-11 (Irinotecan) given in weekly[5] and daily[6] schedules. Comparisons of toxicity and efficacy of these differing schedules in humans are not yet available.

Another important consideration for CPT administration schedules in the clinic are the acute diarrhea and myelosuppression that occur and are the major dose-limiting toxicities with these drugs.[7] We show in this report that acute morbidity can be spared in rapidly proliferating normal tissues when CPT is administered at the most tolerant phase of the mouse activity cycle and that this could potentially allow for safer treatment and even for dose escalation.

MATERIALS AND METHODS

Mice and Tumor

The mice, tumor system, and treatments used in these studies have been described previously.[1] The "circadian" studies were performed on mice housed two to four per cage and allowed to adapt for at least three weeks to a 12-hr light/dark cycle in normal conditions with the light on at 6:00 A.M. (0600 hours) and off at 6:00 P.M. (1800 hours).

---

[a]Address for correspondence: Dr. Tyvin A. Rich, M.D., Department of Radiation Oncology, Box 383, University of Virginia Health System, Charlottesville, VA 22903.
tar4d@virginia.edu

Circadian Toxicity Study

Mice were treated with 9-amino-camptothecin (9-AC) given at six different time points corresponding to the following environmental times: 10:00 A.M., 2:00 P.M., 6:00 P.M., 10:00 P.M., 2:00 A.M., and 6:00 A.M. Two sets of experiments with 9-AC used twice a week i.m. injections for two weeks in a dose of 2 mg/kg of body weight (total of 8.0 mg/kg) or a single injection of 4 mg/kg. At least 12 mice per time point for each drug dose were used. Animals were assessed daily for acute toxicity by measurement of weight loss, evidence of diarrhea, peripheral blood leukocyte counts, and survival. Body weight loss was calculated as the percentage change for each mouse from the first day of treatment. The leukocyte counts were performed by obtaining 25 µl of tail vein blood drawn with a capillary pipette through a microincision of the tail at 10:00 A.M. on days 7, 12, and 15 after the first 9-AC injection. Leukocyte counts were determined with the BD@ Unopette *in vitro* diagnostic system (New Jersey) and calculated as a percentage change for each mouse.

Tumor Growth Delay Assay

The procedure for tumor production has been described previously.[2]

Statistics

The results of the toxicity studies were analyzed by Kaplan-Meier survival with Kwikstat (Cedar Hill, Texas) on a personal computer. Comparisons of percentage body weight loss were analyzed with Sigmaplot (Jandel Scientific Software, San Rafael, CA) by one-way analysis of variance using Student's *t*-test.

RESULTS

Circadian Dependency of 9-AC Normal Tissue Toxicity

Mice treated with fractionated 9-AC (8 mg/kg total dose) at six different times over 24 hours had the highest survival rates at 10:00 A.M., 2:00 P.M., and 6:00 P.M., corresponding to the rest phase of the mouse circadian cycle (FIG. 1). There was a significant decrease in survival in mice treated at 2:00 A.M. (e.g., 90% at 2:00 P.M. versus 15% at 2:00 A.M., $p < 0.00$, Kaplan-Meier). The cause of death for animals treated with either the single or the fractionated 9-AC schedule was gastrointestinal toxicity. Severe diarrhea is preceded by progressive weight loss. The 24 to 32% body weight loss in mice treated during the activity phase was significantly greater than the 12 to 17% body weight loss for mice treated during the rest phase ($p < 0.01$, FIG. 2). We did not observe circadian dependency on the peripheral blood leukocyte count (data not shown).

Radiation Sensitization with Equitoxic 9-AC Doses

Tumor regrowth delay was assessed in the MCa-4 carcinoma using these equitoxic single doses of 9-AC. The results show that average growth delay after irradiation alone depends on the time of irradiation (FIG. 3). For example, there was significant-

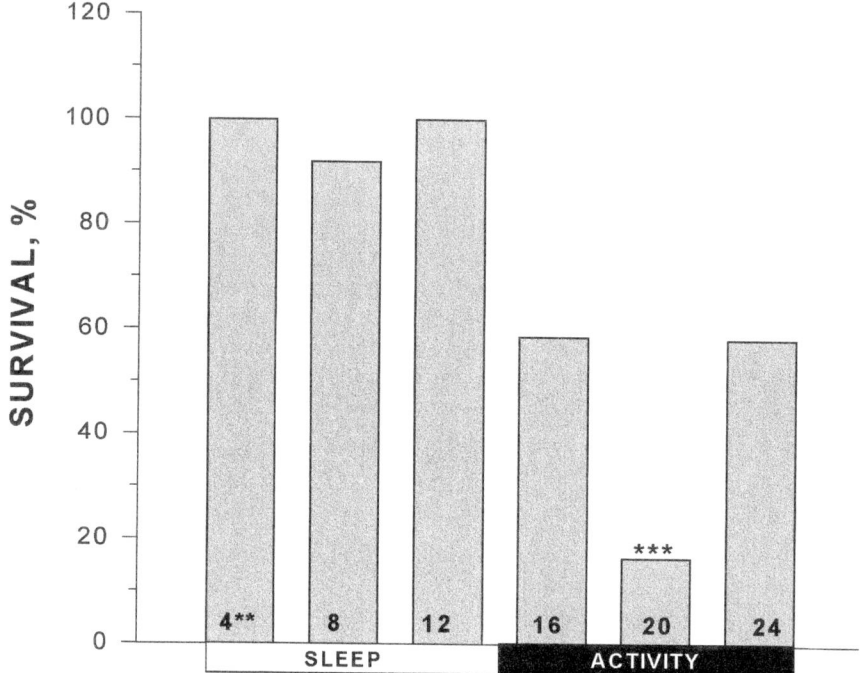

FIGURE 1. Circadian dependency of 9-AC-induced lethal toxicity. Survival of C3H mice treated with repeated 9-AC injections (total dose of 8 mg/kg) delivered at different times of day. In all groups, 9-AC was administered i.m. at 2 mg/kg twice a week for two weeks. ** Numbers inside each bar represent HALO. *** $p < 0.001$ (Kaplan-Meier.)

ly more regrowth delay after irradiation alone given at 2:00 A.M. compared to 2:00 P.M. This accounts for the difference in regrowth delay observed for combined irradiation plus 3 mg/kg of 9-AC given at these two times. The most regrowth delay was observed in the 4 mg/kg group treated at 2:00 P.M. (DMF, 1.12).

DISCUSSION

The data presented here show CPT circadian time dependency for acute toxicity in the gut that is consistent with other S-phase agents.[8] Filipski *et al.* have shown that in BDF2 mice Irinotecan (CPT-11) treatment at 2:00 A.M. results in much higher acute gastrointestinal toxicity compared to other treatment times.[9] Nearly identical results were obtained with CPT-11 in ICR mice.[10] These results are related to circadian cytokinetics of the murine gastrointestinal tract since the peak incorporation of bromodeoxyuridine into S-phase cells in the jejunum occurs around 2:00 A.M.[11] Another factor influencing circadian dependent toxicity of these drugs may be the enzymatic activity of the intestinal flora such as β-glucuronidase or intestinal tissue

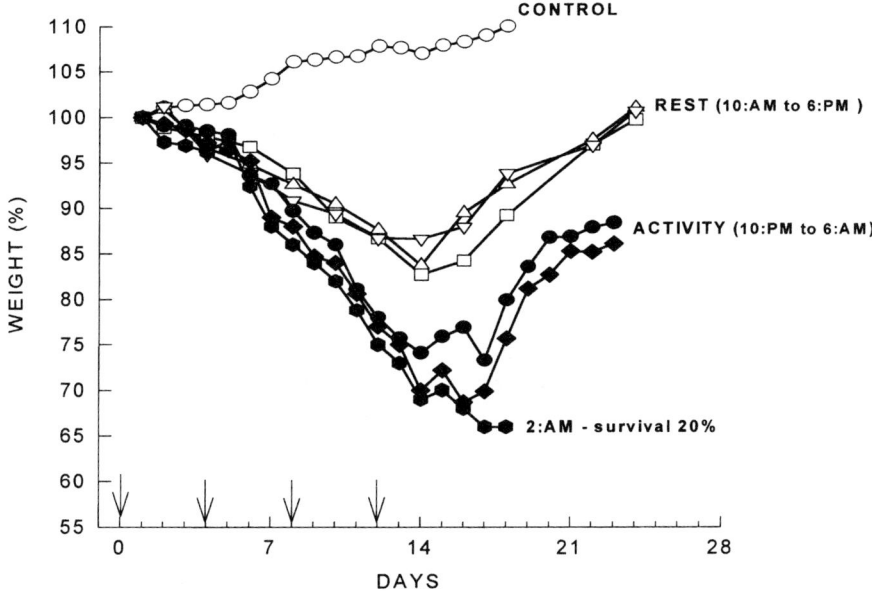

FIGURE 2. Circadian dependency of 9-AC-induced weight loss. Percentage of weight loss as a function of treatment with 9-AC (total dose of 8 mg/kg) delivered at different times of day. ↓ Days of 9-AC injections.

carboxylesterase, which converts CPT-11 into active metabolites in the intestinal lumen.[12] Lastly, a more complete understanding of the chronopharmacology of the CPTs could provide valuable answers that may have clinical relevance.

Circadian dependency of acute toxicity of systemically administered S-phase radiation sensitizers has been demonstrated in a human cancer trial using chronomodulated delivery of 5-fluorouracil.[13] Peak administration of 5-FU during the human rest phase (12 o'clock midnight) is more efficacious compared to treatment with standard 5-FU infusion.[14] These data suggest a rationale for chronomodulated delivery of CPTs as radiation sensitizers, and we hypothesize that administration of CPTs during the human rest phase may even allow dose escalation. Our data show that, when 9-AC is given as a radiation sensitizer during the rest phase, the dose can be escalated by ~30%. A recent report on the treatment of advanced colorectal cancer patients with chronomodulated CPT-11 showed that dose escalation was possible and thus supports this view.[15]

In summary, the optimal scheduling of CPTs with irradiation may be where each is fractionated and there is evidence of circadian-dependent cytotoxicity and radiation sensitization with this class of chemotherapeutic agents. The therapeutic index for these drugs used as radiation sensitizers may be increased by using a chronomodulated delivery schedule.

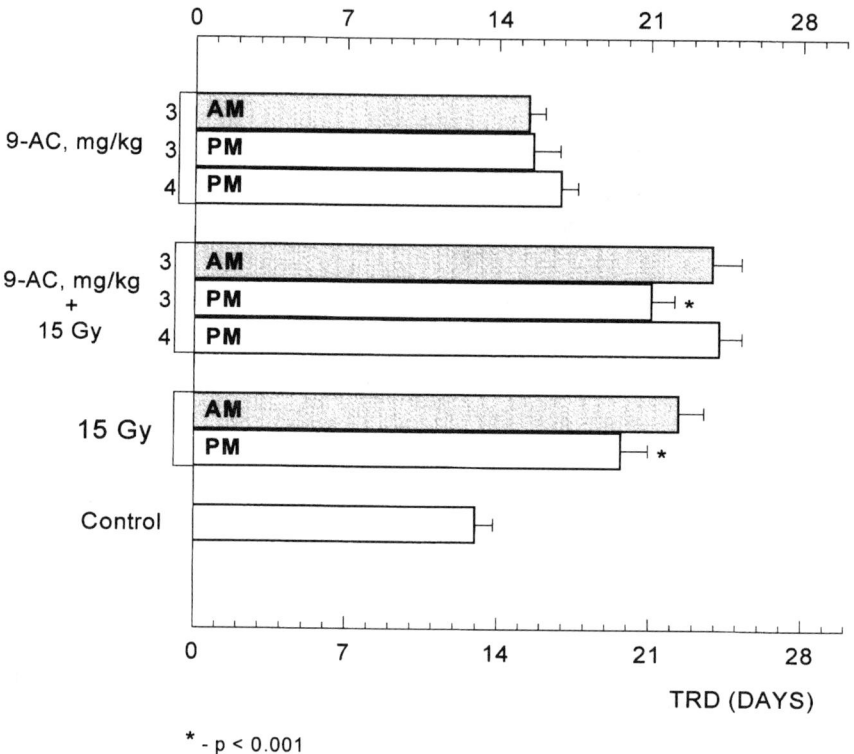

FIGURE 3. Tumor regrowth delay in mice treated with single 9-AC injections alone or in combination with single local irradiation. Radiation sensitization by 9-AC does not depend on the time of administration as shown by regrowth delay. * $p < 0.001$.

ACKNOWLEDGMENTS

This work was supported by The R. W. Fair Foundation and a research and development grant from the University of Virginia School of Medicine.

REFERENCES

1. KIRICHENKO, A.V., T.A. RICH, R.A. NEWMAN & E.L. TRAVIS. 1997. Potentiation of murine MCA-4 carcinoma radioresponse by 9-amino20(S)-camptothecin. Cancer Res. **57:** 1929–1933.
2. LAMOND, J.P., M. WANG, T.J. KINSELLA & D.A. BOOTHMAN. 1996. Concentration and timing dependency of lethality enhancement between topotecan, a topoisomerase I inhibitor, and ionzing radiation. Int. J. Radiat. Biol. **36:** 361–368.
3. COVEY, J.M., C. JAXEL, K.W. KOHN & Y. POMMIER. 1989. Protein-linked DNA strand breaks induced in mammalian cell by camptothecin, an inhibitor of topoisomerase I. Cancer Res. **49:** 5016–5022.

4. HOUGHTON, P.J., C.F. STEWART, W.C. ZAMBONI, et al. 1996. Schedule-dependent efficacy of camptothecin in models of human cancer. Ann. N.Y. Acad. Sci. **803:** 188.
5. KUDOH, S., N. KURIHARA, K. OKISHIO, et al. 1996. A phase I/II study of weekly irinotecan (CPT-11) and simultaneous thoracic radiotherapy for unresectable locally advanced non-small cell lung cancer. Proc. ASCO **15:** 372 (#1102).
6. SALTZ, L., E. EARLY, D. KELSEN, et al. 1997. Phase I study of chronic daily low-dose irinotecan. Proc. ASCO **16:**
7. ROTHENBERG, M.L. 1996. Current status of irinotecan (CPT-11) in the United States. Ann. N.Y. Acad. Sci. **803:** 272.
8. SHEVING, L.E., L.A. SHEVING, J.L. MCCLELLAN & R.J. FENERS. 1995. Experimental basis for circadian cancer chemotherapy. J. Infus. Chemother. **5(1):** 3–7.
9. FILIPSKI, E., F. LEVI, N. VARDOT, et al. 1997. Circadian changes in irinotecan toxicity in mice. Proc. AACR **38:** 305.
10. OHDO, S., T. MAKINOSUMI, T. ISHIZAKI, et al. 1997. Cell cycle–dependent chronotoxicity of irinotecan hydrochloride. J. Pharmacol. Exp. Ther. **283:** 1383–1388.
11. THAMES, H., A. RUIFROK & K. MASON. 1997. The effect of proliferative status and clonogen content on the response of jejunal crypts to split-dose irradiation. Radiat. Res. **147:** 172–179.
12. TAKASUNA, K., T. HAGIWARA, M. HIROHASHI, et al. 1996. Involvement of β-glucuronidase in intestinal microflora in the intestinal toxicity of the antitumor camptothecin derivative irinotecan hydrochloride (CPT-11) in rats. Cancer Res. **56:** 3752–3757.
13. DE W. MARSH, R., N-M. CHU, J-N. VAUTHEY, et al. 1996. Preoperative treatment of patients with locally advanced unresectable rectal adenocarcinoma utilizing continuous chronobiologically shaped 5-fluorouracil infusion and radiation therapy. Cancer **78:** 217–225.
14. WEINSTEIN, G.D., T.A. RICH, C.R. SHUMATE, et al. 1995. Preoperative infusional chemoradiation and surgery with or without an electron beam intraoperative boost for advanced primary rectal cancer. Int. J. Radiat. Oncol. Biol. Phys. **32:** 197–204.
15. MONTEMBAULT, S., F. GOLDWASSER, C. BRESAULT-BONNET, et al. 1998. A pilot study of CPT-11 chronomodulated delivery in patients with metastatic colorectal carcinoma. Proc. AACR **39**.

Rapid Chromatin Reorganization Induced by Topoisomerase I-Mediated DNA Damage

MEI SUN,[a] PU DUANN,[b] CHIN-TAI LIN,[c] HUI ZHANG,[d] AND LEROY F. LIU[a,e]

[a]*Department of Pharmacology, UMDNJ–Robert Wood Johnson Medical School, Piscataway, New Jersey 08854, USA*

[b]*The Cancer Institute of New Jersey, New Brunswick, New Jersey 08901, USA*

[c]*Cooperative Lab., Veterans General Hospital, Taipei 112, Taiwan, R.O.C.*

[d]*Department of Genetics, Yale University, New Haven, Connecticut 06520, USA*

Camptothecin (CPT) induces topoisomerase I (topo I)-mediated DNA damage by specifically blocking the religation step in the topo 1-catalyzed breakage/religation cycles on DNA.[1] Unlike other DNA-damaging agents, CPT causes a highly specific type of DNA damage; the protein-linked single-strand DNA breaks. Little is known about the repair mechanism of topo I-mediated DNA damage.

Compact chromatin is a structural barrier to DNA processes such as DNA replication, RNA transcription, and DNA repair. It is assumed that in order to repair DNA damage, chromatin must undergo some changes for the access of repair proteins to the DNA-damaged site.[2] To monitor the state of chromatin upon CPT treatment, we measured the linking number of SV40 episomal DNA in COS cells. Topo I-mediated DNA damage induced by CPT resulted in a rapid and extensive increase in the linking number of SV40 episomal DNA in COS cells.[3] The linking number increase was shown to be due to topo I-mediated DNA damage induced by CPT, because the inactive S-isomer of CPT, which does not induce topo I-mediated DNA damage, was unable to affect the linking number. The CPT-induced change in linking number was reversible, as removal of CPT from the culture media resulted in a temperature- and time-dependent reversal of the linking number change.[3] CPT-induced linking number increase is probably independent of DNA replication, RNA transcription, and poly(ADP)ribosylation, because aphidicolin (an inhibitor of DNA polymerase α and δ), dichloro-D-ribofuranosylbenzimidazole (DRB) (an RNA polymerase II inhibitor), and 3-aminobenzamide (3-AB) (an inhibitor of poly(ADP)ribose polymerase) do not affect CPT-induced relaxation.

To further study the mechanism of CPT-induced relaxation, we took advantage of yeast genetic system. CPT can similarly induce a large linking number increase in yeast expressing human topoisomerase I (htopoI). Within minutes of CPT treatment, an increase of over 10 linking number was observed on yeast 2μ plasmid DNA. Bleomycin but not etoposide, MMS and cisplatin can similarly induce linking number increase on yeast 2μ plasmid in yeast expressing human DNA topo I. Various yeast mutants have been screened to identify the genes affecting CPT-induced plasmid re-

---

[e]Address for correspondence: Leroy F. Liu, Ph.D., Department of Pharmacology, UMDNJ–Robert Wood Johnson Medical School, 675 Hoes Lane, Piscataway, NJ 08854, USA. Voice: +1 732 235 4592; fax: +1 732 235 4073.

lliu@umdnj.edu

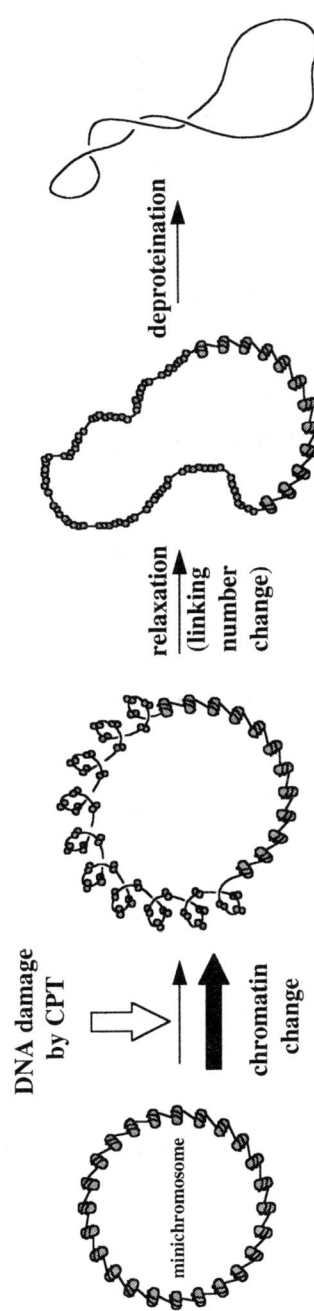

FIGURE 1. A working model for chromatin reorganization induced by topoisomerase I-mediated DNA damage. Chromatin structural alteration induced by CPT may involve disassembly of a group of nucleosomes without the loss of histones. This chromatin structural alteration is detected by the linking number change of the circular episomal DNA due to passive activity of a topoisomerase.

laxation. We show that CPT-induced linking number increase is independent of RNA polymerase II, topoisomerase II (topo II), topoisomerase III (topo III), and a series of repair proteins such as RAD52, RAD6, RAD9, MRE11, TDP (tyrosine-DNA phosphodiesterase),[4] SGS1, TRF4, and TRF5.[5] In addition, CPT-induced linking number increase is not cell-cycle specific; CPT-induced plasmid relaxation was detected in G1, S, and G2 phase of the cell cycle.

The large linking number change on episomal DNA is indicative of chromatin structural alteration. The CPT-induced chromatin structural change was probed by *Staphylococcal aureus* nuclease digestion. No change of the *S. aureus* digestion pattern was observed in either COS cells or yeast upon CPT treatment.[3] This result suggests that chromatin has not completely lost its nucleosomal structure in response to CPT.

In conclusion, our results suggest that topo I-mediated DNA damage may specifically activate a previously uncharacterized process leading to chromatin reorganization. Chromatin structural alteration may involve disassembly of a group of nulceosomes without the loss of histones. This chromatin structural alteration is revealed by the linking number change of the circular episomal DNA due to passive activity of a topoisomerase (FIG. 1).

REFERENCES

1. HSIANG, Y.H. *et al.* 1985. J. Biol. Chem. **260:** 14873–14878.
2. SMERDON, M.J. 1983. Biochemistry **22:** 3516–3525.
3. DUANN, P. *et al.* 1999. Nucl. Acids Res. **27:** 2905–2911.
4. POULIOT, J.J. *et al.* 1999. Science **286:** 552–555.
5. WALOWSKY, C. *et al.* 1999. J. Biol. Chem. **274:** 7302–7308.

NF-κB Activation in Topoisomerase I Inhibitor-Induced Apoptotic Cell Death in Human Non-Small Cell Lung Cancer

MASAHIRO TABATA[a] AND RAM GANAPATHI

Experimental Therapeutics Program, Taussig Cancer Center, Cleveland Clinic Foundation, 9500 Euclid Avenue, Cleveland, Ohio 44195

Activation of the transcription factor NF-κB has been shown to protect cancer cells from the apoptosis induced by cancer chemotherapeutic agents and ionizing radiation.[1,2] However, the functional role of NF-κB in regulating chemotherapy-induced and radiation-induced apoptosis remains controversial.[3,4]

In a human non-small cell lung cancer cell line, NSCLC-3,[5] treatment with a topoisomerase I poison SN-38, an active metabolite of irinotecan,[6] led to apoptotic cell death in a dose-dependent manner. Apoptotic cells defined by typical morphological changes after staining with Hoechst 33342 dye and evaluated by fluorescence microscopy[7] were apparent as early as 4 hours after treatment and maximal at 24–48 hours following drug treatment for 1 hour. In SN-38–treated cells, the enhanced DNA binding activity (activation) of NF-κB was drug concentration-dependent and preceded the induction of apoptosis. Pharmacological inhibition of this NF-κB activation by pretreatment with the proteasome inhibitor MG-132 (20 μM for 30 min) led to a significant decrease in SN-38–induced apoptosis (TABLE 1). These observations suggest a relevant role for NF-κB activation in topoisomerase I poison-induced apoptosis in the NSCLC-3 model system.

To study the functional role of NF-κB activation in the initiation of apoptotic pathways induced by the DNA damaging effect of topoisomerase I poison, NSCLC-3 cells were stably transfected with a super-repressor type mutant IκBα (S32A/S36A). In mutant IκBα-transfected NSCLC-3 cells (NSCLC-3/mIκBα), activation of NF-κB was completely abolished following treatment with a wide concentration range of SN-38 (10–1,000 nM). However, the activation of NF-κB in cells transfected with empty vector control (NSCLC-3/neo) was similar to the parental control cells treated with SN-38. By contrast, no differences in the induction of apoptosis following treatment with SN-38 were observed between NSCLC-3/neo and NSCLC-3/mIκBα (TABLE 2) despite comparable protein-DNA complex formation in both cell lines. Preliminary studies also suggested that following treatment with SN-38, the processing of initiator and effector caspases as well as their activity is similar in the NSCLC-3/neo and NSCLC-3/mIκBα cells. The clonogenic survival in a soft-agar colony assay of the NSCLC-3/neo and NSCLC-3/mIκBα cells after SN-38 treatment were not significantly different.

---

[a]Voice: 216-444-4579 or 216-444-2085; fax: 216-444-7115.
tabatam@cc.ccf.org or ganapar@cc.ccf.org

TABLE 1. Effect of MG-132 (20 μM for 30 min) pretreatment on apoptosis induced by treatment SN-38 for 1 hour

Treatment SN-38 (nM)	% Apoptosis (mean ± SD)	
	MG-132 (−)	MG132 (+)
0	1.7 ± 0.8	2.2 ± 0.3
100	23.2 ± 2.3	16.0 ± 0.9[a]

[a]$p = 0.015$.

TABLE 2. Induction of apoptosis by SN-38 in NSCLC-3 cells transfected with super suppressor mutant IκBα or empty vector control

Treatment SN-38 (nM)	% Apoptosis (mean ± SD)	
	NSCLC-3/neo	NSCLC-3/mIκBα
0	2.0 ± 1.8	1.5 ± 1.5
100	23.5 ± 2.0	21.3 ± 5.1[a]

In conclusion, these results demonstrate that activation of NF-κB following treatment with SN-38 is not required for induction of apoptosis in NSCLC-3 cells.

REFERENCES

1. WANG, C.Y., J.C. CUSACK, JR., R. LIU & A.S. BALDWIN, JR. 1999. Control of inducible chemoresistance: enhanced anti-tumor therapy through increased apoptosis by inhibition of NF-kappa Br. Nat Med. **5:** 412–417.
2. WANG, C.Y., M.W. MAYO & A.S. BALDWIN, JR. 1996. TNF- and cancer therapy-induced apoptosis: potentiation by inhibition of NF-kappa B [see comments]. Science **274:** 784–787.
3. PAJONK, F., K. PAJONK & W.H. MCBRIDE. 1999. Inhibition of NF-kappaB, clonogenicity, and radiosensitivity of human cancer cells [see comments]. J. Natl. Cancer Inst. **91:** 1956–1960.
4. BENTIRES-ALJ, M., A.C. HELLIN, M. AMEYAR, et al. 1999. Stable inhibition of nuclear factor kappaB in cancer cells does not increase sensitivity to cytotoxic drugs. Cancer Res. **59:** 811–815.
5. Ganapathi, M.K., A.K. Weizer, S. Borsellino, et al. 1996. Resistance to interleukin-6 in human non-small cell lung carcinoma cell lines: role of receptor components. Cell Growth Differ. **7:** 923–929.
6. ROTHENBERG, M.L. 1997. Topoisomerase I inhibitors: review and update. Ann. Oncol. **8:** 837–855.
7. MUSCARELLA, D.E., M.K. RACHLINSKI, J. SOTIRIADIS & S.E. BLOOM. 1998. Contribution of gene-specific lesions, DNA-replication-associated damage, and subsequent transcritpional inhibiton in topoisomerase inhibitor-mediated apoptosis in lymphoma cells. Exp. Cell Res. **238:** 155–167.

Phase I Study of 9-Nitro-20(S)-Camptothecin in Combination with Cisplatin for Patients with Advanced Malignancies

C.F. VERSCHRAEGEN,[a,c] M. VINCENT,[a] J.L. ABBRUZZESE,[a] D. SIEGLER,[a] J.J. KAVANAGH,[a] E. LOYER,[a] A.P. KUDELKA,[a] AND E. RUBIN[b]

[a]*The University of Texas, M. D. Anderson Cancer Center, Houston, Texas 77030, USA*

[b]*The Cancer Institute of New Jersey, New Brunswick, New Jersey, USA*

9-Nitrocamptothecin (RFS 2000) is a new, orally administered camptothecin analogue.[1,2] Cisplatin causes DNA damage which employs topoisomerase to repair. Because of the inhibition of topoisomerase I by camptothecins, we postulated that the combination of cisplatin and RFS 2000 may have an additive or synergistic antitumor effect.[3] The objective of this study was to determine the maximum tolerated dose (MTD) and toxicity profile of RFS 2000 and cisplatin.

PATIENTS AND METHODS

Patients were eligible to enter the study if they fulfilled the following criteria: (1) pathologically proven cancer; (2) tumor refractory to standard therapy; (3) evaluable or measurable disease; (4) age ≥ 10 years; (5) PS ≤ 2; (6) expected survival ≥ 12 weeks; (7) adequate liver, renal, and bone marrow functions; (8) no camptothecin allergy; (9) no other concurrent anti-cancer therapy; (10) no symptomatic brain metastases or other severe medical problems; and (11) written, informed consent.

Cisplatin was administered in the outpatient unit, with hydration (minimum 3 liters) as per standard guidelines. RFS 2000 was administered orally, starting on the evening of cisplatin administration, two hours after the last meal or before bedtime with a glass of acidic beverage. Three liters of oral hydration per day were recommended to reduce the possibility of cystitis. Antiemetics were not standardized for this trial. G-CFS was not used prophylactically and could not be used concomittantly with RFS 2000. However, if myelosuppression occurred (requiring discontinuation of RFS 2000), G-CSF was administered according to ASCO guidelines.

Patients could be treated with multiple courses of therapy if they were benefiting medically, absolute granulocyte counts remained $\geq 1,500$ cells/mm^3, and platelets $\geq 100,000$/mm^3. The treatment design is described in TABLE 1.

[c]Address for correspondence: Section of Gynecologic Medical Therapeutics, The University of Texas MD Anderson Cancer Center, 1515 Holcombe Boulevard, Box 401, Houston, TX 77030. Voice: 713-792-7959; fax: 713 7451541.

cverschr@mdanderson.org

TABLE 1. Treatment plan: a two-arm, phase I design

Dose level	Arm 1	Arm 2
Fixed dose	Cisplatin 50 mg/m^2 on day 1	RFS 2000 1.5 mg/day×5 every week×3
Variable dose	RFS 2000 (mg/day×5, every week×3)	Cisplatin (mg/m^2 on day 1)
Level 0	—	—
Level 1	1	30
Level 2	1.25	40
Level 3	1.5	50
Level 4	1.75	60

NOTE: Cycles were repeated every 4 weeks. No intrapatient dose escalation was allowed. Therapy continued until disease progression or development of intolerable side effects.

The statistical approach followed the 3 + 3 patients per cohort design. Dose-limiting toxicity (DLT) was defined as a dose of chemotherapy that produced a reversible grade 3 or 4 hematologic toxicity (lasting more than 7 days) or reversible grade ≥ 3 (grade 2 for neurotoxicity) nonmyelosuppressive toxicity lasting no more than 14 days in > 33% of patients treated at a given dose level. Grades were based on the National Cancer Institute (NCI) Common Toxicity Criteria (CTC Version 2.0, dated 1/30/98). DLTs were based only on patients receiving their first course of treatment. The Phase II dose has been defined as the highest dose for which no more than one of six patients developed a DLT.

RESULTS AND DISCUSSION

Twelve patients were evaluable for toxicity. No toxic effects greater than grade 2 have been observed at dose level 2 and below. The DLT has not yet been reached, and the study is still open to accrual. TABLE 2 describes the current side effects.

Ten patients have received two courses of therapy or more. Thus far, no objective responses have been documented. Eight patients have had progressive disease, and in two patients the disease has remained stable for 4 and 8 months.

CONCLUSIONS

- The combination of cisplatin and RFS 2000 is very well tolerated.
- The MTD has not been reached at doses of 50 mg/m^2 of cisplatin and 1.25 mg/day of RFS 2000.
- Disease stabilization has been noted in one patient with pancreatic cancer and in one patient with cervical cancer.

TABLE 2. Side effects: number of patients experiencing grade 2 side effects (3 patients per cohort)

Cohort	Nausea	Vomiting	Anorexia	Diarrhea	Fatigue	Ototoxicity	Skin rash	Dysgeusia
Arm 1								
Dose level 0	3		1		2			1
Dose level 1	2	2			2			
Dose level 2	1[a]	1[a]						
Arm 2								
Dose level 0	1	1	1	1	1	1	1	

[a]Grade 3 in one patient with peritoneal carcinomatosis. Nausea and vomiting were related to partial bowel obstruction. This cohort will be expanded.

REFERENCES

1. VERSCHRAEGEN, C.F., E.A. NATELSON, B.C. GIOVANELLA, *et al.* 1998. A phase I clinical and pharmacological study of oral 9-nitrocamptothecin, a novel water-insoluble topoisomerase I inhibitor. Anti-Cancer Drugs **9:** 36.
2. VERSCHRAEGEN, C.F., F. GUPTA, E. LOYER, *et al.* 1999. A phase II clinical and pharmacological study of oral 9-nitrocamptothecin in patients with refractory epithelial ovarian, tubal or peritoneal cancer. Anti-Cancer Drugs **10:** 375.
3. GOLDWASSER, F., M. VALENTI, R. TORRES, *et al.* 1996. Potentiation of cisplatin cytotoxicity by 9-aminocamptothecin. Clin. Cancer Res. **2:** 687.

Phase II Study of Intravenous DX-8951f in Patients with Advanced Ovarian, Tubal, or Peritoneal Cancer Refractory to Platinum, Taxane, and Topotecan

C.F. VERSCHRAEGEN,[a] C. LEVENBACK, M. VINCENT, J. WOLF, M. BEVERS, E. LOYER, A.P. KUDELKA, AND J.J. KAVANAGH

Secion of Gynecologic and Medical Therapeutics and Department of Gynecology Oncology, The University of Texas M.D. Anderson Cancer Center, Houston, Texas 77030, USA

In phase I studies of DX-8951f, anti-tumor activity (including partial remissions) was documented with the daily × 5 and the weekly (30-min infusion) regimens. Less gastrointestinal toxicity was observed with the daily × 5 regimen. Therefore, this regimen was selected for phase II studies. The preliminary results of pharmacokinetics studies demonstrated a high concentration of lactone and a prolonged elimination in comparison to topotecan. The objectives of this study are (1) to determine the antitumor activity of DX-8951f when administered as a 30-min intravenous infusion daily for five days every three weeks to patients with advanced ovarian, tubal, or peritoneal carcinoma refractory to platinum, taxane, and topotecan; (2) to evaluate the quantitative and qualitative toxicities of DX-8951f with this schedule in this population; (3) to evaluate the pharmacokinetics of DX-8951f in plasma.

PATIENTS AND METHODS

Patients were eligible if they fulfilled the following criteria: (1) pathologically proven ovarian, tubal, or peritoneal carcinoma; (2) tumor refractory to platinum, taxane, and topotecan; (3) measurable disease ≥2 cm; (4) age ≥18 years; (5) PS ≤2; (6) expected survival ≥ 12 weeks; (7) adequate liver, renal, and bone marrow functions; (8) no camptothecin allergy; (9) no other anti-cancer therapy within 4 weeks of study entry; and (10) written, informed consent. Refractory disease is defined as progressive disease while on chemotherapy, relapse within six months of completing chemotherapy, or failure to achieve a complete response with persistent macroscopic disease after six cycles of chemotherapy if the last two cycles have no measurable change in disease.

---

[a]Address for correspondence: Section of Gynecologic Medical Therapeutics, The University of Texas MD Anderson Cancer Center, 1515 Holcombe Boulevard, Box 401, Houston, Texas 77030. Voice: 713-792-7959; fax: 713-745-1541.
cverschr@mdanderson.org

TABLE 1. Side effects

Side effect	NCI CTC grade			Total
	2	3	4	
Anemia	8	0		8
Neutropenia	4	5	2	11
Thrombocytopenia	1	1		1
Nausea/vomiting	6			6
Diarrhea	5			5
Fatigue	6			6

NOTE: Numbers shown are number of patients with side effects. Highest grade per patient given. Growth factor requirements: Procrit (6 patients) and Neupogen (2 patients).

Treatment is administered daily for five days at a dose of 0.3 mg/m^2 per day if the patient has been heavily pretreated (HP) or at 0.5 mg/m^2 per day if the patient has been minimally pretreated (MP). HP patients are defined as those who had >6 courses of alkylating agent containing chemotherapy (or >4 courses of carboplatin), radiation therapy to >25% of hematopoietic reserves, ≥ 2 courses of mitomycin C or a nitrosourea. Colony-stimulating factors are not used prophylactically to prevent neutropenia. Drugs or food metabolized through the CYP3A enzyme in the human liver are avoided if possible. They include inhibitors (macrolide antibiotics [azithromycin, erythromycin, clarithromycin, troleandomycin, dapsone], azole antibiotics [fluconazole, miconazole, itraconazole, ketoconazole], triazobenzodiazepines [alprazolam, midazolam, triazolam], antidepressants [fluoxetine, sertraline, fluvoxamine, nefazodone], quinolone antimicrobials [ciprofloxacin, ofloxacin], ethinylestradiol, diltiazem, cimetidine, cyclosporin, cisapride, terfenadine, coffee, and grapefruit juice) and inducers (rifampin, imidazole antibiotics [clotrimazole], glucocorticoids, antiepileptics [carbamazepine, phenytoin, phenobarbital], and anti-ulcer agents [omeprazole, lansoprazole]).

The study is a single-arm, nonrandomized phase II trial of DX-8951f in patients with advanced ovarian, tubal, or peritoneal carcinoma refractory to platinum, taxane, and topotecan. The study will enroll up to 37 patients using Simon's optimal two-stage design.

RESULTS AND DISCUSSION

Fourteen patients have been enrolled to date. Out of nine patients assessable for response, stable disease is observed in four patients, who each dropped their CA-125 levels by $\geq 50\%$.

Fourteen patients are assessable for toxicity. Grade ≥ 3 hematologic effects included neutropenia (7 patients) and thrombocytopenia (1 patient). Eight patients had a grade 2 anemia, which was treated with erythropoietin. Grade ≥ 2 nonhematologic effects were nausea and vomiting (6 patients), diarrhea (5 patients), and fatigue (6 patients) (See TABLE 1).

Pharmacokinetics parameters are not available at the time of this update.

CONCLUSIONS

In this refractory patient population, DX-8951f is well tolerated and may stabilize cancer progression in patients with topotecan refractory ovarian cancer. The study is ongoing. If one partial remission is observed in the first 12 evaluable patients, the study will continue to enroll 37 patients.

REFERENCES

1. MITSUI, I., E. KUMAZAWA, Y. HIROTA, et al. 1995. A new water-soluble camptothecin derivative, DX-8951f, exhibits potent antitumor activity against human tumors in vitro and in vivo. Jpn. J. Cancer Res. **86:** 776–786.
2. KUMAZAWA, E. & A. TOHGO. 1998. Antitumor activity of DX-8951f: a new camptothecin derivative. Exp. Opin. Invest. Drugs **7:** 625–632.
3. KUMAZAWA, E., T. JIMBO, Y. OCHI & A. TOHGO. 1998. Potent and broad antitumor effects of DX-8951f, a water-soluble camptothecin derivative, against various human tumors xenografted in nude mice. Cancer Chemother. Pharmacol. **42:** 210–220.

Feasibility, Phase I, and Pharmacological Study of Aerosolized Liposomal 9-Nitro-20(S)-Camptothecin in Patients with Advanced Malignancies in the Lungs

C.F. VERSCHRAEGEN,[a,c] B.E. GILBERT,[b] A.J. HUARINGA,[a] R. NEWMAN,[a] N. HARRIS,[b] F.J. LEYVA,[b] L. KEUS,[b] K. CAMPBELL,[b] T. NELSON-TAYLOR,[a] AND V. KNIGHT[a]

[a]*The University of Texas M. D. Anderson Cancer Center, Houston, Texas 77030, USA*
[b]*Baylor College of Medicine, Houston, Texas, USA*

INTRODUCTION

Topoisomerase-I inhibitors have the capability to eradicate human tumors in xenograft models. Therefore human cancer cells are extremely sensitive to camptothecin.[1] Camptothecin analogues are nevertheless not curative in clinical settings probably because of poor distribution of the camptothecin lactone to the tumor cells growing in humans. We hypothesized that a modification of the formulation and a systemic delivery that avoids first pass in the liver may increase the therapeutic index. Aerosol delivery of liposomal 9-nitrocamptothecin (L-9NC) may possibly delay the opening of the lactone ring through liposomation. We plan to demonstrate that delivery through aerosolization of fine particles is associated with systemic absorption[2] and perhaps with sustained levels of closed ring 9-nitrocamptothecin (9-NC). Animal data (nude mice) show minimal toxicity and no weight loss, with substantial antitumor activity at reduced doses against breast, lung, and colon cancer xenografts.[3] The objective of this study is to determine the feasibility and safety of administering L-9NC by aerosolization for five consecutive days per week.

PATIENTS AND METHODS

Patients with primary or metastatic disease to the lungs were enrolled in this phase I study if they fulfill the following eligibility criteria: (1) pathologic diagnosis of cancer, (2) failure after standard cancer treatment, (3) performance status (Zubrod PS) <3, (4) pulmonary function >50% by spirometry and DLCO, (5) normal organ function, and (6) no symptomatic brain metastasis.

Treatment consisted of 6.7 µg/kg per day by aerosolization with a flow of 10 liters per minute of air. In the feasibility cohort, treatment was given every day for 5 con-

---

[c]Address for correspondence: Section of Gynecologic Medical Therapeutics, The University of Texas MD Anderson Cancer Center, 1515 Holcombe Boulevard, Box 401, Houston, Texas 77030. Voice: 713-792-7959; fax: 713-745-1541.
cverschr@mdanderson.org

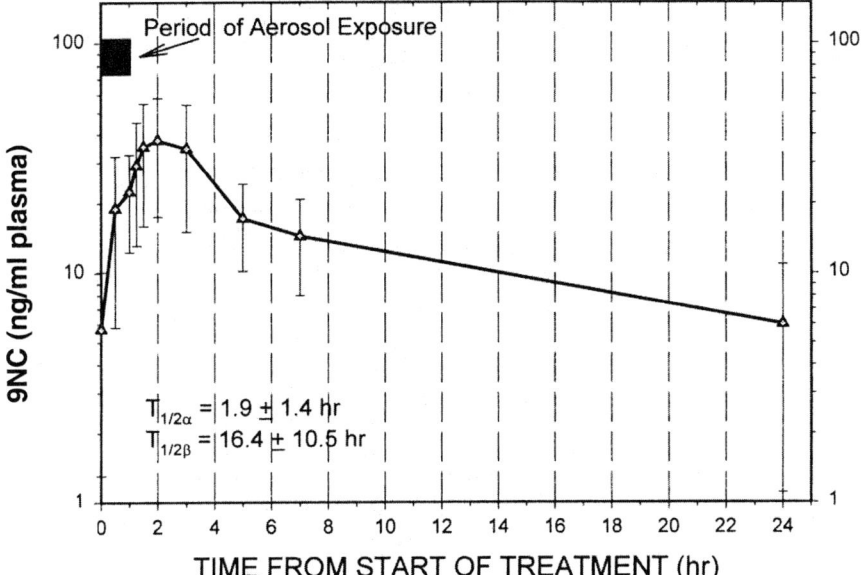

FIGURE 1. Pharmacokinetics of liposomal 9-nitrocamptothecin (9-NC). Mean (±SD) plasma levels in five cancer patients following treatment with 9-nitrocamptothecin liposome aerosol by mouth-only breathing.

secutive days and repeated every 3 weeks if disease remained stable. Plasma was obtained on day 4 or 5 of therapy to determine the pharmacokinetic profile of the drug. Bronchoalveolar lavages to measure the amount of 9-NC were performed on consenting patients. Disease was evaluated by CT scan of the chest every two courses.

RESULTS AND DISCUSSION

Six patients (4 women, 2 men) were treated in the feasibility cohort. Patient characteristics included a median age of 57 years (39–72 years) and a Zubrod PS of 0 (range, 0–1). The median pulmonary function (FEV_1/FVC) was 94% of control. All patients had received a median number of prior treatments of two. Disease sites were cervical cancer (2 patients), leiomyosarcoma, endometrial carcinoma, lung cancer, and melanoma.

Two to fourteen courses have been administered per patient. No side effects higher than grade 2 have been observed at this low dose. 9-NC is absorbed systemically as determined by HPLC and mass spectrometry on the plasma (FIG. 1).

Maximum drug concentration is seen 2 hours after the end of the aerosolization, with a mean concentration of 36.7 ng/ml (4 patients), falling to 4.9 ng/ml 24 hours later. Lactone was detected (<5 ng/ml) but decreased immediately after aerosolization. Stabilization of disease was observed in two patients. This feasibility study has demonstrated that aerosol delivery of liposomal 9-NC for 5 consecutive days is well tolerated and that L-9NC is absorbed systemically. The study will accrue patients at higher doses and longer periods of delivery.

ACKNOWLEDGMENTS

This work was supported in part by The Clayton Foundation.

REFERENCES

1. GIOVANELLA, B.C., J.S. STEHLIN, M.E. WALL, *et al.* 1989. DNA topoisomerase I—targeted chemotherapy of human colon cancer in xenografts. Science **246:** 1046–1048.
2. GILBERT, B.E., C. KNIGHT, F.G. ALVAREZ, *et al.* 1997. Tolerance of volunteers to cyclosporine A–dilauroylphosphatidylcholine liposome aerosol. Am. J. Respir. Crit. Care Med. **156:** 1789–1793.
3. KNIGHT, V., E.S. KLEINERMAN, J.C. WALDREP, *et al.* 2000. 9-Nitrocamptothecin liposome aerosol treatment of human cancer subcutaneous xenograft and pulmonary cancr metastases in mice. Ann. N.Y. Acad. Sci. This volume.

Inhibition of DNA Replication in Camptothecin-Treated Cells Is Regulated by Protein Kinases

XIANG-YANG ZHOU AND YA WANG[a]

Department of Radiation Oncology, Kimmel Cancer Center of Jefferson Medical College, Thomas Jefferson University, Philadelphia, Pennsylvania 19107, USA

INTRODUCTION

Strong inhibition of DNA replication in camptothecin (CPT)-treated cells is a remarkable phenotype. However, the mechanism has yet to be elucidated. It has been suggested that this inhibition is not only a direct consequence of a collision between the advancing replication fork and the cleavable complex of CPT-DNA topoisomerase I (topo I)-DNA, but it might also be an indirect result of CPT-induced DNA damage.[1,2] Here, we show new evidence to support the hypothesis that the inhibition of DNA replication in CPT-treated cells is an active process. Our data indicated that ataxia telangiectasia mutated (ATM) is an important sensor, but not the only one involved in regulation of DNA replication in CPT-treated cells. There might be another caffeine-sensitive kinase which, together with ATM, control the S-phase checkpoint following CPT-treatment. Understanding the roles of these protein kinases in the regulation of DNA replication in CPT-treated cells may offer new ways of intervention for CPT sensitization.

MATERIALS AND METHODS

Drugs, Chemicals, and Antibodies. CPT sodium salt (NCS100800) was obtained from NCI. Caffeine and wortmannin were purchased from Sigma Chemical Co. Antibodies specific for ATM or ATR (ataxia- and rad3-related protein) were purchased from Oncogene Co. PHAS-1 (phosphorylated heat- and acid-stable protein regulated by insulin), the substrate of ATM and ATR, was purchased from Stratagene Co.

Cell Culture and CPT Treatment. HeLa cell culture and CPT treatment are as described.[1] AT5BI and WI38 cells were grown in MEM supplemented with 10% fetal bovine serum (Hyclone). MO59J and MO59K cells were grown in DMEM supplemented with 10% iron-supplemented bovine serum (Sigma).

DNA Synthesis Assays. Assays were performed as described previously.[3] Samples were counted by dual label liquid scintillation and [^{3}H] values were normalized using [^{14}C] count.[3] Inhibition of DNA synthesis was calculated as the ratio of

---

[a]Voice: 215-955-2045; fax: 215-955-2052.
ya.wang@mail.tju.edu

$[^3H]:[^{14}C]$ in the treated samples over the $[^3H]:[^{14}C]$ ratio in the untreated control samples.

Immune Complex Kinase Assays. Assays were performed as described in Sarkaria et al.'s publication.[4]

RESULTS AND DISCUSSION

ATM is an important factor for S-phase checkpoint control following DNA damage,[6,7] and DNA-dependent protein kinase (DNA-PK) might also be involved in the control pathway.[2,8] To study whether ATM and DNA-PK are involved in the active process controlling the inhibition of DNA replication following CPT treatment, we used ATM mutant (AT5BI) and DNA-PK mutant (MO59J) cell lines to examine regulation of DNA replication following CPT treatment. Data are shown in FIGURE 1A. Following CPT treatment, AT5BI cells showed much less inhibition than did their normal counterparts, and MO59J cells showed similar inhibition of DNA replication than did their normal counterparts. Data indicated that as the common pathway of S-phase checkpoint, ATM is also an important factor involving inhibition of DNA replication in CPT-treated cells. It has been reported that 3 mM of caffeine could completely inhibit the kinase activity of ATM, but it had only a small effect on the kinase activity of DNA-PK[5] and that 20 μM wortmannin could completely inhibit the kinase activities of both ATM and DNA-PK.[4] To further study the involvement of ATM and DNA-PK in the regulation of DNA replication, we used caffeine and wortmannin, the inhibitors of protein kinases, to test their effects on DNA replication in CPT-treated HeLa cells. Data are shown in FIGURE 1B. After the cells were treated with CPT for 3 hours, their DNA replication was strongly inhibited. Wortmannin 20 μM partially released the inhibition of DNA replication induced by CPT, whereas 3 mM caffeine almost completely released this inhibition. FIGURE 2A shows that ATM kinase activity increased following CPT treatment and that it was more strongly inhibited by 20 μM wortmannin than by 3 mM caffeine. Recently, it was reported that DNA-PK could facilitate the recovery from inhibition of DNA replication following DNA damage at the late stage, but it had no effect on the initial inhibition.[9] We considered whether DNA-PK could facilitate the recovery from the initial inhibition of DNA replication following CPT treatment. Data obtained from MO59J cells excluded this possibility (FIG. 1D). MO59J cells have no DNA-PK activity, but wortmannin still could not completely recover the DNA replication activity following CPT treatment. On the other hand, although AT5BI cells showed reduced inhibition of DNA replication following CPT treatment, caffeine could still efficiently release residual inhibition of DNA replication in ATM-deficient cells (FIG. 1C). These results indicated that another factor besides ATM might regulate the S-phase checkpoint following DNA damage. This factor should be caffeine sensitive and wortmannin resistant, because inhibition of DNA replication in CPT-treated HeLa cells was completely released when the dose of wortmannin was increased to 200 μM (data not shown). To distinguish whether the factor is a promoter or an inhibitor in the regulation of DNA replication in CPT-treated cells, we further tested the combined effects of 3 mM caffeine and 20 μM wortmannin on the DNA replication in CPT-treated cells. The combined effects were similar to those observed with caffeine alone; the activity of DNA replication recovered completely (data not shown). Therefore, the factor is not like

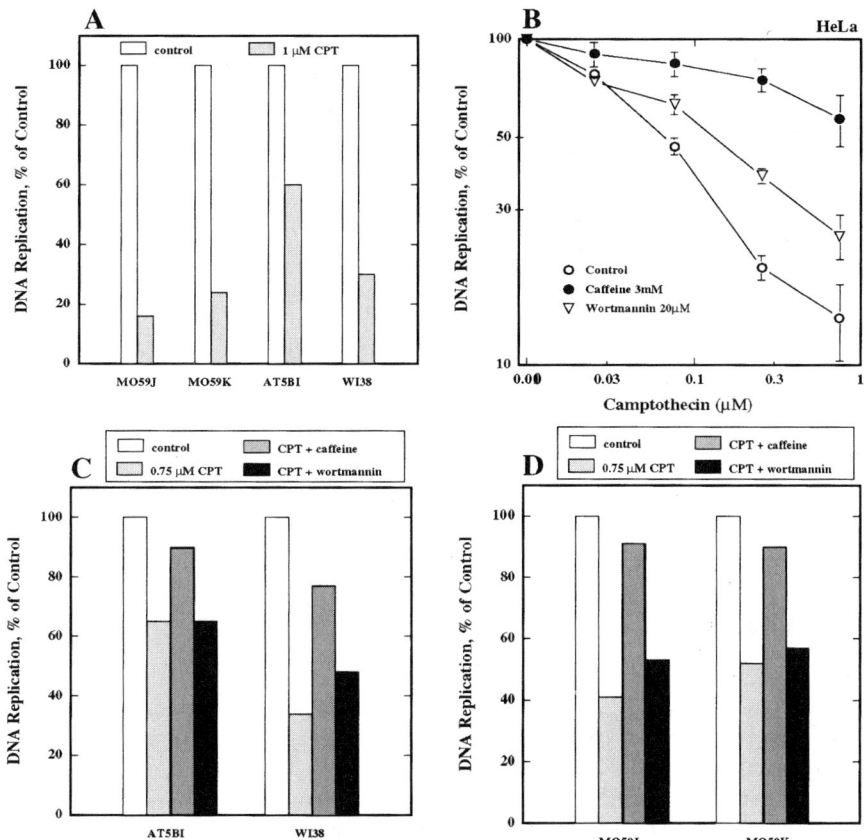

FIGURE 1. DNA synthesis in camptothecin (CPT)-treated cells. (**A**) DNA synthesis in CPT-treated AT5BI, WI38, MO59J, and MO59K cells. Cells were plated in 60 mm dishes (1×10^5 cells + 3 ml medium/dish) with 0.01 µCi ^{14}C-thymidine/ml of medium for 3 days. Cells were changed with fresh medium plus different concentrations of CPT for 3 hours, and ^{3}H-thymidine was added to the medium (0.1 µCi/ml) for 1 hour, and then the cells were stopped before DNA replication as previously described.[3] (**B**) DNA synthesis in CPT-treated HeLa cells with caffeine or wortmannin. As described in **A**, when the cells were treated with CPT for 2.5 hours, caffeine (3 mM) or wortmannin (20 µM) was added to the medium for 30 minutes, then the ^{3}H-thymidine was added as described in **A**. (**C**) DNA synthesis in CPT-treated AT5BI and WI38 cells with caffeine or wortmannin. (**D**) DNA synthesis in CPT-treated MO59J and MO59K cells with caffeine or wortmannin. Mean and SE are from three independent experiments.

a promoter. We previously reported that DNA-PK plays an important inhibitory role in SV40 *in vitro* DNA replication observed in extracts of CPT-treated cells.[8] Data shown in this study could not demonstrate a similar role for DNA-PK in intact cells. It is possible that different mechanisms control DNA replication *in vitro* and *in vivo*. ATR is another ATM-related protein kinase, which plays important roles in checkpoint after DNA damage,[10] compared to ATM; ATR activity is less sensitive to caf-

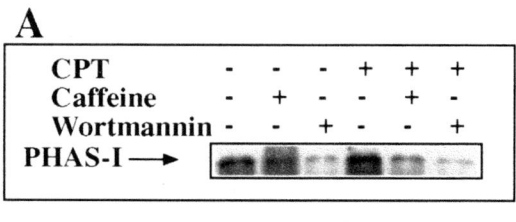

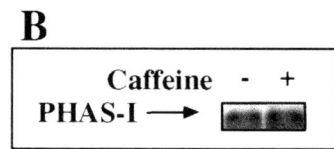

FIGURE 2. ATM and ATR kinase activities in HeLa cells. (A) ATM kinase activity in HeLa cells. ATM immunoprecipitates from HeLa cells were preincubated with 2 × final concentrations of kinase buffer. Kinase reactions were initiated with the addition of an equal volume of kinase buffer containing PHAS-I, $MnCL_2$, and $[\gamma\text{-}^{32}P]$ ATP. The reaction products were resolved by SDS-PAGE, and incorporation of ^{32}Pi into PHAS-I was quantitated with a Molecular Dynamics Storm Phosphorimaging system and ImageQuant software. (B) ATR kinase activity in HeLa cells. ATR activity was measured with ATR immunoprecipitates from HeLa cells. The kinase reaction components and the condition were identical to those used in ATM activity assay.

feine and more resistant to wortmannin.[4,5] Therefore, ATR might be the candidate. Although ATR activity in cells treated with 3 mM caffeine did not show much change (FIG. 2B), we still could not exclude the role of ATR in the inhibition of DNA replication in CPT-treated cells. Caffeine presumably functions as a reversible inhibitor of ATM and ATR; it is expected to recover catalytically active ATM and ATR when caffeine is removed during the process of immunoprecipitation.[5] ATR is less sensitive than ATM to caffeine: therefore, ATR activity might show less change than ATM in our experimental condition (FIG. 2). In conclusion, this study indicates that ATM plays an important role in the inhibition of DNA replication in CPT-treated cells and also suggests that there is another factor to facilitate ATM function in S-phase checkpoint.

ACKNOWLEDGMENTS

We wish to thank Dr. Allalunis-Turner for MO59J and MO59K cells, Dr. Iliakis for helpful discussions, and Nancy Mott for secretarial help. This work was supported by Grants CA76203, T32-CA09137, and P30-CA56036 from the National Institutes of Health.

REFERENCES

1. WANG, Y. *et al.* 1997. Down-regulation of DNA replication in extracts of camptothecin-treated cells: activation of an S-phase checkpoint? Cancer Res. **57:** 1654–1659.

2. SHAO, R.G. *et al.* 1999. Replication-mediated DNA damage by camptothecin induced phosphorylation of RPA by DNA-dependent protein kinase and dissociates RPA:DNA-PK complexes. EMBO J. **18:** 1397–1406.
3. WANG, Y. & G. ILIAKIS. 1992. Prolonged inhibition by X-rays of DNA synthesis in cells obtained by transformation of primary rat embryo fibroblasts with oncogenes H-*ras* and v-*myc*. Cancer Res. **52:** 508–514.
4. SARKARIA, J.N. *et al.* 1998. Inhibition of phosphoinositide 3-kinase related kinases by the radiosensitizing agent wortmannin. Cancer Res. **58:** 4375–4382.
5. SARKARIA, J.N. *et al.* 1999. Inhibition of ATM and ATR kinase activities by the radiosensitizing agent, caffeine. Cancer Res. **59:** 4375–4382.
6. PAINTER, R.B. & B.R. YOUNG. 1980. Radiosensitivity in ataxia-telangiectasia: A new explanation. Proc. Natl. Acad. Sci. USA **77:** 7315–7317.
7. ZAKIAN, V.A. 1995. *ATM*-related genes: what do they tell us about functions of the human gene? Cell **82:** 685–687.
8. WANG, Y. *et al.*. 1999. Roles of replication protein A and DNA-dependent protein kinase in the regulation of DNA replication following DNA damage. J Biol. Chem. **274:** 22060–22064.
9. Guan, J. *et al.* 2000. The catalytic subunit DNA-dependent protein kinase (DNA-PKcs) facilitates recovery from radiation-induced inhibition of DNA replication. Nucl. Acids Res. **28:** 1183–1192.
10. Hall-Jackson, C.A. *et al.* 1999. ATR is a caffeine-sensitive, DNA-activated protein kinase with a substrate specificity distinct from DNA-PK. Oncogene **18:** 6707–6713.

Concluding Remarks

CLAIRE VERSCHRAEGEN

M.D. Anderson Cancer Center, Houston, Texas 77030, USA

To conclude this conference, "The Camptothecins: Unfolding Their Anticancer Potential," I would like to summarize the topics that have been presented, offer a few thoughts, and express my hope that most cancers will be cured one day.

The second conference on camptothecins organized by the New York Academy of Sciences has focused on a clinical puzzle that the scientific and medical community will need to solve at the dawn of the 21st century. Camptothecins have the potential to cure cancer. Human cancer cells are completely eradicated after treatment with most camptothecin analogues in nude mouse models bearing xenografts. However, in clinical settings, camptothecins fail to eliminate neoplastic tumors. One explanation that has been proposed is that the pharmacokinetics of camptothecin in the presence of human albumin favors the lactone form, or open-ring form, of the drug. Yet, if the lactone form is the active form, it may also be the toxic form, as Dr. Giovanella demonstrated through his experiments. The human metabolism of camptothecins yields a poor therapeutic index, which in turn may explain the low response rate of human cancers treated with camptothecins. Dr. Liu's excellent lecture clarified the catabolic pathway of camptothecins. The understanding of the cellular fate of camptothecins and their interaction with the DNA and other nuclear proteins may lead to better therapeutic modulations during clinical administration. Understanding the biochemistry of camptothecins in the context of the biology of human cancers is a crucial step in selecting a camptothecin candidate.

Many authors presented an excellent review of the chemistry of different analogues. Many new analogues have been designed, a few have been tested forward, and none have proven better to date.

Clinical investigative reports related studies of alternative administration of camptothecins in order to maximize the exposure to the lactone form. Studies of continuous infusion, oral administration, and other routes of administration were presented. Again, results have been disappointing.

Combination treatments utilizing the known mechanism of action to promote synergy with other classes of cytostatic agents or radiotherapy have yielded some promises, but again are far from curing patients.

Let me hope that the common effort of basic scientists and clinicians working in the field of topoisomerase I inhibitors will be effectively supported by pharmaceutical companies. Only by utilizing sound scientific strategies will we be able to one day cure more cancers. I wish for a third conference on camptothecins entitled, "Camptothecins: The Cure for Cancer."

Index of Contributors

Abbruzzese, J.L., 345–348
Ahmed, A.E., 216–223
Ahmed, F., 195–204
Ahn, S.K., 324–325

Bang, Y.J., 324–325
Beijnen, J.H., 188–194
Beran, M., 247–259
Bernacki, R.J., 293–297
Bevers, M., 349–351
Bhatt, R., 136–150
Bigg, D., 100–111, 301–302, 303–305, 314–316
Bjornsti, M.-A., 65–75
Bom, D., 36–45, 112–121, 317–319
Boothman, D.A., 274–292
Bornmann, W.G., 274–292
Boven, E., 175–177
Brun, Y., 293–297
Burke, T.G., 36–45

Camara, J., 301–302
Campbell, K., 352–354
Cao, Z., 27–35, 122–135
Carlson, M., 303–305
Champoux, J.J., 56–64
Chauvier, D., 314–316
Chen, A.Y., 298–300
Cheverton, P., 260–273
Chourpa, I., 314–316
Chow, D.S-L., 164–174
Cook, T., 195–204
Coulomb, H., 301–302, 303–305
Coyle, J., 260–273
Curran, D.P., 112–121, 317–319

De Cesare, M., 330–333
De Jager, R., 260–273
de Vries, P., 136–150
Demarquay, D., 100–111, 301–302, 303–305

Desai, S.D., 1–10, 306–308
Downey, A., 178–187
Du, W., 112–121, 317–319
Duann, P., 340–342
Ducharme, M., 260–273
DX-8951f Investigators, 260–273

Early, J., 122–135
Edwards, T.K., 46–55

Fiorani, P., 65–75

Gabarda, A.E., 112–121, 317–319
Gambacorta, P., 293–297
Ganapathi, R., 343–344
Geng, L., 298–300
Gilbert, B.E., 151–163, 237–246, 352–354
Giovanella, B.C., xi–xii, 27–35, 122–135, 151–163, 164–174, 216–223, 237–246, 320–323
Gong, L., 164–174
Greco, W.R., 293–297
Gupta, E., 195–204

Hallahan, D.E., 298–300
Hamilton, A., 178–187
Harris, N.J., 27–35, 122–135, 216–223, 352–354
Hecht, S.M., 76–91
Hochster, H., 178–187
Hong, C.I., 324–325
Hoogsteen, I., 175–177
Hornreich, G., 178–187
Huang, T.T., 274–292
Huaringa, A.J., 352–354
Huchet, M., 301–302, 303–305

Jaeckle, K., 237–246

Jonker, J.W., 188–194
Josien, H., 112–121

Kancherla, R., 326–329
Kantarjian, H.M., 247–259
Kasprzyk, P.G., 100–111, 303–305
Kavanagh, J.J., 345–348, 349–351
Kemp, K.R., 320–323
Keus, L., 352–354
Kim, J.K., 324–325
Kinsella, T.J., 274–292
Kirichenko, A.V., 334–339
Klein, P., 136–150
Kleinerman, E.S., 151–163
Knight, V., 151–163, 237–246, 352–354
Kohn, K.W., 11–26
Koshkina, N.V., 151–163
Kozielski, A., 122–135
Kudelka, A.P., 345–348, 349–351

Lauer, J., 303–305
Lavergne, O., 100–111, 301–302, 303–305
Lee, J.H., 324–325
Lee, J.M., 324–325
Lesueur-Ginot, L., 301–302
Levenback, C., 349–351
Lewis, R.A., 136–150
Leyva, F.J., 352–354
Li, C., 136–150
Li, T.-K., 1–10, 306–308
Liebes, L., 178–187
Liehr, J.G., xi–xii, 27–35, 122–135, 216–223, 320–323
Lim, K.H., 324–325
Lin, C.-T., 340–342
Liu, L.F., 1–10, 306–308, 340–342
Loyer, E., 345–348, 349–351

Maliepaard, M., 188–194
Manfait, M., 314–316
Mao, Y., 1–10, 306–308
Mendoza, J., 27–35, 122–135, 216–223
Milas, L., 136–150

Miller, S.E., 309–313
Miyamoto, S., 274–292
Muggia, F., 178–187

Nair, J.S., 326–329
Nelson-Taylor, T., 352–354
Newman, R., 352–354

Pantazis, P., 122–135
Pera, P., 293–297
Pinedo, H.M., 175–177
Pilch, D.S., 309–313
Pink, J.J., 274–292
Pommier, Y., 11–26
Potmesil, M., 178–187
Pratesi, G., 330–333

Rasheed, Z., 46–55
Rich, T.A., 334–339
Rivory, L.P., 205–215
Rothenberg, M.L., 298–300
Rubin, E.H., 46–55, 195–204, 345–348

Saijo, N., 92–99
Sakamoto, N., 260–273
Saleem, A., 46–55
Satomi, M., 260–273
Scheffer, G.L., 188–194
Schellens, J.H.M., 188–194
Scheper, R.J., 188–194
Schinkel, A.H., 188–194
Schlüper, H.M.M., 175–177
Scruggs, P.B., 298–300
Seiter, K., 326–329
Siegler, D., 345–348
Sim, S.-P., 1–10
Singer, J.W., 136–150
Sinko, P., 195–204
Smit, J.W., 188–194
Sorich, J., 178–187
Stehlin, J.S., 27–35, 122–135
Sun, M., 1–10, 306–308, 340–342
Suzuki, M., 260–273

INDEX OF CONTRIBUTORS

Tabata, M., 343–344
Tagliarino, C., 274–292
Takimoto, C.H., 224–236
Tamanoi, K., 260–273
Thomas, R., 224–236
Traganos, F., 326–329
Tse-Dinh, Y.-C., 326–329
Tulinsky, J., 136–150

Van Hattum, A.H., 175–177
Vardeman, D., 122–135
Verschraegen, C.F., 237–246, 345–348, 349–351, 352–354, 360
Vincent, M., 345–348, 349–351

Vyas, V., 195–204

Waldrep, J.C., 151–163
Wallace, S., 136–150
Wang, Y., 355–359
Wasserstrom, H., 178–187
Wolf, J., 349–351
Wolfe, M.D., 164–174
Wu, J., 306–308
Wuerzberger-Davis, S., 274–292

Zhang, H., 340–342
Zhou, X.-Y., 355–359
Zunino, F., 330–333

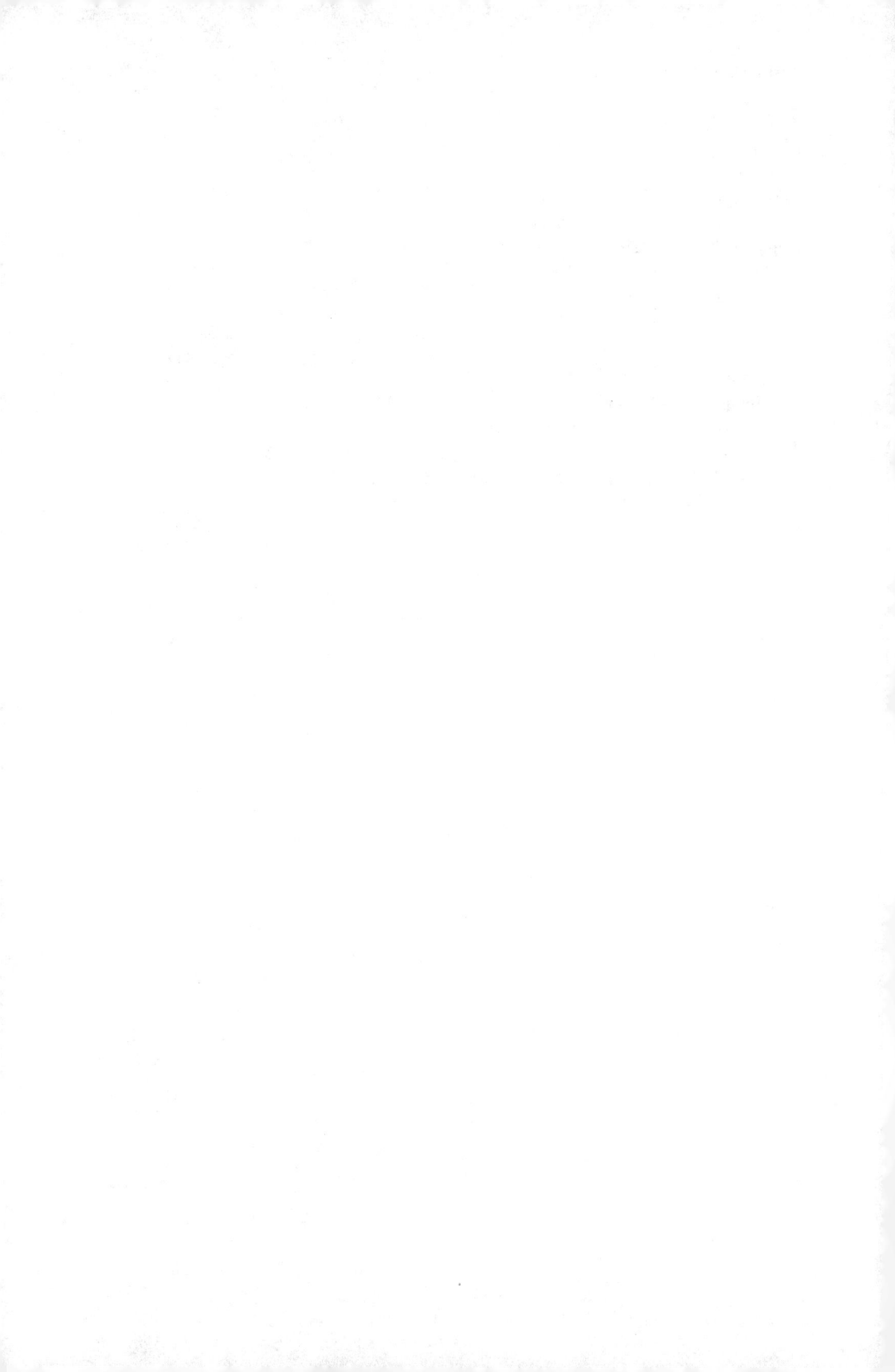